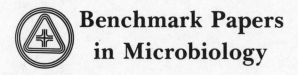

Benchmark Papers
in Microbiology

Series Editor: Wayne W. Umbreit
Rutgers University

Published Volumes and Volumes in Preparation

MICROBIAL PERMEABILITY
  John P. Reeves
CHEMICAL STERILIZATION
  Paul M. Borick
MICROBIAL GENETICS
  Morad Abou-Sabé
MICROBIAL PHOTOSYNTHESIS
  June Lascelles
MICROBIAL METABOLISM
  H. W. Doelle
ANIMAL CELL CULTURE AND VIROLOGY
  R. J. Kuchler
MICROBIAL GROWTH
  P. S. S. Dawson
MARINE MICROBIOLOGY
  C. D. Litchfield
MICROBIAL VIRUSES
  S. P. Champe
INFLUENCE OF TEMPERATURE ON MICROORGANISMS
  J. L. Stokes
MOLECULAR BIOLOGY AND PROTEIN SYNTHESIS
  Robert Niederman
ANTIBIOTICS AND CHEMOTHERAPY
  M. Solotorovsky
INDUSTRIAL MICROBIOLOGY
  Richard W. Thoma

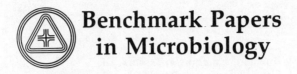

Benchmark Papers in Microbiology

—— A *BENCHMARK* ® Books Series ——

MICROBIAL METABOLISM

Edited by
H. W. DOELLE
University of Queensland, Australia

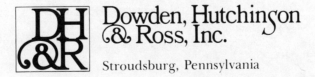

Dowden, Hutchinson
& Ross, Inc.
Stroudsburg, Pennsylvania

Library of Congress Cataloging in Publication Data

Doelle, H   W   comp.
   Microbial metabolism.

   (Benchmark papers in microbiology, v. 5)
   1. Microbial metabolism--Addresses, essays, lectures.
I. Title. [DNLM: 1. Microbiology--Collected works.
QW52 D615m 1974]
QR88.D63   576'.11'3308   73-16370
ISBN 0-87933-063-5

Acknowledgments and Permissions

ACKNOWLEDGMENTS
National Academy of Sciences—*Proceedings of the National Academy of Sciences*
"The Role of Transcarboxylation in Propionic Acid Fermentation"

PERMISSIONS
The following papers have been reprinted by permission of the authors and copyright holders.
Academic Press, Inc.—*The Harvey Lectures*
"The Enzymatic Synthesis of the Purine Nucleotides"

Académie des Sciences—*Comptes rendus hebdomadaires des Scéances de l'Académie des Sciences*
"Chemoautotrophic Carbon Metabolism: Cycle for Carbon Dioxide Assimilation"

American Association for the Advancement of Science—*Science*
"Biological Sulfate Activation and Transfer"
"The Bacterial Oxidation of Tryptophan: A Study in Comparative Biochemistry"
"Mechanisms of Oxygen Metabolism"

American Chemical Society—*Journal of the American Chemical Society*
"Mechanism of the Pyrocatechase Reaction"
"Oxygen Transfer and Electron Transport by the Phenolase Complex"

American Society for Microbiology
Bacteriological Reviews
"Pathways of Biosynthesis of Aromatic Amino Acids and Vitamins and Their Control in Micro-
organisms"
Journal of Bacteriology
"Simultaneous Adaptation: A New Technique for the Study of Metabolic Pathways"

American Society of Biological Chemists, Inc.—*Journal of Biological Chemistry*
"Heavy Carbon As a Tracer in Bacterial Fixation of Carbon Dioxide"
"Glucose and Gluconic Acid Oxidation of *Pseudomonas saccharophila*"
"Coenzyme A Function in and Acetyl Transfer by the Phosphotransacetylase System"

The Biochemical Society—*Biochemical Journal*
"The Chemical Reactions by Which *Cl. sporogenes* Obtains Its Energy"
"The Bacterial Formation of Methane by the Reduction of One-Carbon Compounds by Molecular
Hydrogen"

Cambridge University Press—*Journal of General Microbiology*
"The Reduction of Sulphur Compounds by *Desulphovibrio desulphuricans*"

Elsevier Publishing Company—*Biochimica et Biophysica Acta*
"Enzymes of Fatty Acid Metabolism"

Federation of American Societies for Experimental Biology—*Federation Proceedings*
"Amino Acid Metabolism in Mutant Strains of Microorganisms"

D. W. Junk, Publishers, The Hague—*Enzymologia*
"The Role of Citric Acid in Intermediate Metabolism in Animal Tissues"

Macmillan (Journals) Ltd.—*Nature*
"Structure of Coenzyme A"
"Synthesis of Cell Constituents from C_2-Units by a Modified Tricarboxylic Acid Cycle"
"Growth of 'Knallgas' Bacteria (*Hydrogenomonas*) Using Direct Electrolysis of the Culture Medium"

The Physiological Society—*Journal of Physiology*
"Some New Forms of Apparatus for the Analysis of the Gases of the Blood by the Chemical Method"

The Royal Society, London—*Proceedings of the Royal Society, London*
"The Alcoholic Ferment of Yeast-juice. Part II. The Coferment of Yeast-juice"

Springer-Verlag, Berlin-Heidelberg—*Klinische Wochenschrift*
"Über die intermediären Vorgänge bei der Glykolyse in der Muskulatur"

Series Editor's Preface

Microbial metabolism is a vast and complex field that had its origins in the late 1880s and made its most spectacular advances in the 1930s. These were exciting times and Dr. Doelle has captured some of the thrill and excitement of the era by his selection of papers, including his masterly translations of classical texts. Most students have heard of the Meyerhof–Embden–Parnas system, the citric acid cycle; most have heard of Buchner's preparation of cell-free enzymes; most have some acquaintance with autotrophic and heterotrophic CO_2 fixation; but here are the classic papers (translated into English when necessary, but retaining the flavor of the originals). The basic elements of microbial metabolism are all here. More recent contributions are based on these fundamentals. If the fundamentals are understood, the present mass of detailed information becomes more manageable.

In the advance of science, and in what has been called "the jungle of journals and the tangle of tongues," there is a real danger that the fundamental contributions will become so buried in the avalanche of subsequent work that they will be lost forever and the assumptions implicit in them forgotten. Dr. Doelle makes it possible for us to study these essential papers, which ought to be part of the background of today's research.

Even more important, perhaps, this selection of papers indicates the sameness of metabolic pathways from one cell to another. One notes that the data about human muscle fit with information about bacteria; streptococcus and human muscle have much in common. And as more information is provided, it becomes clear that in many of its metabolic aspects, the "ground plan" of most, if not all, organisms is strikingly similar. Evidently the basic process of altering usable substances to provide necessary intermediates and energy is so fundamental that the evolutionary process has not tampered with it; it has remained a constant, stable portion of each living cell. In a real sense, only the preliminary maneuvers and possibly the final disposition of the fragments is different; the core of metabolic pathways remains the same for all cells. Many of the papers in this book provide direct evidence for this concept; indeed, the results demonstrate what Kluyver called "the unity of biochemistry in the cell."

Much of today's work in the field of metabolism is concerned with such things as the metabolic paths of unusual materials, the methods of control of metabolism, and the properties of specific enzymes concerned with peripheral steps, but the main core, represented by the papers selected here, is still valid and very vital—so much so that it is taken for granted. For the young worker in the field it will be refreshing to be able to see, in a convenient fashion, the methods, concepts, and working methods of the masters of the field, who laid the basis for, and still play a significant role in, modern work.

W. W. Umbreit

Contents

III. METABOLISM OF INORGANIC COMPOUNDS

IV. AROMATIC CARBON METABOLISM

V. ANAEROBIC FERMENTATION

Contents by Author

Introduction

This volume of the Benchmark series has been created out of the desire to preserve the outstanding work performed from the early days of microbial metabolism research to the present time. It is a difficult task indeed to make a choice as to what contributions to select, as the field of microbial metabolism has expanded rapidly in the last 50 years. Apart from this difficulty of selection, there exists a problem in evaluating the early work, as the methodology of the nineteenth century is so vastly different from that of today, yet forms the basis of our current research. In studying the early literature concerning microbial metabolism one is also struck by the different approach of the researchers toward their work. First it was mainly a "one-man job," perhaps that of an idealist who studied natural phenomena. Then it became more specifically directed research carried out by research teams. This development alone shows the tremendous advances and specialization that has occurred during the 140 years of the investigation of microbial metabolism. This specialization has to be taken into account and thus this volume looks at five areas of development:

1. The early stages of microbial metabolism research to 1900
2. Carbohydrate metabolism
3. Metabolism of inorganic compounds
4. Aromatic carbon metabolism
5. Anaerobic fermentation

Apart from this separation, great emphasis has to be given to the dependence of the research progress on newly developed methods. As examples one can easily pick three main techniques: (1) the preparation of cell-free extracts (yeast juice) in 1897, (2) the construction of the Warburg respirometer in 1906–1910, and (3) the introduction of radioisotopes about 1940. However, one should never forget the tremendous work done in the field of growth and nutrition of these microorganisms (another volume in this series), which made it possible to investigate metabolic events.

A further aspect of selection was taken into consideration. The difficulties encountered in obtaining literature from the early days of microbiology, as well as the

1

recognition of the work at that time, led to stressing this era more than was originally anticipated. In view of this preference, it was decided to cite as many appropriate publications as possible not only to preserve a certain number of publications, but also to provide a guide for all those who wish to study the history of microbial metabolism research. The need for such an additional reference list was found to be of advantage, as a number of previous history books (Dubos, 1950; Winslow, 1950; Waksman, 1953; Bryson, 1959; Doetsch, 1960; Vallery-Radot, 1960; Brock, 1961) lacked such a guide. The aim is therefore to present the reader with a historical development of five different streams of microbial metabolism research in chronological order, emphasizing the most significant contribution by a full or partial reproduction of its original form.

The start of microbial metabolism investigation occurred well after Antonie van Leeuwenhoek developed his microscope. It took the best part of 150 years before Theodore Schwann and Charles Cagniard-Latour had a closer look at the fermentation of wine. (The word "ferment" was used as the term for "boiling" or "bubbling," which we now know to be caused by carbon dioxide production. Only when one is reminded of the original meaning of this word can one understand why this terminology has been used for all metabolic events for such a long time.) Both research workers, now generally forgotten as founders of microbial metabolism research, observed that the fermentation of sugar to alcohol and carbon dioxide was caused by yeasts. Since they saw the yeast in a budding stage, they mistakenly assigned them to the plant kingdom.

The first outstanding microbial chemist was, however, Louis Pasteur. A number of books have been written about his life (e.g., Dubos, 1950; Valleroy-Radot, 1960) and attention is drawn to these biographies. It is most entertaining to read about this great man and his battle with the main opponent of his theories, the outspoken German organic chemist Justus Liebig. Pasteur laid the foundations for research in the fields of fermentation and aerobic respiration. He was able to distinguish between facultative anaerobes and strict anaerobes. His quantitative approach to his studies led him to discover the effect of oxygen on microbial metabolism, the effect that carries his name (Pasteur effect) and has not as yet been fully elucidated. It was also Pasteur who recognized that not only yeasts carry out fermentation, but also "animalcules," which are much smaller. We assume that he discovered the lactic acid bacteria, which are so important in the malolactic fermentation of wine. Other prominent areas of study were the anaerobic butyric acid fermentation and the aerobic oxidation of ethanol by acetic acid bacteria (vinegar production).

The next period of great activity began about 1900. Although Schloesing and Müntz, as well as Warrington, were the forerunners of what we now call soil microbiology, names like Sergei Winogradsky and M. W. Beijerinck come to everyone's mind. These two outstanding microbiologists initiated the era of soil microbiology, which is so important for agriculture and also for the potential of our mineral resources (e.g., ore leaching). The establishment of the nitrogen and sulfur cycles are some of the examples of importance for agriculture. The early years of the 1900s also marked the start of the microbiology of hydrocarbon breakdown, with Kaserer and Söhngen laying the foundation for this now almost independent stream in microbial metabolism.

Until that time, most of the work was concerned with observations and establishing the attack on certain compounds and thus exploring the capacity of the organism to utilize a variety of organic or inorganic compounds. The outstanding work of Buchner in 1897 certainly marked the start of the tremendous development of microbial biochemistry. His method of breaking the cell, together with the observation that the "yeast juice," or cell-free extract, is able to perform the same fermentative reactions as a whole cell, stimulated interest in the mechanisms and the substances responsible for these transformations. E. Buchner and coworkers (1897, 1898, 1899, 1900, 1901, 1904, 1905, 1906, 1907, 1908, 1909, 1910, 1912), A. Lebedev (1909, 1911, 1912, 1913, 1926, 1927), A. Harden and coworkers (1906, 1909, 1910, 1912, 1914, 1917, 1927, 1929), C. Neuberg and his research team (1911, 1914, 1915, 1917, 1918, 1920, 1923, 1925, 1928, 1930), and H. v. Euler and his research group (1905, 1911, 1912, 1913, 1917, 1918, 1923, 1924, 1926, 1927) certainly made a tremendous impact in this field. A. H. Harden summarized these activities in his excellent book on alcoholic fermentation in 1932.

O. Meyerhof and Otto Warburg and their respective research groups carried on evaluation of the breakdown mechanisms. Meyerhof not only contributed to the study of nitrification (1916), but also established, together with Embden and Parnas, the nature of the glycolytic pathway, which bears the name of all three men (Embden–Meyerhof–Parnas pathway). Otto Warburg, on the other hand, turned his work more toward aerobic respiration. Making use of the Warburg respirometer, he and his team established the second pathway of glucose utilization, which is often referred to as the Warburg–Dickens pathway, or, more commonly, the hexosemonophosphate pathway. This was possible through the discovery of the coenzyme nicotinamide adenine dinucleotide phosphate (NADP) and the enzyme glucose 6-phosphate dehydrogenase (Zwischenferment). By the late 1930s we have, in other words, two coenzymes, NAD and NADP, and the two corresponding pathways of glucose utilization. The Warburg respirometer was, however, helpful not only in finding a number of different enzymes, but mainly for investigations into the respiration of microorganisms (see volume on respiration). Glucose utilization during this time period was therefore expressed mainly in the form of respiration rates, or P/O ratios. As this ratio reflects the existence of the electron transport chain, great emphasis was given to the energy relations in metabolic events. It was at that time that the School of Delft evolved under the leadership of Albert Jan Kluyver, who developed the idea of biochemical unity (Kamp et al., 1959). The concept of biochemical unity, mentioned by S. Winogradsky, implies that all microorganisms, plants and animals, follow common rules in nature.

During this time of energy considerations there was great interest in the mechanisms by which microorganisms break down pyruvate. Neuberg had already established the branch-off toward acetaldehyde and ethanol and Lohmann and Schuster found the carboxylase that decarboxylates pyruvate. There was, however, no indication of the aerobic breakdown of pyruvate. Hans Krebs made the breakthrough by establishing, in 1937, the tricarboxylic acid cycle in muscle tissue. Not long afterward, another outstanding research group, under the guidance of F. Lipmann, found it present in microorganisms. It was this research group that was responsible for the discovery of coenzyme A and phosphotransacetylase, thus establishing the connection between pyruvate and the tricarboxylic acid cycle.

3

During their investigations of glucose breakdown by *Pseudomonas saccharophila,* Entner and Doudoroff found that the labeled carbon distribution did not agree with either of the two suggested pathways and thus established, in 1952, a third pathway, still unique to microorganisms, which bears their names. Radioactive-tracer work also led to the discovery that amino acid biosynthesis is linked to the tricarboxylic acid cycle. Thus, if certain members of this cycle are being continuously withdrawn from the cycle, there would not be enough oxalacetate available for citric acid formation. Again it was the research group of Hans Krebs and H. Kornberg who found the glyoxylate cycle, which is able to replenish oxalacetate.

Other aspects of microbial metabolism research developed at the same rate. Once the initial problems of cultivation were solved, investigations into sulfur metabolism, nitrogen metabolism, and hydrocarbon metabolism got under way. Since 1950 a tremendous number of publications have appeared. The outstanding teams in these areas are under the leadership of J. Postgate, H. D. Peck, Jr., A. Nason, M. I. H. Aleem, P. A. Trudinger, and H. Kelly. In the field of hydrocarbon metabolism, O. Hayaishi, G. Hegemann, R. Stanier, M. Doudoroff, and J. Mandelstam have certainly contributed most. One should not forget the recent upsurge in clarifying the position of the "Knallgas" bacteria, or *Hydrogenomonas,* by H. G. Schlegel and his research team.

The endeavor to cover the past history of microbial metabolism research results in unavoidable omissions. Selection was indeed difficult, especially when one would have liked to include a greater number of outstanding papers. It is hoped, however, that objectivity was maintained, although it is almost impossible to avoid bias toward certain research fields.

The history presented could be separated into three main developmental time periods:

1. The period of observation, which encompassed the initial observations and the discoveries by Buchner in 1897.

2. The period of exploration, which started with the discoveries by Buchner and the development of the Warburg respirometer and end between 1955 and 1960.

3. The period of determination, which began around 1955 with the development of microbial chemistry at the molecular level. We are still in this third period of development.

The immediate question, of course, is where do we go in the near and distant future. My personal opinion is that for a number of years the determination and collection of data will continue. We need still more information as to how the living cell works on the molecular level. This can be obtained by using cell-free extracts, thus employing the microbe as a tool for exploring its own chemistry. However, the day must come when we will sit back, look at the massive collection of data, and try to visualize how the whole cell implements the various mechanisms under different conditions. We may have to go back to the stage of observation in order to be able to cope with this problem. Comparisons will be made between the unicellular and multicellular organisms with the goal of understanding life. The introduction of continuous cultivation using the chemostat or turbidostat or both opens a new era, as we can subject the microorganisms to almost every possible environmental condition. By altering the conditions of growth in regard to energy source, air, carbon dioxide, nitrogen, etc., we can study the reactions of a microbe and ultimately try to fit these observations into schemes obtained during the developmental stage of determination. We may then also be able to classify microbes in a much more satisfactory way than is possible at the present moment. Some problems facing the world at the moment (e.g., pollution and food shortages) involve areas that we can enter more confidently once such considerations have been carried out. I am convinced that the future brings us back to the microbe itself and its function in nature, as we certainly will understand its biochemical potential more fully. It may then be possible to draw parallels with higher organisms, with the ultimate aim of understanding life processes.

I

The Early Stages
of Microbial Metabolism

Editor's Comments on Paper 1

1 **Schwann:** Vorläufige Mittheilung, betreffend Versuche über die Weingährung und Fäulniss
   English Translation: A Preliminary Report Concerning Experiments on the Fermentation of Wine and Putrefaction
   Ann. Physik Chem., **11**, 184–193 (1837)

Theodore Schwann was one of the first to associate a fermentation process with microorganisms. His paper on alcoholic fermentation is thus the first report in the field of microbial metabolism. In this almost forgotten publication, Schwann made the observation that yeast was able to grow in the process of alcohol fermentation.

In his article, Schwann clearly noted that the appearance of yeast is absolutely necessary for the process of alcoholic fermentation. He also stated that oxygen or air is not necessary for the fermentation process, but that air contains "something" [*Ed. Note:* the yeast] which causes the fermentation. His experiments and findings could be summarized as follows:

1. A boiled organic substance, or a boiled, previously fermentable liquid, neither putrifies nor ferments if the air introduced has been heated.

2. In putrefaction, fermentation, or other processes in which animals or plants appear, there must be either unboiled organic matter or unheated air.

3. In grape juice, gas development is a sign of fermentation and is connected with a filamentous fungus which can be called a sugar fungus [*Ed. Note:* = *Saccharomyces*]. Throughout the process these plants grow and increase in numbers.

4. If ferments that already contain plants are placed in a sugar solution, fermentation begins very quickly, much more so than when these plants must first develop.

5. Poisons effective against infusoria, but not lower plants (Extractum Nucis vomicae spirituosum), inhibit putrefaction phenomena characteristic of infusoria. They do not inhibit fermentation or putrefaction caused by fungi; poisons toxic to animals and plants (arsenic) inhibit putrefaction as well as fermentation.

Reprinted from *Ann. Physik Chem.*, **11**, 184–193 (1837)

184

XVI. *Vorläufige Mittheilung, betreffend Versuche über die Weingährung und Fäulniß; von Dr. Th. Schwann in Berlin.**

Bei der letzten Versammlung der Naturforscher in Jena habe ich Versuche über *generatio aequivoca* mitgetheilt, aus denen hervorgeht, daſs, wenn eine verschlossene Glaskugel, die mit atmosphärischer Luft gefüllt ist, und auſserdem ein wenig einer Infusion von Muskelfleisch enthält, der Siedhitze des Wassers ausgesetzt wird, so daſs Flüssigkeit und Luft der Glaskugel bis 80° R. erwärmt werden, nachher in der Flüssigkeit innerhalb mehrerer Monate keine Infusorienbildung und keine Fäulniſs stattfindet, und zwar selbst dann nicht, wenn die Quantität der in der Glaskugel enthaltenen thierischen Substanz so gering ist, daſs an eine vollständige Verschluckung des Sauerstoffs aus der Luft der Glaskugel nicht zu denken ist. Es war indessen doch wünschenswerth den Versuch in der Art zu modificiren, daſs eine Erneuerung der Luft möglich würde, doch so, daſs die neu hinzugeführte Luft, wie in den vorigen Versuchen, vorher einer höheren Temperatur ausgesetzt würde. Dieſs habe ich nun auf folgende Weise bewirkt.

Ein Fläschchen, welches einige Stückchen Muskelfleisch enthielt und bis zu Einem Drittel mit Wasser gefüllt war, wurde mit einem Stöpsel geschlossen, der von zwei dünnen Glasröhren durchbohrt war. Diese Glasröhren wurden in einer Strecke von ungefähr drei Zoll durch eine leichtflüssige Metallmischung geleitet, welche anhaltend in einer dem Siedepunkt des Quecksilbers nahe liegenden Temperatur erhalten wurde. Die eine dieser Glasröhren wurde mit ihrem aus dem Metall hervorragenden Ende mit einem Gasometer in Verbindung gesetzt. Nun wurde die Flüssigkeit in dem Fläschchen stark gekocht, so daſs alle Luft, die in dem

*An English translation of this paper follows.

Fläschchen und in den Glasröhren enthalten war, theils
ausgetrieben, theils bis zum Siedpunkt des Wassers
erwärmt wurde. Nach dem Erkalten wurde mehre
Wochen lang ein anhaltender Strom atmosphärischer
Luft aus dem Gasometer durch das erste Glasröhr-
chen in das Fläschchen, und, nachdem so hierin die
Luft erneuert worden war, durch das zweite Glasröhr-
chen wieder fortgeleitet. Die hinzugeleitete Luft aber
wurde, indem sie durch die in dem erhitzten Metallbad
liegende Glasröhre strich, vorher stark erwärmt. Auch
in diesen Versuchen, deren mehrere angestellt wurden,
zeigte sich nach mehren Wochen keine Infusorien- oder
Schimmelbildung und keine Fäulnifs, sondern das Fleisch
blieb unverändert, und die Flüssigkeit so klar wie sie
nach dem Kochen war [1]).

Ob sich aus diesen Versuchen, zu deren Vervoll-
ständigung noch viele andere Versuche angestellt wurden, ein Schlufs über *generatio aequivoca* ziehen lasse

[1]) Da dieser Versuch zu viel Sorgfalt bei der Unterhaltung der
Lampe erfordert, so habe ich später folgende Methode ange-
wandt: Ein Gläschen von 3 Unzen Inhalt wurde zum vierten
Theil mit Wasser und Fleisch gefüllt, und mit einem dichten
Kork verschlossen, der mit Draht darauf fest gebunden wurde.
Der Kork war von zwei dünnen Glasröhren durchbohrt, von
denen die erste sich sogleich abwärts bog und in eine kleine
Schale mit Quecksilber tauchte, welches mit Oel bedeckt war.
Die zweite Glasröhre bog sich, so wie sie aus dem Kork hervorkam, zuerst horizontal, dann 1½ Zoll weit abwärts, machte
dann ein Paar enge Spiralwindungen, stieg wieder aufwärts, dann
wieder horizontal und wurde zuletzt in eine Spitze ausgezogen.
Der ganze Kork wurde dann mit einer dicken Auflösung von
Kautschuck in kochendem Leinöl, die mit Terpenthinöl verdünnt
war, mehrmals überzogen. Dann wurde die Flüssigkeit des Gläs-
chens so stark gekocht, dafs der Dampf an beiden Glasröhren
stark hervorkam, und auch das Quecksilber und Oel so stark
erwärmt wurden, dafs sich die Wasserdämpfe nicht mehr darin
condensirten. Damit aber in dem zwischen dem Oel und Quecksilber sich condensirenden Wasser keine Infusorien sich bildeten, wurden zur Vorsicht einige Stückchen Sublimat auf das
Quecksilber gelegt. Während des Kochens wurde unter die Spi-

oder nicht, werde ich an einem anderen Orte auseinandersetzen, und bemerke hier nur, dafs diese Versuche, wenn man sie vom Standpunkte der Gegner der *generatio aequivoca* betrachtet, sich so erklären lassen, dafs die Keime des Schimmels und der Infusorien, die nach dieser Ansicht in der atmosphärischen Luft vorhanden sind, beim Ausglühen der Luft zerstört werden. Alsdann mufs die Fäulnifs [1]) so erklärt werden, dafs diese

ralwindung der zweiten Glasröhre eine Spiritusflamme gesetzt, die zur Verhütung des Wegblasens der Flamme mit einem Kamin versehen war. Die Hitze dieser Flamme wurde so stark unterhalten, dafs die Glasröhre sich erweichte. Die sich in den kühlen Stellen der Glasröhre condensirenden Wassertropfen wurden durch eine andere Spiritusflamme, zur Verhütung des Springens der Glasröhre, sogleich wieder in Dampf aufgelöst. Nachdem das Kochen etwa eine Viertelstunde gedauert hatte, wurde damit aufgehört, und beim Erkalten des Fläschchens drang die Luft durch die zweite Glasröhre in das Fläschchen, wurde aber zuvor in der Spiralwindung ausgeglüht. Nach dem völligen Erkalten des Fläschchens wurde die Spitze der zweiten Glasröhre zugeblasen, der zwischen dieser Spitze und der glühenden Spiralwindung liegende Theil der Glasröhre, der nicht ausgeglühte Luft enthielt, besonders ausgeglüht, und dann auch die Weingeistlampe unter der Spiralwindung entfernt. Das Fläschchen enthielt nun blofs gekochtes Fleisch und ausgeglühte Luft. Um diese zu erneuern, wurde von Zeit zu Zeit die Spirale abermals bis zur beginnenden Schmelzung der Glasröhre erhitzt, die Spitze dieser Glasröhre abgebrochen und neue Luft langsam hineingeblasen; während die alte durch das Quecksilber entwich. Dann wurde die Glasröhre wieder zugeschmolzen, ihr freies Ende wieder besonders ausgeglüht und dann der Apparat wieder sich selbst überlassen. Auf diese Weise habe ich bei einer Temperatur von 14^0 bis 20^0 R. solche Gläschen mit Fleisch 6 Wochen ohne Fäulnifs oder Infusorien- und Schimmelbildung aufbewahrt. Nach Oeffnung des Fläschchens faulte die Flüssigkeit innerhalb einiger Tage, als ob sie eben erst gekocht worden wäre. Das vollkommen dichte Schliefsen des Stöpsels und der Glasröhren in demselben erfordert aber die gröfste Vorsicht.

1) Es kann hier natürlich nur die Rede seyn von der gewöhnlichen, bald nach dem Tode eintretenden Fäulnifs, und zwar zunächst gekochter organischer Substanzen, nicht von all den man-

Keime, indem sie sich entwickeln und auf Kosten der
organischen Substanz ernähren, eine solche Zersetzung
in dieser hervorbringen, wodurch die Phänomene der
Fäulnifs entstehen: eine Ansicht, für die auch der Um-
stand spricht, dafs gerade diejenigen Stoffe, welche für
Infusorien und Schimmel nachweisbar starke Gifte sind,
z. B. Arsenik oder Sublimat, auch am besten die Fäulnifs
verhüten, und dafs diejenigen Stoffe, die nur für Infusorien Gifte sind, z. B. *Extractum Nucis vomicae spirituosum*, nicht für den Schimmel, alle Erscheinungen, unter denen sich die mit Infusorienbildung verbundene
Fäulnifs kund giebt, namentlich den Schwefelwasserstoff-
geruch verhindern, und blofs die Reihe von Erscheinungen gestatten, welche der mit Schimmelbildung ver-
bundenen Fäulnifs angehören.

Ich führe indessen diefs hier nur an, da es mich
auf Versuche über die Weingährung geleitet hat, welche geeignet scheinen den Untersuchungen über diesen
Procefs eine andere Wendung zu geben. In der Ab-
sicht nachzuweisen, dafs bei anderen Processen, bei denen atmosphärische Luft mitwirkt, bei denen aber, so
viel bekannt war, keine Bildung neuer Thiere oder
Pflanzen stattfindet, es gleichgültig ist, ob die Luft vorher geglüht wird oder nicht, stellte ich Versuche über
die Respiration und über die Weingährung an. Es
zeigte sich auch, dafs ein Frosch in ausgeglühter Luft
sehr gut fortlebte.

Mit der Weingährung machte ich den Versuch auf
folgende Weise. Eine Auflösung von Rohrzucker wurde
mit Bierhefe vermischt und vier Fläschchen damit ganz
angefüllt und verkorkt. Die Fläschchen wurden alsdann
gleich lange (etwa **10** Minuten lang) in siedendes Wasser gestellt, so dafs die ganze Flüssigkeit in denselben
die Siedhitze erreichte. Dann wurden sie herausgenom-

nichfaltigen Processen, die man unter dem Namen Fäulnifs zu-
sammengefafst, z. B. Moderbildung, Braun- und Steinkohlenbil-
dung etc.

men, unter Quecksilber umgestülpt, und nach dem Erkalten in alle vier Fläschchen atmosphärische Luft hineingeleitet, die etwa $\frac{1}{3}$ bis $\frac{1}{4}$ vom Volumen der ganzen
Flüssigkeit betrug. Diefs geschah bei zweien durch eine
dünne Glasröhre, die an einer Stelle bis zur Rothglühhitze erwärmt war, bei den beiden andern durch ·dieselbe, aber nicht erwärmte Glasröhre. Eine Analyse,
mit Hülfe eines Platinkügelchens, ergab, dafs atmosphärische Luft, die durch eine glühende Glasröhre geleitet
worden ist, noch ungefähr 19,4 Proc. Sauerstoff enthält.
Dem Einwurf, der sich aus dieser geringen Sauerstoffgasverminderung hernehmen liefse, wurde dadurch vorgebeugt, dafs in eines der Gläschen, welche ausgeglühte Luft enthielten, etwas mehr von dieser hineingeleitet wurde als in die übrigen. Die Fläschchen wurden dann verkorkt und bei einer Temperatur von 10°
bis 14° R. umgekehrt hingestellt. Nach 4 bis 6 Wochen trat in den beiden Fläschchen, welche nicht ausgeglühte Luft enthielten, die Gährung ein, und zeigte
sich dadurch, dafs die Fläschchen, da sie umgestülpt
waren, weggeschleudert wurden. Die beiden andern
Fläschchen stehen auch jetzt noch, nach der doppelten
Zeit, ganz ruhig [1]).

1) Spätere Wiederholungen dieses Versuches zeigten mir, dafs
   derselbe nicht immer so gut gelingt, und zuweilen in keinem
   der Gläschen Gährung eintritt (wenn man sie nämlich zu lange.
   gekocht hat), zuweilen auch in den Gläschen, die ausgeglühte
   Luft enthalten, die Flüssigkeit gährt. Diefs wird indessen
   leicht erklärlich durch die Art wie die Versuche angestellt
   wurden, indem von der Oberfläche des Quecksilbers, obgleich
   diefs unmittelbar vorher stark erhitzt worden war, und namentlich bei dem Lüften und Wiederaufsetzen des Stöpsels
   leicht etwas ungekochte organische Substanz eindringen konnte.
   Die bei der Fäulnifs angewandte Methode war hier nicht anwendbar, weil dazu langes Kochen erforderlich ist. Ich würde
   deshalb das obige Resultat nicht aussprechen, wenn nicht, nachdem einmal die Existenz einer Pflanze sich herausgestellt hat,
   dieses Resultat aus der Analogie mit der Fäulnifs- und Schim-

Es ist also auch bei der Weingährung wie bei der Fäulnifs nicht der Sauerstoff, wenigstens nicht allein der Sauerstoff der atmosphärischen Luft, welcher dieselbe veranlafst, sondern ein in der atmosphärischen Luft enthaltener, durch Hitze zerstörbarer Stoff.

Es drängte sich sofort der Gedanke auf, dafs vielleicht auch die Weingährung eine Zersetzung des Zukkers sey, welche durch die Entwicklung von Infusorien oder irgend einer Pflanze veranlafst werde. Da *Extr. Nucis vom. spir.* ein Gift für Infusorien, nicht für Schimmel ist, Arsenik aber nicht nur Infusorien, sondern auch die meisten Schimmelarten tödtet, so wurden zunächst diese Stoffe angewandt, um vorläufig auszumitteln, ob ich meine Aufmerksamkeit mehr auf Infusorien oder auf Pflanzen zu richten hätte. Es ergab sich, dafs nicht das *Extr. Nucis vom.*, wohl aber einige Tropfen einer Auflösung von arsenichtsaurem Kali die Weingährung aufheben. Es war also wahrscheinlicher eine Pflanze zu erwarten.

Bei der mikroskopischen Untersuchung der Bierhefe zeigten sich darin die bekannten Körnchen, welche das Ferment bilden; allein ich sah zugleich die meisten derselben in Reihen zusammenhängen. Es sind theils runde, gröfstentheils aber ovale Körnchen von gelblichweifser Farbe, die theils einzeln vorkommen, gröfstentheils aber in Reihen von zwei bis acht oder noch mehreren zusammenhängen. Auf einer solchen Reihe stehen gewöhnlich ein oder mehrere andere Reihen schief auf. Häufig sieht man auch zwischen zwei Körnchen einer Reihe seitwärts ein kleines Körnchen aufsitzen, als Grundlage einer neuen Reihe, und meistens befindet sich an dem letzten Körnchen einer Reihe ebenfalls ein kleines, zuweilen etwas in die Länge gezogenes Körperchen. Kurz das Ganze

melbildung höchst wahrscheinlich wäre. Die Sache wird sich indessen durch eine andere sichrere Methode entscheiden lassen.

hat grofse Aehnlichkeit mit manchen gegliederten Pilzen, und ist ohne Zweifel eine Pflanze.

Hr. Prof. Meyen, der diese Substanz auf meine Bitte ebenfalls zu untersuchen die Güte hatte, war ganz derselben Meinung, und äufserte sich dahin, dafs man nur zweifelhaft seyn könne, ob es mehr für eine Alge oder für einen Fadenpilz zu halten sey, welches letztere ihm wegen des Mangels an grünem Pigment richtiger schien.

Die Bierhefe besteht fast ganz aus diesen Pilzen. In frisch ausgeprefstem Traubensaft ist nichts der Art vorhanden. Setzt man denselben aber einer Temperatur von ungefähr 20° R. aus, so finden sich schon nach 36 Stunden einige solcher Pflanzen darin, die aber erst aus wenigen solcher Körner bestehen. Diese wachsen sichtbar unter dem Mikroskop, so dafs man schon nach $\frac{1}{2}$ bis 1 Stunde die Zunahme des Volumens eines sehr kleinen Körnchens, welches auf einem gröfseren aufsitzt, beobachten kann. Erst einige Stunden später, als man die ersten dieser Pflanzen beobachtet, zeigt sich die Gasentwicklung, weil die erste Kohlensäure im Wasser aufgelöst bleibt. Die Bildung solcher Pflanzen nimmt nun im Verlauf der Gährung sehr zu, und nach Beendigung derselben setzen sie sich in grofser Quantität als ein gelblichweifses Pulver zu Boden. Sie zeigen gröfstentheils einige geringe Verschiedenheiten von den Pilzen in der Bierhefe. Nur einige stimmen ganz mit denselben überein; bei den meisten andern nähern sich die Körncher mehr der runden Form, liegen nicht so regelmäfsig in geraden Linien; endlich ist die Zahl der einzelnen Körnchen und solcher, wo aus einem einzelnen Körnchen nur noch ein zweites kleines Körnchen hervorwächst, weit gröfser als diefs in der Bierhefe der Fall ist. Die Beobachtung ihres Wachsens läfst aber über ihre Natur als Pflanzen keinen Zweifel [1]).

1) Wird Zuckerauflösung mit Muskelfleisch, Urin oder Leim län-

Aus diesen Versuchen lassen sich demnach folgende
Thatsachen als die Hauptsache festsetzen:

1) Eine gekochte organische Substanz, oder eine gekochte, vorher gährungsfähige Flüssigkeit geräth
nicht in Fäulniſs, resp. in Gährung, wenn auch
hinlänglicher Zutritt von atmosphärischer Luft, die
aber ausgeglüht worden ist, stattfindet.

2) Zur Fäulniſs wie zur Gährung, überhaupt zu Processen, wobei neue Thiere oder Pflanzen zum Vor-
schein kommen, muſs entweder ungekochte organische Substanz da seyn, oder nicht ausgeglühte
atmosphärische Luft zugeführt werden [1]).

3) In ausgepreſstem Traubensaft tritt die sichtbare
Gasentwicklung als Zeichen der Gährung ein, bald
nachdem die ersten Exemplare eines eigenthümli-
chen Fadenpilzes, den man Zuckerpilz nennen
könnte, sichtbar geworden sind. Während der
Dauer der Gährung wachsen diese Pflanzen und
vermehren sich der Zahl nach.

4) Wird Ferment, welches schon gebildete Pflanzen
enthält, in eine Zuckerauflösung gebracht, so treten
die Erscheinungen der Gährung sehr bald ein, viel
schneller, als wenn sich diese Pflanzen erst bilden
müssen.

5) Gifte, die nur für Infusorien, nicht für niedere
Pflanzen tödtlich sind (*Extr. Nucis vom. spir.*),
hindern die Erscheinungen, welche die mit Infu-
sorienentwicklung verbundene Fäulniſs charakteri-
siren, nicht die Weingährung und die Fäulniſs mit

gere Zeit hingestellt, so entstehen darin ähnliche Pflanzen, aber
in geringerer Zahl, meistens kleiner und gleichsam verkrüppelt.

[1]) Es scheint selbst, daſs Blut (ungekocht), unmittelbar aus den
Gefäſsen eines lebenden Thieres in ein Gefäſs geleitet, welches
atmosphärische Luft enthält und vorher der Siedhitze des Wassers ausgesetzt war, nicht fault. Doch bedarf dieser Versuch
noch einer mehrmaligen Wiederholung.

Schimmelbildung; Gifte, die für Thiere und Pflanzen tödtlich sind (Arsenik) hindern die Fäulnifs sowohl als die Weingährung [1]).

Der Zusammenhang zwischen der Weingährung und der Entwicklung des Zuckerpilzes ist also nicht zu verkennen, und es ist höchst wahrscheinlich, dafs letzterer durch seine Entwicklung die Erscheinungen der Gährung veranlafst. Da aber zur Gährung, aufser dem Zucker, ein stickstoffhaltiger Körper nothwendig ist, so scheint es, dafs dieser ebenfalls eine Bedingung zum Leben jener Pflanze ist, wie es denn an und für sich schon wahrscheinlich ist, dafs jener Pilz Stickstoff enthält. Die Weingährung wird man sich demnach so vorstellen müssen, als diejenige Zersetzung, welche dadurch hervorgebracht wird, dafs der Zuckerpilz dem Zucker und einem stickstoffhaltigen Körper die zu seiner Ernährung und zu seinem Wachsthum nothwendigen Stoffe entzieht, wobei die nicht in die Pflanze übergehenden Elemente dieser Körper (wahrscheinlich unter mehren andern Stoffen) vorzugsweise sich zu Alkohol verbinden. Aus dieser Erklärung ergeben sich die meisten über die Weingährung gemachten Beobachtungen sehr natürlich. Doch beschränke ich mich hier, da die Untersuchung noch nicht beendigt ist, auf diese vorläufigen Mittheilungen, und verweise über das Weitere, sowohl die Gährung als die Fäulnifs und *generatio aequivoca* betreffend, auf meine bald herauszugebenden »physiologischen Beiträge.«

Der Text des hier gegebenen Aufsatzes ist der unveränderte Abdruck einer Abhandlung, die in den ersten Tagen des Februar d. J. vom Hrn. Prof. Müller in

[1]) Die künstliche Verdauung von Eiweifs wird durch arsenichtsaures Kali in solcher Quantität, wie es hinreicht zur Verhinderung der Fäulnifs, nicht gehindert.

in meinem Namen in der hiesigen Gesellschaft naturforschender Freunde vorgelesen wurde. Bald darnach erhielt ich das *Institut* vom 23. Nov. 1836, woraus ich ersah, dafs Cagniard-Latour ähnliche, mir bis dahin unbekannte Beobachtungen über die Gährung des Biers gemacht hatte. Er beobachtete in der Maische, eine halbe Stunde nach dem Zusatz der Hefe, isolirte Kügelchen, denen der Hefe ähnlich. Eine Stunde später fanden sich einige doppelte Kügelchen, d. h. solche, an denen ein secundäres Kügelchen wie durch Expansion des Hauptkügelchens hervorgetrieben zu seyn schien. Später waren gar keine einfachen Kügelchen mehr zu sehen, die doppelten Kügelchen waren gleich grofs, und endlich hingen selbst drei, vier und mehr Kügelchen zusammen. Zugleich vermehrte sich die Zahl der Kügelchen sehr bedeutend, und die ganze Masse der Hefe hatte um das Siebenfache der zuerst zugesetzten Hefe zugenommen. Er schliefst ferner aus der Vergleichung der Kügelchen der Maische mit denen in gährendem Johannisbeer- und Rosinensaft, wo keine Hefe zugesetzt war, dafs die Kügelchen der Maische *jünger* sind als die der Hefe, und dafs letztere *während ihrer Wirkung auf die Maische Samen ausschicken, die sich sogleich entwickeln.* Auch sah er wirklich zwei Mal dieses Ausströmen von etwas Flüssigkeit aus einem solchen Kügelchen. Diefs ist die Hauptsache der von Cagniard-Latour damals gemachten Mittheilungen über die Gährung. Vor Kurzem hat der hochgeachtete französische Gelehrte ein Werk über die Gährung des Biers herausgegeben, welches aber noch nicht hierher gekommen ist, und über dessen Inhalt ich bis jetzt nur aus den politischen Blättern Kenntnifs habe. Ich kann daher nicht beurtheilen, in wiefern unsere in der Hauptsache übereinstimmenden Ansichten im Detail zusammentreffen.

———————

1

A Preliminary Report Concerning Experiments on the Fermentation of Wine and Putrefaction

T. SCHWANN

Translated expressly for this Benchmark volume by H. W. Doelle from "Vorläufige Mittheilung, betreffend Versuche über die Weingährung und Fäulniss," Ann. Physik Chem., **11**, *184–193 (1837)*

At the last gathering of scientists in Jena I reported on experiments related to a "generatio aequivoca." These experiments demonstrated that in a closed glass vessel containing atmospheric air and an infusion from muscles heated at 80°R over boiling water, no growth or putrefaction occurs for several months. This occurs even when the quantity of animal tissue is so small that a complete disappearance of the oxygen from air in the glass vessel is thought to be impossible. I had, however, hoped to modify the experiment in such a way as to be able to introduce fresh air that had been preheated. This I was able to do in the following way.

A small flask, which contained a few pieces of muscle tissue and was one-third filled with water, was closed with a stopper through which two thin glass tubes were bored. These glass tubes passed through an approximately 3 Zoll metal mixture that was heated to a temperature approximating the boiling point of mercury. One of the glass tubes was connected to a gas meter. The fluid in the small flask was boiled briskly to drive all air out of the flask and the glass tubes or to heat it to the boiling point of water. After cooling, a long, continued stream of atmospheric air was led through the gas meter and the first glass tube and into the flask for a period of several weeks. After the air inside the flask was replenished, it was let out through the second glass tube. As it passed through the glass tube into the heated metal mixture, the inflowing air was strongly heated. In these experiments, which were repeated a number of times, there was no formation of "infusorien" or mold, and no putrefaction occurred. The tissue was unchanged and the fluid as clear as it was after the boiling process.[1]

---

[1]Since this experiment required that too much attention be given to the maintenance of the lamp, I later used the following method: A small, 4-oz flask was one-quarter filled with water and meat and closed tightly with a stopper, which was secured with wire. The cork contained two thin glass tubes, the first of which was immediately bent downward and led through a

Whether it is possible to draw conclusions about the generatio aequivoca with these and additional experiments I will discuss at another gathering; I only wish to note that these experiments could be explained from the point of view of enemies of generatio aequivoca in this way: that the seeds of the mold and the infusorien, which are present in the atmospheric air, must have been killed during the burning of the air. Putrefaction[2] must be explained thus: that these seeds in developing and living from the organic substances cause the decay that leads to putrefaction, an opinion supported by the fact that those substances which are poisonous to infusorien and mold (e.g., arsenic or mercuric chloride) also prevent putrefaction, and those substances which are poisonous for infusorien alone and not for mold (e.g., Extractum Nucis vomicae spirituosum) prevent only those types of putrefaction connected with infusorien (i.e., the formation of hydrogen sulfide) and allow only those types of putrefaction to occur which are connected with mold.

I mention this only because it led me to experiments on wine fermentation that appear to give these investigations a different turn. To demonstrate that in other processes, where air plays a role, but as far as it is known, no formation of new animals or plants occur, and where it is not important whether or not air has been burnt, I undertook experiments on respiration and wine fermentation. It was also shown that a frog continued to live very happily in previously heated air.

---

small dish containing mercury covered with oil. The second glass tube was bent horizontally outside the cork for 1½ Zoll, bent downward in a number of closely wound spirals, then upward, horizontally, and finally ended as a drawn-out capillary. The cork was then covered with a thick layer of a suspension of rubber in boiling linseed oil that was thinned with turpentine oil. The fluid in the flask boiled so strongly that the steam came through both glass tubes and warmed the mercury and the oil to such extent that no condensation occurred inside the glass tube. A piece of mercuric chloride was added to the mercury to prevent infusorien growth in the condensing water between the oil and mercury. During the boiling process, a spirit flame was placed under the spirals of the second glass tube, which was protected by a chimney to avoid misdirection of the flame. The heat of the flame was kept so strong that the glass tube softened. The use of a second spirit flame was used to avoid glass breakage due to water condensation at the cooler spots of the glass tubes. After 15 minutes the boiling was stopped, and during the cooling of the flask, air was sucked through the second glass tube into the flask after being heated in the glass spirals. Once the flask was completely cooled, the end of the second glass tube was closed by melting the ends. The spirit flames were taken away. The flask contained only the cooked meat and the burnt air. Occasionally, to renew the air, the spiral was heated until the glass softened. Then the ends of the tube were broken off and new air slowly introduced while the old air left the flask through the mercury. After this process the glass tube was again closed by melting the ends together. With this method, I was able to keep such flasks at 14 to 20°R for 6 weeks without the formation of infusorien or mold or putrefaction. After the flask was opened, the fluid decayed within a few days. Special care must be taken during complete closure of the flask and the glass tube.

[2]Of course, one can only be concerned about the usual putrefaction of the cooked organic substances and not about all the other processes that go under the name "putrefaction" (e.g., rotting, coal formation).

I carried out the wine fermentation experiments in the following way. Solubilized sugar was mixed with beer yeast and four flasks were completely filled and stoppered. The flasks were transferred into boiling water (approximately 10 minutes) in order to obtain the same temperature inside the flask. After their removal, they were put upside down under mercury, and, after cooling, air was introduced into all four flasks until it occupied one-third to one-fourth of the total volume of the fluid. This was done in the case of two flasks via a thin glass tube that was heated until it was glowing red, whereas no heating of the glass tubes was carried out in the other two flasks. Analysis using a platinum ball showed that the heated air contained approximately 19.4 percent oxygen. Because of this, the amount of air introduced into the flasks was increased in one of the flasks in which glass tubes were heated. The flasks were stoppered and left upright at a temperature of 10–14°R. Fermentation (demonstrated by the blowing off of the stoppers) occurred after 4–6 weeks in the flasks that had air introduced without previous heating. After twice the period of time, the two other flasks were still quiet.[3]

In the wine fermentation, as in the case of putrefaction, it is not the oxygen, at least not solely the oxygen in the air, which is the cause, but a substance that is in the air and can be destroyed by heat.

Immediately the thought arises that perhaps wine fermentation is a decomposition of sugar caused by a plant or by the development of infusorien. Since Extractum Nucis vomicae spirituosum is a poison for infusorien and not for mold, and arsenic is a poison for both, I used those substances to find out whether I should turn my attention more to the infusorien or to the plants. The experiments showed that potassium arsenate stopped the fermentation but that Extractum Nucis vomicae did not. Thus a plant had to be suspected as being the cause.

During microscopic investigations of beer yeast, the seeds known to form the ferment were observed; most of them that I saw occurred in chains. They were partly round but mostly ellipsoid yellowish-white seeds. They can be arranged singly but are usually chained in rows of two to eight or more. On top of such a row there are others that come from the side. One also often observes between two seeds in a row a small seed placed sideways which serves as the basis for a new row. A small, often stretched, body is observed, usually on the last seed of a row. In short, the picture is very similar to that of many fungi and thus is undoubtedly that of a plant.

---

[3]Successive experiments were not always successful. Occasionally no fermentation occurred (if cooked too long), and sometimes fermentation occurred in flasks that contained pre-heated air. This is easily explained, however; uncooked organic substances could be introduced from the surface of the mercury during the aeration or replacement of the stopper. The method used to produce putrefaction was not employed because it necessitates a longer boiling period. I would not mention these results if they could not be obtained by analogy with the formation of mold and putrefaction after the existence of a plant has been established. However, this will surely be decided finally by another, more secure method.

21

Meyen, who studied the substance at my request, came to the same conclusion but commented on the difficulty of deciding whether it is an alga or a fungus, although the latter appeared to him to be correct since there was no green pigment.

The beer yeast consists entirely of these fungi. Freshly pressed grape juice does not contain anything of that kind, but they begin to appear after 36 hours at 20°R. One can see them grow under the microscope; thus after ½ to 1 hour one observes the growth in volume of a small seed that sits on top of a large one. It takes a few hours from the first observation of these seeds until gas development occurs, since the first parts of carbon dioxide will be solubilized in the water. During fermentation, the growth of these plants increases rapidly, and after fermentation ceases they appear in large quantities as a yellowish-white powder [*Ed. Note:* sediment] on the bottom. They show, in most cases, small differences from the beer yeast. Only a few are identical; most of them are rounder and do not appear in rows; the number of single seeds and those from which a small second seed grows is much larger than in the case of beer yeast. The observation of its growth leaves no doubt as to its plant nature.[4]

From all these experiments the following conclusions can be drawn:

1. A cooked organic substance, or a cooked, previously fermentable fluid, does not show putrefaction or fermentation, even if aeration with previously heated air occurs.

2. For putrefaction or fermentation, or in general for all processes whereby new animals or plants appear, an uncooked substance has to be present or the air should not be heated.[5]

3. In pressed grape juice, gas development is a sign of fermentation that occurs soon after the appearance of the fungus, which one could call sugar fungus. During fermentation these plants grow and multiply.

4. If one adds the ferment, which already contains these plants, to a sugar solution, fermentation starts very rapidly—much faster compared with solutions where these plants have first to develop.

5. Poisons that are deadly for infusorien but not for lower plants (Extractum Nucis vomicae spirituosum) inhibit those phenomena connected with infusorien development but not the wine fermentation and putrefaction caused by fungi; poisons for animals and plants (arsenic) inhibit putrefaction as well as wine fermentation.[6]

There is no doubt about the connection between wine fermentation and the growth of the sugar fungus, and it is highly probable that the development of the latter causes the fermentation. Since fermentation requires, apart from sugar, a nitrogen source, it appears that this is also a requirement for the life of the plant,

---

[4]If a sugar solution containing muscle, urine, or glue is left standing for longer periods of time, similar plants, which are smaller in numbers and usually smaller and crippled, appear.
[5]It also appears that blood (uncooked) that has been immediately transferred from the vessel of a living animal into a flask that contains air and was previously heated to the boiling point of water does not putrefy. However, this experiment still requires a number of repetitions.
[6]The artificial digestion of albumin is not inhibited by those quantities of potassium arsenate, which inhibits putrefaction.

since the fungus contains nitrogen. The wine fermentation process therefore is a decomposition that is caused by the sugar fungus withdrawing from the sugar and a nitrogenous substance those substances necessary for its nutrition and growth, whereby those substances that are not taken up by the plant are converted (preferably) to alcohol. This explanation would justify all observations made about wine fermentation. However, since this research has not been completed, I am not content with this preliminary report and refer to my later-to-be-published "physiological contributions."

Editor's Comments on Paper 2

2 **Cagniard-Latour:** Report on the Fermentation of Wine
  Ann. Chim. Phys., **68**, 206–207, 220–222 (1838)

At the same time as Schwann, Charles Cagniard-Latour was concerned with the same problem in France. However, his main emphasis was on the physiology of the yeast itself, particularly the beer yeast. In principle, Cagniard-Latour supported Schwann's discovery and his results could be summarized as follows:

1. The beer yeast is a mass of small globules that are able to reproduce. Consequently, they are organized and are not a simple organic or chemical substance, as has been supposed.

2. These bodies appear to belong to the plant kingdom.

3. They seem to cause a decomposition of sugar only when they are alive, and one can conclude that it is very probable that the production of carbon dioxide and the decomposition of sugar and its conversion to alcohol are effects of their growth.

Apart from these statements it is also of interest to read of the physiological aspect of these investigations, which firmly established that yeasts are able to grow anaerobically and that they withstand freezing and dessication.

2

Report on the Fermentation of Wine

C. CAGNIARD-LATOUR

Translated expressly for this Benchmark volume by G. Gordon of the University of Queensland, Australia, from "Mémoire sur la fermentation vineuse," Ann. Chim. Phys., **68**, *206–207, 220–222 (1838)*

In the year VIII, the physical and mathematical sciences group of the Institute proposed, as the subject of a prize, the following question: In plant and animal materials, what are the characters that distinguish substances which assist fermentation from those that experience fermentation? The prize was a medal worth 1 kilogram of gold (i.e., a little more than three thousand francs). This prize was again proposed in the year X but was later withdrawn in the year XII, just as were all those for other groups, because of an unexpected occurrence that deprived the Institute of funds from which these prizes would have been paid.

The question concerning fermentation, having been left unsolved, can still be considered interesting, even though it was formerly made the object of a competition. According to this incentive and before believing that the competition had fermentation in view as the most important aspect, that is, the effect of converting sugared material into alcohol and carbon dioxide (in a word, wine fermentation), I have undertaken a series of experiments concerning it, although proceeding differently than had previously been done, that is, by studying the phenomena of this action with the aid of a microscope.

Chemists know that, having mixed fresh beer yeast with a sugar solution and having introduced this mixture into a well-closed vessel (for example, a flask provided with a Voulf tube) if one exposes this flask to about 25 degrees centigrade, the solution ordinarily begins to ferment after several minutes; progress is rapid if the proportion of yeast is not large. However, wine fermentation does not occur, under the same circumstances, even after a long period of time, when the solution does not contain yeast and if the sugar of this solution is pure.

It was, therefore, expedient to make a microscopic examination first of the material that causes the fermentation of sugar. This examination, as can be seen from the letter I had the honor of addressing to the Academy on April 27, 1835, led me

25

to recognize that the particles of which it is composed have a globular shape, from which I have concluded that these particles were very probably organized.[1]

Whatever attention I devoted to observing the globules, which are, in general, single, translucent, spherical or slightly oblong, and nearly colorless, I have never seen them execute anything which could be considered as signs of exterior willingness [*Ed. Note:* motility?]. On the other hand, yeast globules, as I will soon remark, are able to appear in a liquid where they have not been seen before wine fermentation had begun. When bodies of globular form (i.e., other than crystals) happen to be produced in a mucous liquor, which, before being altered, did not allow the observation of globules, and when these bodies appear to have no locomotive movements, then microscopists normally consider these bodies to be as simple as plants. It is this observation that Monsieur Turpin has made regarding the protospheres that had developed in a gelatinous product, and that I reported in the previously cited letter in the *Journal l'Institut,* No. 103.

It is, then, highly probable that yeast globules are organized, and that they belong to the plant kingdom. Furthermore, these conjectures seem to be confirmed by various observations that are going to be related later.

These plants, if indeed one can give this name to these simple vesicles, are extremely small, for among the globules of diverse dimensions which comprise yeast, the diameter of those that appear to have attained the final stage in their development does not ordinarily exceed 1/100 of a millimeter. For the most part they are smaller than this, with the result that in only 1 cubic millimeter of firm yeast paste, there are probably about 1 million of these individual globules.

Presuming that yeast globules must have the ability to reproduce themselves, I have performed various experiments in order to clarify my own thinking. The first attempt failed spectacularly, but the same is not true for one or two others that I made. One experiment was performed with a vat holding about 10 hectoliters of wort (thanks to Monsieur Leperdriel, owner of the English brewery situated at No. 19 Avenue de Neuilly, who has been kind enough to make the method easy for me) and the other on a smaller quantity of similar wort.

I add here a note in which I have indicated the diverse observations to which

---

[1] It is more than 28 years since I first occupied myself with better methods of producing alcohol by fermentation of boiled liquids from various grass substances. I was curious to examine fresh yeast microscopically. The instrument I used was very imperfect, so I believed that this yeast was like a very fine sand composed of crystalline grains, but it is now evident that I had inferred in error.

Most of the microscopic observations indicated in the present report have been made with a microscope constructed by Monsieur Georges Oberhauser. The magnifications I used most often were 300 to 400 times. In order to measure the size of the globules, I introduced into this instrument an ocular micrometer constructed by Monsieur Charles Chevalier. I will add that this optician was willing to put at my disposal one of his Amici microscopes, which has been useful to me for examining these globules with magnifications superior to the preceding ones.

these experiments have led me,[2] the principal results of which are: first that yeast globules, by the effect of gaseous liberation that they bring about in beer wort, rise to the surface, and many of these globules remain suspended in the abundant foam produced by the fermentation, where one easily distinguishes them correctly with the aid of a microscope by the brilliance that characterizes them; and second that during their action on beer wort, these yeasts diminish in volume and during this contraction most probably emit spores or reproductive bodies that are cloudy, although fairly large. These globules, which are unnoticed at first, are peculiar in that they appear to have the ability to reproduce by buds or by prolongation of their natural tissue. The ability to form multiple globules in this way, initially in twos, threes, or sometimes in a greater number, seems to confirm my hypothesis that yeast globules are organized, and that they belong to the plant kingdom.

Having found it rather extraordinary that the yeast globules may be prevented from regenerating by extension of their tissue, while younger individuals may possess this ability, I have asked Monsieur Turpin if he knew if a similar distinction had been observed with regard to other microscopic growths composed of isolated globules. However, according to the response of this academic, it appears that my observations may be novel.

In the note I am going to speak of, I report that, having examined attentively some samples taken hour-by-hour in proportion to their extraction from the vat, I recognized that the wort already contained double globules at the end of the first hour after adding yeast, that is, on each globule one noticed a smaller secondary globule; that a little later the latter appeared to have increased, since several pairs of double globules were almost the same size; and finally that the fourth sample offered scarcely any double globules. I will add that in order to assure myself that these pairs of globules are united and not simply close together, I applied, with a small point, impacts on the glass covering the globules placed under the microscope. These impacts, although they produce great concussions among the globules, do not destroy the joints. However, it appears that these bodies come apart naturally as they grow older, since in commercial yeast they are generally single, as I have already remarked. This subsequent disunion can hardly be attributed to a vital force, and it seems to me that it eliminates the idea of the formation of these globules as merely an effect of crystallization or of albuminous coagulation. In the course of various fermentations I have performed with beer yeast, I have sometimes distinguished, after the disunion that I have just questioned, a round or oval speck between several granular globules that is presumed to be a cicatricule or an umbilical mark that is sometimes central and sometimes lateral.

I have supposed that yeast, although nitrogenous, belongs to the plant kingdom on the principal basis that the globules have no locomotary movements. On this subject I have been reproached with the fact that certain animals are deprived of similar movements. It seems permissible to presume that analogous types are found

[2]See *Journal l'Institut*, No. 185.

among the microscopic animalcules, and that perhaps the ferment globules are of this type. However, it does not appear probable that yeast belongs to the animal kingdom when one considers, first, that by acting on sugar this substance uses its nitrogen [as discovered a long time ago by Monsieur Thenard (*Annales de Chimie,* year XI, page 313)], and, second, that all plants in the rudimentary state give ammonia directly upon distillation. Furthermore, the nitrogenous material can be eliminated entirely to leave the plant tissue isolated (Report by Monsieur Payen, Collection of foreign scientists, 1834).

I will add that, having attentively followed the various alterations happening unexpectedly in white currant juice, which I closed in a flask with a stopper ground to fit and having filtered the liquid, I noticed a few days after introduction of the yeast many rather large animalcules in the liquid, which were very active at first but which became languid after the wine fermentation started and which have not disappeared. This further disproves the idea that the globules of ferment must belong to the animal kingdom. After this observation I am inclined to believe that the minute corpuscles which comprise Tavel's deposit, which I have spoken of in my letter to the Academy, are inert or almost amorphous particles and not animalcules, as I had supposed after their small movements.

It appears from this that the globules of ferment are capable of developing very readily, for having examined yeast microscopically 8 hours after the addition of a little wort from the contents of the vat that I have spoken of, 80 to 100 globules were already present in the field of the instrument magnifying 300 times, while immediately after the introduction of yeast, one saw only an average of 18.

Furthermore, after harvesting the total quantity of yeast that the contents of the vat had been able to produce during fermentation, I found that this quantity was almost seven times the weight of yeast used, which agrees with the results of my microscopic examination.

After the speed with which the excess of yeast has been obtained, there is reason to believe that this surplus has resulted principally from the reproduction of yeast globules; that is, these globules are found in the liquid that contained food favorable to their reproduction. No brewer is unaware that beer wort normally produces a weight of yeast superior to that of ferment used for inoculation, but it was supposed that this augmentation arises principally from a precipitation of plant albumin which comprises the wort; this explanation appeared well founded, as wort and strong beers generally produced more yeast than those of ordinary beer.

Although beer wort is a medium in which reproduction of ferment globules can take place very easily, it does not appear to be the same as simple sugar solutions, since yeast acting in these solutions does not increase in weight, and, furthermore, it loses its activity.

Wishing to find a reason for this impoverishment, I examined microscopically a yeast with which I accomplished two successive sugar fermentations in closed vessels. I recognized that this yeast, which had only a very moderate fermentation, contained a certain amount of amorphous debris, arising, no doubt, from disorganized globules, and that the globules had, in general, something of a dull and faded outline. It would now appear that the yeast is less active after having acted on the sugar although it diminished very little in weight. This is because it contained healthy globules endowed with life. From this one can conclude that it is very probably by some effect of their growth that the ferment globules destroy the equilibrium of the main constituents of sugar and, in this way, gradually bring about its conversion to alcohol and carbon dioxide. Let us add that these globules appear to be of the plant family that does not perish upon deprivation of water, since air-dried yeast ceases to be a very good ferment, as one knows.

Monsieur Gay-Lussac, in the extract of his report on fermentation, remarked that it still appeared to be one of the most mysterious processes of chemistry—above all, because it only takes place in succession (*Ann. de Chimie*, 1810). It can now be judged how this scientist was actually thinking, since after my research one is led to think that wine fermentation results from a plant phenomenon.

The same scholar demonstrated by the results of various experiments that oxygen exercises a large influence on the development of fermentation in certain liquids, especially grape juice; although if this oxygen is necessary for development, it is not for continuation. After this discovery (that beer yeast is able to produce fermentation of sugared materials without the influence of oxygen), Monsieur Gay-Lussac expressed the opinion that the ferment will be lasting in a large number of substances but in a particular way different from that of beer yeast.

With the idea of obtaining data on the nature of this difference, I made the following experiment, the results of which seem to demonstrate that the opinion of this scholar is justified.

Following his procedure, I preserved under mercury for 2 weeks some grape juice I had squeezed from a bunch of grapes kept under a bell jar filled with hydrogen gas. At the end of this time, I examined microscopically a little of the deposit that had settled out of the juice and found it to be almost amorphous. After the introduction of a little oxygen under the bell I made a suitable examination; wine fermentation had been induced in the grape juice, and I found many globules in the deposit. One would then be tempted to suspect that, first, the grains of this small plant form a part of the deposited material; second, they still have not germinated when they are enclosed in the grapes; and third, germination begins as soon as they are exposed to the influence of oxygen, and that it is by the commencement of this development that they become capable of acting as beer yeast.

At this point, I will report that Monsieur Thenard, by filtering currant juice that had just been squeezed from the fruit by a tightened cloth, has collected on the filter a material that contains almost one-sixth of its weight as ferment, although it had been subjected to several washings before being analyzed in a sugar solution. According to this result and those of my microscopic observations of the ferment, there is hardly reason to doubt that the globules observed in the deposit of grape juice, of which I have just spoken, can be formed along with the elements contained in the same material of the deposit—at least in part, if not totally.

After the information I previously reported concerning yeast globule reproduction in wort, it seems that this reproduction is hardly to be called into question. However, a learned physician has reproved me by noting that, according to Monsieur Milne Edwards, by heating eggwhite diluted in water to a suitable temperature, one is able to determine the appearance of globules which previously did not exist.[3] It would, therefore, be permissible, he added, to suppose that the yeast, being a nitrogenous material, is formed by the coagulation of some plant–animal material contained in beer wort; consequently, the globules of which yeast consists have no more vital organization than that obtained with the aid of eggwhite coagulated by the action of heat.

In order to enlighten myself on this point I put a mixture of 50 g of water and 1 g of eggwhite in a capsule and placed it on a sandbath heated to about 90°C. When a portion of albumin had been coagulated by heat, I removed the capsule, and, after cooling it, I microscopically examined a small part of the very thin pellicle that was formed on the surface of the liquid. I found that this pellicle contains a type of globule. Their diameter was on an average 1/100 of a millimeter, but they had, in general, a crystalline property, and one could distinguish neither granules nor an umbilical spot in any of them. It now seems to me that the objection that I have just mentioned is not sufficient to permit one to think that the ferment globules are analogous to those of coagulated eggwhite.

Furthermore, I have fermented wort spontaneously in a closed apparatus without the addition of yeast. As expected from the experiments of Monsieur Thenard and those to which I will return in an instant, this wort, although it had been filtered, produced a yeast deposit by wine fermentation. Upon microscopic examination of this deposit, I found that it was composed of globules analogous to those of ordinary yeast. Since this fermentation has taken place more slowly than those performed by brewers, the hypothesis that these globules are formed by a sort of albuminous coagulation would require that some must be very large, or at least slightly crystalline —almost like the globules of coagulated eggwhite. This has not taken place. Furthermore, one finds that in this deposit the globules are not the same size as those of ordinary yeast, which would be more favorable to the supposition of an organization, for one imagines that in a ferment produced over a long period of time the globules must be of many different ages.

I performed the same experiment in a flask that had been filled with carbon dioxide. The fermentation developed a little more slowly, but the deposit obtained had almost the same microscopic appearance.

From the work of Monsieur Thenard, it is known that the juice of ripe fruit, and in general the liquors that undergo wine fermentation, form deposits possessing the same properties as yeast (*Annales de Chimie,* year II). It is also known that a sugar solution, to which eggwhite has been added, is able to undergo wine fermentation and produce a yeast deposit when held at a temperature of about 35 degrees for a period of time.

According to these analogies, I thought that the similar deposits must offer the same traces of organization under the microscope as those of beer yeast. Consequently, I carried out various fermentations in closed vessels, notably with currant juice, raisin juice, and prune juice, as well as with a sugar solution mixed with eggwhite. All

---

[3]*Annales des Sciences Naturelles,* 1826.

liquids had been filtered before introduction into their respective apparati. Upon microscopic examination of the deposits obtained, I recognized that each of these deposits was composed in large part[4] of globules analogous to those of beer yeast. As can be seen, these results are in remarkable accordance with the observations of Monsieur Thenard.

Those who are customarily occupied in large-scale fermentation (i.e., brewers and distillers of grain spirit) know that in spite of all the care they take in their operations, the results are extremely variable. These irregularities could even be more favorable to the hypothesis that wine fermentation is induced by bodies endowed with life, because who knows how many different types of similar bodies can be affected.

Since the work by Monsieur Thilorier, it is known that carbon dioxide can be solidified by cooling to a certain temperature, and that in this state of condensation its temperature is much lower than that at which mercury freezes.[5] Having had a quantity of his solidified carbon dioxide by the kindness of this capable and ingenious experimenter, put at my disposal, I mixed it with dry yeast ground to a very fine powder. Although it was exposed to an extremely low temperature (more than 60° below zero centigrade), this yeast has not been less active in the decomposition of sugar than similar yeast powder which has not been chilled.

Recently I froze some fresh yeast reconstituted with water at a temperature of 5°C, and I noted that after this cooling it was as able to act on sugar solution as ordinary fresh yeast.

Summary

I have considered the principal works which deal with wine fermentation, but I have not seen any proposal that attempted to use the microscope for studying the phenomena on which it depends.[6]

As can be seen from the studies that have just been described, this attempt was useful, since it has provided several new observations, the principal results of which are: first, beer yeast, this ferment which is used so much and for this reason is suitable for close examination, is an accumulation of small, consistently organized bodies capable of reproducing themselves—not merely an organic or chemical substance, as

---

[4]Apart from the globules, one could distinguish some other bodies in certain deposits, for example crystals in the deposit from raisin juice and amorphous floccules in the deposit produced during the experiment with albumin.

[5]*Comptes Rendus de l'Academie des Sciences*, October 12, 1835.

[6]In 1680, Leeuwenhoek, having already seen with the aid of the microscope that beer yeast was composed of globules, attributed their origin to the flour employed in the production of beer wort. But this observation, of which I had knowledge for more than a year after the presentation of my report to the Academy, had not led its author to the most important point, which was to realize that the globules are capable of germination and growth in beer wort during its fermentation. See the report by Monsieur Turpin in *Comptes Rendus de l'Academie des Sciences*, August 20, 1838, p. 396.

has been supposed. Second, these bodies appeared to belong to the plant kingdom and regenerate by two different methods. And third, they seem to act on a sugar solution when they are alive, from which it can be concluded that they probably liberate carbon dioxide from this solution and convert the solution into an alcoholic liquor by some effect of their growth.

In addition I will note that the consideration of yeast as an organized material perhaps merits the attention of physiologists; first, because it is able to form and develop quickly under certain circumstances, even in the midst of carbon dioxide, as in brewer's vats. Second, because its mode of regeneration presents peculiarities of a type that had not been observed in other microscopic growth composed of isolated globules. Third, because it lives even after considerable cooling or dehydration.

In conclusion, I will add that the question previously proposed by the Institute appears now to be resolved by the results that I have just explained and by various others that I have communicated to the Société Philomathique during the years 1835 and 1836.[7] The results agree with the conclusion that ferments (at least those which produce wine fermentation in the yeast manner) are generally composed of very simple organized microscopic bodies, and that the materials with which they undertake this fermentation are purely chemical substances, since, as it is known, they are sugar and compounds related to it.

---

[7]See the *Journal l'Institute*, Nos. 158, 159, 164, 165, 166, 167, 185 and 199.

Editor's Comments on Paper 3

3 Liebig: About the Occurrence of Fermentation, Putrefaction, and Decay, and Their Causes
Ann. Physik Chem., **48**, 120–122, 130–136, 142–144 (1839)

In his classical paper, the outspoken organic chemist from Germany, Justus Liebig, disputes the participation of living matter in alcoholic fermentation and attempts to consider this process as a purely chemical phenomenon. The weight of his authority almost forced scientists to forget the two previously discussed publications. Liebig's main argument was that organic chemistry recognizes two separate types of phenomena for the behavior of its compounds:

1. Substances develop from newly developed properties, in which the elements of many atoms of simple compounds become transformed into molecules of a high order.

2. Molecules of a higher order can decompose into molecules of a lower order as a result of a neutralization of the equilibrium in the attraction of their elements.

Although some historians (Brock, 1961) have stated that Liebig's theories are incorrect and lacked experimentation, this author has often wondered whether Liebig was ahead of his time and had already indicated the importance of enzymes in the alcoholic process. If one regards the word "substance" as being "enzyme," his theory would be in accordance with our present knowledge of the role of these "chemical substances" in biological systems. This thought gains support from Liebig's statement that heat, contact with different substances, and the influence of a substance which is in the process of changing are the main factors that bring about decomposition.

3

About the Occurrence of Fermentation, Putrefaction, and Decay, and Their Causes

J. LIEBIG

*Translated expressly for this Benchmark
volume by H. W. Doelle from Über die
Erscheinungen der Gährung, Fäulniss
und Verwesung, und ihre Ursachen,"*
Ann. Physik Chem., **48**, *120–122,
130–136, 142–144 (1839)*

By decay (Eremacausie: ἠρέμα, gradual, and καῦσις, burn) one generally means changes that organic substances undergo at normal or above-normal temperatures. These changes take place only in moist conditions; they stop when water freezes and do not occur in the absence of oxygen.

If the air supply is cut off by the addition of water during the decaying process, the process continues as putrefaction.

Decay is a combustion at low temperatures, in which the elements of a substance take part depending upon their relation to oxygen.

Putrefaction is a decaying process in which the oxygen of the air does not take part; it is a combustion of one or more elements of a substance with the oxygen of that substance, or of water, or of both.

If access of oxygen and water is cut off, putrefaction and decay both occur, a decaying process called rotting (Aposepsie).

Fermentation (fermentatio) is a putrefaction of plant substances that do not develop an uncomfortable odor during the decaying process.

According to the known behavior of the elements of organic substances, one has to assume the basic fact that, in a decaying body containing carbon, hydrogen, and oxygen, part or all of the hydrogen reacts first with the oxygen of the air and forms water; the oxygen of the substance either stays with the other elements in form of oxides, starved of hydrogen, or reacts with part of the carbon to form carbon dioxide, which separates from the other elements.

The carbon of a substance does not react with the oxygen of the air until all hydrogen present in the substance is converted to water.

Substitution of an equivalent amount of oxygen for the hydrogen does not occur during the decaying process.

If the oxygen uptake is higher than the amount of hydrogen present during the decaying process, hydrogen-starved oxides, which have the potential to take up more oxygen and thus form a higher oxidation state, occur.

These rules have been developed from those decaying processes that have been studied most and are now well known: the formation of acetic acid from alcohol and the formation of humus from decaying plants. Further experience is required, however, to correct and enlarge those rules.

In the case of alcohol decay, the oxygen of the air converts two hydrogen equivalents to water, and a hydrogen-starved oxide, the aldehyde, which contains all the oxygen of the alcohol, is formed.

If the oxygen supply is continued, the aldehyde takes up two oxygen equivalents and forms acetic acid. A substitution of the hydrogen that has been shown by Dumas to occur in isomorphic substances with chlorine, iodine, and bromine, does not occur during acetic acid formation.

$$* \quad * \quad * \quad * \quad * \quad * \quad *$$

The "ferment" develops as a result of a metamorphosis which starts as soon as air is introduced into a sugar-rich plant sap and can continue without interruption up to a point if oxygen is removed; the ferment contains all the nitrogen of the plant sap, which is known as protein, glue, and mucilage. The ferment develops, therefore, as a result of changes that occur in these substances; in most cases it has a uniform constitution.

If one summarizes all the observations made by Thénard, Colin, and others, it can be said that the ferment is a labile substance that is in a continuous progressive metamorphosis, putrefaction, decay, or fermentation, or whatever one wishes to call this process.

I will try to explain these observations so that it will be seen that the ferment is not a mysterious seed, but that putrefaction and fermentation are the result of changes that occur in the ferment itself.

The ferment is a putrefying and decaying body; it converts the oxygen of the air into CO_2 and forms more CO_2 from its own mass; it continues to produce CO_2 underwater; after some days it develops an evil-smelling gas (Thenard) and will have changed finally to a mass similar to old cheese (Proust); its fermentation potential ceases as soon as the decaying process is completed.

The presence of water is essential to maintain the characteristics of the ferment (for maintaining its putrefaction). The characteristics of fermentation are slowed down by pressing the water out and are destroyed after drying out. These characteristics are also destroyed by heat, alcohol, NaCl, an excess of sugar, mercuric oxide, arsenic, sulfuric acid, $AgNO_3$, oil (in other words, all substances that prevent putrefaction).

The insoluble body that is called ferment does not start fermentation. If one washes beer and wine yeast carefully with boiled, cold, distilled water, making sure that the solids are completely covered with water, the residue does not cause fermentation in a sugar solution. However, the wash water now has this potential, although it loses it a few hours after air is added.

The potential for fermentation that the soluble part of the yeast in the water possesses is not based on contact; yeast loses its potential for fermentation on contact as soon as alcohol is added. A hot, clear, and aqueous extract of ferment in a closed flask containing sugar solution does not start fermentation; it is caused by the soluble part that appears during decay of the ferment itself. If the hot extract is cooled in air and left in air for several hours, strong fermentation occurs (Colin); without the air supply, no fermentation occurs (Colin). The contact with air causes oxygen absorption and the extract contains a remarkable amount of carbon dioxide after several hours.

During the fermentation of sugar with the ferment, two decaying processes occur. If 1 ml of an aqueous suspension of beer yeast and 10 g of a sugar solution that contains 1 g of pure sugar are added to a mercury-filled graduated flask, one finds, after 24 hours (if the flask was stored at 20–25°C), a volume of CO_2 that at 0°C and 0.76^m B [*Ed. Note:* atmospheric pressure] is equal to 245–250 ml, or 0.485–0.495 g. Since 11 ml of fluid contains an equal volume of CO_2, the total obtained would thus be 255–259 ml or 50.3–51.27 percent CO_2.

Thenard obtained 57.2 parts ethanol of 39°B [*Ed. Note:* Baume], which is equivalent to 52.62 parts ethanol, from 100 parts sugar.

100 parts sugar thus give 51.27 parts CO_2 plus 52.62 parts alcohol equals 103.89 parts total.

One finds all carbons of the sugar in the amounts of CO_2 and alcohol produced.

The analysis of sugar revealed that it unmistakably contains 4 atoms of CO_2, 2 atoms of ether, and 1 atom of water.

From the products of fermentation one can see that alcohol is two-thirds CO_2 and one-third the carbon of the sugar; however, these products contain 2 atoms of hydrogen and 1 atom of oxygen more than sugar. It is thus obvious that 1 atom of water must have participated in the change.

According to the ratios by which sugar combines with equivalent bases, as well as to the analyses of its oxidation products (the sugar acids), one must agree that 1 atom of sugar contains 12 carbons. None of these are present in the form of CO_2; treatment with $KMnO_4$ produces oxalic acid and it is impossible to obtain oxalic acid by an oxidative process from CO_2. The hydrogen of the sugar does not bind in the form of ether; treatment with concentrated HCl gives a brown coal and water, and it is known that no ether is able to react this way.

Thus sugar does not contain ready-formed CO_2, alcohol, ether, or any other product. Its behavior characterizes it as a complex organic atom that decays into alcohol and CO_2 as a result of a metamorphosis of its elements.

Therefore, as can be seen from the endproducts obtained during the fermentation of sugar, the elements of the ferment do not play any part; it is the split of a complex atom, similar to the results of the metamorphosis that organic atoms undergo during heating, with the difference that it occurs in water and that the elements of water react with one of the formed products. During fermentation of the sugar, the ferment also undergoes changes; it is reduced in quantity. If one uses the insoluble part from the fermentation and transfers it into a fresh sugar solution, its quantity will be reduced further. The insoluble part of this second fermentation does not react again in a fresh sugar solution.

Thenard obtained, after complete fermentation, 13.7 parts insoluble residue from 20 parts fresh beer yeast and 100 parts sugar. After a second fermentation this quantity was reduced to 10 parts. These 10 parts were white, possessed the characteristics of wooden fiber, and were completely inert in a fresh sugar solution.

The above description reveals that, during the fermentation of sugar with ferment, both decay in a way that will eventually cause both to disappear; their elements re-form to produce new compounds. One knows that CO_2 and alcohol (compounds the elements of which are always present, with the exception of 1 atom water, which can be found in the alcohol) are formed from the sugar. What products are formed during the transformation of the ferment have not been investigated; one knows only that the nitrogen content can be found as ammonia in the fermentation fluid.

The ferment is therefore a decaying body; it obtains its potential by contact with oxygen. The insoluble ferment, which loses its characteristics by being washed with air-free water, can recapture this during the decaying process (Colin).

If one adds sugar to a ferment that is in metamorphosis, the gradual decomposition process begins. If the amount of ferment is too small in relation to the sugar, the decaying process of the ferment stops before that of the sugar. Undecomposed sugar is retained since the cause of the decay, the contact with a decaying body, is lost. The condition of the ferment, its insolubility in water, causes less decay. If the amount of ferment is greater, the decay of the sugar is completed before that of the ferment. One portion of ferment has disappeared; another, still in the decaying stage, is left behind. In a fresh sugar solution this portion can continue to ferment until it goes through its own metamorphosis.

A given amount of ferment is necessary to ferment a given portion of sugar; however, its influence is not an influence of its mass but is restricted to its presence until the time that the last sugar atom is decomposed. The ferment, as cause of the fermentation, therefore, does not exist. The insoluble part does not possess this characteristic; the soluble part, which develops during the decay, also loses this characteristic. Both substances together cause fermentation from the moment they start to decay under the influence of oxygen and water, which results in their complete destruction. It is, therefore, no mysterious body, no substance, that causes decomposition; they are only the carriers of an activity that reaches over the sphere of the decaying body.

* * * * * * *

Carbon dioxide and hydrogen gas develop during the decay of glue under anaerobic conditions, which means that water is decomposed and its oxygen forms a new compound (Saussure, Proust).

The fermentation of sugar, in contact with the ferment, is therefore completely different from the fermentation of glue or wort; in the first case the ferment disappears with the sugar, while in the latter, the ferment is formed during meta-morphosis of the sugar.

The form and nature of these insoluble precipitates has led to strange opinions among physiologists about the fermentation.

In water, separated beer and wine yeast appear under a good magnifying glass as translucent flat balls that occasionally occur in rows and take the form of vegetation; in the eyes of others they are similar to infusorien.

It would be quite remarkable if glue and protein, which separate into different constituents during fermentation of beer and plant sap, would take on a geometrical form during their separation or precipitation, since they have never been obtained in crystallized form. Indeed this is not the case; they precipitate, like any other substance that does not possess a crystalline structure, in the form of round balls that either swim around freely or stick together.

These scientists have been lured by these forms to consider the ferment as living organic compounds, declaring them plants or animals that require sugar for their development, use it, and excrete CO_2 and alcohol; with this they explain the decomposition of sugar and the increase in mass of the added ferment during the fermentation.

This opinion is contradictory. In a pure sugar solution the "seed" disappears with the plants during fermentation; the fermentation takes place; and the de-composition of sugar and ferment occurs without the development or reproduction of seed, plant, or animal, which are described by these scientists as the cause of the chemical processes.

During decay, the elements of animal tissue are in a state of continuous change, a state of disturbed equilibrium that is changed and modified by even the weakest influence, such as other substances and heat. Such a condition appears to be the most fruitful one for the development of the incomplete and lowest animal classes, the microscopic animals, whose eggs can spread anywhere (a well-known fact); they develop in the decaying material and multiply using the new products from the fermentation for their nutrition.

Some scientists consider the chemical processes of putrefaction a result of the development of these animals; this would be equal to saying that the cause of wood decay and rotting comes from the plants that use the decayed material and soil for their nutrition.

These animals do not originate in the decaying material if one removes the contact with air, just as no worms develop in decaying cheese if one keeps the flies away.

This opinion proves false if one considers that the animals die as soon as the decaying bodies disappear, that after their death a cause should be known which destroys the organisms, which determines the parts of the muscle or organs that change into new solid and gaseous products. This cause is finally a chemical process.

In the behavior of its compounds organic chemistry offers two entirely different appearances:

1. Bodies with new, changed characteristics develop, since the elements of a number of atoms of a single compound change and combine to an atom of higher status.

2. Complex atoms of higher status can decompose into two or more less complex atoms of lower status by suspending the equilibrium of their attracting elements.

These disturbances can be caused by heat, by contact with a different substance, and by the influence of a body that is in the state of metamorphosis.

Editor's Comments on Paper 4

4 **Pasteur:** Report on Alcoholic Fermentation
   Ann. Chim. Phys., **58**, 381–393 (1860)

Louis Pasteur is regarded as the first outstanding microbial biochemist. A very large collection of letters and biographies indicate (see Valleroy-Radot, 1960) that he and J. Liebig fought vigorously about the cause of fermentation. The reproduced extracts are from Pasteur's original publication on alcoholic fermentation (Paper 4). Credit has to go to Pasteur for his carefully planned experimentation. For the first time, quantitative methods were employed. In doing so, Pasteur was able not only to confirm the observations of Schwann and Cagniard-Latour, but also to demonstrate that yeast actually increased in weight, nitrogen, and carbon content during the fermentation. Of further significance in his work was the introduction of synthetic media. Whereas all previous scientists used rather rich media for their study, Pasteur carried out his experiments in a solution containing sugar, ammonium tartrate, and trace elements. After inoculation, he observed the growth of yeast and fermentation of sugar occurring concurrently, with ammonia being transformed to albumin. The experiments of Pasteur, without any doubt, provided the first evidence for the cause of fermentation and the close relationship between the carbon source (sugar), nitrogen source (ammonia), and the living yeast cell. These quantitative experiments laid the foundation for the study of microbial metabolism.

Pasteur in this paper also deals with Liebig's theory. One can read that Pasteur strongly objected to the idea that an "unstable substance," rather than a living cell, causes fermentation.

4

Report on Alcoholic Fermentation

L. PASTEUR

*Translated expressly for this Benchmark
volume by G. Gordon of the University
of Queensland, Australia, from "Mémoire sur la fermentation alcoolique,"*
Ann. Chim. Phys., **58**, *381–393*
(1860)

III. Yeast Production in a Medium Formed
from Sugar, an Ammonium Salt, and Phosphates

Unpublished experiments at the beginning of my studies on gaseous fermentation products in grain and beet-root distilleries have proved to me that carbon dioxide
is almost completely absorbed by potash. In several efforts, where each time I have
collected 60 to 70 liters of gas in several hours with the aid of a potash apparatus that
dissolves the gas in proportion to its release, I have found that the carbon dioxide
produced by these large industrial fermentations, completed in the presence of
natural ammonium salts contained in the liquor, comprises about one ten-thousandth
of its volume as nitrogen.[1] A residue of 7 to 8 cubic centimeters that is not absorbed
by potash is left by 60 to 70 liters of gas. These experiments merit reconsideration
under the experimental conditions of the preceding paragraph. Nevertheless, I can
infer from these results without other verification that the nitrogen in the ammonia
that disappears during alcoholic fermentation is not released as a gas.

Guided by these indications and somewhat justified by what appeared from this
assumption, I asked myself, "If, under fermentation conditions, ammonia was not
formed from albuminous material by combination with sugar in such a way as to enter

---

[1] The description of the apparatus that was used on this occasion (see Fig. 2) will perhaps be of
some use. B is a round-bottomed flask with a capacity of ½ to 1 liter filled with a very concentrated solution of caustic potash. F is a flask that receives potash during the arrival of carbon
dioxide bubbles, dissolution of which is not immediate. E is a funnel inverted in the fermentation vat, which conducts the gaseous carbon dioxide into vessel B through the rubber tube *abc*
and the glass tube *def*. R is a safety valve for the manipulation of the apparatus. The rubber
tube is fitted to the safety valve when potash fills tube *fed* and after all the air has been driven
out of the funnel and tube *abc*. The exact quantity of carbon dioxide is determined by the

into the composition of yeast, what would explain its disappearance as ammonia?"

Thus I have been led to note the following results, which will show all the organized power of yeast and which will, I hope, put an end to discussions of its nature. In a solution of pure candied sugar, I place 1 part of an ammonium salt (for example, tartrate of ammonia), a like amount of the mineral material that enters into the composition of beer yeast, and finally a batch of fresh yeast globules. Remarkably, the globules sown in these conditions develop; they multiply and the sugar ferments, while the mineral material dissolves gradually and the ammonia disappears. In other words, ammonia is transformed into a complex albuminous material that is incorporated into the yeast; at the same time, phosphates provide the new globules with necessary minerals. Carbon is evidently supplied by sugar. For example, here is the composition of one of the liquors used: 10.000 g of pure candied sugar; ashes of 1 g of yeast obtained by a system of pulleys from a cup furnace; 0.100 g of dextrotartrate of ammonia; and traces of fresh, washed beer yeast, about the size of a pinhead, moist, losing 80 percent water at 100°C.

Fermentation takes place in a similar mixture, in a flask filled to the neck and well sealed or provided with a gas tube immersed in pure water. After 24 to 36 hours the liquor begins to display appreciable signs of fermentation, indicating by a release of microscopic bubbles that the liquid is already saturated with carbon dioxide. I do not believe that fermentation manifests itself by an obvious release of gas before this condition of saturation has been reached.

In the following days, the turbidity of the liquor progressively increases, while the release of gas becomes sufficiently perceptible and foam fills the neck of the flask. A deposit gradually covers the bottom of the vessel. When observed microscopically, a drop of this deposit is seen as a fine, very branched yeast, extremely young in

---

difference in weight of the apparatus before and after the experiment. The apparatus cannot readily be used for small fermentations, because the liberation of gas and gas pressure are too slight to allow the movement of potash from *d* to *c* through the valve.

Figure 2.

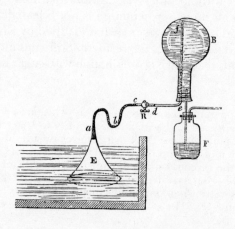

appearance; that is, the globules are swollen, translucent, ungranulated, and one can distinguish among them quite easily every globule of the small quantity of yeast originally sown. These globules have a thick cover, breaking off in blacker circles; their contents are yellowish and granular, but the manner in which they are some- tmes surrounded by young globules clearly indicates that they have given birth to the latter, which form a string of beads.

These interesting observations are necessarily made during the first days; the old globules are distinguished from the infinitely more numerous young ones in the evening by gaslight as easily as one distinguishes a small black ball in the middle of many white ones.

Gradually differences disappear and the newly separated globules lose all branched appearance; one no longer sees buds. The globules are very granular, similar to full-grown or exhausted beer yeast.

Fermentation is just as active if one makes use of an appropriate albuminous material, such as that of grapes, of beet-root, or of the soluble part of normal beer yeast instead of ammonia for the nitrogenous nutrition of the sown yeast. If one places globules of fresh yeast in sugared water mixed with a little of these albuminous materials, the general phenomena will always be the same as those I have just described, although the fermentation will probably be more active. For example, instead of becoming visible after 36 to 48 hours, the first small bubbles of carbon dioxide appear at the end of 12 to 24 hours. Furthermore, the quantity of yeast formed and deposited in the same length of time is much greater, but this is propor- tional to the greater amount of energy, and the products formed are the same.

This influence of the nitrogenous and mineral nature of the medium on the activity of fermentation is very strange. I have performed multiple experiments concerning it, several results of which I will report. One of the more interesting relates to the use of albumin from eggwhite. I have been quite surprised to find this material entirely unable to nourish the beer-yeast globules. If some sugar is dissolved in egg- white albumin diluted in water, filtered (so that it is neutral or slightly acid), and a small quantity of beer yeast added, the globules will not develop at all, and there will be no trace of fermentation.[2]

However, it is known, from the experiments of Monsieur Collin and Monsieur Thénard, that a concoction of sugared albumin left to itself ferments, and that, according to Monsieur Turpin, it forms ordinary alcoholic yeast. But, as noted by Messieurs Thénard and Collin, this effect is evident only after 3 weeks to 1 month at a temperature of 30 to 35°C; from the very beginning this fermentation is always very slow. By examining the liquor during the interval that precedes alcoholic fermenta- tion, it is easy to verify that various products (infusoria or molds) are formed, and I have no doubt that the albumin, slightly modified in its nature by these materials, becomes slightly suited to nourish the beer yeast.

---

[2]See the similar experiments of Monsieur Bouchardat in Volume XVIII of *Comptes Rendus de l'Academie.*

Materials decompose quite differently in blood serum or the liquids squeezed from muscles. Sugar and some yeast globules are added to the clear, colorless serum, permitting the yeast to develop with remarkable ease; the sugar ferments almost as easily as if one used a naturally sugared juice or clear yeast water. I do not think that the serum albumin has a nature different from that of eggwhite; rather I believe that the difference is due to other albuminous materials that accompany blood albumin and are individually suitable for the nutrition of yeast globules. Here is what led me to adopt this opinion.

I coagulated colorless serum and boiled it with water. After filtration to perfect clarity to separate the coagulated albumin, I dissolved some sugar in the filtered liquid and added several fresh globules. These multiplied and very definite alcoholic fermentation occurred.

I have performed the same experiment with boiled water on eggwhite, but have not obtained any fermentation. These experiments have been repeated many times and have always given the same results.

Whatever causes it, is it not remarkable to see an ammonium salt being used to nourish yeast globules, supplying their albuminous elements, while the pure eggwhite albumin is completely unsuitable? Therefore, one understands that the distance between the diverse species of this generic group can be great, as indicated by the expression of albuminous or proteinaceous materials. I have also observed that certain proteinaceous materials are more favorable than others to the development of lactic yeast; for example, the soluble parts of gluten and casein, and the nitrogenous materials of liquids that have experienced alcoholic fermentation. Even though globules of beer yeast are sown in aqueous sugar solutions of these products, it is not rare to see alcoholic fermentation accompanied by lactic fermentation; that is, it develops spontaneously (as a result of contact with air at the beginning) due to lactic yeast that acts on sugar parallel to alcoholic yeast.

The influence of the medium and the appropriation of the nitrogenous material and the mineral materials into the life of the yeast are further demonstrated in another way, which is no less dramatic; I speak of the spontaneous fermentation of sugared liquid without the addition of a given yeast.

Everyone knows that grape juice left alone for several hours undergoes alcoholic fermentation, and it is extremely rare for it to be complicated by another fermentation (for example, lactic fermentation). The same thing happens to beet-root juice if it has been made acid by Monsieur Dubrunfaut's method. But here one encounters quite frequently (I have many proofs of it) the production of parallel, simultaneous fermentation by the individual yeasts.

When use is made of yeast water (i.e., the soluble part of beer yeast filtered to perfect clarity, supplemented with sugar, and left to stand), alcoholic fermentation (i.e., spontaneous formation of beer yeast) will almost always occur if there was contact with air at the beginning. Although I have seen several examples of it in the course of my research, fermentation is very rarely produced only by lactic, butyric, or other yeasts. As is frequently the case under these conditions, fermentation is due to the simultaneous formation of alcoholic yeast and lactic yeast, and one can cause any of these yeasts to predominate by employing either fresh or old yeast water. Although perfectly clear after boiling, old yeast water is much more suited to the formation of lactic yeast.

These results would be even more remarkable if the conditions of neutrality or of alkalinity of the media (either primordial or permanent) had been altered.

It could be suggested that the nature of the albuminous material plays the principal role in these phenomena independent of any combination with mineral substances. But here are some facts which clearly show that the presence and quality of mineral elements are no less essential than the organic elements. Essentially, if one eliminates mineral material from the composition of the medium formed from sugared water, an ammonium salt, and yeast ash, the sown globules do not multiply at all, and there is no sign of fermentation. What is more, if the nature of the principal minerals is modified, by removing the alkaline phosphates, for example, the progress of fermentation is appreciably modified and retarded.

Phosphate of magnesium, when used alone, does not produce the same results as crude yeast ash. Some alterations become evident when use is made of ash from yeast either fused at white heat (which partly removes the alkalis) or merely roasted by moderate heat. It is during these latter conditions that the progress of fermentation is most rapid and regular.

In the same way one is able to ascertain that the ammonium salt is indispensable. Yeast globules sown in some sugared water mixed with yeast ash cause no perceptible fermentation. However, fermentation is not entirely absent, for sometimes a fraction of a cubic centimeter of gas is formed. This must be due to ammonia from the distilled water or to the infinitely small amount of albuminous material that is carried across in the inoculation.

The necessity of the presence of sugar, which alone can provide the carbon of yeast globules, is sufficiently proven in the experiments so that I am not dwelling on it. Therefore, everything (sugar, nitrogenous material, and mineral material) cooperates in the fermentation phenomenon.

The influence of inoculation is no less certain. If inoculation is suppressed, its influence is so marked that there is a similar fermentation, but I have never seen a single yeast globule being formed, instead only some small infusoria and some lactic yeast with which fermentation is correlative with their development.

Where does this complete absence of beer yeast in the latter experimental orders come from? The facts I have previously reported are reply enough. The answer is that the medium is not sufficiently suited to the propagation of this yeast. There is no material barrier to the formation of beer yeast, except that none of it has been sown. It appears spontaneously by contact with air in grape must, in beet-root juice, and soon, but the medium formed from sugar, phosphates, and an ammonium salt is not really suitable, so spontaneous production may be impossible, although the same medium can maintain the viability and development of the adult yeast that is sown in it. This particular medium appears more appropriate to lactic yeast and infusoria; all the mineral agents support the formation of these products if the liquor has been in contact with normal air.

If one boils the mixture for several minutes and exposes it to heated air, no organism or any kind of fermentation activity appears.

It seems to me that all these facts, which further illuminate the phenomena of fermentation, will help us to understand an extraordinary peculiarity of the fermentations that take place in a medium of sugared water, an ammonium salt, phosphates, and seeds of beer yeast: namely, the spontaneous appearance of lactic yeast and infusoria. The latter are seen only during the first days and promptly disappear, while the lactic yeast persists, multiplies, and frequently ends by acting almost alone because the acidity that it causes in the liquor is harmful to many beer yeasts. Although only beer yeast has been sown, the fact that there is a mixture of two yeasts is due to the nature of the medium, which is more suitable to the development of lactic yeast than alcoholic yeast (alcoholic yeast never occurs in the case of spontaneous fermentation).

That being so, I am going to give the detailed analysis of a fermentation carried out in a medium composed of water, pure candied sugar, tartrate of ammonia, and white, fused, powdered yeast ashes.

At midday on December 10, 1858, I placed in an oven 10 g of sugar, 100 cubic centimeters of water, 0.100 g of dextrotartrate of ammonia, ash from 1 g of yeast, and traces of fresh yeast (the size of a pinhead).

At 4 o'clock in the evening of the 11th, by attentively observing the place where the small fragments of added yeast had fallen to the bottom of the vessel, one could see gaseous bubbles of an extreme thinness being continually produced. This phenomenon continued there. Elsewhere on the bottom of the flask, only small gas bubbles are produced intermittently. Furthermore, several small floccules are suspended in the bulk of the liquid by very small gas bubbles adhering to them.

At 7 o'clock in the evening of the same day, fermentation is quite appreciable, although still weak. There is already a small amount of foam in the neck of the flask at the liquid's surface. The bubbles are released from various points at the bottom of the vessel. On the 12th, fermentation is very active, with much foam and a deposit on the bottom of the flask. The liquid is clouded by yeast in suspension.

On the 13th, 14th, and 15th, fermentation was active, but on the following days its rate gradually abated, although it still continued.

From periodic examination of the liquid in January, it became apparent that lactic yeast had formed and that it continued to increase, as did the acidity of the liquor.

Since lactic fermentation interferes with alcoholic fermentation, I terminated the experiment and studied the liquor. One part provided a perceptible amount of alcohol which had not been determined.

The analysis, by the copper solution method, of the quantity of sugar remaining has shown that 4.5 g of sugar was fermented and 5.5 g remained.

By saturating 10 cubic centimeters with standardized limewater, I found that a quantity of acid was formed equivalent to 0.597 sulfuric acid (i.e., almost 1 g of organic acids), which is a considerable quantity that amply demonstrates that the alcoholic fermentation has deviated from its original direction.

I determined the quantity of ammonia by analyzing 50 cubic centimeters of the fermented liquid. I found that 0.0062 g of ammonia disappeared. All the harvested yeast, dried at 100°C on a calibrated filter, weighed 0.043 g. I am sure that all the yeast ash used was dissolved during the procedure. This weight (0.043 g) is, then, the dry weight of the yeast formed.

In order to identify the nature of the acid, a portion of the fermented liquid was evaporated, redissolved several times in ether, evaporated again, saturated with lime water, evaporated again, and treated with alcohol. This gives a very faint crystalline precipitate (which is probably succinate of lime) from which I have extracted crystalline succinic acid, which is so easy to identify even when working with a very small quantity.

The alcoholic liquid produced abundant crystals of lactate of lime mixed with a small amount of the lime salt of succinic acid. From the crystallization volume of lactate of lime, it is certain that most of the liquor is lactic acid.

I transformed a portion of this salt into lactate of zinc, which is easily characterized by its crystalline form.

Finally, in the residue treated with ether and left insoluble by it, I distinguished very clearly with a microscope a crystalline precipitate having the exact form of mannitol and a sugary taste, which removes the doubt arising from the presence of tartaric acid in the residue. Glycerine is present in the residue after treatment with a mixture of alcohol and ether.

All these results have been obtained by acting mainly on very small materials with the most rigorous accuracy, and they prove the production of alcoholic and lactic yeasts by their particular fermentations in a unique medium of sugar, an ammonium salt, and mineral elements.

All the evidence in this article supports this conclusion.

Later I will publish a special work on alcoholic fermentation occurring under these conditions, and I will then study the unique nature of the albuminous yeast materials formed with the aid of sugar and ammonia.[3]

---

[3]Monsieur Dumas, when I had the honor of speaking to him about the first results, which have been presented in this chapter, was very impressed with the necessary individual roles of ammonium salts, phosphates, and hydrocarbon materials in the viability and multiplication of yeast globules. Comparing yeast and the youngest plant tissues, he said to me, "I understand that sugar, ammonium salts, and phosphates have always been collected with plant sap. It must be with their aid that the cell forms itself." In the course of my work I have had the occasion to reread the remarkable works by Monsieur Payen on plant composition, and I acknowledge that the numerous relationships that one can establish between yeast and young plant organs stuck in my mind.

The reader will also do well to compare the research that preceded the work of Monsieur Mirbel on cambium and the more recent writings on the role of phosphates in the life of plants.

Editor's Comments on Papers 5, 6, and 7

5 **Pasteur:** Mémoire sur la fermentation appelée lactique
English Translation: Report on Lactic Fermentation
Compt. Rend. Acad. Sci., Paris, **45**, 913–916 (1857)

6 **Pasteur:** Animalcules infusoires vivant sans gaz oxygène libre et déterminant des fermentations
English Translation: Infusorial Animalcules Living Without Free Oxygen and Causing Fermentation
Compt. Rend. Acad. Sci., Paris, **52**, 344–347 (1861)

7 **Pasteur:** Influence de l'oxygène sur le développement de la levûre et la fermentation alcoolique
English Translation: Influence of Oxygen on Yeast Development and Alcoholic Fermentation
Bull. Soc. Chim. Paris, **28**, 79–80 (1861)

Louis Pasteur not only studied the process of sugar fermentation by yeast, he also investigated lactic and butyric acid fermentation. The first two papers (Papers 5 and 6) are of particular interest, as Pasteur recognized that these fermentations are carried out, not by yeast, but in the first instance by "tiny globules of small objects" and in the second (Paper 6) by "infusoria." As he demonstrated his malolactic fermentation (Paper 5) in a medium containing yeast extract, sugar, and chalk, it can well be assumed that he not only discovered malolactic acid fermentation, but also what we now understand as homofermentation by lactic acid bacteria. The "small objects" were possibly streptocci, which require chalk to neutralize acid production.

Using strict anaerobic conditions, by excluding air, Pasteur discovered butyric acid production (Paper 6). Although it is not known, it can be assumed that either a *Clostridium* species or butyribacterium was involved. The great significance of this publication is, however, that it is the first report of an anaerobic microorganism, which can live and grow under complete exclusion of air.

This finding that microorganisms are able to grow with air, facultatively or under strict anaerobic conditions, caught Pasteur's particular interest. His subsequent studies with yeast under anaerobic conditions led to those experiments, the mechanisms of which have not been solved as yet, that carry his name as the Pasteur effect (Paper 7). In the complete absence of oxygen, yeast forms small buds and multiplies slowly, while a large amount of sugar disappears (60–80 parts sugar/1 part yeast formed). Under aerobic conditions, Pasteur observed the disappearance of 4–10 parts sugar per 1 part yeast being formed. The yeast reproduces vigorously, but its fermentation character tends to disappear. Unknowingly, Pasteur actually established the existence of the two main types of energy metabolism: fermentation and respiration.

Louis Pasteur, through his quantitative approach, thus laid the foundation for the study of yeast fermentation and discovered homolactic fermentation, respiration, butyric acid fermentation, and the fact that some microorganisms can tolerate oxygen, whereas others require the complete absence of air for their existence.

5

Reprinted from *Compt. Rend. Acad. Sci.*, *Paris*, **45**, 913–916 (1857)

MÉMOIRES LUS.

CHIMIE ORGANIQUE. — *Mémoire sur la fermentation appelée lactique;* par **M. L. PASTEUR**. (Extrait par l'auteur.)*

(Renvoi à l'examen de la Section de Chimie.)

« J'ai été conduit à m'occuper de la fermentation à la suite de mes recherches sur les propriétés des alcools amyliques et sur les particularités cristallographiques fort remarquables de leurs dérivés. J'aurai l'honneur de présenter ultérieurement à l'Académie des observations qui offriront une liaison inattendue entre les phénomènes de la fermentation et le caractère de dissymétrie moléculaire propre aux substances organiques naturelles...

» Les conditions matérielles de la préparation et de la production de l'acide lactique sont bien connues des chimistes. On sait qu'il suffit d'ajouter à de l'eau sucrée de la craie, qui maintient le milieu neutre, plus une matière azotée, telle que le caséum, le gluten, les membranes animales, etc., pour que le sucre se transforme en acide lactique. Mais l'explication des phénomènes est très-obscure; on ignore tout à fait le mode d'action de la matière plastique azotée. Son poids ne change pas d'une manière sensible. Elle ne devient pas putride. Elle se modifie cependant et elle est continuellement dans un état d'altération évidente, bien qu'il serait difficile de dire en quoi il consiste.

» Des recherches minutieuses n'ont pu jusqu'à présent faire découvrir dans ces opérations le développement d'êtres organisés. Les observateurs qui en ont reconnu ont établi en même temps qu'ils étaient accidentels et nuisaient au phénomène.

» Les faits paraissent donc très-favorables aux idées de M. Liebig (1). A ses yeux, le ferment est une substance excessivement altérable qui se décompose et qui excite la fermentation par suite de l'altération qu'elle éprouve elle-même, en ébranlant par communication et désassemblant le groupe moléculaire de la matière fermentescible. Là, selon M. Liebig, est la cause première de toutes les fermentations et l'origine de la plupart des maladies

---

(1) Il résulte des recherches historiques récentes de M. Chevreul, insérées au *Journal des Savants,* que Stahl avait déjà émis des idées analogues à celles de M. Liebig sur les causes de la fermentation alcoolique.

*An English translation of this paper follows.

contagieuses. Cette opinion obtient chaque jour un nouveau crédit. On peut à cet égard consulter le Mémoire de MM. Fremy et Boutron sur la fermentation lactique, les pages qui traitent de la fermentation et des ferments dans le bel ouvrage que M. Gerhardt a laissé en mourant, enfin le Mémoire tout récent de M. Berthelot sur la fermentation alcoolique. Ces travaux s'accordent à rejeter l'idée d'une influence quelconque de l'organisation et de la vie dans la cause des phénomènes qui nous occupent. Je suis conduit à une manière de voir entièrement différente.

» Je me propose d'établir dans la première partie de ce travail que, de même qu'il existe un ferment alcoolique, la levûre de bière, que l'on trouve partout où il y a du sucre qui se dédouble en alcool et en acide carbonique, de même il y a un ferment particulier, une levûre lactique toujours présente quand du sucre devient acide lactique, et que, si toute matière plastique azotée peut transformer le sucre en cet acide, c'est qu'elle est pour le développement de ce ferment un aliment convenable.

» Il y a des cas où l'on peut reconnaître dans les fermentations lactiques ordinaires, au-dessus du dépôt de la craie et de la matière azotée, des portions d'une substance grise formant quelquefois zone à la surface du dépôt. Son examen au microscope ne permet guère de la distinguer du caséum, du gluten désagrégés, etc., de telle sorte que rien n'indique que ce soit une matière spéciale, ni qu'elle ait pris naissance pendant la fermentation. C'est elle néanmoins qui joue le principal rôle. Je vais tout d'abord indiquer le moyen de l'isoler, de la préparer à l'état de pureté.

» J'extrais de la levûre de bière sa partie soluble en la maintenant quelque temps à la température de l'eau bouillante avec quinze à vingt fois son poids d'eau. La liqueur est filtrée avec soin. On y fait dissoudre environ 50 grammes de sucre par litre, on ajoute de la craie et l'on sème dans le milieu une trace de la matière grise dont j'ai parlé tout à l'heure, en la retirant d'une bonne fermentation lactique ordinaire. Dès le lendemain, il se manifeste une fermentation vive et régulière. Le liquide, parfaitement limpide à l'origine, se trouble, la craie disparaît peu à peu, en même temps qu'un dépôt s'effectue et augmente continûment et progressivement au fur et à mesure de la dissolution de la craie. En outre, on observe tous les caractères et tous les accidents bien connus de la fermentation lactique. On peut remplacer dans cette expérience l'eau de levûre par la décoction de toute matière plastique azotée, fraîche ou altérée selon les cas. Voyons maintenant les caractères de cette substance dont la production est corrélative des phénomènes compris sous la dénomination de *fermentation lactique*. Son aspect rappelle celui de la levûre de bière quand on l'étudie en masse et égouttée ou pressée. Au microscope, elle est formée de petits globules ou de petits articles très-courts, isolés ou en amas constituant des flocons irréguliers. Ses globules, beaucoup plus petits que ceux de la levûre de bière, sont agités vivement du mouvement brownien. Lavée à grande eau par décantation, puis délayée dans de l'eau sucrée pure, elle l'acidifie immédiatement, progressivement mais avec une grande lenteur, parce que l'acidité gène beaucoup son action sur le sucre. Si l'on fait intervenir la craie qui maintient la neutralité du milieu, la transformation du sucre est fort accélérée ; et lors même que l'on opère sur très-peu de matière, en moins d'une heure le dégagement du gaz est manifeste et la liqueur se charge de lactate et de butyrate de chaux. Il faut très-peu de cette levûre pour transformer beaucoup de sucre. Ces fermentations doivent s'effectuer de préférence à l'abri de l'air, sans quoi elles sont gênées par des végétations ou des infusoires parasites.....

» La fermentation lactique est donc aussi bien que la fermentation alcoolique ordinaire un acte corrélatif de la production d'une matière azotée qui a toutes les allures d'un corps organisé mycodermique probablement très-voisin de la levûre de bière. Mais les difficultés du sujet ne sont qu'à moitié résolues. Sa complication est extrême. L'acide lactique est bien le produit principal de la fermentation à laquelle il a donné son nom. Il est loin d'être le seul. On le trouve constamment accompagné d'acide butyrique, d'alcool, de mannite, de matière visqueuse. La proportion de ces matières est soumise aux plus capricieuses variations. Il y a une circonstance mystérieuse relative à la mannite. Non-seulement la proportion qui s'en forme est sujette aux plus grandes variations ; M. Berthelot vient d'établir, en outre, que si l'on remplace le sucre par la mannite dans la fermentation lactique, toutes les autres conditions demeurant sensiblement les mêmes, la mannite fermente en donnant de l'alcool, de l'acide lactique et de l'acide butyrique. Comment dès lors concevoir qu'il puisse y avoir formation de mannite dans des cas de fermentation lactique, puisque, peut-on croire, elle devrait se détruire au fur et à mesure de sa production?

» Étudions avec plus de soins que nous ne l'avons fait les propriétés chimiques de la nouvelle levûre. J'ai dit que lavée à grande eau et placée dans de l'eau sucrée pure, elle acidifiait progressivement la liqueur. La transformation du sucre devient, dans ces conditions, de plus en plus pénible, à mesure que le liquide prend lui-même une plus grande acidité. Or, si l'on analyse la liqueur, ce qui ne peut être accompli avec succès qu'après la saturation des acides par la craie et la destruction ultérieure du sucre en excès par la levûre de bière, on trouve dans le liquide évaporé, et en proportion variable, la mannite d'une part, de l'autre la matière visqueuse. Ainsi donc la levûre lactique lavée mise en présence du sucre le transforme en divers produits parmi lesquels il y a toujours de la mannite, mais c'est à la condition que le liquide puisse devenir promptement acide ; car si l'on répète exactement la même expérience avec la précaution d'ajouter un peu de craie afin que le milieu reste constamment neutre, ni gomme, ni mannite ne prennent naissance, ou mieux ne peuvent persister, parce que, on va le voir, les conditions de leur propre transformation se trouvent réunies.

» J'ai rappelé tout à l'heure que M. Berthelot avait prouvé qu'en substituant la mannite au sucre dans la fermentation lactique, cette matière fermentait. Or il est facile de se convaincre que dans les cas nombreux de fermentation de la mannite, c'est la levûre lactique qni prend naissance et produit le phénomène. Si l'on mêle à une solution de mannite pure de la craie en poudre et de la levûre lactique fraîche et lavée, au bout d'une heure déjà le dégagement gazeux et la transformation chimique de la mannite commenceront. Il se forme de l'acide carbonique, de l'hydrogène, et la liqueur renferme de l'alcool, de l'acide lactique, de l'acide butyrique, tous les produits de la fermentation de là mannite.

» Quant à l'acide butyrique, l'expérience prouve que la levûre lactique agit directement sur le lactate de chaux en donnant du carbonate de chaux et du butyrate de chaux. Mais l'action s'exerce d'abord sur le sucre, et tant qu'il y en a dans la liqueur, la levûre le fait fermenter de préférence à l'acide lactique.

» Dans des communications très-prochaines, j'aurai l'honneur de présenter à l'Académie l'application des idées générales et des nouvelles méthodes d'expérimentation de ce travail à d'autres fermentations. »

5

Report on Lactic Fermentation

L. PASTEUR

Translated expressly for this Benchmark volume by G. Gordon of the University of Queensland, Australia, from "Mémoire sur la fermentation appelée lactique," Compt. Rend. Acad. Sci., Paris, **45**, *913–916 (1857)*

I have been led to concern myself with fermentation following my research on the properties of amyl alcohols and the remarkable crystallographic properties of their derivatives. Later I will have the honor of presenting to the Academy observations that will offer an unexpected connection between the fermentation phenomena and the molecular dissymmetric character of natural organic substances.

Chemists have long known the material conditions for the preparation and production of lactic acid. Also they have known that it is only necessary to add chalk (to maintain the neutrality of the medium) and a nitrogenous material, such as casein, gluten, animal membranes, etc., to a sugared medium for the sugar to be transformed into lactic acid. But the explanation of these phenomena is very obscure if one completely ignores the mode of action of plastic nitrogenous material. Its weight does not change in an appreciable way. It does not become putrid. It is modified, however, and is continually in an obvious state of alteration, although it would be difficult to say what it consists of.

Until the present time, detailed research has not been able to elucidate the development of organized beings by these operations. Observers who have examined it have, at the same time, established that any organized beings were occasional and interfered with the phenomenon.

These facts then appeared to substantiate the ideas of Monsieur Liebig.[1] In his opinion, the ferment is a readily alterable substance that decomposes itself and consequently excites fermentation by that alteration. It proves itself by disassembling the molecular grouping of fermentable material. According to Monsieur Liebig, this is the major cause of all fermentation and the origin of most contagious maladies. This

---

[1] It appears from the recent journalistic study in the *Journal des Savants* (by Monsieur Cherreul) that Stahl had previously expressed analogous ideas to those of Monsieur Liebig on the cause of alcoholic fermentation.

opinion gathers new credit each day. In this regard one is able to consult the report of Messieurs Fremy and Boutron on lactic fermentation, the pages that deal with fermentation and ferments in the fine piece of work by the late Monsieur Gerhardt, and finally, the recent report by Monsieur Berthelot on alcoholic fermentation. These workers agree in rejecting the idea of a given influence on organization and life as the cause of the phenomena with which we are occupied. I am led to an entirely different point of view.

I propose to establish in the first part of this work that, just as beer yeast exists with alcoholic fermentation (which I have found wherever sugar is split into alcohol and carbon dioxide), there is a particular ferment, a lactic yeast, always present when sugar becomes lactic acid; and that, if all plastic nitrogenous material is able to transform sugar into this acid, then this material is a suitable food for the development of this ferment.

There were some occasions when I was able to recognize, beneath the deposit of chalk and nitrogenous material in normal lactic fermentation, some portions of a gray substance that occasionally formed at the surface of the deposit. My microscopic examination just barely permitted the distinction of casein, disintegrated gluten, etc., so it is neither a special material, nor does it originate during fermentation. Nevertheless, it is this substance that plays the principal role. I am going to indicate, from the very first step, the method for its isolation and for its preparation in the pure state.

I extracted the soluble part from beer yeast by maintaining it, with 15 to 20 times its weight of water, for a time at the temperature of boiling water. The liquid was carefully filtered. About 50 g of sugar per liter was dissolved in it, chalk was added, and a trace of the gray matter of which I have spoken was sown in the medium. This produced a good, normal lactic fermentation. As early as the next day, a spirited, regular fermentation is evident. The liquid, which is clear at the start, becomes cloudy; the chalk disappears little by little while a deposit is formed that grows in proportion to the dissolution of the chalk. However, I observed all the characters and well-known symptoms of lactic fermentation. In this experiment the yeast water could be replaced by extracting all soluble plastic nitrogenous material, either fresh or altered.

Let us now examine the character of this substance, production of which is related to the phenomenon known as lactic fermentation. Its appearance recalls that of beer yeast when it is studied in mass and when strained or pressed. Under the microscope, these take the form of small globules or small, very short units, isolated or accumulated into irregular floccules. The globules, much smaller than those of beer yeast, vibrate quickly by Brownian movement. Washed in water by decantation, they are then diluted in pure sugared water and acidified immediately (but progressively and slowly because acidity hinders yeast action on the sugar). If the chalk (which maintains neutrality of the medium) is interfered with, transformation of sugar is greatly accelerated. Even though it acts on very small amounts of material, gas evolution is evident in less than 1 hour and the liquor becomes charged with lactate and butyrate of lime. It takes very little of this yeast to transform a large amount of sugar. These fermentations take place, by preference, in the absence of air; otherwise they are hindered by vegetation or parasitic infusoria.

Lactic fermentation, as well as normal alcoholic fermentation, is then an act related to the production of a nitrogenous material that has the behavior of an organized mycodermic body, probably very similar to beer yeast. But the difficulties of the subject are only half determined, as it is extremely complicated. Lactic acid is the principal product of the fermentation that bears its name. It is far from being the only one, for butyric acid, alcohol, mannitol, and viscous materials are constantly found to accompany it. The proportions of these materials are subject to the most capricious variations, and there is a mysterious circumstance relating to mannitol. Not only is the proportion in which it is formed subject to great variation, but Monsieur Berthelot has just established that if mannitol replaces sugar in the lactic fermentation, then all other conditions remain appreciably the same, with mannitol fermentation giving rise to alcohol, lactic acid, and butyric acid. Since, as one would believe, mannitol is formed during lactic fermentation, why must it destroy itself in proportion with its production?

More careful studies revealed the chemical properties of the new yeast. I have said that, when washed with water and placed in pure sugared water it progressively acidifies the liquor. Under these conditions, sugar transformation becomes more and more laborious as the liquid becomes more acid. If the liquor is analyzed, which can be done after saturation of the acids with chalk and the subsequent destruction of excess sugar by beer yeast, mannitol and the viscous material are found in variable proportion in the evaporated liquid. Thus washed lactic yeast transforms sugar into diverse products, included among which is always mannitol. The liquid, however, always becomes predominantly acid. If the same experiment is repeated except for the addition of a little chalk so that the medium remains neutral, no gum or mannitol is formed, or, rather, none persists, because the conditions for proper transformation have been created.

I have just recalled how Monsieur Berthelot has proven that mannitol is formed by substituting it for sugar in lactic fermentation. But it is easy to argue that in numerous cases of mannitol formation it is the lactic yeast which is formed and which produces this phenomenon. If a solution of pure mannitol, powdered chalk, and fresh, washed, lactic yeast is mixed, gas formation and chemical transformation of mannitol will begin after 1 hour. Carbon dioxide and hydrogen are formed, and the liquid contains alcohol, lactic acid, and butyric acid, which are all products of mannitol fermentation.

With respect to butyric acid, the experiments prove that lactic yeast acts directly on lactate of lime to give carbonate of lime and butyrate of lime. But the action is exerted first on sugar and, as long as there is some of it in the liquor, the yeast ferments it preferentially to lactic acid.

In communications to be released very soon, I will have the honor of presenting to the Academy the application of the general ideas and new experimental methods of this work to other fermentation.

6

Reprinted from *Compt. Rend. Acad. Sci., Paris,* **52,** 344–347 (1861)

MEMOIRES PRÉSENTÉS.

PHYSIQUE. — *Animalcules infusoires vivant sans gaz oxygène libre et déterminant des fermentations; par* **M. L. Pasteur.** *

(Commissaires précédemment nommés : MM. Chevreul, Milne Edwards, Decaisne, Regnault, Claude Bernard.)

« On sait combien sont variés les produits qui se forment dans la fermentation appelée *lactique.* L'acide lactique, une gomme, la mannite, l'acide butyrique, l'alcool, l'acide carbonique et l'hydrogène, apparaissent simultanément ou successivement en proportions extrêmement variables et tout à fait capricieuses. J'ai été conduit peu à peu à reconnaître que le végétal-ferment qui transforme le sucre en acide lactique est différent de celui ou de ceux (car il en existe deux) qui déterminent la production de la matière gommeuse, et que ces derniers à leur tour n'engendrent pas d'acide lactique. D'autre part j'ai également reconnu que ces divers végétaux-ferments ne pouvaient dans aucune circonstance, s'ils étaient bien *purs,* donner naissance à l'acide butyrique.

» Il devait donc y avoir un ferment butyrique propre. C'est sur ce point

*An English translation of this paper follows.

56

que j'ai arrêté depuis longtemps toute mon attention. La communication que j'ai l'honneur d'adresser aujourd'hui à l'Académie se rapporte précisément à l'origine de l'acide butyrique dans la fermentation appelée lactique.

» Je n'entrerai pas ici dans tous les détails de cette recherche. Je me bornerai d'abord à énoncer l'une des conclusions de mon travail : c'est que *le ferment butyrique est un infusoire.*

» J'étais bien éloigné de m'attendre à ce résultat, à tel point que pendant longtemps j'ai cru devoir appliquer mes efforts à écarter l'apparition de ces petits animaux, par la crainte où j'étais qu'ils ne se nourrissent du ferment végétal que je supposais être le ferment butyrique, et que je cherchais à découvrir dans les milieux liquides que j'employais. Mais n'arrivant pas à saisir la cause de l'origine de l'acide butyrique, je finis par être frappé de la coïncidence que mes analyses me montraient inévitable, entre cet acide et les infusoires, et inversement entre les infusoires et la production de cet acide, circonstance que j'avais attribuée jusque-là à l'utilité ou à la convenance que l'acide butyrique offrait à la vie de ces animalcules.

» Depuis lors, les essais les plus multipliés m'ont convaincu que la transformation du sucre, de la mannite et de l'acide lactique en acide butyrique, est due exclusivement à ces infusoires, et qu'il faut les considérer comme le véritable ferment butyrique.

» Voici leur description : Ce sont de petites baguettes cylindriques, arrondies à leurs extrémités, ordinairement droites, isolées ou réunies par chaînes de deux, de trois, de quatre articles et quelquefois même davantage. Leur largeur est de $0^{mm},002$ en moyenne. La longueur des articles isolés varie de $0^{mm},002$ jusqu'à $0^{mm},015$ ou $0^{mm},02$. Ces infusoires s'avancent en glissant. Pendant ce mouvement, leur corps reste rigide ou éprouve de légères ondulations. Ils pirouettent, se balancent ou font trembler vivement la partie antérieure et postérieure de leur corps. Les ondulations de leurs mouvements deviennent très-évidentes dès que leur longueur atteint $0^{mm},015$. Souvent ils sont recourbés à une de leurs extrémités, quelquefois à toutes deux. Cette particularité est rare au commencement de leur vie.

» Ils se reproduisent par fissiparité. C'est évidemment à ce mode de génération qu'est due la disposition en chaînes d'articles qu'affecte le corps de quelques-uns. L'article qui en traîne d'autres après lui s'agite quelquefois vivement comme pour s'en détacher.

» Bien que les corps de ces Vibrions aient une apparence cylindrique, on les dirait souvent formés d'une suite de grains ou d'articles très-courts à peine ébauchés. Ce sont sans nul doute les premiers rudiments de ces petits animaux.

» On peut semer ces infusoires comme on sèmerait de la levûre de bière. Ils se multiplient si le milieu est approprié à leur nourriture. Mais ce qui est bien essentiel à remarquer, on peut les semer dans un liquide ne renfermant que du sucre, de l'ammoniaque et des phosphates, c'est-à-dire des substances cristallisables et pour ainsi dire toutes minérales, et ils se reproduisent corrélativement à la fermentation butyrique qui apparaît très-manifeste. Le poids qui s'en forme est notable, bien que toujours minime, comparé à la quantité totale d'acide butyrique produit, comme cela se passe pour tous les ferments.

» L'existence d'infusoires possédant le caractère des ferments est déjà un fait qui semble bien digne d'attention ; mais une particularité singulière qui l'accompagne, c'est que ces animalcules infusoires vivent et se multiplient à l'infini sans qu'il soit nécessaire de leur fournir la plus petite quantité d'air ou d'oxygène libre.

» Il serait trop long de dire ici comment je me suis arrangé pour que les milieux liquides où ces infusoires vivent et pullulent par myriades ne renferment absolument pas d'oxygène libre dans leur intérieur ou à leur surface, ce que j'ai d'ailleurs soigneusement constaté. J'ajouterai seulement que je n'ai pas voulu présenter mes résultats à l'Académie sans en avoir rendu témoins plusieurs de ses Membres, qui m'ont paru reconnaître la rigueur des preuves expérimentales que j'ai mises sous leurs yeux.

» Non-seulement ces infusoires vivent sans air, mais l'air les tue. Que l'on fasse passer dans la liqueur où ils se multiplient un courant d'acide carbonique pur pendant un temps quelconque, leur vie et leur reproduction n'en sont aucunement affectées. Si, au contraire, dans des conditions exactement pareilles, on substitue au courant d'acide carbonique un courant d'air atmosphérique, pendant une ou deux heures seulement, tous périssent, et la fermentation butyrique liée à leur existence est aussitôt arrêtée.

» Nous arrivons donc à cette double proposition :

» 1° *Le ferment butyrique est un infusoire.*

» 2° *Cet infusoire vit sans gaz oxygène libre.*

» C'est, je crois, le premier exemple connu de ferments animaux, et aussi d'animaux vivant sans gaz oxygène libre.

» Le rapprochement du mode de vie et des propriétés de ces animalcules avec le mode de vie et les propriétés des ferments végétaux qui vivent
également sans le concours du gaz oxygène libre, se présente de lui-même,
aussi bien que les conséquences qu'il est permis d'en déduire, relativement
à la cause des fermentations. Cependant je veux réserver les idées que ces
faits nouveaux suggèrent jusqu'à ce que j'aie pu les soumettre à la lumière
de l'expérience. »

6

Infusorial Animalcules Living Without Free Oxygen and Causing Fermentations

L. PASTEUR

*Translated expressly for this Benchmark
volume by G. Gordon of the University
of Queensland, Australia, from
"Animalcules infusoires vivant sans
gaz oxygène libre et déterminant des
fermentations,"* Compt. Rend. Acad.
Sci., Paris, **52**, *344–347 (1861)*

The varied nature of products formed in lactic fermentation is well known. Lactic acid, gum, mannitol, butyric acid, alcohol, carbon dioxide, and hydrogen appear simultaneously or successively in extremely variable proportions and all are formed inconsistently. I have gradually been led to discover that the plant ferment that transforms sugar to lactic acid is different from those (for there are two) which determine the production of the gummy material, and that the latter do not form lactic acid. I have also established that the various plant ferments, if they are indeed pure, are unable to produce butyric acid under any circumstance.

Accordingly there must be a butyric ferment. I have focused my attention on this point for a long time. The communication that I have the honor of addressing to the Academy today relates precisely to the origin of butyric acid during lactic fermentation.

I shall not enter here into all the details of this study. At first I shall limit myself to the announcement of the conclusions of my work—that butyric ferment is an infusorium.

For a long time I believed it necessary to ignore the apparition of these tiny animals, fearing that they were not nourished by the plant ferment that I have supposed to be the butyric ferment, and for which I was searching in the liquid media used. But failing to discover the origin of butyric acid, I was struck by my analyses which showed coincidences with those circumstances that so far I had attributed to the usefulness or convenience that butyric acid was offering to the life of these animalcules.

Since then, multiple tests have convinced me that transformation of sugar, mannitol, and lactic acid into butyric acid is due exclusively to these infusoria, and that it is necessary to consider them as the true butyric ferment. They are small cylindrical rods, rounded at the ends; normally straight; single or joined in chains of two, three, or four, or sometimes even more. Their width averages 0.002 mm. The length of the single objects varies from 0.002 to 0.015 or 0.02 mm. These infusoria

60

move by sliding. During this motion, their body remains rigid or experiences slight undulations. They whirl round and round, balancing themselves or vibrating the anterior or posterior part of their body. The undulatory movements become very noticeable when the length of the infusoria reaches 0.015 mm. They are frequently curved at one end, sometimes at both; but this peculiarity is rare at the beginning of growth.

They reproduce by fission. Evidently the disposition of the units in chains is due to this method of generation. Ultimately the trailing unit wriggles sharply several times to break away.

Although these vibrioid bodies have a cylindrical appearance, one could often say that they were formed from a series of particles or from newly formed, very short units. Without doubt these are the first rudiments of the small animals.

These infusoria can be sown as beer yeast is sown. They multiply if the medium is appropriate to their nutrition. It is indeed essential to note that their reproduction results in unmistakable butyric fermentation when they are sown in a liquid containing only sugar, ammonia, and phosphates (i.e., crystallizable or mineral substances). The weight of infusoria that are produced is considerable, although always insignificant compared to total butyric acid produced, as is the case for all ferments.

The existence of infusoria possessing the character of ferments is already a fact worthy of attention, but there is another accompanying peculiarity: these infusorial animalcules live and multiply *ad infinitum* without it being necessary to supply the smallest quantity of air or free oxygen to them.

It would be too detailed to tell here how I prepared the liquid media that contained no free oxygen either internally or at the surface (where these infusoria live and grow rapidly to myriad numbers), although I have carefully proven it. I will add only that I did not wish to present my results to the Academy without having presented several items of evidence to its members, who appeared to recognize the rigor of the experimental arguments I have put before them.

Not only do these infusoria live without air, but air kills them. If a stream of pure carbon dioxide is passed through the liquor where they are multiplying for a time, their life and reproduction are not affected in any way. However, if, under exactly parallel conditions, a stream of atmospheric air is substituted for carbon dioxide for only 1 or 2 hours, all perish, and the butyric fermentation coupled to their existence is also arrested.

We now arrive at this double proposal:

1. The butyric ferment is an infusorium.
2. This infusorium lives without free oxygen.

I believe that this is the first known example of animal ferments and also of animals living without free oxygen.

The correlation of their mode of life and the properties of these animalcules with this particular mode of life with the peculiar qualities of the plant ferments that also live without the aid of free oxygen, as well as those products that have allowed deduction to be made appear to explain the real cause of fermentation. However, I wish to reserve the ideas which these new facts suggest until I have been able to subject them to experiment.

61

Reprinted from *Bull. Soc. Chim. Paris*, **28**, 79–80 (1861)

Influence de l'oxygène sur le développement de la levûre et la fermentation alcoolique, par M. PASTEUR. *

M. Pasteur expose les résultats de ses recherches sur la fermentation du sucre et le développement des globules de levûre suivant que cette fermentation s'opère à l'abri ou au contact du gaz oxygène libre. Ces expériences n'ont d'ailleurs rien de commun avec celle de Gay-Lussac sur le moût de raisin écrasé à l'abri de l'air, puis amené au contact de l'oxygène.

La levûre toute formée peut bourgeonner et se développer dans un liquide sucré et albumineux en l'absence complète d'oxygène ou d'air. Il se forme peu de levûre dans ce cas, et il disparaît comparativement une grande quantité de sucre, 60 ou 80 parties pour une de levûre formée. La fermentation est très-lente dans ces conditions.

Si l'expérience est faite au contact de l'air et sur une grande surface, la fermentation est rapide. Pour la même quantité de sucre disparu, il se fait beaucoup plus de levûre. L'air en contact cède de l'oxygène qui est absorbé par la levûre. Celle-ci se développe énergiquement, mais son caractère de ferment tend à disparaître dans ces conditions. On trouve en effet que pour 1 partie de levûre formée, il n'y aura que 4 à 10 parties de sucre transformé. Le rôle de ferment de cette levûre subsiste néanmoins et se montre même fort exalté si l'on vient à la faire agir sur le sucre en dehors de l'influence du gaz oxygène libre.

Il paraît dès lors naturel d'admettre que lorsque la levûre est ferment, agissant à l'abri de l'air, elle prend de l'oxygène au sucre, et que c'est là l'origine de son caractère de ferment.

M. Pasteur explique le fait d'une activité tumultueuse à l'origine des fermentations par l'influence de l'oxygène de l'air qui est en dissolution dans les liquides quand l'action commence. L'auteur a reconnu en outre que la levûre de bière, semée dans un liquide albumineux, tel que l'eau de levûre de bière, se multiplie encore lorsqu'il n'y a pas trace de sucre dans la liqueur, pourvu toutefois que l'oxygène de l'air soit présent en grande quantité. A l'abri de l'air et dans ces conditions, la levûre ne bourgeonne pas du tout. Les mêmes expériences peuvent être répétées avec un liquide albumineux mêlé à une dissolution de sucre non fermentescible comme le sucre de lait cristallisé ordinaire. Les résultats sont du même ordre.

La levûre formée ainsi en l'absence du sucre n'a pas changé de na-

*An English translation of this paper follows.

ture; elle fait fermenter le sucre si on la fait agir sur ce corps à l'abri de l'air. Il faut remarquer toutefois que le développement de la levûre est très-pénible lorsqu'elle n'a pas pour aliment une matière fermentescible.

En résumé la levûre de bière se comporte absolument comme une plante ordinaire, et l'analogie serait complète si les plantes ordinaires avaient pour l'oxygène une affinité qui leur permît de respirer a l'aide de cet élément enlevé à des composés peu stables, auquel cas, suivant M. Pasteur, on les verrait être ferments pour ces matières.

M. Pasteur annonce qu'il espère réaliser ce résultat, c'est-à-dire rencontrer des conditions dans lesquelles certaines plantes inférieures vivraient à l'abri de l'air en présence du sucre, en provoquant alors la fermentation de cette substance à la manière de la levûre de bière.

7

Influence of Oxygen on Yeast Development and Alcoholic Fermentation

L. PASTEUR

Translated expressly for this Benchmark volume by G. Gordon of the University of Queensland, Australia, from "Influence de l'oxygène sur le développement de la levûre et la fermentation alcoolique," Bull. Soc. Chim. Paris, **28**, 79–80 (1861)

Monsieur Pasteur explains the results of his investigations into sugar fermentation and yeast development that takes place in the presence or the absence of free gaseous oxygen. Furthermore, these experiments have nothing in common with those of Gay-Lussac on grape juice crushed in the absence of air and then brought into contact with oxygen.

All the yeast that is formed can bud and develop in a sugary, albuminous medium in the complete absence of oxygen or air. Small quantities of yeast are formed under these conditions, while comparatively large quantities of sugar are broken down: 60 to 80 parts sugar per part of yeast formed. Fermentation is very slow under these conditions.

Fermentation is rapid if the experiment is conducted in the presence of a large surface area of air. Much more yeast is produced for the breakdown of the same quantity of sugar. Oxygen is withdrawn from the surrounding air and is absorbed by the yeast. The latter develops energetically, but its fermentative nature tends to vanish under these conditions. Four to 10 parts of sugar are transformed for the production of 1 part of yeast. Nevertheless, the fermentative action of the yeast remains, and even appears greatly magnified, if it is set in motion on sugar without the influence of free gaseous oxygen.

Consequently, it appears natural to acknowledge that, when yeast is actively fermenting in the absence of air, it takes oxygen from sugar, and that this is the source of its fermentable character.

Monsieur Pasteur explains that the violent activity at the beginning of fermentation is due to the atmospheric oxygen that is dissolved in the liquids at the time activity commences. Furthermore, the author recognizes that beer yeast sprinkled into an albuminous liquid, such as yeast water, increases until there is no trace of sugar in the liquor, provided that atmospheric oxygen is present in large quantities. Under these conditions, and in the absence of air, the yeast does not bud at all. The same experiment is repeated with a mixture of albuminous liquid and a nonfermentable sugar, such as ordinary crystalline milk sugar [*Ed. Note:* lactose]. The results are of the same order.

Hence the yeast formed in the absence of sugar has not changed, since it ferments sugar in the absence of air if set in motion. Still, it is necessary to note that yeast development is very laborious when no fermentable material is available for nutrition.

In summary, beer yeast definitely behaves as an ordinary plant, and the analogy would be complete if ordinary plants had an affinity for oxygen that allowed them to respire by removing this element from less stable compounds. In that case, if we are to be guided by Monsieur Pasteur, they could be seen as ferments for these substances.

Monsieur Pasteur declares that he hopes to find the conditions under which certain lower plants would live on sugar in the absence of air, thus causing the fermentation of this substance in the same manner as beer yeast.

Editor's Comments on Paper 8

8 **Buchner:** Alkoholische Gährung ohne Hefezellen
English Translation: Alcoholic Fermentation Without Yeast Cells
Chem. Ber., **30**, 117–124 (1897)

   The discovery that alcoholic fermentation can be obtained in the absence of living cells by extracting the proteinaceous material from the cell was made by Edward Buchner. He succeeded for the first time in obtaining "yeast juice" [*Ed. Note:* cell-free extract]. These experiments opened up possibilities for the development of two disciplines, biochemistry and microbial metabolism. Being able to disrupt living cells made it possible to study in more detail how the living organism works and thus to study "ferments," which are now called enzymes. At last J. Liebig and L. Pasteur proved to be right in their early statements (see Papers 3 and 4). This discovery by Buchner merged microbiology and organic chemistry, creating biochemistry; further development in microbial metabolism is so closely linked with biochemistry that a separation is very often impossible.

8

Reprinted from *Chem. Ber.*, **30**, 117–124 (1897)

19. **Eduard Buchner:** Alkoholische Gährung ohne Hefezellen.*
[Vorläufige Mittheilung.]
(Eingegangen am 11. Januar.)

Eine Trennung der Gährwirkung von den lebenden Hefezellen ist bisher nicht gelungen; im Folgenden sei ein Verfahren beschrieben, welches diese Aufgabe löst.

1000 g für die Darstellung von Presshefe gereinigte. aber noch nicht mit Kartoffelstärke versetzte Brauereibierhefe[1]) wird mit dem

[1]) Dieselbe ist von oberflächlich anhaftendem Wasser soweit befreit, dass bei einem Druck von 25 Atmosphären kein Wasser mehr abgeht.

*An English translation of this paper follows.

gleichen Gewichte Quarzsand[1]) und 250 g Kieselguhr sorgfältig ge-
mengt und sodann zerrieben, bis die Masse feucht und plastisch geworden ist. Man setzt dem Teige nun 100 g Wasser zu und bringt
ihn, in ein Presstuch eingeschlagen. allmählich unter einen Druck von
4—500 Atmosphären: es resultiren 300 ccm Presssaft. Der rück-
ständige Kuchen wird abermals zerrieben, gesiebt und mit 100 g
Wasser versetzt; von Neuem in der hydraulischen Presse dem gleichen
Drucke unterworfen, giebt er noch 150 ccm Presssaft. Aus einem
Kilo Hefe gewinnt man also 500 ccm Presssaft, welche gegen 300 ccm
Zellinhaltssubstanzen enthalten. Zur Entfernung einer spurenhaften
Trübung wird der Presssaft endlich noch mit 4 g Kieselguhr ge-
schüttelt und unter mehrmaligem Aufgiessen der ersten Antheile durch
ein Papierfilter filtrirt.

Der so erhaltene Presssaft stellt eine klare, nur opalisirende.
gelbe Flüssigkeit von angenehmem Hefegeruch dar. Das spec. Ge-
wicht wurde einmal zu 1.0416 (17° C.) gefunden. Beim Kochen tritt
starke Ausscheidung von Gerinnsel ein, so dass die Flüssigkeit fast
vollständig erstarrt; die Bildung von unlöslichen Flocken beginnt
bereits bei 35—40°; schon vorher wird Aufsteigen von Gasbläschen,
nachweislich Kohlensäure bemerkt, mit welcher die Flüssigkeit demnach gesättigt ist[2]). Der Presssaft enthält über 10 pCt. Trockensubstanz. In nach einem früheren, weniger guten Verfahren her-
gestelltem Presssaft waren 6.7 pCt Trockensubstanz. 1.15 pCt. Asche
und, nach dem Stickstoffgehalt zu schliessen, 3.7 pCt. Eiweissstoffe
vorhanden.

Die interessanteste Eigenschaft des Presssaftes besteht darin, dass
er Kohlenhydrate in Gährung zu versetzen vermag. Beim Mischen
mit dem gleichen Volumen einer concentrirten Rohrzuckerlösung tritt
schon nach $1/4$ - 1 Stunde regelmässige Kohlensäureentwickelung ein.
die Tage lang andauert. Ebenso verhalten sich Trauben-, Frucht-
und Malz-Zucker: keine Gährungserscheinungen treten dagegen in Ge-
mischen des Presssaftes mit gesättigter Milchzucker-, sowie mit Man-
nit-Lösung auf, wie ja diese Körper auch durch lebende Bierhefezellen
nicht vergohren werden. Mehrere Tage in Gährung befindliche, im
Eisschrank aufgestellte Mischungen von Presssaft und Zuckerlösung
trüben sich allmählich, ohne dass mikroskopisch Organismen auf-
zufinden sind; dagegen zeigen sich bei 700facher Vergrösserung ziem-
lich zahlreiche Gerinnsel von Eiweissstoffen, deren Ausscheidung

---

[1]) Glaspulver ist wegen seiner Wirkung als schwaches Alkali weniger
geeignet.
[2]) Die Pflanzenphysiologen mögen entscheiden. ob diese Kohlensäure
etwa von den mit der Athmung zusammenhängenden Oxydationsprocessen
herstammt.

wahrscheinlich durch bei der Gährung entstandene Säuren bedingt wurde. Sättigen des Gemisches von Presssaft und Saccharoselösung mit Chloroform verhindert die Gährung nicht, führt aber frühzeitig zu geringer Eiweissausscheidung. Ebenso wenig vernichtet Filtriren des Presssaftes durch ein sterilisirtes B e r k e f e l d t - Kieselgubrfilter, welches sicher alle Hefezellen zurückhält, die Gährkraft; das Gemisch des ganz klaren Filtrates mit sterilisirter Rohrzuckerlösung geräth, wenn auch unter Verzögerung, nach etwa einem Tag, selbst bei der Temperatur des Eisschrankes, in Gährung. Beim Einhängen eines mit Presssaft gefüllten Pergamentpapierschlauches in 37-proc. Rohrzucker-lösung bedeckt sich nach einigen Stunden die Oberfläche des Schlauches mit zahllosen, winzigen Gasbläschen; natürlich war auch im Innern infol geHineindiffundirens von Zuckerlösung lebhafte Gasentwickelung zu bemerken. Weitere Versuche müssen entscheiden, ob thatsächlich der Träger der Gährwirkung durch das Pergamentpapier zu diosmiren vermag, wie es den Anschein hat. Das Gährvermögen des Presssaftes geht mit der Zeit allmählich verloren; fünf Tage in Eiswasser in halbvoller Flasche aufgehobener Presssaft erwies sich als inactiv gegenüber Saccharose. Es ist merkwürdig, dass dagegen mit Rohr-zucker versetzter, also gährthätiger Presssaft die Gährwirkung im Eis-schrank mindestens zwei Wochen lang behält. Man muss dabei wohl zunächst an eine günstige, den Luftsauerstoff abhaltende Einwirkung der bei der Gährung gebildeten Kohlensäure denken; es könnte aber auch der leicht assimilirbare Zucker zur Erhaltung des Agens bei-tragen.

Um über die Natur der wirksamen Substanz im Presssaft Aufschluss zu erhalten, sind bisher nur wenige Versuche ausgeführt. Beim Erwärmen von Presssaft auf 40—50⁰ tritt zunächst Kohlen-säureentwickelung, dann allmählich Ausscheidung von geronnenem Eiweiss auf; nach einer Stunde wurde unter mehrmaligem Zurück-giessen abfiltrirt. Das klare Filtrat besass gegenüber Rohrzucker bei einem Versuch noch schwache Gährkraft, bei einem zweiten jedoch nicht mehr: die wirksame Substanz scheint demnach entweder ihre Wirkung schon bei dieser auffallend niederen Temperatur einzubüssen oder zu gerinnen und auszufallen. Ferner wurden 20 ccm Auspress in das dreifache Volum absoluten Alkohols eingetragen, der Niederschlag ab-gesaugt und über Schwefelsäure im Vacuum getrocknet; es resultirten 2 g trockne Substanz, welche sich beim Digeriren mit 10 ccm Wasser nur zum kleinsten Theil wieder auflösten. Das Filtrat davon besass auf Rohrzucker keine Gährwirkung. Diese Experimente müssen wieder-holt werden; insbesondere soll ferner die Isolirung der wirksamen Substanz mittels Ammonsulfat versucht werden.

Für die T h e o r i e der G ä h r u n g sind bisher etwa folgende Schlüsse zu ziehen. Zunächst ist bewiesen, dass es zur Einleitung des Gährungsvorganges keines so complicirten Apparates bedarf, wie ihn die Hefezelle vorstellt. Als Träger der Gährwirkung des Presssaftes ist vielmehr eine gelöste Substanz, zweifelsohne ein Eiweisskörper zu betrachten; derselbe soll als Zymase bezeichnet werden.

Die Anschauung, dass ein den Hefezellen entstammender, besonders gearteter Eiweisskörper die Gährung veranlassse, ist als Enzym- oder Ferment-Theorie bereits 1858 von M. Traube ausgesprochen und später insbesondere von F. Hoppe-Seyler vertheidigt worden. Die Abtrennung eines derartigen Enzymes von den Hefezellen war aber bisher nicht geglückt.

Es bleibt auch jetzt noch fraglich, ob die Zymase direct den schon länger bekannten Enzymen zugezählt werden darf. Wie schon C. v. Nägeli[1]) betont hat, bestehen zwischen Gährwirkung und der Wirkung der gewöhnlichen Enzyme wichtige Unterschiede. Die letzteren sind lediglich Hydrolysen, welche durch einfachste chemische Mittel nachgeahmt werden können. Wenn auch A. v. Baeyer[2]) den chemischen Vorgang bei der alkoholischen Gährung unserem Verständnisse näher gebracht hat, indem er ihn auf verhältnissmässig einfache Principien zurückführte, so gehört der Zerfall von Zucker in Alkohol und Kohlensäure doch immer noch zu den complicirteren Reactionen; es werden dabei Kohlenstoffbindungen gelöst, wie es in dieser Vollständigkeit durch andere Mittel bisher nicht erreicht wird. Auch in der Wärmetönung besteht ein bedeutender Unterschied[3]).

Das Invertin lässt sich aus den durch trockene Hitze getödteten (eine Stunde auf 150° erhitzten) Hefezellen mittels Wasser ausziehen und durch Fällen mit Alkohol als in Wasser leicht lösliches Pulver isoliren. Auf die gleiche Weise ist der die Gährung bewirkende Stoff nicht zu erhalten. In den so hoch erhitzten Hefezellen wird er wohl überhaupt nicht mehr vorhanden sein; er geht durch Alkoholfällung, wenn der oben angeführte Versuch einen Schluss gestattet, in eine in Wasser unlösliche Modification über. Man wird deshalb in der Annahme kaum fehlgehen, dass die Zymase zu den genuinen Eiweisskörpern gehört und dem lebenden Protoplasma der Hefezellen noch viel näher steht als das Invertin.

Aehnliche Ansichten hat der französische Bacteriologe Miguel bezüglich der Urase, des von den Bacterien der sogen. Harnstoffgährung ausgeschiedenen Enzymes geäussert; er bezeichnet dieselbe direct als Protoplasma, das des Schutzes der Zellhaut entbehre, ausserhalb derselben wirke und sich hauptsächlich nur dadurch von dem-

[1]) Theorie der Gährung. München 1879. S. 15.
[2]) Diese Berichte 3, 73.
[3]) Die bei der alkoholischen Gährung durch Sprosshefe auftretende Wärmeentwickelung hat kürzlich A. Bouffard wieder bestimmt, Compt. rend. 121, 357.

jenigen des Zellinhaltes unterscheide [1]). Auch die Erfahrungen von
E. Fischer und P. Lindner [2]) bezüglich Einwirkung des Hefe-
pilzes Monilia candida auf Rohrzucker gehören hierher. Dieser
Sprosspilz vergährt Saccharose; es war aber weder Ch. E. Hansen
noch den genannten Autoren gelungen, aus frischer oder aus getrock-
neter Hefe ein invertinartiges Enzym, welches die vorhergehende
Spaltung in Trauben- und Fruchtzucker besorgen würde, durch
Wasser zu extrahiren. Ganz anders verlief der Versuch, als
Fischer und Lindner frische Monilia-Hefe benutzten, in welcher
durch sorgfältiges Zerreiben mit Glaspulver zuerst ein Theil der
Zellen geöffnet wurde. Die invertirende Wirkung war nun unverkenn-
bar. »Das invertirende Agens scheint allerdings hier kein beständiges
in Wasser lösliches Enzym, sondern ein Bestandtheil des lebenden
Protoplasma zu sein.

Die Vergährung des Zuckers durch die Zymase kann nun innerhalb der Hefezellen stattfinden [3]); wahrscheinlicher aber scheiden die
Hefezellen diesen Eiweisskörper in die Zuckerlösung aus, wo er die
Gährung bewirkt [4]). Der Vorgang bei der alkoholischen Gährung ist
dann vielleicht nur insofern als physiologischer Akt aufzufassen, als es
die lebenden Hefezellen sind, welche die Zymase ausscheiden. Dass
aus Hefezellen in anfänglich schwach alkalisch reagirender (durch
K_3PO_4), später neutral werdender Nährlösung bei 30° schon nach
15 Stunden beträchtliche Mengen von durch Kochen gerinnbaren
Eiweisskörpern herausdiosmiren, haben Nägeli [5]) und O. Löw gezeigt. In der That scheint auch, wie der oben erwähnte Versuch
zeigt, die Zymase durch Pergamentpapier hindurchzugehen.

[1]) Bemerkt muss hierbei allerdings werden, dass die sogen. Harnstoffgährung, der Zerfall des Harnstoffs in Ammoniak und Kohlensäure, chemisch
sich ausserordentlich von den eigentlichen Gährungsvorgängen unterscheidet
und deshalb von vielen überhaupt nicht als Gährung betrachtet wird. Es ist
einfache Hydrolyse, schon durch Wasser bei 120° zu erreichen.

[2]) Diese Berichte 28, 3037.

[3]) Die diosmotischen Verhältnisse lassen dies als möglich erscheinen.
Vergl. v. Nägeli, l. c. S. 39.

[4]) Damit sind wahrscheinlich auch die Versuche von J. de Rey-
Pailhade (Compt. rend. 118, 201) zu erklären, welcher aus frischer Bierhefe unter Zusatz von etwas Traubenzucker einen schwach alkoholischen
(22-procentigen) Auszug bereitet hat. Nach Befreiung von Mikroorganismen
mittels Filtriren durch eine sterile Arsonval-Kerze entwickelte dieser zucker-
haltige Auszug bei Sauerstoffabschluss spontan Kohlensäure.

[5]) loc. cit. S. 94. Die Versuche wurden mit demselben Erfolge wieder-
holt; nur ergab sich, dass sie ebenso wie in Saccharose-, auch in Lactose-
Lösungen verlaufen. Die Diffusionsvorgänge sind demnach nicht an die Aus-
übung der Gährthätigkeit gebunden, wie die genannten Autoren annahmen.

Gährversuche.

No.	Presssaft ccm	Kohlenhydrat-lösung ccm	Gesammt-Procent-gehalt an Zucker pCt.	Versuchs-temperatur	Beobachtungen
1	30	Saccharose 30	37	Eisschrank	Nach 1 Stunde deutliche Gase wickelung, die nach 14 Tagen noch ni beendet ist. Die Schaumschicht trägt schliesslich 1 cm.
2	50	50	37		Starke Gasentwickelung u. Schau schicht. Die erst klare Lösung opali nach 3 Tg. ohne Eintritt einer Fällu
3	150	150	37		Die Schaumschicht beträgt na 3 Tagen ³⁄₄ cm.
4	20	20	37		Die Gasentwickelung wird nach zv Stunden sichtbar u. ist nach 14 Tag noch nicht beendet: die anfangs kl Flüssigkeit zeigt am Schluss nur minim Trübung; Schaumschicht $1\frac{1}{2}$ cm hc
5	30	» 30	37		Gasentwickelung beginnt nach 1 T und ist nach 1 Woche noch nicht endet: dabei ist die Lösung noch v ständig klar.
6	20	» 20	37	Zimmer-temperatur	Nach 1 Stunde lebhafte Gase wickelung: auch nach 2 Wochen n geringe Blasenbildung bei nur m maler Trübung.
7	20	» 20	37	40⁰	Nach 2 Stunden bereits 10 cm h Schaumschicht: nach 1 Tag starke rinnselausscheidung; die Gasentwic lung ist beendet.
8	30	30	12	Eisschrank	Nach 6 Tagen noch starke G entwickelung: ferner Trübung, die feinst vertheiltem Gerinnsel besteht
9	5	Maltose 5	33	»	Nach 1 Stunde Beginn der Gase wickelung, die auch nach 12 Tagen n andauert.
10	10	5	26		Die Gasentwickelung ist schon na 3 Stunden ausserordentlich stark.
11	10	Glucose 10	33		Erst nach 20 Std. starke Gase wickelung, die aber nach 12 Tagen n andauert; Schaumschicht ³⁄₄ cm ho
12	10	10	26		Schon nach ¹⁄₂ Stunde zieml starke Gasentwickelung, die 12 T anhält; die Lösung wird dabei tri und setzt etwas Niederschlag ab (s.
13	10	Fructose 10	37		Die Gasentwickelung ist schon na ¹⁄₄ Stunde sehr stark u. nach 3 Ta noch lebhaft im Gang; die Lös bleibt dabei klar.
14	10	10	25		Die Schaumschicht ist nach 15 nuten schon beträchtlich und misst na 3 Tagen 1 cm.
15	10	Lactose 10	gesättigte Lösung	Zimmer-temperatur	Keine Gasentwickelung, auch ni nach 6 Tagen.
16	10	Mannit 10	»	»	Wie bei Lactose.

Bemerkungen. Bei Versuch 1) wurde das entweichende Gas 4 Stunden nach Beginn der Entwickelung in Kalkwasser geleitet und als Kohlensäure identificirt. Bei 2) und 3) erfolgte nach 3 Tagen Bestimmung des durch Gährung gebildeten Alkohols; es waren bei 2) 1.5 g, bei 3) 3.3 g Aethylalkohol vorhanden; hiervon sind die Mengen in Abzug zu bringen, welche der verwendeten Hefe noch von der Bierbereitung her anhafteten. Bei 2) war die Hefe vor Herstellung des Presssaftes mit je 5 L Wasser noch 4 mal gewaschen worden; dann wurde in 2/3 des Ganzen der Alkohol bestimmt, das Uebrige auf Presssaft verarbeitet; nach den Ergebnissen war in der verwendeten Hefe höchstens 0.3 g Alkohol vorhanden. Bei 3) wurde für die Presshefefabrikation gereinigte, aber noch nicht mit Stärke versetzte Bierhefe des Handels direct verarbeitet; der Alkoholgehalt der zur Herstellung von 150 ccm Presssaft nöthigen Hefe berechnet sich nach der ausgeführten Bestimmung zu 1.2 g. Sonach war bei 2) 1.2 g, bei 3) 2.1 g Alkohol durch Gährung entstanden. In allen Fällen wurde der Alkohol durch die Jodoformreaction identificirt und schliesslich mittels Pottasche aus der wässrigen Lösung ausgesalzen. Die bei 3) erhaltene Abscheidung ging vollständig zwischen 79—81° (734 mm) über, das Destillat war farblos, brennbar und besass den Geruch des Aethylalkohols.

Mikroskopisch untersucht wurden die Versuche 2) und 3), nachdem sie 3 Tage im Gange waren, ferner 8) nach 6tägiger Dauer und von 12) nach 12 Tage währender Gährung der geringe Bodensatz: in allen Fällen fanden sich keine Organismen. sondern lediglich Eiweissgerinnsel als Ursache der mehr oder minder starken Trübung. Von Versuch 3) wurden ausserdem bei seiner Unterbrechung nach im Ganzen 3 tägiger Dauer noch 6 Plattenculturen angelegt. Je 1 ccm Flüssigkeit kam zur Aussaat in 3 Röhrchen mit verflüssigter Bierwürzegelatine, und je 1 ccm in 3 Röhrchen mit verflüssigter Fleischwasserpeptongelatine. Nach 6 Tagen zeigte eine Würzegelatineplatte 11 Colonieen, die beiden anderen waren steril geblieben; die 3 Peptongelatineplatten wiesen gleichmässig je 50 -- 100 Colonieen auf und waren verflüssigt worden. In Anbetracht der bei diesen Versuchen zur Aussaat gelangten grossen Flüssigkeitsmengen beweisen die Ergebnisse, dass die Gährwirkung nicht von Mikroorganismen ausgegangen ist, was übrigens schon durch das rasche Auftreten der Gährungserscheinungen beinahe ausgeschlossen ist.

Endlich wurde bei den Versuchen 4) und 5) der Presssaft durch sterilisirte Berkefeldt-Kieselguhrfilter gesaugt. Bei 5) war ausserdem auch noch die Rohrzuckerlösung im Autoklaven sterilisirt worden, und wurde die Mischung der beiden Flüssigkeiten unter allen aseptischen Vorsichtsmaassregeln vollzogen.

Es hat sich ergeben, dass die oben geschilderte Auspressmethode auch zur Gewinnung des Inhalts von Bacterienzellen geeignet ist, und sind Versuche darüber, namentlich auch mit pathogenen Bacterien, im hygienischen Institute zu München im Gang.

Tübingen, den 9. Januar 1897.

8

Alcoholic Fermentation
Without Yeast Cells

E. BUCHNER

Translated expressly for this Benchmark
volume by H. W. Doelle from "Alko-
holische Gährung ohne Hefezellen,"
Chem. Ber., **30**, *117–124 (1897)*

A separation of the action of fermentation from living yeast cells has so far been unsuccessful; a method will be described that solves this problem.

One thousand g of cleaned brewing yeast[1] (to which potato starch has not yet been added) was mixed with an equal amount of quartz sand[2] and 250 g of Kieselguhr and ground until the mass became moist and plastic. To this plastic mass 100 g of water was added; the whole mixture was transferred into a cloth and gradually exposed to a pressure of 4000–5000 atmospheres. The result was 300 ml of sap. The residue in the cloth was again ground and sieved, and 100 g of water was added. Under pressure, an additional 150 ml of sap was obtained. Thus 1 kg of yeast produces 500 ml of sap, which contains approximately 300 ml of cell substance. In order to remove the slight turbidity, the sap was shaken out with 4 g of Kieselguhr and filtered through a paper filter.

The resulting sap is a clear, opalescent yellow fluid that had a pleasant yeast odor. Its specific weight was 1.0416 (17°C). During boiling, the precipitate obtained was so thick that the fluid became almost solid. The formation of insoluble particles started at 35–40°C, but before this occurred the development of gas bubbles indicated the release of CO_2, with which the fluid was apparently saturated.[3] The sap contained more than 10 percent dry substance. According to an earlier, less efficient method, the sap contained 6.7 percent dry substance, 1.15 percent ash, and, according to the nitrogen content, 2.7 percent protein.

The most interesting feature of the sap was that it was able to initiate the

---

[1] The surface water has been removed in such way that under 25 atm pressure no water is released.
[2] Glass powder is not suitable because of its weak alkaline nature.
[3] The plant physiologists may decide whether this amount of CO_2 comes from the oxidation processes in respiration.

fermentation of carbohydrates. If sap and a concentrated sugar solution were mixed in equal volume, regular carbon dioxide release started after ¼ to 1 hour and lasted for days. Grape, fruit, and malt sugars reacted in the same way; no fermentation occurred in mixtures of the sap with saturated milk sugar, or with mannitol solutions, since these substances are not fermented by living cells of beer yeast either. Mixtures of sap and sugar solution gradually become turbid without the appearance of microscopic organisms after several days fermentation and storage in a refrigerator; however, at 700 times magnification a large number of protein particles were observed, the precipitation of which was probably caused by the acid formation during fermentation. A saturation of the sap–saccharose mixture with chloroform does not prevent fermentation, but leads to an early protein precipitation. Filtration of the sap through a sterilized Berkefeldt–Kieselguhr filter, which filters out the yeast cells, does not destroy the fermentation ability; the completely clear filtrate mixture begins fermentation after approximately 1 day, even at refrigeration temperature. Small gas bubbles also occur at the surface of a dialysis tube containing the sap that was immersed in a 37 percent sugar solution; gas development occurred, of course, also inside the tube, since the sugar solution diffused into the dialysis tube. Further experiments are needed to decide whether the sources of the fermentation are able to diffuse through the dialysis tube. The fermentation capability of the sap is gradually lost; storage of the sap in ice water for 5 days inactivated the sap against saccharose. This is amazing because normally the sap and saccharose mixture is able to keep its fermentation ability for at least 2 weeks. It is probable that CO_2 formation prevents the access of oxygen; it could also be that the sugar protects the reagent.

Very few experiments that give an indication of the nature of the active substance in the sap have been carried out. On heating of the sap to 40–50°C, carbon dioxide develops first, followed by precipitation of denatured protein; after 1 hour, filtration was carried out. The clear filtrate possessed weak fermentation ability with saccharose in the first experiment, but none in the second; the active substance appeared either to lose its activity at these low temperatures, or to denature and precipitate. Twenty ml of sap was introduced into three times that volume of absolute alcohol; the precipitate was separated by suction and dried over sulfuric acid under vacuum; of the 2 g of dry substance obtained, only a very little was soluble in 10 ml of water. The filtrate of this suspension had no fermentation ability. These experiments have to be repeated, and, in particular, the isolation of the active substance with ammonium sulfate should be tried.

As far as the theory of fermentation is concerned, the following conclusions can be drawn. First, evidence that the initiation of the fermentation process does not require such a complicated apparatus as the yeast cell should be obtained. The source of the fermentation activity of the sap is a soluble substance, doubtlessly a protein; it should be called zymase.

The opinion that a protein in the yeast cell is the cause of fermentation, known as the enzyme or ferment theory, was proposed by M. Traube in 1858 and later strongly defended by F. Hoppe-Seyler. The separation of such enzymes from the yeast cells, however, was so far unsuccessful.

It is still questionable whether zymase can be added to the known enzymes. As C. v. Nägeli[4] has already mentioned, important differences exist between the action of fermentation and the action of the normal enzyme. The latter is just hydrolysis, which can be improvised with the simplest chemical material. Although A. v. Baeyer[5] explained the chemical process of the alcoholic fermentation in simple terms, the decomposition of sugar to alcohol and carbon dioxide still belongs to the more complicated reactions; carbon compounds are decomposed in an unknown way, and cannot be carried out with other methods yet. A distinct difference also exists in the heat development.[6]

Invertin can be isolated easily from dead (1 hour at 150°C) yeast cells mixed with water followed by alcohol precipitation as a soluble powder. The active substance of fermentation cannot be obtained in this way. It probably will not remain after such heat treatment; the substance is converted into a form insoluble in water by alcohol precipitation. It can thus be assumed that the zymase belongs to the genuine proteins and is probably more attached to the living cell than invertin.

A very similar opinion was expressed by the French bacteriologist Miguel in regard to urease, an enzyme excreted from bacteria during urea fermentation; he labeled the enzyme protoplasm that does not require the cell membrane and is able to act outside the cell, which is its only distinction from the cell content.[7] The observations of E. Fisher and P. Lindner[8] in regard to the influence of the yeast fungus *Monilia candida* on sugar should also be mentioned. This fungus ferments saccharose; neither Ch. E. Hansen nor previously mentioned authors succeeded in the extraction of an invertin-like enzyme, which was able to split grape and fruit sugar, from fresh or dried yeast. The experimental results were different when Fischer and Lindner used fresh Monilia yeast, in which part of the cells were opened by carefully grinding them with glass powder first. The action of invertin was noticeable. The invertin agent does not appear to be a stable, water-soluble enzyme but part of the living protoplasm.

The fermentation of sugars by the zymase now appears to occur inside the yeast cell[9]; the yeast cell probably excretes these proteins into the sugar solution, where they ferment.[10] The process of alcoholic fermentation is probably, therefore, a

---

[4]*Theorie der Gährung.* München, 1879, p. 15.

[5]*Ber. Deut. Chem. Gesellschaft*, **3**, 73.

[6]The heat development that occurs during alcoholic fermentation of budding yeast has been determined recently by A. Bouffard, *Compt. Rend.*, **121**, 357.

[7]It should be noted that in urea fermentation the decomposition of urea to ammonia and carbon dioxide is distinctly different from normal fermentation processes and, therefore, one may dispute that the chemical process should be called a fermentation. It is a single hydrolysis, which can be obtained with water at 120°C.

[8]*Ber. Deut. Chem. Gesellschaft*, **28**, 3037.

[9]The osmotic conditions appear to make this possible. See also v. Nägeli, *loc. cit.*, p. 39.

[10]This could also explain the experiments of J. de Rey-Pailhade (*Compt. Rend.*, **118**, 201), who produced a weak alcoholic extract (22 percent) after adding fresh beer yeast to some dextrose. After separation from the microorganisms by filtration through a sterile Arsouval candle, the sugar containing extract spontaneously produced carbon dioxide under exclusion of oxygen.

physiological process only, since it is the living yeast cell that excretes the zymase. Nägeli[11] and O. Löw have shown that significant amounts of protein, which are denatured by heating, are excreted from yeast cells after 15 hours incubation at 30°C first in weak alkaline and later in neutral nutrient solution. It appears that zymase, as was reported above, is also able to penetrate dialysis tubing.

Remarks

In Experiment 1 (see the table) the gas was absorbed into $Ca(OH)_2$ 4 hours after the start and identified as carbon dioxide. In Experiments 2 and 3, alcohol determinations were carried out after 3 days; 1.5 g of ethanol (Experiment 2) and 3.3 g of ethanol (Experiment 3) were present. One must, of course, subtract those amounts that had been carried into the experiment with the yeast. In the case of Experiment 2, the yeast was washed 4 times with 5 liters of water each time before the sap was produced; the alcohol content of two-thirds of the material was then determined and the rest was used for the sap. The results revealed that not more than 0.5 g of ethanol was present in the yeast used. In Experiment 3, clean yeast that had no potato starch added was used. The ethanol content of the yeast used for the production of 150 ml sap was 1.2 g. Thus the ethanol production due to fermentation in Experiment 2 was 1.2 g and in Experiment 3, 2.1 g. The alcohol was identified, in all cases, by the iodoform reaction followed by the salt precipitation with potassium carbonate. The precipitate was distilled at 79–81° (734 mm in the case of Experiment 3). The distillate was colorless, burned, and had the characteristic odor of ethanol.

Experiments 2 and 3 were microscopically investigated after 3 days of fermentation, Experiment 8 after 6 days, and Experiment 12 after 12 days; in all cases no organisms were found in the sediment, only protein particles, which caused the more or less strong turbidity. Plate cultures were also made from Experiment 3. Three test tube containing wort gelatine and three test tubes containing peptone meat extract gelatine were each inoculated with 1 ml of the fluid. After 6 days, only one wort gelatine plate showed colonies (11), while the other two remained sterile. In the case of the peptone meat extract gelatine plates, 50–100 colonies appeared on the plates, which were liquified. Considering the large inoculum, the results indicate that the fermentation is not caused by microorganisms, which actually was a false hypothesis because of the rapid initiation of fermentation.

Finally, in Experiments 4 and 5, the sap was sucked through a sterilized Berkefeldt–Kieselguhr filter. In Experiment 5 even the sugar solution was sterilized in an autoclave; and both fluids were mixed under the most stringent aseptic conditions.

It was proved that the press method described above can be used to obtain the content of the bacterial cell and experiments are in progress (with pathogenic bacteria) in the Institute of Hygiene at Munich.

---

[11]*Loc. cit.*, p. 94. The experiments were repeated with the same result; it was shown that these occur in saccharose and lactose solutions. The diffusion process is not, therefore, dependent on the fermentation activity, as was originally thought by these authors.

Experiment No.	Sap, ml	Carbohydrate solution, ml		Sugar content, %	Incubation temperature, °C	Remarks
1	30	Saccharose	30	37	Refrigerated	Gas developed after 1 hr which had not stopped after 14 days. Froth layer was finally 1 cm.
2	50	Saccharose	50	37	Refrigerated	Strong gas development and froth layer. Clear solution, becomes opalescent after 3 days without precipitation.
3	150	Saccharose	150	37	Refrigerated	Froth layer after 3 days is ¾ cm.
4	20	Saccharose	20	37	Refrigerated	Gas development can be seen after a few hours and has not stopped after 14 days. Clear solution shows only minimal turbidity. Froth 1½ cm.
5	30	Saccharose	30	37	Refrigerated	Gas development starts after 1 hr and has not ceased after 1 week; solution is still clear.
6	20	Saccharose	20	37	Room temperature	Vigorous gas development after 1 hr; after 2 weeks still small bubble production by minimal turbidity.
7	20	Saccharose	20	37	40	10-cm froth layer after 2 hr; strong precipitation after 1 day; gas development ceased.
8	30	Saccharose	30	12	Refrigerated	Still strong gas development after 6 days; turbidity consisting of fine particles.
9	5	Maltose	5	33	Refrigerated	Gas development starts after 1 hr and has not ceased after 12 days.
10	10	Maltose	5	26	Refrigerated	Gas development very strong after 3 hr.
11	10	Glucose	10	33	Refrigerated	Strong gas development only after 20 hr, not ceased after 12 days; froth layer ¾ cm.
12	10	Glucose	10	26	Refrigerated	Strong gas development after ½ hour, continues 12 days; solution becomes turbid; precipitation occurs.
13	10	Fructose	10	37	Refrigerated	Very strong gas development after ¼ hr and after 3 days; solution stays clear.
14	10	Fructose	10	25	Refrigerated	Froth strong after few minutes, after 3 days, 1 cm.
15	10	Lactose	10	Sat.	Room temperature	No gas after 6 days.
16	10	Mannitol	10	Sat.	Room temperature	Same as lactose.

II

Carbohydrate Metabolism

Editor's Comments on Papers 9 and 10

9 **Barcroft and Haldane:** A Method of Estimating the Oxygen and Carbonic Acid in Small Quantities of Blood
   J. Physiol., **28**, 232–240 (1902)

10 **Brodie:** Some New Forms of Apparatus for the Analysis of the Gases of the Blood by the Chemical Method
   J. Physiol., **39**, 391–396 (1909)

   The initial work of Buchner (Paper 8) inspired scientists to explore the "yeast juice" for those chemical substances which bring about the anaerobic and aerobic conversion of glucose. This exploration was possible only because of the development of a new method of gas analysis. In 1902, Barcroft and Haldane developed a new apparatus (Paper 9) for the estimation of oxygen and carbonic acid. This apparatus was altered a few years later by Brodie (Paper 10) to measure gases by a chemical method. In its final form, the apparatus became known as the Warburg respirometer, as Warburg (Paper 15) and his research group made most use of this new method in their respiratory studies. Both articles were included because of their tremendous impact on the development of research in microbial metabolism and enzymology in later years. Details of the method itself can be found in the book by Umbreit et al. (1964).

9

Reprinted from *J. Physiol.*, **28**, 232–240 (1902)

A METHOD OF ESTIMATING THE OXYGEN AND CARBONIC ACID IN SMALL QUANTITIES OF BLOOD. By JOSEPH BARCROFT, M.A., B.Sc., *Fellow of King's College, Cambridge,* AND J. S. HALDANE, M.D., F.R.S., *Fellow of New College, Oxford.* (Three Figures in Text.)

(*From the Physiological Laboratories of Oxford and Cambridge.*)

IN the investigation of the blood-gases in small animals, or in individual organs such as the salivary glands, it is desirable to have a method which will permit of obtaining results with very small amounts of blood. The method now described was designed with the special object of fulfilling this requirement, but it may also be conveniently made use of even where large samples are available, or when it is desired to make a number of determinations of the blood-gases of a single animal. The apparatus needed is considerably simpler and the time required much shorter than with the ordinary method of extracting the oxygen and carbonic acid by a vacuum pump and subsequently analysing them.

The apparatus consists of a small glass vessel attached by tubing to a pressure-gauge of narrow bore. The vessel is so arranged that the oxygen in the sample of blood can be liberated within it by ferricyanide and the resulting increase of pressure measured by means of the gauge. From the increase of pressure the volume of the oxygen can be calculated. By similar manipulation with the use of tartaric acid in the place of ferricyanide the carbonic acid is subsequently determined.

The whole apparatus is shown in Fig. 1. Two gauges, one connected with the blood-gas vessel, and the other with a precisely similar control vessel, are fixed on a wooden stand, the front of which is painted white to form a convenient background for reading the graduations on the tubes. Each gauge is graduated on both limbs in millimetres etched on the glass, the length graduated being about 350 mm. The limbs of each gauge are connected below by a piece of india-rubber tubing of about 1·25 cm. bore, which can be compressed by a screw clamp (3cm. broad), so as to adjust the levels. The gauges are filled with water which may be tinged with a suitable dye. The bore of the gauges is 2 to 2·5 mm. and must be even, though it need not be the same in different limbs. The evenness can be ascertained by means of a column of mercury in the usual way. One limb of each gauge is provided with

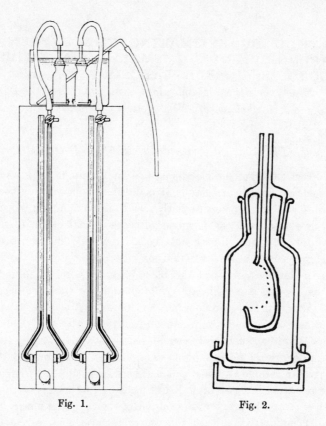

Fig. 1.   Fig. 2.

a 3-way tap close to the top. The gauges should be thoroughly cleaned before being filled, otherwise the readings will be unreliable, as shown by the fact that the water does not ascend or descend to equal distances on the two sides on compressing or relaxing the rubber tube with the taps open.

The blood-gas vessel and control vessel are of the form shown in Fig. 2. They each have a capacity of about 25 c.c. The stopper is perforated by a glass tube of narrow bore; which passes below into an open pocket capable of holding about ·3 c.c. of liquid. The pocket is so arranged that any liquid in it can easily be emptied by tilting the vessel. To this end the orifice above the pocket should be at least 1·8 cm. in height and as broad as possible.

Before the sample of blood is collected, 1·5 c.c. of the alkaline solution (2 c.c. of strong ammonia, ·88 sp. gr., to 1000 c.c. of distilled water) used in carrying out the ferricyanide[1] method is measured with a pipette into the blood-gas vessel, and ·25 c.c. of saturated potassium ferricyanide solution is placed in the glass pocket of the stopper, which has previously been greased with resin ointment or some other adhesive lubricant.

Blood entirely deprived of its power of clotting may be collected in a pipette which delivers 1 c.c. between two marks. The pipette should be a tube of uniform bore, graduated in hundredths of a c.c. A cubic centimetre of fluid should form a column 15—20 cm. in height.

In such a tube there is no perceptible gaseous exchange except at the very surface of the column. It has already been shown that saliva and blood collected in such tubes do not lose CO_2[2], nor does a change of colour take place away from the meniscus. As the exposed portion of blood is never delivered from the pipette no error is introduced from aeration.

For the collection of coagulable blood a hypodermic syringe with special adjustments is used. This instrument is shown in Fig. 3. The syringe, which is entirely made of glass[3], should have a capacity of 1·2 to 1·5 c.c. It contains a flat glass bead, pierced with a large

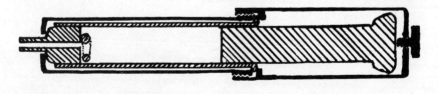

■■ **BRASS**
▨▨ **GLASS**

Fig. 3.

hole. The syringe is screwed into a brass case, which is so made that the distance from the shoulder of the nozzle to the end of the plunger when pulled out as far as possible is a constant quantity. The syringe

[1] This *Journal*, xxv. p. 205. 1900.
[2] This *Journal*, xxvii. p. 37. 1901.
[3] We have used an "All-glass" syringe of Burroughs and Wellcome.

has three fixed points, which will be referred to as positions I. II. and III :

Position I. when the plunger is pressed against the bead,

Position II. when the plunger is touching the back of the brass case, and

Position III. when the screw at the back of the case is screwed home and the plunger is touching the tip of the screw.

The collection of blood is carried out as follows :

(1) A 1 % solution of potassium oxalate is sucked into the syringe and all the air-bubbles expelled. Oxalate is then expelled till the plunger is in position I. The syringe now contains a known quantity of oxalate.

(2) Blood is sucked in till the plunger is in position II. The blood and the oxalate are mixed by means of the bead. (The blood in the nozzle, which is quite trivial in amount, less than ·02 c.c., does not mix with the oxalate.) A mixture containing blood and oxalate in known proportions has now been obtained.

(3) The screw is screwed up till the plunger is in position III. The blood in the nozzle has now been expelled and a little of the mixture has been expelled.

(4) The mixture is expelled into the bottle, the plunger returning to position I. A known volume of a mixture of blood and oxalate of known composition, and hence a known volume of blood, has been put into the bottle.

The volume of blood delivered by the syringe is ascertained by weighing it :

    (1) When empty.
    (2) With nozzle just filled with water.
    (3) Filled with water in position I.
    (4)   „   „   „ II.
    (5)   „   „   „ III.

The mixture is discharged cautiously into the bottom of the blood-gas vessel, care being taken that the blood lies under the ammonia solution. The blood-gas vessel is then closed and placed in the water beside the control vessel as shown in Fig. 1, care being taken not to mix the blood with the ammonia solution or spill the ferricyanide. The water is stirred two or three times by blowing air through it by means of a tube shown in Fig. 1, and the gauge is watched till the temperature of the two vessels is found to be exactly the same. In making these and other observations it is necessary first to squeeze the rubber tubing connecting the limbs of the gauges, so as to insure that the glass above each meniscus should be wet. The two gauges are now adjusted by opening the three-way taps, so that they are both level and stand at zero. The blood-gas bottle is taken out and the blood and ammonia solution mixed without spilling any ferricyanide. When this solution is completely transparent the vessel is tilted so as to empty out the ferricyanide, and then shaken for a few minutes to liberate all the oxygen. During these manipulations it should be held either in a cloth or by the lead stand, to avoid warming the glass. It is now replaced in the water, which is stirred. When the temperature of the two vessels has again come even the gauges are adjusted so that the levels in the limbs connected with the bottles are at zero. The heights on the other limbs are read off; and if, as is usual, the temperature has risen since the original reading, so that the level is now higher in the open limb of the control tube gauge, the reading of this gauge is deducted from the reading of the other gauge.

A further correction is also necessary. If a blank experiment be made in which no ferricyanide is added, but all the other manipulations are gone through it will be found that a slight negative reading amounting to about 3·5 mm. is obtained. This is apparently due to the tension of ammonia vapour being less after the blood and ammonia solutions are mixed or to absorption of the minute amount of carbonic acid in the air within the bottle. Hence a constant determined for the ammonia solution used must be added to the reading.

The temperature of the vessel of water is now read off. As the specific gravity of mercury at 0° is 13·59 and of water at 15° ·999 it is evident that the normal barometric pressure equals that of a column of water $760 \times \dfrac{13\cdot59}{\cdot999} = 10340$ mm. high.

Hence the volume at 760 mm. pressure of oxygen given off equals the volume of air in the blood-gas tube and its connections multiplied by the corrected reading of the gauge in millimetres and divided by 10340. Thus if the total capacity of the blood-gas vessel and its connections to the zero of the gauge = 23·35 c.c. and that of the fluids which have been put in is 2·75 c.c. the volume of air will be 20·6 c.c. If now, the reading of the gauge = 100·0 mm. the oxygen given off will be $20\cdot6 \times \dfrac{100}{10340}$ c.c. = ·201 c.c. If the temperature were 14° this would correspond to ·191 c.c. of oxygen at 0°. If this came off 1 c.c. of blood the combined oxygen of the blood would be 19·1 %.

The capacity of the blood-gas vessel is previously ascertained by weighing it first empty and then full of water. That of the connecting tubing is determined by adjusting the gauge to zero and then raising the pressure to a certain definite amount, first with the vessel connected and afterwards with a stopper inserted into the end of the rubber tube in place of the glass tube of the vessel. The capacity of the vessel and the connecting tubing will be to that of the connecting tubing alone, as the first reduction in volume of the closed limb as read off on the gauge is to the second.

To estimate the carbonic acid the stopper of the blood-gas vessel is removed after the estimation of the oxygen and ·25 c.c. of 20 % tartaric acid solution is placed in the glass pocket; the stopper is then replaced and the gauge adjusted to zero in the same way as before. The acid is then spilt and the bottle shaken till all the CO_2 is set free, which takes a very short time. The gauge is again read off and the volume of the CO_2 calculated.

The determinations should always be made in a well-ventilated room, as the presence of an abnormally high percentage of CO_2 in the air enclosed in the bottle at the beginning of the experiment might evidently give rise to error both in the oxygen and CO_2 determinations.

A correction is necessary for any CO_2 which may be present in the solutions employed or is absorbed from the air enclosed in the bottle. This correction is obtained by previously doing a complete blank experiment, using boiled distilled water in place of blood to mix with the ammonia solution and ferricyanide. After the correction has been obtained the ammonia solution should be kept in a stoppered bottle.

A further complication is introduced by the fact that CO_2 is very soluble in water or the acid mixture of water and precipitated proteid etc. present in the bottle. To ascertain the solubility of CO_2 in this mixture as compared with its solubility in water we used a vessel of 340 c.c. capacity, provided with a mercury gauge, and immersed in water at a constant temperature. In successive experiments we filled this vessel with pure CO_2 and then forced into it 50 c.c. of boiled distilled water or 50 c.c. of blood diluted with water, ferricyanide, and acid in the proportions used for the blood-gas determinations, and after this mixture had been freed from CO_2 by shaking with air and boiling *in vacuo*. On thoroughly shaking up the liquid with the CO_2, and observing the final reading of the gauge, the relative solubilities of CO_2 in the water and in the mixture could be calculated. The mean of several closely concordant experiments gave at 15° a coefficient of absorption of 1·001 for water, and 0·900 for the mixture. The solubility of carbonic acid in the mixture was thus 90 % of its solubility in water.

At a temperature of 13° one volume of water dissolves 1·065 volumes of CO_2 reduced to a temperature of 0°, or 1·11 volumes measured at 13°. Hence at the same temperature one volume of the blood mixture would dissolve 1·00 volume of CO_2 measured at 13°. There would therefore be no error at that temperature if in calculating the CO_2 given off by the blood the blood-gas vessel were regarded as containing no liquid. Within the ranges of temperature commonly met with the solubility of CO_2 diminishes by about 10 % for every four degrees of rise of temperature. With a bottle of about 25 c.c. capacity this would cause an error in a CO_2 determination of about 1 % for every four degrees above 13° if the vessel were regarded as containing no liquid. The simplest way of calculating the percentage of CO_2 in the blood is thus to regard the blood-gas vessel as containing no liquid, and to deduct 0·25 % from the final result for every degree C. by which the temperature of the water-bath exceeds 13°. Thus if the temperature of the bath were 17°, and the uncorrected result were 40·0 .volumes of CO_2 per 100 c.c. of blood, the corrected result would be 39·6 volumes.

To test the method we have made a variety of experiments:

In the first place it was necessary to see that the gauges acted with sufficient sharpness. This was tested by the simple plan of opening both limbs and screwing up the clamp so as to raise the level of the liquid. It was found that the gauges were always practically level provided that the tube had been well cleaned with ether, nitric acid, and water before being set up. The two gauges also showed the same differences of pressure when the temperature of the bath was raised provided that the volume of the air in the vessels and connections was the same.

In order to ascertain whether any error arose from diffusion of oxygen through the ammonia solution to venous blood, we placed in the apparatus blood which had been completely deprived of its oxygen by commencing putrefaction. It was found that after the temperature had become equal in the blood-gas and control vessels the gauges kept perfectly together for a far longer time than would be needed for an analysis, hence no error arises from diffusion.

To test directly the accuracy of the determinations we took defibrinated blood, saturated with air, and determined the oxygen capacity with the apparatus and by Haldane's method[1] with a carefully standardised hæmo-globinometer. The results were as follows:

A. *Ox-blood.*

	(1)	(2)	Mean
By hæmoglobinometer	19·60	19·80	19·70
By new apparatus	19·87	19·61	19·74

B. *Cat's blood.*

By hæmoglobinometer	12·25	12·25	12·25
By new apparatus	12·3	12·1	12·2

It is thus evident that the oxygen determinations are very accurate with saturated blood. With unsaturated blood, however, there is an evident source of slight error in the fact that the blood contains practically no dissolved oxygen when put into the apparatus, but an appreciable quantity at the end of the analysis, since at ordinary temperatures blood takes up 0·6 % of oxygen from the air. It is therefore necessary to add about that amount to the result when the blood is venous.

To test the carbonic acid determinations we employed in place of blood, 1 c.c. of a 0·200 % solution of Na_2CO_3 (which had been well heated in a platinum crucible before being weighed out). The results were as follows:

Calculated 42·1 %

Found { First series 41·6, 42·5, 42·0   Mean 42·0 %
Second „   42·7, 42·2, 42·6, 41·9, 42·3   Mean 42·3 %

Further we have allowed the CO_2 to stay for a considerable time in the apparatus and have found that no measurable quantity is absorbed by the rubber tubing in the time taken for a determination. We have also ascertained that no appreciable change in volume is caused by the precipitation of proteids, etc. which occurs on mixing the acid with the blood and ferricyanide.

We have tested arterial blood taken directly from two cannulæ placed in the carotid and femoral arteries respectively of a dog. The former was attached to the measuring burette of Barcroft's blood-gas apparatus and 8 c.c. of blood withdrawn: the latter to a pipette containing oxalate; the former was analysed for CO_2 with the pump, the latter with the new apparatus:

CO_2 by pump   42·0 %
by new apparatus   43·5 %

[1] This *Journal*, XXVI. p. 501. 1901.

Finally, to test the consistency of the apparatus we have made three analyses of defibrinated blood from the same vessel which gave the following results:

	(1)	(2)	(3)	Mean
O	18·5	18·5	18·8	18·6
CO_2	52·4	52·7	51·2	52·1

It is thus evident that the apparatus is capable of giving sufficiently accurate results in spite of the small volume of blood used; and provided sufficient pains are taken to avoid errors due to temperature differences and to the reagents employed it is not much less accurate than the blood-pump with much larger quantities of blood.

(The expenses of this research have been taken from grants placed at the disposal of the authors by the Royal Society.)

10

Copyright © 1909 by The Physiological Society

Reprinted from *J. Physiol.*, **39**, 391–396 (1909)

SOME NEW FORMS OF APPARATUS FOR THE ANALYSIS OF THE GASES OF THE BLOOD BY THE CHEMICAL METHOD. By T. G. BRODIE, M.D., F.R.S.

(*From the Physiological Laboratories of the London School of Medicine for Women and the Brown Institution, University of London.*)

IN the course of investigations in which I have used the Barcroft-Haldane apparatus for the estimation of the gases of the blood I have introduced several modifications which, I think, simplify the use of the apparatus and increase the rapidity with which the analyses can be made. As, in most experiments, several analyses have to be made, and as, too, it is very essential that they should be carried out rapidly I have gradually introduced a number of time-saving devices for the collecting and measuring of the various volumes of blood and liquid used in the method. These are described in the following sections.

The modified blood gas apparatus. Each pair of manometer tubes is mounted on a small wooden base (see Fig. 1) in such a way that the tubes can be easily removed for cleaning purposes. The two tubes are united at the bottom and at the lowest part of the bend a wider tube is fused in. To this a piece of rubber tubing is attached. This tubing can be compressed by a screw clamp, *E*, and thus the level of the fluid in the manometer tubes adjusted. The most important modification in the apparatus is in the form of the bottle. Since each apparatus is small it is now possible to have the bottle rigidly attached instead of being fitted in position by rubber tubing. In this way the volume of the air space in the apparatus is always quite constant. The contents of the bottle can be vigorously shaken by shaking the whole apparatus without running any risk of endangering the manometer reading. I have discarded the little glass cup into which the ferricyanide solution was placed because this was difficult to clean and was frequently broken.

The following arrangement takes its place. The stopper, F (Fig. 2), of the bottle is made of good size and the manometer tube is attached to it at one side. Fused into the side of the stopper is a small bent glass tube, G, which opens through the side. The neck of the bottle has a small recess, so that when the bottle is placed on the stopper the lower end of the tube, G, is closed in all positions of the bottle except when the recessed part faces the lower end of the internal tube. By removing the small stopper, J (Fig. 2), the ferricyanide solution can be placed in the tube G, when the bottle is in position. The proximal manometer tube has a single mark, L, upon it; the other tube is graduated in

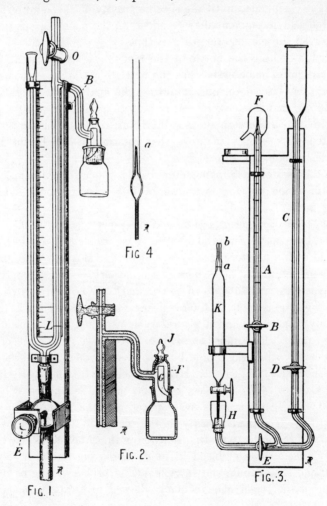

FIG 4

FIG. 2.

FIG. I.

FIG. 3.

millimetres, or the tubes are mounted on a glass mirror graduated in millimetres. The capacity of the bottle and of the tube down to the mark *L* is determined by filling with mercury and then weighing the mercury.

I at first experienced considerable difficulty in getting the manometer tubes sufficiently clean to give the readings accurately. This difficulty was at last overcome by employing a dilute solution of bile salt wherewith to fill the manometer and it then does not matter if the tubes are not perfectly clean. The solution I use consists of a 0·5 % solution of bile salt in which a little toluol is dissolved. Sodium chloride is then added until the specific gravity of the solution is 1,034. If desired a little pigment may be added to the solution, but it is quite easy to read the manometer without this.

When attaching the bottle to the manometer tubes for an analysis great care must be observed that the bottle is pushed well home on the stopper, otherwise in turning it during the analysis an alteration may occur in the manometer zero. It is best to use a very small amount of thin vaseline on the stopper as a lubricant, and each apparatus should be tested while empty to prove that rotation of the bottle does not alter the manometer zero.

On the back of each manometer there is a bent metal support, *B*, by means of which the apparatus can be suspended from the side of the cooling bath.

The blood sampling pipette. This pipette is illustrated at *K*, Fig. 3. It consists of a tube of about 6 c.c. capacity. Its lower end is provided with a tap terminating in a long fine nozzle. The upper end has a constriction and here there is a fine mark, *a*, encircling the tube. The capacity of the tube down to the mark *a* is accurately determined. When the tube is to be used for collecting a blood sample it is first held vertically in a clamp and a Hg reservoir attached to the lower end by rubber tubing. The upper end is connected by a short piece of rubber tubing with a fine glass tube bent so as to project downwards. The tube is now nearly filled with Hg and then a solution of hirudin (1 %) in Na Oxalate (4 %) is drawn into the tube. When about 1 c.c. has entered the Hg reservoir is again raised and the hirudin solution run out until the Hg stands exactly at the mark *a*. This leaves a known quantity of the anticoagulating solution in the tube. It is now ready for receiving the sample of blood. The clamp on the vein or artery is first opened and the cannula and short length of rubber tubing is filled with blood from the vessel, enough being allowed to escape to wash out the

27—2

tube thoroughly. The sampling tube is then attached to the cannula by rubber tubing, and by opening the tap mercury is run out slowly into a small measure until a sufficient amount of blood (about 4 c.c.) has been drawn into the tube. The vessel is then clamped and the tube removed. A finger is at once placed over the open orifice, b, the tube inverted and by a sharp downward swinging movement Hg is driven into the capillary orifice to seal off that end. The tube is then turned upwards and downwards a few times to mix blood and anti-coagulating fluid thoroughly. It is then placed upper end downwards in a vessel containing Hg which seals up the open end until the blood is required for the analysis.

The amount of Hg collected gives the volume of blood taken into the tube. The capacity of the tube down to the mark, a, being known the amount of dilution of the blood is known and allowance for this dilution can be made when calculating the blood gases.

The automatic pipette for delivering the blood into the analysis bottle. This pipette is shown in Fig. 3. It consists of a long tube, A, 43 cms. in length, the upper half of which is graduated for 1 c.c. in 1/100 c.c. The upper end is closed in by a small cover, F, to catch any mercury which escapes when filling. On this tube there is a tap, B. A second vertical tube, C, is provided above with a receiver to hold mercury. It also is provided with a tap, D, and a little lower turns horizontally and shortly after the first tube joins it as in the figure. A little further there is a third tap, E, and finally the end is turned up and has a short length of thick walled rubber tubing on it. Over this again is a glass cup, H. It is used in the following way. The whole of the tubing and cups being filled with mercury the sampling tube containing the blood is attached so that the fine nozzle of the tap end of the tube fits into the rubber tubing under the mercury until the two glass ends lie in apposition (see Fig. 3). To the upper end of the sampling tube a bent glass tube of capillary bore is attached, and on opening taps D and E mercury is run in and the mercury seal and a little blood discharged from the sampling tube, enough blood being run out to wash out this fine tube thoroughly. The tap D is then turned. The bottle of the analysing apparatus is now held so that the orifice of the fine tube delivering the blood touches the bottom of the bottle and by opening tap B exactly 1 c.c. of blood is displaced into the bottle.

Before receiving the blood 2 c.c. of dilute NH_3 solution (3 c.c. NH_3 ·880 in 1 l. distilled water) is run into the bottle. This is delivered by means of a somewhat similar pipette to that just described. In placing this NH_3 solution in the bottle great care must be taken to protect it. It should be done in front of an open window and a glass plate of good size should be placed in front so that the expired air of the operator cannot by any possibility be blown into the bottle. The two bottles are only filled immediately before being required. The blood is then at once run in and the bottles quickly attached to their proper manometers.

When attaching the bottle to the manometer the tap O at the top of the manometer tube must be open and the little stopper J removed. The bottle is then ground well home and left in such a position that the lower end of tube G is closed. The proper quantity of ferricyanide solution is then put in by a choked pipette (Fig. 4) with a very fine capillary orifice at a.

The volume of fluid this delivers is previously carefully estimated by weighing. The fluid is drawn up and discharged by a small syringe, not by the mouth, so as to prevent any possible inclusion of expired air in the apparatus. The stopper J is then inserted and the apparatus placed in the cold water bath.

The water bath. This consists of a long copper trough 93 cms. long, 9·5 cms. wide and 11·5 cms. deep. Along the back and lower angle runs a metal tube with a large number of fine holes bored through it. One end of this tube is closed and the other is attached to the water supply and the water is then driven into the bath through the fine holes. The bath is thus filled, excess of water escaping through a side tube at the top of the bath. In this way there is a continuous stream of water coming in from the main water supply by a number of fine jets. These jets are directed obliquely upwards so that they impinge on the bottoms of the bottles on the manometers and in this way there is a continuous stirring of the water of the bath. The temperature too very rarely varies, and if it does it is only to a very small extent.

The bath is long enough to receive a row of 20 manometers. It stands upon a wooden support with a longitudinal strip at the base to steady the lower ends of the manometers. In most experiments eight samples of blood, 4 venous and 4 arterial have been analysed. Each is done in duplicate, thus 16 manometers are necessary. A seventeenth is also used to act as a temperature control and to estimate the amount of CO_2 in the ammonia solution. For this purpose the experiment is carried out in this apparatus just in the same way as in all the others with the exception that no blood is placed in it. As soon as the taps of two manometers are closed to commence the observation, that of the temperature control is also closed and read. Each time a fresh reading of a manometer is made a temperature reading is also taken so that the necessary correction, if any, may be made. The analysis is carried out as described in the paper by Barcroft and Haldane[1]. After the temperature has become constant the tap O is turned, the blood is laked and allowed to stand for 1 min. The bottle is then rotated and the ferricyanide allowed to run in. It is then well shaken. I find that shaking for 1 min. is usually sufficient to disengage all the oxygen. The apparatus is then cooled and read. If the manometers have been sorted out into pairs of nearly equal capacity, the readings for the same blood ought to agree. This is a great convenience in determining if all the O_2 has been disengaged. After the readings have been taken the taps, O, are opened, the manometers taken out, the bottles wiped and the stopper J removed. The saturated tartaric acid solution is then run in from the pipette as before and the whole operation repeated for the CO_2 determination. With two workers it is possible to carry out an experiment including the 16 blood analyses in five hours. It is best to get the blood into the apparatus as quickly as possible. Usually with two workers this is done within 2 or 3 minutes after each sample has been taken.

The apparatus described in this paper may be obtained from Messrs F. E. Becker & Co., Hatton Wall, Hatton Gardens, London, E.C.

[1] This *Journal*, XXVIII. p. 232. 1902.

Editor's Comments on Paper 11

11 **Harden and Young:** The Alcoholic Ferment of Yeast-juice. Part II. The Coferment of Yeast-juice
Proc. Roy. Soc., London, **B 78**, 369–375 (1906)

The first major breakthrough in the study of glucose utilization must be credited to the research group of A. Harden, who, in 1905, discovered cozymase, which is now known under the name of nicotinamide adenine dinucleotide (NAD). Of the two publications involved (Harden and Young, 1906), the second part was chosen (Paper 11), as it gives a very detailed description of their experiments. It took almost 10 more years before Meyerhof (1918) found this coenzyme in muscle tissue. With the discovery of NAD, Harden and Young established the first steps of anaerobic glucose utilization. They established the Harden–Young ester (fructose 1,6-diphosphate, Harden and Young, 1909) as an important intermediate. Another 30 years passed before the sequence of the glycolytic pathway was fully elucidated.

Neuberg and his coworkers continued the work and established pyruvate as a key intermediate. With the discovery of the enzyme carboxylase (Neuberg and Hildesheimer, 1911; Neuberg and Tir, 1911; Neuberg and Reinfurth, 1918), a first mechanism for the breakdown of glucose to alcohol was suggested.

11

Reprinted from *Proc. Roy. Soc., London*, **B 78**, 369–375 (1906)

The Alcoholic Ferment of Yeast-juice. Part II.—The Coferment of Yeast-juice.

By Arthur Harden, D.Sc., Ph.D., and William John Young, M.Sc.

(Communicated by Dr. C. J. Martin, F.R.S. Received June 14,—Read June 28, 1906.)

(From the Chemical Laboratory, Lister Institute.)

In a previous communication* it was shown that the fermentation of glucose by yeast-juice is dependent upon the presence of a dialysable substance which is not destroyed by heat. This substance is contained in the active yeast-juice prepared by disintegrating living yeast, and, therefore, most probably exists in the yeast cell side by side with the zymase.

The occurrence of an analogous activating substance has been described by Magnus† in the case of the lipase of the liver. He observed that the active juice of this organ became inactive when dialysed into water, but regained its activity when the dialysate or boiled liver juice was added. The term *coferment* was suggested by Bertrand‡ to denote substances of this kind, and he applied it in two instances—to the calcium salt, which he considered was necessary for the action of pectase on pecten substances, and to the manganese of laccase, which he supposed to be essential for the activity of this enzyme. Although not entirely satisfactory, this term may be provisionally applied to activating substances such as those present in liver lipase and yeast-juice, until further knowledge of their nature and function permits of a more rational terminology.

(1) *Preparation of the Inactive Residue from Yeast-juice in the Dry State.*

In the previous communication§ it was shown that when yeast-juice is filtered through a Martin gelatin filter, both the residue and the filtrate are incapable of fermenting sugar, whereas a mixture of the two produces a vigorous fermentation.

In carrying out the experiments which established this result, the residue left on the filter was always dissolved in water as soon as the filtration and washing were completed, and the activity of the solution was examined without delay. It has since been found possible to obtain the inactive

---

* 'Roy. Soc. Proc.,' B, vol. 77, 1906, p. 410.
† 'Zeit. Physiol. Chem.,' 1904, vol. 42, p. 149.
‡ 'Compt. Rend.,' 1897, vol. 124, p. 1032.
§ *Loc. cit.*

residue in the solid form, in which condition it retains its properties for a considerable time.

This is accomplished by spreading the sticky mass left on the filter over a large watch-glass, and exposing it over sulphuric acid in a vacuum. The residue dries up in a few hours to a brittle mass, which is converted by grinding into a light yellow powder.

Complete removal of the coferment is generally not effected by a single filtration, and the powder prepared as above is usually found to be slightly active. A completely inactive residue may, however, be obtained by redissolving in water and repeating the filtration and desiccation. The powder prepared in this way and dried over sulphuric acid in a vacuum for 15 hours only loses its potential activity slowly. The following examples show the original inactivity of the powder, its fermentative power in presence of boiled yeast-juice, and the loss of this power with lapse of time :—

I. 200 c.c. of yeast-juice were filtered in quantities of 50 c.c. through Martin filters and yielded 17·6 grammes of dry solid. This was dissolved in 50 c.c. of water and again filtered, yielding 9·2 grammes of dry solid residue.

The following experiments were then made at 26° in presence of toluene :—

1. March 8, 1906. One gramme of dry residue was dissolved in 15 c.c. of water and 1·5 grammes glucose added. No evolution of carbon dioxide was observed ; 12 c.c. of boiled yeast-juice containing 1·2 grammes of glucose were then added. Fermentation at once commenced, and 108 c.c. of carbon dioxide were evolved in 20 hours, when the experiment was discontinued.

2. Two months later (May 18, 1906) a similar experiment was carried out, a sample of the same boiled yeast-juice being employed. As before, 1 gramme of the residue dissolved in sugar solution was quite inactive. On the addition of the boiled juice fermentation at once commenced ; the rate was, however, only about one-third of that attained in the previous experiment, and fermentation ceased when only 42 c.c. of carbon dioxide had been evolved.

Although the fermentation in the first experiment was not continued to the end, the comparison shows clearly that the potential activity of the dry residue had greatly diminished.

II. In the case of another sample of dry residue, with which two similar experiments were made with the interval of a week, it was found that in the first experiment 364 c.c. of carbon dioxide were produced, and in the second 344 c.c., a difference of only about 5·5 per cent.

(2) *Disappearance of the Coferment from Yeast-juice during Fermentation and Autolysis.*

When a small amount of boiled yeast-juice is added to a solution of the inactive residue in 10-per-cent. glucose solution, fermentation commences and continues for a period which varies with the amount added. The cessation of fermentation appears in such a case to be due to some change in the coferment, since the addition of a further quantity of boiled yeast-juice again sets up fermentation, and if the quantity of boiled juice added on each occasion be small enough, this process can be repeated a third time.

The following experiments, made at 26° in presence of toluene, illustrate this point :—

1. One gramme of dry inactive residue was dissolved in 15 c.c. of 10-per-cent. glucose solution, and three quantities of 3 c.c. of boiled juice were then successively added, the fermentation being allowed to come to an end before each addition.

Carbon dioxide evolved.

1st addition	....	8·2 c.c.
2nd „	....	6 „
3rd „	....	6 „

2. Two grammes of dry inactive residue were dissolved in 15 c.c. of 10-per-cent. glucose solution, and two quantities of 15 c.c. of a diluted boiled juice containing 10 per cent. of glucose were successively added.

Carbon dioxide evolved.

1st addition	....	54 c.c.
2nd „	....	41·2 „

This phenomenon has been frequently observed in the course of experiments on the filtration of the juice through the Martin filter. The first residue obtained is generally slightly active, and produces a small amount of fermentation with glucose solution. The evolution of carbon dioxide, however, soon stops, but is again renewed when boiled yeast-juice is added. One instance of this was quoted in our previous communication,[*] and many more have been observed, some of which are tabulated below.

Carbon dioxide evolved from residue + glucose.	Boiled juice added.	Subsequent evolution of carbon dioxide.
c.c.	c.c.	c.c.
8 ·6	20	72
13 ·2	16	364 ·3
16 ·4	20	368 ·8

[*] *Loc. cit.*, p. 410.

The cessation of fermentation in any particular mixture of inactive residue and coferment may, therefore, be due to the disappearance either of ferment or coferment from the liquid. If the amount of coferment present be relatively small, it is the first to disappear, and fermentation can then only be renewed by the addition of a further quantity, whilst the addition of more ferment produces no effect. If, on the other hand, the amount of coferment be relatively large, the inverse is true ; the ferment is the first to disappear, and fermentation can only be renewed by the addition of more ferment, a further quantity of coferment producing no effect. This is illustrated by the following experiment made at 26°:—

Two solutions were made up, each containing 0·5 gramme of dry inactive residue + 10 c.c. of 10-per-cent. glucose solution and toluene, and to each of these 2 c.c. of boiled juice containing 10 per cent. glucose were added. As soon as fermentation had ceased, 0·5 gramme of dry residue in 10 c.c. of glucose solution was added to one solution (a), and 2 c.c. of boiled juice diluted to 10 c.c. with glucose solution to the other (b). Two other solutions were also prepared, each containing 0·4 gramme of the same dry inactive residue + 10 c.c. of 10-per-cent. glucose solution + toluene, and 25 c.c. of the same boiled juice containing glucose were added to each.

As soon as fermentation had ceased, 0·4 gramme of residue dissolved in 10 c.c. of glucose solution was added to one (c), and 10 c.c. of boiled juice containing glucose to the other (d). The following were the results :—

	Boiled juice added.	Fermentation produced.	Subsequent addition.	Additional fermentation.
	c.c.	c.c.		c.c.
(a)	2	9·4	0·5 gr. residue	0
(b)	2	7·6	2 c.c. boiled juice	8·9
(c)	25	56·8	0·4 gr. residue	36·8
(d)	25	50	10 c.c. boiled juice	0

(3) *Rate of Disappearance of the Coferment from Yeast-juice.*

The following experiments were made to ascertain approximately the rate at which the coferment disappears from yeast-juice both in the absence and presence of added glucose. For this purpose a quantity of yeast-juice was preserved at 25° in presence of toluene, and samples were removed, boiled and filtered, at the commencement of the incubation and after various intervals. In one case a parallel experiment was made with yeast-juice to which 10 grammes of glucose per 100 c.c. had been added. The filtrates were then all rendered neutral to litmus and tested with equal quantities of an inactive residue and glucose, care being taken to keep the concentration of glucose the same throughout.

Material digested.	Time of digestion.	Volume of filtrate taken.	Fermentation produced.
	days.	c.c.	c.c.
1. *a.* Yeast-juice alone	0	20	168·5
b. „	9	20	0
2. *a.* „	0	16	364·3
b. „	2	16	2·6
c. „	4	16	0
3. *a.* „	0	15	62·9
b. „	1	15	2·1
c. „	2	15	0
d. „	4	15	0
e. Yeast-juice + glucose..............	0	15	62·9
f. „	1	15	15·6
g. „	2	15	4·5
h. „	4	15	8·3

In two cases in which a negative result was obtained (1*b* and 2*c*) an equal volume of the same fresh boiled juice was added and in both cases a vigorous fermentation was produced, thus proving that the autolysed juice had not exerted any specific detrimental effect on the ferment:—

	Fresh boiled juice added.	Carbon dioxide evolved.
1. *b*............	20 c.c.	112 c.c.
2. *c*............	16 „	297 „

It appears from this that the coferment disappears from the juice less rapidly in the presence of glucose than in its absence. In yeast-juice to which no addition of glucose has been made the coferment usually disappears at 26° in about 48 hours; in the presence of 10 per cent. of glucose coferment was still present at the end of four days, although only in a small amount. (The observation that the fermentation after four days' incubation is somewhat greater than that given after two days is probably to be explained by the presence of a greater amount of phosphate in the juice which had been digested for the longer period.)

4. *Soluble Phosphates do not Render the Inactive Residue Capable of Fermenting Glucose.*

In view of the fact that soluble phosphates, as described in the previous communication, exert a remarkable effect on the fermentation of glucose by yeast-juice, experiments were made to ascertain whether the addition of a soluble phosphate to a solution of the inactive residue in glucose is sufficient to set up fermentation. All the attempts hitherto made to effect this have yielded entirely negative results, although both the kind of phosphate and the amount added have been varied.

Dipotassium hydrogen phosphate, a mixture of this with the dihydrogen phosphate, disodium hydrogen phosphate, diammonium hydrogen phosphate, microsmic salt, and a mixed phosphate of potassium and magnesium obtained by boiling a solution of potassium dihydrogen phosphate with magnesium carbonate, were employed, all of which are capable of producing the characteristic effect of phosphates on the fermentation of glucose by yeast-juice.

Although these substances did not set up fermentation when added to an inactive filtered residue and glucose, they did not affect the potential activity of the residue. This is evident from the fact that the subsequent addition of boiled juice produced an immediate fermentation.

In every case the solution of the phosphate was saturated with carbon dioxide at 26° and added to the solution of the inactive residue in glucose solution also saturated with carbon dioxide at 26°, and in no case was any evolution of gas observed after the cessation of the slight disturbance which inevitably occurs when the solutions are mixed. The phosphate solutions were all of 3/10 molar strength, with the exception of the mixed phosphate of magnesium and potassium, 5 c.c. of which yielded 0·1594 gramme $Mg_2P_2O_7$.

In those cases in which the residue employed was slightly active, incubation was continued until all fermentation had ceased before the phosphate solution was added, and the amount of carbon dioxide evolved in this preliminary period is given in the table. The amount of glucose, both in the solution of the residue and in that of the phosphate, was throughout 10 grammes to 100.

	Amount of residue.	Preliminary fermentation.	Phosphate added.	Carbon dioxide produced.	Subsequent evolution of carbon dioxide after the addition of boiled juice.
1	25 c.c.	41 ·2	2 ·5 c.c. KMg phosphate ...	0	18 ·4
2	25 ,,	47 ·7	5 ,, ,, ...	0	—
3	25 ,,	0 ·6	3 ,, K₂HPO₄	0	268 ·8
4	1 ·6 gr.	21 ·5	3 ,, KMg phosphate ...	0	159 ·2
5	1 ·2 ,,	10 ·7	5 ,, ,, ...	0	—
6	0 ·5 ,,	0	2 ,, mixture of K₂HPO₄ and KH₂PO₄	0	3 c.c. per hour
7	0 ·5 ,,	0	2 ,, (NH₄)₂HPO₄	0	4 ·2 ,, ,,
8	0 ·5 ,,	0	2 ,, (NH₄)NaHPO₄ ...	0	3 ·8 ,, ,,
9	0 ·5 ,,	0	2 ,, Na₂HPO₄	0	3 ·6 ,, ,,

The foregoing conclusion is confirmed by the observation, made in the experiments on the disappearance of the coferment from yeast-juice, that boiled autolysed juice does not set up fermentation in a mixture of the inactive residue with glucose, although it itself contains a large amount of phosphate precipitable by magnesia mixture. The following numbers were obtained by the analysis of three specimens of boiled autolysed juice employed in those experiments, two of which were quite inactive, whilst the other only produced a fermentation of 2·6 c.c.

No. of experiment.	Volume of juice.	Carbon dioxide evolved.	Phosphate present in grammes of $Mg_2P_2O_7$.
	c.c.	c.c.	
1. *b*	20	0	0 ·3400
2. *b*	16	2 ·6	0 ·3011
3. *c*	15	0	0 ·1893

These experiments throw no light on the actual chemical nature of the coferment, but show that most probably it does not consist of a phosphate precipitable by yeast-juice. They also indicate that substances, which, like phosphates, increase the total fermentation produced by yeast-juice, are not necessarily capable of setting up fermentation when added to a mixture of inactive residue and glucose.

Further experiments are in progress with the hope of obtaining more information on these points.

Editor's Comments on Papers 12, 13, and 14

12   **Embden, Deuticke, and Kraft:** Über die intermediären Vorgänge bei der Glykolyse in der Muskulatur
English translation: About the Intermediary Processes During Glycolysis of the Muscle
Klin. Wochschr., **12**, 213–215 (1933)

13   **Meyerhof and Lohmann:** About the Enzymatic Equilibrium Reaction Between Hexosediphosphoric Acid and Dioxyacetone Phosphoric Acid

14   **Parnas, Ostern, and Mann:** About the Linkage of Chemical Processes in the Muscle
Biochem, Z., **272**, 64–70 (1934)

The final elucidation of the pathway of anaerobic glucose fermentation was made possible by the observation of Robison (1922) that hexosemonophosphates participate in the form of the equilibrium mixture of glucose 6-phosphate and fructose 6-phosphate (Robison ester). The classical experiments which followed, by G. Embden, O. Meyerhof, and J. K. Parnas and their respective research groups (Papers 12–14), established the Embden–Meyerhof–Parnas (EMP) pathway of glucose utilization. The evidence for the existence of this pathway was based extensively on enzymatic studies (Lohmann, 1933; Meyerhof, 1935, 1942; Lohmann and Meyerhof, 1934; Meyerhof and Lohmann, 1934; Meyerhof and Kiessling, 1935; Meyerhof et al., 1936; Parnas et al., 1935; Parnas, 1938), inhibitory studies (Nilsson and Westerberg, 1940; Nilsson and Alm, 1940), and kinetic studies (Meyerhof, 1945, 1949). Although the pathway was established (see Racker, 1954), enzymatic, kinetic, and particularly, regulatory problems were dealt with later in an ever-increasing number of publications.

12

Copyright © 1933 by Springer-Verlag

Reprinted from *Klin. Wochschr.*, **12**, 213–215 (1933)

ORIGINALIEN.

ÜBER DIE INTERMEDIÄREN VORGÄNGE BEI DER GLYKOLYSE IN DER MUSKULATUR.*

Von

Prof. G. Embden, Privatdozent Dr. H. J. Deuticke
und Gert Kraft.

Aus dem Institut für vegetative Physiologie der Universität Frankfurt.

In längere Zeit zurückliegenden Untersuchungen aus dem hiesigen Institut wurde gezeigt, daß durch Muskelpreßsaft und Muskelbrei unter der Einwirkung bestimmter Salze große Mengen von anorganischer Phosphorsäure zum Verschwinden gebracht werden. Durch Zusatz von Kohlehydrat in Form von Glykogen oder Stärke wurde dies Verschwinden von Phosphorsäure gesteigert, und in den Preßsaftversuchen gelang es, eine Hexosediphosphorsäure zu isolieren, die in ihren Eigenschaften völlig mit dem bei der Hefegärung entstehenden Harden-Youngschen Ester übereinstimmte.

Bei einer Nachprüfung dieser Untersuchungen durch Lohmann zeigte sich, daß die Verhältnisse in Wahrheit verwickelter liegen. Lohmann stellte nämlich fest, daß das Gemisch der entstandenen Phosphorylierungsprodukte nicht mit der gleichen Leichtigkeit wie der Harden-Youngsche Ester unter der Einwirkung von Säure in der Hitze Phosphorsäure abspaltet, sondern weit schwerer hydrolysierbar ist. Es mußte sonach die Hauptmenge der in seinen Versuchen gebildeten Phosphorsäureester aus einer von der bekannten Form der Hexosediphosphorsäure abweichenden Substanz bestehen. Isolierungsversuche führten Lohmann zu der Anschauung, daß es sich bei der schwer hydrolysierbaren Substanz um eine von dem Harden-Youngschen Ester verschiedene Hexosediphosphorsäure handle.

Im Verlaufe kürzlich mit ganz anderem Ziel begonnener neuer Untersuchungen über die ional bedingte Kohlehydratphosphorsäuresynthese fiel uns in großer Menge ein schön krystallisierendes Bariumsalz in die Hände, das als das sekundäre Bariumsalz eines Monophosphorsäureesters der l-Glycerinsäure identifiziert werden konnte.

Die Verfolgung dieses Befundes ergab, wie wir glauben möchten, weitgehende Aufschlüsse über die bei der glykolytischen Milchsäurebildung in der Muskulatur sich abspielenden Vorgänge, wenigstens soweit die Glykolyse unter intermediärer Phosphorylierung erfolgt.

Es zeigte sich zunächst, daß unter anaeroben Bedingungen Muskelbrei aus zugesetztem Hexosediphosphat in noch viel höherem Maße als aus Stärke Phosphoglycerinsäure bildet, daß also trotz der ional bedingten Hemmung der Dephosphorylierung des Hexoseesters der Zerfall der Sechskohlenstoffkette in 2 Bruchstücke mit je 3 Kohlenstoffatomen weiter verläuft. Wir möchten glauben, daß auch in den analogen Versuchen Lohmanns der schwer hydrolysierbare Ester zum guten Teil aus Phosphoglycerinsäure bestanden hat.

Wir beobachteten bisher die Bildung dieser Substanz unter der Einwirkung von Natriumlactat, Natriumfluorid und Natriumoxalat.

Unsere Vermutung, daß die neu aufgefundene Substanz ein normalerweise bei der Glykolyse in der Muskulatur auftretendes Intermediärprodukt sei, konnte durch weitere Untersuchungen gestützt werden.

Hierbei ergab sich nämlich zunächst, daß frischer Muskelbrei zugesetzte Monophosphoglycerinsäure mit größter Leichtigkeit in Phosphorsäure und Brenztraubensäure spaltet. Die letztere Substanz konnte ohne Verwendung eines Abfangmittels an der Hand einer sicher nicht verlustlos arbeitenden Methode in einer Ausbeute bis zu 80% der theoretisch möglichen isoliert werden. Nicht mit Phosphorsäure veresterte Glycerinsäure bildete unter den gleichen Bedingungen keine nachweisbare Menge von Brenztraubensäure.

Die Glycerinsäure und die aus deren Monophosphorsäureester durch Muskulatur abspaltbare Brenztraubensäure

sind höher oxydierte Substanzen als die Sechskohlenstoffzucker und die aus diesen bei der Glykolyse gebildete Milchsäure. Das Auftreten dieser Oxydationsprodukte erfolgt unter anaeroben Bedingungen in größtem Ausmaße, und dieser oxydative Vorgang ist natürlich nur unter gleichzeitigem Auftreten von reduktiven Prozessen möglich.

Auf Grund der bisher mitgeteilten experimentellen Ergebnisse bildeten wir uns die Vorstellung, daß die der Milchsäurebildung vorangehende Spaltung der Sechskohlenstoffkette in der Mitte unter Erhaltung der Phosphorylierung erfolgt derart, daß hierbei aus 1 Molekül Hexosediphosphorsäure 2 Moleküle Triosemonophosphorsäure entstehen. Für die *Fructose*diphosphorsäure müßte dieser Vorgang folgendermaßen formuliert werden*:

Formel 1.

Fructosediphosphorsäure   Glycerinaldehydphosphorsäure

Durch einen Dismutationsvorgang nach Art der Cannizzaroschen Reaktion könnten diese beiden Triosephosphorsäuremoleküle in ein Molekül *Glycerinphosphorsäure* und ein Molekül *Phosphoglycerinsäure* umgewandelt werden nach folgender Formel:

Formel 2.

Von den beiden angenommenen Dismutationsprodukten konnte die Glycerinphosphorsäure, deren reichliches Vorkommen in der Leber übrigens kürzlich von Fiske nachgewiesen wurde, bisher noch nicht isoliert werden**.

Nach unseren eben mitgeteilten Befunden wird die Phosphoglycerinsäure unter Phosphorsäureabspaltung in Brenztraubensäure umgewandelt. Wir untersuchten nunmehr, ob die so entstandene Brenztraubensäure dadurch zu Milchsäure hydriert werden kann, daß gleichzeitig die bei der erwähnten Dismutation etwa entstandene Glycerinphosphorsäure wieder zu Triosephosphorsäure dehydriert wird.

In der Tat ließ sich zeigen, daß die geringfügige, im Muskelbrei auftretende Milchsäurebildung aus *Phospho-*

---

* In Übereinstimmung mit dieser Vorstellung konnten Embden und Jost in jüngster Zeit zeigen, daß unter den in der vorliegenden Arbeit angewandten Bedingungen synthetisch hergestellte d-l-Glycerinaldehydphosphorsäure reichlich Milchsäure bildet.

** Würde eine Glykosediphosphorsäure nach dem gleichen Schema gespalten werden, so würde eines der beiden Dismutationsprodukte nicht am endständigen, sondern am mittelständigen C-Atom phosphoryliert sein, es würde also z. B. statt der α-Glycerinphosphorsäure deren β-Form entstehen können.

*An English translation of this paper follows. **107**

glycerinsäure allein und aus *Glycerin*phosphorsäure allein bei *gleichzeitigem* Zusatz *beider* Substanzen gewaltig gesteigert wird. Der Beteiligung der Phosphoglycerinsäure an dieser Milchsäurebildung entspricht die Feststellung, daß in den Versuchen mit gleichzeitigem Zusatz beider Substanzen der Gehalt an Brenztraubensäure viel geringer ist, als in den Versuchen mit Phosphoglycerinsäure allein, und die Mitbeteiligung der Glycerinphosphorsäure kommt darin zum Ausdruck, daß der Mindergehalt an Brenztraubensäure in den Mischversuchen zur Deckung der in diesen Versuchen mehrgebildeten Milchsäure bei weitem nicht ausreicht.

Ein *Beispiel* möge dies erläutern:

50 g Muskelbrei eines mit Adrenalin vorbehandelten Hungerkaninchens enthielten unmittelbar nach der Gewinnung 173 mg Milchsäure (Versuch A). Nach 2stündigem Aufenthalt der Muskulatur in Natriumbicarbonatlösung bei 40° stieg der Milchsäuregehalt auf 213 mg an (Versuch B_1). Bei Zusatz einer bestimmten Menge von Phospho*glycerinsäure* in Form ihres Natriumsalzes und nachfolgender Exposition wurde nur wenig mehr Milchsäure als im Leerversuch B_1 gefunden (244 mg, Versuch B_2). Eine äquimolekulare Menge des Natriumsalzes der *Glycerin*phosphorsäure bewirkte nur eine minimale Vermehrung des Milchsäurewertes gegenüber dem Leerversuch (218 mg, Versuch B_3).

Wurden aber die gleichen Mengen *beider* Substanzen wie in den Versuchen B_2 und B_3 *zusammen* vor der Exposition zugesetzt (Versuch B_4), so stieg nunmehr der Milchsäurewert auf 402 mg an.

Der im Ansatz mit beiden Substanzen gegenüber dem Versuch mit Phosphoglycerinsäure allein erfolgten Mehrbildung von 158 mg *Milchsäure* entsprach ein Mindergehalt von nur 105 mg *Brenztraubensäure*, dem Äquivalent von 107 mg Milchsäure. Der Rest von 51 mg Milchsäure hat wohl seinen Ursprung in der Glycerinphosphorsäure, deren Fähigkeit zur Brenztraubensäurebildung unter Einwirkung von Muskelbrei übrigens bereits von AMANDUS HAHN festgestellt wurde. Eine Brenztraubensäurebildung aus Glycerin konnte der gleiche Autor nicht beobachten. In *unseren* Versuchen kam es weder zur Milchsäurebildung aus allein zugesetztem Glycerin, noch trat bei gleichzeitigem Zusatz von Phosphoglycerinsäure und Glycerin vermehrte Milchsäurebildung auf.

Die *Phosphorsäure* wird aus der *Phosphoglycerinsäure* unter der Einwirkung der Muskulatur quantitativ abgespalten, wie aus den Versuchen mit alleinigem Zusatz dieser Substanz hervorgeht.

Die Phosphorsäurebildung aus *allein* zugesetzter *Glycerinphosphorsäure* ist demgegenüber nur geringfügig, doch wird sie durch gleichzeitigen Zusatz von Phosphoglycerinsäure erheblich gesteigert, wie wir glauben möchten, eben deswegen, weil die *Hydrierung* der aus Phosphoglycerinsäure entstandenen Brenztraubensäure zu Milchsäure auf Kosten gleichzeitiger *Dehydrierung* von Glycerinphosphorsäure bis zur Phosphoglycerinsäurestufe erfolgt. Ein Teil der so entstandenen Phosphoglycerinsäure geht dann weiterhin über Brenztraubensäure in Milchsäure über.

Die Tatsache, daß die fermentative Abspaltung von Phosphorsäure aus Phosphoglycerinsäure so außerordentlich viel leichter als aus Glycerinphosphorsäure erfolgt, erscheint uns jedenfalls als sehr bemerkenswert.

Unsere gesamten bisherigen Versuchsergebnisse führen zu folgendem Bilde der glykolytischen Milchsäurebildung, soweit die Glykolyse überhaupt unter Mitbeteiligung von Phosphorylierungsvorgängen erfolgt (s. hierüber BUMM und FEHRENBACH).

Erste Phase: Synthese von Hexosediphosphorsäure aus 1 Molekül Hexose und 2 Molekülen Phosphorsäure oder aus 1 Molekül Hexosemonophosphorsäure* und aus 1 Molekül Phosphorsäure.

Zweite Phase: Zerfall des Hexosediphosphorsäuremoleküls in 2 Moleküle Triosephosphorsäure (s. oben Formel 1).

Dritte Phase: Dismutation von 2 Molekülen Triosephosphorsäure in 1 Molekül Glycerinphosphorsäure und 1 Molekül Phosphoglycerinsäure, wobei je nachdem, ob die Hexosediphosphorsäure Ketose- oder Aldosecharakter hatte, α- oder β-Glycerinphosphorsäure entstehen könnte (Formel 2).

Vierte Phase: Spaltung der Phosphoglycerinsäure in Phosphorsäure und Brenztraubensäure nach der untenstehenden Formel 3:

Formel 3.

$$CH_2{-}O{-}P{\overset{O}{\underset{OH}{<}}}OH \quad CH_3$$
$$CHOH \qquad\qquad = \quad C{=}O \quad + H_3PO_4$$
$$COOH \qquad\qquad\qquad COOH$$

Phosphoglycerinsäure   Brenztraubensäure

In dieser Formel kommt zum Ausdruck, daß bei der Spaltung Glycerinsäure als Intermediärprodukt *nicht* auftritt, daß die Spaltung also ohne Wasseraufnahme von außen erfolgt.

Fünfte Phase: Reduktive Umwandlung der Brenztraubensäure in Milchsäure auf Kosten oxydativer Triosephosphorsäurebildung aus Glycerinphosphorsäure nach der Formel 4:

Formel 4.

$$CH_3 \quad CH_2{-}O{-}P{\overset{O}{\underset{OH}{<}}}OH \quad CH_3 \quad CH_2{-}O{-}P{\overset{O}{\underset{OH}{<}}}OH$$
$$C{=}O + CHOH \qquad = CHOH + CHOH$$
$$COOH \quad CH_2OH \qquad COOH \qquad C{\overset{O}{\underset{H}{}}}$$

Brenztraubensäure   Glycerinphosphorsäure   Milchsäure   Triosephosphorsäure

An der Triosephosphorsäure wiederholen sich die Vorgänge, die wir als 3. bis 5. Phase schilderten.

Wie man sieht, fehlt in diesem Bilde der Glykolyse das Methylglyoxal, das bekanntlich von NEUBERG ebenso wie für die Hefegärung auch für die glykolytische Milchsäurebildung im Tierkörper als Intermediärprodukt angenommen wird.

Das Auftreten dieser Substanz als Vorstufe der vom tierischen Organismus anscheinend ausschließlich gebildeten *rechtsdrehenden* Milchsäure wurde in einer lange zurückliegenden Arbeit aus unserem Institut deswegen für unwahrscheinlich gehalten, weil diese Substanz durch tierisches Material nach dem Ergebnis der damals vorliegenden Untersuchungen nicht in reine d-Milchsäure*, sondern in ein Gemisch der optischen Antipoden umgewandelt wird, in dem die l-Milchsäure überwiegt, und in jüngster Zeit wurde von LOHMANN die wichtige Tatsache festgestellt, daß die Wirksamkeit der Methylglyoxalase — des Methylglyoxal *unmittelbar* in Milchsäure umwandelnden Fermentes — an die Anwesenheit von Glutathion gebunden ist, während die fermentative Milchsäurebildung aus Glykogen durch Muskulatur auch ohne Glutathion erfolgt.

Wenn auch nicht mit voller Sicherheit ausgeschlossen werden kann, daß, entsprechend einer zuerst von NEUBERG geäußerten Anschauung, die im intermediären Stoffwechsel auftretende Form des Methylglyoxals von der synthetisch zugänglichen verschieden ist, und daß dieses alloiomorphe Methylglyoxal im Stoffwechsel unabhängig vom Glutathion in Milchsäure, und zwar in deren rechtsdrehende Form, umgewandelt werden könnte, so wird es doch auf Grund der oben mitgeteilten Befunde nunmehr notwendig sein, als Hauptweg des unter intermediärer Phosphorylierung verlaufenden anaeroben Kohlehydratabbaues im Tierkörper den im vorstehenden gekennzeichneten in Betracht zu ziehen.

EMBDEN und M. OPPENHEIMER konnten vor bald 2 Jahrzehnten zeigen, daß Brenztraubensäure in der künstlich

---

* In der frischen Muskulatur der bisher untersuchten Tierarten findet sich nach EMBDEN und MARGARETE ZIMMERMANN ausschließlich Hexose*mono*phosphorsäure, und diese ist deswegen als die nächste im Muskel *vorgebildete* Vorstufe der Milchsäure von den genannten Autoren als „*Lactacidogen*" bezeichnet worden. Die Umwandlung der Hexosemonophosphorsäure in Hexosediphosphorsäure erfolgt nicht nur unter der Einwirkung bestimmter, besonders zugesetzter synthesebegünstigender Salze, sondern wie kürzlich gezeigt wurde, schon beim Verreiben von Muskelbrei mit großen Mengen Kieselgur (EMBDEN, JOST und MARGARETE LEHNARTZ). Das Fehlen der Hexose*di*phosphorsäure in der frischen Muskulatur ist vielleicht gerade darauf zurückzuführen, daß sie viel leichter als die Hexosemonophosphorsäure abgebaut wird. Die Vorstellung, daß dem Abbau der Hexosemonophosphorsäure ihr Übergang in Hexosediphosphorsäure vorausgeht, wurde bereits von MEYERHOF und seinen Mitarbeitern geäußert.

* Bekanntlich gehört die rechtsdrehende Milchsäure ihrem sterischen Bau nach der l-Reihe an.

durchströmten Leber ausschließlich in d-Milchsäure übergeht, und das gleiche dürfte auch für die entsprechende Umwandlung der Brenztraubensäure in der Muskulatur gelten (Untersuchungen darüber sind im Gange).

Die Tatsache, daß der normale Stoffwechsel verschiedenster Lebewesen verschiedenartigste Substanzen mit asymmetrischem Kohlenstoffatom nur in *einer* der möglichen stereoisomeren Formen entstehen läßt, und daß gerade die Milchsäure eine Ausnahme von dieser Regel bildet, würde verständlich, wenn die Bildung der beiden optischen Antipoden stets auf zwei verschiedenen Wegen erfolgte. Bei der Methylglyoxalasewirkung scheint ausschließlich l-Milchsäure gebildet zu werden, und der kürzlich von EMBDEN und METZ erhobene Befund, daß eine aus roten Blutkörperchen durch Hämolyse mittels destilliertem Wasser gewonnene zellfreie Fermentlösung Methylglyoxal ausschließlich in l-Milchsäure umwandelt, dürfte ebenso wie das früher von WIDMANN im Neubergschen Laboratorium gefundene gleichartige Verhalten bestimmter Bakterien darauf zurückzuführen sein, daß es sich in beiden Fällen um reine Methylglyoxalasewirkung, also um *direkte* Umwandlung des Methylglyoxals in Milchsäure handelte.

Da das Methylglyoxal aber außer auf diesem *direkten* Wege auch auf dem Umwege über Brenztraubensäure in Milchsäure verwandelt werden kann, erscheint es ohne weiteres als verständlich, daß Organismen, für die das Methylglyoxal mehr als für den Tierkörper ein normales Intermediärprodukt ist, beide Formen der Milchsäure bilden. Andererseits spricht das bisher fast ausschließlich beobachtete Auftreten von rechtsdrehender Milchsäure bei der Glykolyse im Tierkörper dafür, daß das Methylglyoxal im normalen Stoffwechsel des Tieres überhaupt nicht, oder doch nicht in irgend in Betracht kommenden Mengen auftritt*.

Wenn das von uns gezeichnete Bild der glykolytischen Milchsäurebildung durch Muskulatur von den bisherigen Vorstellungen auch stark abweicht, so erscheint uns doch der Hinweis darauf als notwendig, daß vielfältige Beobachtungen früherer Forscher mit den von uns entwickelten Anschauungen durchaus vereinbar sind. Wir denken dabei in erster Linie an manche Feststellungen NEUBERGs bei seinen grundlegenden Untersuchungen über den Verlauf der Hefegärung. So sei namentlich auf die in neuerer Zeit von NEUBERG gemeinsam mit MARIA KOBEL festgestellte Tatsache hingewiesen, daß es unter gewissen abnormen Bedingungen bei der Hefegärung zur Bildung äquimolekularer Mengen von Brenztraubensäure und Glycerin kommen kann, und auf die viel ältere Feststellung von NEUBERG und J. KERB, daß Zusatz von Glycerin bei der Spaltung von Brenztraubensäure durch Hefecarboxylase neben Kohlendioxyd an Stelle von Acetaldehyd Äthylalkohol entstehen läßt.

Doch wollen wir die Frage, inwieweit der von uns für die Glykolyse angenommene Weg auch für die alkoholische Hefegärung Geltung haben könnte, nicht weiter erörtern. Nur sei ausdrücklich darauf hingewiesen, daß NILSSON nach der Einwirkung von Fluorid auf Hefe eine Substanz als amorphes neutrales Bariumsalz und als krystallisiertes Strychninsalz gewinnen konnte, die er für Monophosphoglycerinsäure hielt, wenngleich in seinen Untersuchungen deren endgültige Identifizierung noch nicht gelang**.

Schon früher hatte GREENWALD aus Blutkörperchen die zweifach phosphorylierte Glycerinsäure isoliert und in ihrer Konstitution aufgeklärt, und in einer aus unserem Institut veröffentlichten Untersuchung konnte H. JOST zeigen, daß diese Substanz bei der anaeroben Glykolyse durch Blutkörperchen entsteht. Schon damals wurde für die Bildung der Diphosphoglycerinsäure ein Weg angenommen, der dem für die Entstehung der Monophosphoglycerinsäure von uns eben gezeichneten sehr ähnlich ist, wenn auch noch nicht

daran gedacht wurde, daß die glykolytische Milchsäurebildung über Phosphoglycerinsäure und Brenztraubensäure führt.

Der *Rockefeller Foundation*, die die Durchführung dieser Arbeit in wirksamster Weise unterstützte, sagen wir unseren aufrichtigen Dank.

---

* Wir halten es übrigens für nicht ausgeschlossen, daß weitere Untersuchungen Formen der Glykolyse durch tierische Zellen aufdecken werden, bei denen auch l-Milchsäure — unter intermediärer Bildung von Methylglyoxal — entsteht.
** NEUBERG, WEINMANN und M. VOGT sowie M. VOGT haben vor einigen Jahren auf synthetischem Wege Monophosphoglycerinsäure hergestellt und ein schwer lösliches krystallinisches Bariumsalz erhalten, das mit dem von uns in optisch einheitlicher Form gewonnenen weitgehende Ähnlichkeit zeigt.

12

About the Intermediary Processes During Glycolysis of the Muscle

G. EMBDEN, H. J. DEUTICKE, and G. KRAFT

Translated expressly for this Benchmark volume by H. W. Doelle from "Über die intermediären Vorgänge bei der Glykolyse in der Muskulatur," Klin. Wochschr., **12**, *213–215 (1933), with permission from Springer-Verlag*

Earlier investigations carried out in this Institute showed that muscle sap and muscle paste are able to remove large quantities of inorganic phosphoric acid under the influence of certain salts. By adding carbohydrates in form of glycogen or starch to these, the disappearance of phosphoric acid was accelerated and it was possible to isolate a hexosediphosphate that was identical to the Harden–Young ester from the experiments with pressed juice.

A reinvestigation by Lohmann showed that the relationship is more complicated. Lohmann showed that the mixture of phosphorylated products did not split phosphoric acid under the influence of acid and heat as easily as the Harden–Young ester; however, it was much harder to hydrolyze. Thus the main proportion of the phosphoric ester formed must consist of a substance different from that of the known hexosediphosphate. Isolation experiments led Lohmann to the opinion that the difficult-to-hydrolyze substance must be a hexosediphosphate different from that of the Harden–Young ester.

During recent investigations (which had an entirely different goal since they were concerned with investigations about the ion-dependent carbohydrate phosphoric acid synthesis), a large amount of a crystalline barium salt, which was identified as the secondary barium salt of the monophosphoric ester of 2-glyceric acid, was obtained.

A follow-up of this discovery revealed new ideas about the mechanism of glycolytic lactic acid formation in the muscle, at least as far as the glycolysis under intermediary phosphorylation is concerned.

It could be demonstrated that the sap formed significantly larger quantities of phosphoglyceric acid under anaerobic conditions if hexosediphosphate was added instead of starch; and that despite ional inhibition of the dephosphorylation of hexose ester, the six-carbon chain was broken into two parts of three-carbon chains. We like to believe that the ester that Lohmann found so difficult to hydrolyze consisted mainly of phosphoglyceric acid.

We observed the formation of this substance under the influence of sodium lactate, sodium fluoride, and sodium oxalate. Our assumption that the new product is an intermediary product of the glycolysis of muscle was supported by further studies. These investigations revealed that fresh muscle paste split the monophosphoglyceric acid into phosphoric acid and pyruvic acid with ease. Eighty percent of the theoretically possible amount of the latter substance was recovered without the use of a trapping agent. Normal glyceric acid did not form pyruvic acid under the same conditions.

The glyceric acid and pyruvic acid obtainable from the monophosphoric ester of glyceric acid are more highly oxidized substances than the six-carbon sugar and the end product, lactic acid. The appearance of these oxidation products occurs under anaerobic conditions to a significant extent and must be accompanied by reductive processes.

From these experimental results we assume that the split of the six-carbon chain, which occurs before lactic acid is produced, occurs under preservation of phosphorylation in the middle of the chain in such a way that one molecule of hexosediphosphate forms two molecules of triose monophosphate. In the case of fructosediphosphate, this step would occur as follows*:

Formula 1

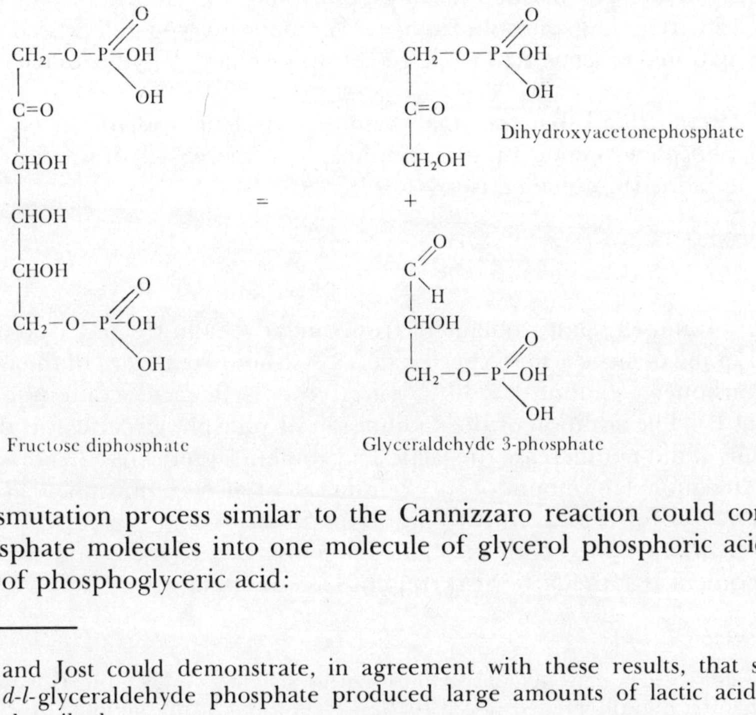

Fructose diphosphate   Glyceraldehyde 3-phosphate

A dismutation process similar to the Cannizzaro reaction could convert both triosephosphate molecules into one molecule of glycerol phosphoric acid and one molecule of phosphoglyceric acid:

---

*Embden and Jost could demonstrate, in agreement with these results, that synthetically produced *d-l*-glyceraldehyde phosphate produced large amounts of lactic acid under the conditions described.

Formula 2

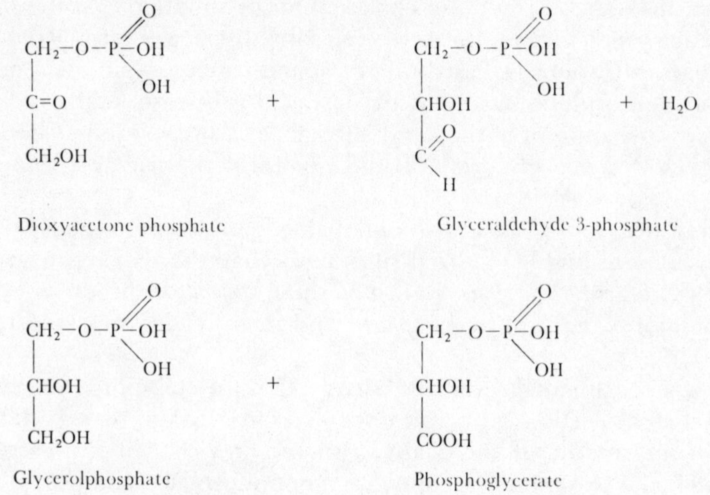

Dioxyacetone phosphate   Glyceraldehyde 3-phosphate

Glycerolphosphate   Phosphoglycerate

Of the two assumed dismutation products, glycerolphosphate (which was identified by Fiske from liver) has not yet been isolated.*

According to abovementioned findings, phosphoglycerate can now be converted to pyruvic acid, releasing phosphoric acid. We now investigated whether pyruvic acid can be hydrated to lactic acid while glycerolphosphate dehydrates back to triose-phosphate.

It was demonstrated that the small amounts of lactic acid produced in muscle paste from phosphoglycerate or glycerolphosphate increased dramatically if both substances are added simultaneously.

Example

Fifty g of muscle paste obtained from an adrenalin-treated, starved rabbit contained 173 mg of lactic acid (Experiment A). A 2-hour treatment of the muscle in a sodium bicarbonate solution at 40°C raised the lactic acid content to 213 mg (Experiment B). The addition of the sodium salt of phosphoglyceric acid during the above treatment did not increase the lactic acid content significantly (244 mg, Experiment B_2). An equimolar amount of the sodium salt of glycerolphosphate also did not give higher values for lactic acid (218 mg, Experiment B_3).

However, if one added both substances together before the 2-hour treatment at 40°C (Experiment B_4), the lactic acid content rose to 402 mg.

---

*If a diphosphoric acid were split according to this scheme, one of the two dismutation products would be phosphorylated not at the last carbon but at the middle C carbon of the molecule. One would arrive at a β-form and not the α-form.

The difference between results obtained with the phosphoglycerate alone and combined with glycerolphosphate resulted in an increase of 158 mg of lactic acid from phosphoglycerate, which corresponds to a deficit of only 105 mg of pyruvic acid, which is equivalent to 107 mg of lactic acid. The remaining 51 mg of lactic acid must have its origin in glycerolphosphate, which has a potential, according to A. Hahn, for forming pyruvic acid. He has not observed pyruvic acid formation from glycerol. Our experiments showed also that glycerol alone combined with phosphoglycerate had no influence on lactic acid formation.

The experiments revealed that phosphoric acid is quantitatively removed from phosphoglycerate. Thus the phosphoric acid formation from glycerolphosphate is small; it can be increased, however, by the addition of phosphoglycerate. The reason, we like to believe, is that the hydration of pyruvic acid to lactic acid requires the dehydration of glycerolphosphate to phosphoglycerate. Part of the phosphoglycerate thus formed can, therefore, be metabolized to lactic acid via pyruvic acid.

The fact that the fermentative release of phosphoric acid from phosphoglycerate is so easy in comparison with release from glycerolphosphate was found especially worthy of note.

Our results on the glycolysis can be summarized as follows:

Phase 1: Hexosediphosphate is synthesized either from one molecule of hexose and two molecules of phosphoric acid or from one molecule of hexosemonophosphate* and one molecule of phosphoric acid.

Phase 2: Hexosediphosphate splits into two molecules of triosephosphates.

Phase 3: Dismutation of two molecules of triosephosphate produces one molecule of glycerolphosphate and one molecule of phosphoglycerate, whereupon α- or β-glycerolphosphate can be obtained depending upon whether hexosediphosphate has ketose or aldose character (Formula 2).

Phase 4: Transformation of phosphoglyceric acid into pyruvic acid with the release of phosphoric acid:

$$
\begin{array}{ccc}
\begin{array}{l}
CH_2-O-\overset{\displaystyle O}{\underset{\displaystyle OH}{P}}-OH \\
| \\
CHOH \\
| \\
COOH
\end{array}
& = &
\begin{array}{l}
CH_3 \\
| \\
C=O \\
| \\
COOH
\end{array}
\quad + \quad H_3PO_4
\end{array}
$$

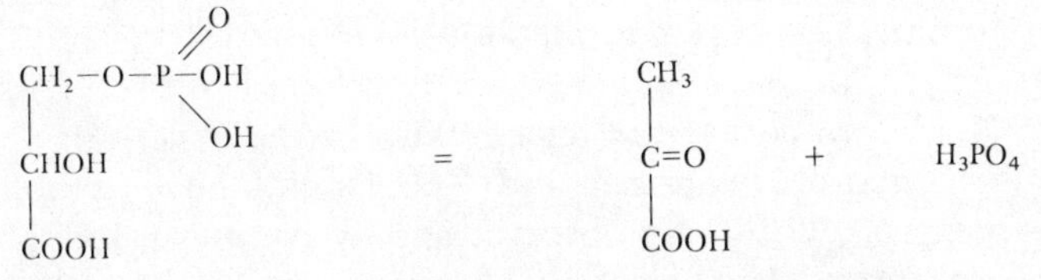

Phosphoglyceric acid   Pyruvic acid

---

*In fresh muscles of all animals studied so far, only hexosemonophosphoric acid has been found according to Embden and M. Zimmermann. Both authors call it "Lactacidogen," since it is seen as the precursor for lactic acid. The transformation of hexosemonophosphoric acid into hexosediphosphoric acid occurs not only under influence of certain specially added salts, but also, as was demonstrated recently, during the grinding of the muscle paste with large amounts of Kieselguhr (Embden, Jost, and M. Lehnartz). The absence of hexosediphosphoric acid in the fresh muscle may be due to the fact that it can be broken down more easily than hexosemonophosphoric acid. The concept that hexosemonophosphoric acid is converted to hexosediphosphoric acid has already been proposed by Meyerhof and his coworkers.

113

This reaction shows that glyceric acid is not an intermediate and that the split occurs without an additional water molecule.

Phase 5: Reductive transformation of pyruvic acid to lactic acid with the help of glycerolphosphate conversion to triosephosphate:

$$
\begin{array}{ccccc}
\mathrm{CH_3} & \mathrm{CH_2-O-P{\overset{O}{\underset{OH}{\diagdown}}}OH} & & \mathrm{CH_3} & \mathrm{CH_2-O-P{\overset{O}{\underset{OH}{\diagdown}}}OH}\\
| & | & & | & |\\
\mathrm{C{=}O} \quad + & \mathrm{CHOH} & = & \mathrm{CHOH} \quad + & \mathrm{CHOH}\\
| & | & & | & |\\
\mathrm{COOH} & \mathrm{CH_2OH} & & \mathrm{COOH} & \mathrm{C{=}O}\\
& & & & \diagdown\mathrm{H}
\end{array}
$$

Pyruvic acid   Glycerolphosphate   Lactic acid   Triosephosphate

In regard to the formation of triosephosphate, phases 3, 4, and 5 would be repetitive.

As one can see, this glycolytic scheme omits methylglyoxal, which has been assumed by Neuberg to be an intermediate in yeast fermentation, as well as animal glycolysis.

The appearance of this substance as precursor of the L(+)-lactic acid, which is apparently formed predominantly in animals, has been questioned in earlier papers from this Institute, since it was found that methylglyoxal produces not only this isomer, but a mixture in which D(−)-lactic acid is predominant. Lohmann demonstrated very recently that the activity of methylglyoxalase—the ferment that converts methylglyoxal into lactic acid—depends on the presence of glutathion, while the fermentative lactic acid formation from glycogen by muscles also occurs in the absence of glutathion.

* * * * * * *

Although the glycolytic lactic acid formation by muscles described above seems to be different from previous opinions, it should be noted that many observations of earlier scientists agree with the scheme we have developed. We refer specifically to the observations of Neuberg about yeast fermentation (under certain abnormal conditions of yeast fermentation, Neuberg and Kobel obtained equimolar amounts of pyruvic acid and glycerol) and the observations by Neuberg and J. Kerb that the addition of glycerol causes the formation of ethanol (instead of acetaldehyde) from pyruvic acid by yeast carboxylase.

However, we do not wish to pursue the comparison between the alcoholic yeast fermentation and our glycolysis. It should be noted that Nilsson obtained an amorphous barium salt, which he assumed to be monophosphoglycerate, after adding fluoride to the yeast, although he was not able to identify the compound.

Greenwald isolated the double phosphorylated glyceric acid from red blood cells and clarified its structure; H. Jost demonstrated that this substance occurred during glycolysis of red blood cells. The formation of this diphosphoglycerate was shown to be very similar to the formation of our monophosphoglyceric acid, although it was not known at the time that the glycolytic lactic acid formation pathway led through phosphoglyceric acid and pyruvic acid.

13

About the Enzymatic Equilibrium Reaction Between Hexosediphosphoric Acid and Dioxyacetone Phosphoric Acid

O. MEYERHOF and K. LOHMANN

Translated expressly for this Benchmark volume by H. W. Doelle from "Über die enzymatische Gleichgewichtsreaktion zwischen Hexosediphosphorsäure und Dioxyacetonphosphorsäure," Biochem. Z., 271, 89–110 (1934), with permission from Springer-Verlag

III. Characteristics of the "Zymohexase"

We call the ferment that catalyzes the reaction hexosediphosphate ⇌ dioxyacetonephosphate, zymohexase. It is present in such excessive amounts that an equilibrium must be reached immediately between these compounds, either in the living muscle or wherever hexosediphosphate occurs in the tissue. This means that dioxyacetonephosphate should always be present in measurable amounts.

A rabbit muscle extract, which represents the fermentation solution, is obtained using three parts distilled water and two parts muscle,[1] is inactivated for 3 hr at room temperature, followed by 20 hr of dialysis with distilled water. The latter should free the extract from adenylpyrophosphate and magnesium. The substrate is Na-hexosediphosphate (not Mg-hexosediphosphate). Lohmann[2] has shown that the presence of Mg^{2+} can cause the removal of one phosphoric acid group from the hexosediphosphate. In order to obtain the equilibrium accurately it is important that the described enzyme present is the only one that influences the transformation of hexosediphosphate.

A. Dilution

A 4-fold dilution of the muscle extract brings the transformation of hexosediphosphate at 20°C to three-fourths completion after 15 sec and almost finishes it in 1 min. Further dilution causes a delay in reaching the equilibrium until it can never be reached. We chose $4.2 \times 10^{-3} M$ bound phosphate as the most convenient substrate concentration and 20°C as the temperature.

---

[1] Further extractions also produce acceptable active extracts.
[2] K. Lohmann, *Biochem. Z.*, **262**, 137 (1933).

115

In this case the equilibrium would correspond to

$$\frac{0.33 \text{ triose-P}}{0.67 \text{ hexose-P}}$$

(A variation between 31 and 36 percent triose-P is within experimental error.) The concentration is related to M phosphate and not to the phosphate ester. The limits of enzyme activity also depend, of course, on the preparation and the age of the extract. The latter were used after 1–8 days storage in the refrigerator. From Table II [*Ed. Note:* Table II is not reproduced here.] it can be observed that the equilibrium of a 160-fold diluted extract is reached in 15 min, whereas a 400-fold dilution requires 45 min.

The concentration of the enzyme is much lower in the maceration sap as experiments 9–12 in Table IV indicate. This occurs despite the fact that maceration sap (4 parts water and 1 part dry yeast) is 2.5 times as concentrated in relation to the cell substance. The equilibrium situation, however, is the same as in the muscle extract.

Table IV. Triose ester in diluted ferment extracts

No.	Date 1934	Extract	n-fold dilution	Percent reached in minutes: 1	3	15	45
1	12.2	Dialyzed muscle	4	31.5			
2	13.2		4		30.7		
3	13.2		16		31.5		
4	13.2		40		20.5	33	
5	13.2		160		14	31	
6	19.2		160		14.4	30.5	
7	19.2		400		6	15.2	25
8	19.2		800		4		13
9	13.2	Dialyzed maceration	16		33.6		
10	14.2		16		31		
11	14.2		40		22.4		
12	14.2		160		8	18.5	

B. Thermostability

The ferment is relatively thermostable. No effect occurs after 10 min at 50°C. After 10 min at 60°C, the catalysis is slower, but a 4-fold dilution of the extract still reaches equilibrium in 15 min. Heating the extract for 30 min at 60°C or for 10 min at 70°C causes the ferment to become inactive.

C. Precipitation and Adsorption of the Ferment

The ferment can be precipitated with acetone (and also with alcohol) and can be stored as powder after drying with ether. This powder shows no loss of activity after

116

5 weeks. An aqueous extract that corresponds to a 16-fold dilution of the extract reaches its equilibrium (34 percent triose-P) in 3 min and does not differ from the original extract.

The ferment is easy soluble in water; thus adsorption is difficult. "Willstättersche Tonerdepräparate B and C" and "Fasertonerde von Merck" were used as adsorption material. If a 4-fold diluted muscle extract is mixed with one-eighth of its volume of a "Tonerde" suspension, it can be demonstrated that the solution, which corresponds to a 1:40 dilution of the original extract, forms 14.4 percent triose-P in 3 min and 31 percent in 15 min which corresponded with the results of a 160-fold dilution of the original extracts. The adsorbent contains less, as it forms 5.6 percent triose ester after 3 min and 28 percent after 15 min. At higher dilutions, equivalent to 1:100 of the original extract, the adsorbent becomes inactive, whereas the centrifuged supernatant at a dilution of 1:200 reached equilibrium (31 percent triose-P) in 45 min, which compares with a 400-fold dilution of the original extract. In weak acidic solutions (addition of acetate to pH 5), the adsorbent is useless. Nor was a concentration obtained with "negative adsorption." The Kjeldahl-N remains constant in relation to activity. A 400-fold diluted original extract and a 200-fold diluted extract treated with Al_2O_3 contains 6–7 μg of N.

D. Effects on the Ferment

The ferment is relatively unaffected by changes in pH. A 4-fold dilution reaches its equilibrium between pH 6 and 10 after 1 min, whereas at pH 5 and pH 11, the transformation is still incomplete after 15 min. Iodoacetic acid, NaF, and Na-oxalate, which inhibit lactic acid formation, do not alter the equilibrium nor the rate of reaction of a 160-fold dilution. Fluoride inhibits the release of phosphoric acid from phosphoglycerate[3]; oxalate does the same by a different mechanism[4]; iodoacetate inhibits the conversion of triosephosphate. The equilibrium can, however, also be obtained in nondialyzed extracts after iodoacetate poisoning. An iodoacetate poisoned muscle contains (apart from hexosemonophosphate and hexosediphosphate) a certain amount of triosephosphate that corresponds to the equilibrium according to the hexosediphosphate concentration. Thus 2 mg of P_2O_5-hexosediphosphate in 1 ml of aqueous muscle solution could contain about 10 percent triosephosphate at 20°C. In nonpoisoned muscle, no hexosediphosphate can be found and, therefore, no measurable amount of triosephosphate.[5]

Because of the rapid formation of triosephosphate and the slower transformation of this compound, nondialyzed and nonpoisoned muscle and yeast extract always contain a certain amount of triosephosphate during the decomposition of glycogen, hexose, and hexosediphosphate; under all circumstances hexosediphosphate can be found in the presence of the ferment. The triosephosphate is formed faster, then further metabolized. This correlation will be considered in another paper.

---

[3]O. Meyerhof and W. Kiessling, *Biochem. Z.*, **264**, 72 (1933).
[4]Unpublished results of O. Meyerhof and K. Lohmann.
[5]The monoesters do not form triosephosphate directly.

IV. The Hexosediphosphate $\rightleftharpoons$ Dioxyacetonephosphate Equilibrium

In regard to the equilibrium, the following rules exist:

1. For each temperature a true thermodynamic equilibrium exists, following the equation

$$K = \frac{c^2 \text{ (dioxyacetone phosphoric acid)}}{c \text{ (hexosediphosphoric acid)}}$$

K, which is independent of the amount of ferment, varies under the studied conditions between 7.5×10^{-4} and 6.8×10^{-2} mole bound phosphate (e.g., at a concentration of 1:100 the variation is 1:2, which is within the experimental error).

2. The establishment of an equilibrium with a constant amount of ferment occurs with the same speed from either side, which demonstrates that the same ferment causes utilization and synthesis of the hexosediphosphate. This is in contrast to the characteristics of glyceraldehyde phosphoric acid.

3. The value of K increases with temperature and is equal to 22×10^{-3} at 70°C, 13×10^{-3} at 60°C, 1.5×10^{-3} at 20°C, 0.3×10^{-3} at 0°C, and 0.18×10^{-3} at −7°C. This almost 100-fold change within a range of 80°C can be explained on thermodynamic grounds. According to van't Hoff's isotherm equation, such change should correspond to the value of $U = -12$ kcal/mole of hexosediphosphate split. Direct measurements reveal, in fact, a negative free energy of −5.4 kcal. It can be established that the equilibria are really temperature dependent; a change in temperature causes the equilibrium to change to its approximate value. These three observations will now be considered in detail with the help of experiments.

A. Establishment of Equilibrium at a Certain Temperature

Table V combines all determinations of equilibrium conditions that reached the endpoint, irrespective of the pretreatment, dilutions of the ferment, or whether the establishment occurred from hexosediphosphate or dioxyacetonephosphate. The average has been given for every concentration. Most of the available measurements are for the concentration of 4.25×10^{-3} mole bound phosphate (2.5 mg of P_2O_5 in 8.3 ml of solution). Table V contains the results for 70°C, 60°C, 20°C, 0°C, and −7°C and Fig. 1 for 60°C and 20°C. With temperatures of 60°C and 70°C, the time chosen for the experiment was between 45 sec and 1 min, because longer incubation times caused the release of inorganic phosphate. At 20°C, the establishment of the equilibrium took 1–2 min for the normal, 1:4 diluted extract; measurements were therefore taken after 3 min and, for more dilute extracts, after 3 and 15 min. As lowest temperature, −7°C was chosen. If the enzyme mixture was first cooled to 0° and then further to −7°C, an undercooling was obtained. The period of time before the solution freezes is long enough to demonstrate that reactions from either side give identical values.

118

Table V. Equilibrium constant $K = (^c\text{diox.})^2/(^c\text{hexph.})$ at different temperatures

Temp., °C	No.	Total concn. ester in M phosphate	% triose ester	No. experiments	$M \times 10^{-3}$ hexose diphosphoric acid	$M \times 10^{-6}$ (dihydroxy-acetone–P)	$K \times 10^{-3}$	Av. value $K \times 10^{-3}$
70	1	0.85	90	1	0.0425	0.585	13.8	
	2	4.25	79	3	0.468	11.0	23.5	22
	3	17	55	2	4.4	78	22.8	
60	1	0.75	88	1	0.045	0.435	9.7	
	2	1.06	83	1	0.090	0.78	8.7	
	3	4.25	70.5	7	0.63	9.0	14.3	13
	4	17	36.8	1	5.4	39.2	7.3	
	5	68	26.7	1	24.9	33.0	13.2	
20	6	0.75	68	1	0.118	0.26	2.20	
	7	0.85	58	2	0.178	0.244	1.37	
	8	1.06	52	2	0.255	0.304	1.19	
	9	3.5	41	3	1.03	2.06	2.0	
	10	4.25	32.5	12	1.43	2.00	1.40	1.5
	11	5.95	29	2	2.11	2.97	1.41	
	12	17	15.0	2	7.24	6.5	0.90	
	13	68	8.0	2	31.3	29.0	0.95	
0	14	0.53	44	1	0.15	0.054	0.36	
	15	3.5	18.4	1	1.44	0.416	0.29	0.30
	16	4.25	16	1	1.79	0.46	0.26	
7	17	4.25	13	4	1.85	0.305	0.165	
	18	17.0	8	1	7.8	1.85	0.24	0.18
	19	37.5	4.9	1	17.8	3.36	0.19	

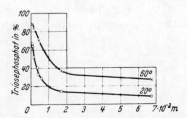

Figure 1. Equilibrium (2-triosephosphoric acid $\rightleftharpoons$ 1-hexose diphosphoric acid) at variable total concentrations of bound phosphate. Ordinate: Triosephosphoric acid; Abscissa: $10^{-2} M$ bound phosphate. ×—×—×: Adjustment of equilibrium at 60°C; o—o—o: Adjustment of equilibrium at 20°C.

Na-hexosediphosphate was obtained for the experiments by the treatment of a calcium salt (candiolin) with oxalic acid and NaOH, which gave a 93 percent pure preparation according to the hydrolysis curve; it contains only 1 percent triosephosphate. The concentration value included the total amount of organically bound phosphate. As triosephosphoric acid, either the barium salt isolated from the enzyme reaction described in Chapter IV, whose organically bound phosphate could be saponified to 80–95 percent, or the synthetic calcium salt that Dr. Kiessling produced for us, which also could be saponified to 90 percent were utilized. Since these preparations were extremely labile, the concentration was determined at the start of the experiments.

Proof that the obtainable distribution of a certain concentration does, in fact, represent the equilibrium was obtained not only by the identical results received from both sides of the reaction but also from the dilution experiments. If, for example, an enzyme mixture of a known equilibrium is diluted with water, the new obtainable distribution is identical with that of the concentrated one. Addition of muscle extract to the excess of ferment does not effect this distribution. No reaction occurred if the ferment is added to a solution containing the appropriate mixture of triosephosphate and hexosediphosphate that would be expected at that temperature and concentration. Table V contains the average values for K. It does not include the experiments with dialyzed maceration sap. At 20°C and an average ester concentration, the equilibrium is identical to that of the muscle extract at higher concentrations, and at a lower temperature the amount of triosephosphate observed was lower; however, there is a possibility that the reaction may not have reached equilibrium. The difference at 60°C is of importance, since the ferment of the maceration sap is not stable at this temperature, and the reaction remains incomplete. At the same time, inorganic phosphate is released. The conclusion can be reached, however, that muscle and yeast extracts have identical equilibria if the ferment is active enough.

B. Rate for Obtaining Equilibrium

Figure 2 represents the results of an experiment to determine the rate at which an equilibrium can be obtained by using either hexosediphosphate or triosephosphate as a substrate under conditions of equal ferment solution and phosphoric ester

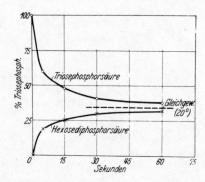

Figure 2. Adjustment of equilibrium 2-triose-P $\rightleftharpoons$ hexosedi-P; $4.2 \times 10^{-3}\,M$ organic phosphate. Ordinate: Percent triosephosphoric acid; Abscissa: time, seconds.

120

concentration. Both reactions not only reached the same end value but also exhibited equal rates. The experiment is also presented in Table VI.

These results, of course, do not apply for different ferment solutions. It is, however, important to note that the synthetic dioxyacetonephosphate is transformed at the same rate as the natural triosephosphate under the same conditions, while the rate for glyceraldehyde phosphate is much slower. Such a comparison is presented in Table VII. The reaction of the glyceraldehyde ester has not been determined. This ester reacts more than an optimal component and probably with different rates. During this reaction, hexosediphosphate is formed only as one part. Of particular interest is the slow start of the reaction.

Table VI. Rate of obtaining equilibrium

	Hexosediphosphate			Triosephosphate		
Time, sec	mg saponifiable P_2O_5	mg hexosediphosphate	Transformation, %	mg saponifiable P_2O_5	mg hexosediphosphate	Transformation, %
0	0	2.5		2.5		
5	0.49	2.01	58	1.50	1.0	60
15	0.63	1.87	74	1.20	1.30	79
30	0.75	1.71	88	1.04	1.46	88
60	0.79	1.71	93	0.95	1.55	94
180	(0.85)	(1.65)		(0.85)	(1.65)	

The same extract was used for hexosediphosphate and triosephosphate transformations. In both cases a 4-fold extract + 4.25×10^{-3} mole of bound phosphate (2.5 mg of ester P_2O_5 in 8.3 ml) was used.

Table VII. Rate of synthetic dioxyacetonephosphate and glyceraldehydephosphate transformation

	Dioxyacetonephosphate			Glyceraldehydephosphate	
Time	mg saponifiable P_2O_5	mg hexosediphosphate formed	Transformation, %	mg saponifiable P_2O_5	mg saponifiable P_2O_5 transformed
0 sec	2.43			4.69	
6 sec	1.69	0.74	49		
8 sec				4.51	0.81
30 sec	1.47	1.26	83	4.15	0.54
1 min	1.03	1.40	92	3.60	1.09
3 min	0.91	1.52		3.02	1.67
15 min				1.91	2.78

121

The same, 4-fold diluted extract (4.2×10^{-3} mole in relation to the fermentable component) was used.

The experimental results in Table VII indicate that in 8 sec only 10 percent and in 30 sec, 20 percent of one component is transformed, while 83 percent of the end value of dioxyacetonephosphate has already been reached. However, the transformation continues for more than 15 min, and 60 percent of the total saponifiable phosphorus disappears. The disappearance of methylglyoxal, formed by acid hydrolysis, parallels the disappearance of the saponifiable P and of the iodine-oxidized substance. Glyceraldehyde phosphate conversion results in small amounts of an ester that is difficult to hydrolyze, but even the easily hydrolyzable part consists only partially of hexosediphosphate. The presence of the latter can be determined, since a warmer enzyme mixture can again produce saponifiable phosphorus. Despite the slow and incomplete transformation of glyceraldehyde phosphate, the latter ferments as fast as both the natural and the synthetic dioxyacetonephosphate, which could be explained by the fact that zymohexase is present in greater amounts than all other fermentation enzymes.

It is particularly important to realize the different biological behavior of dioxyacetonephosphate and glyceraldehyde phosphate. It follows that hexosediphosphate is broken down enzymatically into two dioxyacetonephosphates without a recognizable formation of glyceraldehydephosphate. The rate toward the equilibrium of hexosediphosphate to triosephosphate increases with temperature. At 60°C, equilibrium is reached in 5 sec under the conditions described in Table VI.

C. Equilibrium Shifts Due to Changes in Temperature

In order to investigate the shifts occurring as a result of temperature changes, special precautions had to be taken (particularly at high temperatures where the reaction rates toward equilibrium are so fast). It is important to avoid temperature changes due to the addition of trichloroacetic acid (to stop the reaction of the ferment) and thus to avoid a new distribution of the phosphoric ester. Trichloroacetic acid has to be brought to exactly the same temperature as ferment solution before its addition, and it should be made certain that no temperature change occurs. If one follows these conditions strictly, each incubation temperature has its own equilibrium, as is demonstrated in Fig. 3. Three different systems with the same concentration of esterified phosphate ($4.2 \times 10^{-3} M$) are used (i.e., Na-hexosediphosphate, synthetic dioxyacetonephosphate from W. Kiessling, and natural triosephosphate). Each system was brought to 60°C, −7°C, and partly to 20°C in turn, and a sample was taken at each temperature. In order to allow for the reaction time necessary at the appropriate temperatures, the systems were left at 60°C for 20 sec to 1 min, at 20°C for 3 min, and at −7°C for 10 min. The equilibrium distribution obtained for identical temperatures was within the experimental error.

The position of the equilibria for certain concentrations, dependent on temperature, is demonstrated in Fig. 4.

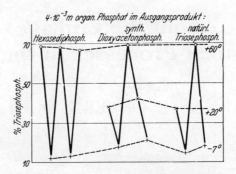

Figure 3. $4 \times 10^{-3} M$ organic P in original product. Changes in equilibrium at different temperatures. Ordinate: percent triosephosphoric acid.

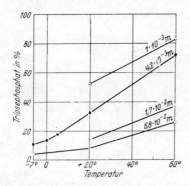

Figure 4. Equilibrium–temperature curves at varying concentrations of organic phosphate. Ordinate: percent triosephosphoric acid; abscissa: temperature.

14

About the Linkage
of Chemical Processes in the Muscle

J. K. PARNAS, P. OSTERN, and T. MANN

*Translated expressly for this Benchmark
volume by H. W. Doelle from "Über die
Verkettung der chemischen Vorgänge im
Muskel,"* Biochem. Z., **272**, *64–70
(1934), with permission from
Springer-Verlag*

I

During our investigations into the factors that inhibit the formation of ammonia, the following observations were made. Muscle paste, which is obtained by grinding fresh tissue with equal volumes of water at 12–14°C, does not produce ammonia; if larger quantities of water are used, ammonia production begins immediately, as described by Parnas and Mozolowski,[1] and ceases after 2–5 minutes. It can be concluded that the "traumatische" [*Ed. Note:* injury-like] formation of ammonia is linked to the diluting out of a factor that inhibits the process in the tissue. This factor is phosphate; it was observed that the addition of M/10 potassium phosphate (pH 7) suppresses the formation of ammonia for 30–60 minutes during the grinding of the muscles. Potassium chloride or borate buffers produce no effect.

This inhibition is curious because it exists only for a brief period, after which ammonia formation is very vigorous. This indicates that it cannot be an enzyme inhibition; rather, it is an interference with the substrate of the deamination. It is noteworthy that the addition of adenylic acid to the concentrated muscle paste causes a rapid deamination of this acid. This observation confirms our assumption, which we received from the results of Mozolowski and Sobozuk[2] and T. Mann[3] that the muscle deaminates only the adenylic acid, not the ATP.

So far, no method exists for the determination of ATP; the usual determination based on the phosphoric acid release by 1 mole of HCl (P_7—P_0)——(P_{30}—P_7) gives only the total for ribose polyphosphoric acids. We developed a method whereby the barium salt of ATP was precipitated with trichloroacetic acid and (after decomposition with H_2SO_4 and incubation with muscle paste according to G. Schmidt[5]) the release of ammonia was determined. With this method we were able to demonstrate that the ATP content remains constant in the muscle paste in which ammonia formation does not occur; with the formation of ammonia, the content of ATP is reduced. The rate of deamination is determined by the release of phosphate.

The inhibition of ammonia formation by M/10 phosphate can be reversed by the addition of N/1000 iodoacetic acid or N/200 sodium fluoride. This indicates that lactic acid formation is the cause of the phosphate inhibition of ammonia production. Lactic acid formation occurs, initially, at a rapid and, later, at a slower rate in the muscle paste, while little change is observed in the rate in phosphate paste. We were able to demonstrate for the first time that the addition of phosphate to the muscle paste causes lactic acid formation without ammonia release. The latter (without lactic acid production) had been observed during fluoride[6] and iodoacetate poisoning.[7,8] Experiments employing a phosphate–iodoacetate paste exhibited the same relationship between ammonia formation and ATP disappearance as was observed in the experiments performed without the addition of iodoacetic acid.

These observations indicate that only adenylic acid is deaminated in the muscle. In the concentrated muscle paste, as well as in the phosphate paste, ATP is continuously regenerated by a mechanism that is driven by the lactic acid formation, the most important compound of which must occur in the reaction[9] between adenylic acid and phosphocreatine. Earlier experiments of Mozolowski, Mann, and Lutwak (Table IV, Abb. 1[7]) have already explained how ammonia can be liberated in iodoacetate poisoned muscles by splitting creatine phosphate. According to Lohmann[9] and other workers, the mechanism appears to be clear; the "big ammonia production" starts as soon as creatine phosphate is split and ATP cannot be regenerated.

We are not yet sure how higher phosphate concentrations are able to influence the mechanism. They certainly do not increase lactic acid production but could, perhaps, stimulate the resynthesis of phosphocreatine and ATP. In symmetrical muscles one finds, for example, 128 mg percent phosphocreatine-P in the phosphate paste and only 37 mg percent in the aqueous paste.

The inhibition of the deamination by phosphate (or in concentrated muscle paste) disappears after a time. This observation is related to those of Mann,[3] who observed an increase in ammonia release with the age of the muscle extract. What the mechanism is, is not known; however, during the interplay between phosphate release and ATP formation, it was observed that, for example, after 1 hour, one-fourth of the original amount of ATP could still be formed in the aqueous paste. This ATP eventually disappears due to the deamination of adenylic acid and thus lactic acid production is arrested. This is in contrast to the effect of the presence of iodoacetic acid; ATP has disappeared completely within minutes in the phosphate—and also in the aqueous paste under release of ammonia and the complete release of the $(P_2 \text{——} P_0)$ ——$(P_{30} \text{——} P_7)$-labile phosphates that can be precipitated in barium hydroxide.

The formation of ammonia from ATP occurs only at the adenylic acid step and plays no part in the energy-producing cycle of this substance. That it occurs under physiological conditions can only be explained by an earlier assumption[10] that it is important to block certain parts of the muscle mechanism. This would allow an oxidative recovery, which in turn allows the synthesis of the glycolytic substrate and the specific element of the coferment.

II

Further experiments have shown that a definite relationship exists between maintenance and resynthesis of ATP and ammonia formation in the phosphate–muscle paste. If one adds adenylic acid to such muscle paste and leaves the mixture for 10 minutes (at 12°C), a ratio of ⅔ ATP to ⅓ ammonia can be determined; after 1 hour, this ratio changes to ⅓ ATP to ⅔ ammonia. Adenylic acid is labile in the muscle; it will either form ATP or be deaminated. These facts lead to the following role of ammonia release in the mechanism of the muscle: after adenylic acid has been set free from its two phosphates during the first step of the anaerobic recovery step, Lohmann's reaction,[1] where adenylic acid is transformed back to ATP at the cost of phosphocreatine decomposition, occurs. These steps occur if the anaerobic recovery, including the sugar utilization, occurs in an ideal, completely reversible way. However, if this sequence fails to operate this way, the unconverted adenylic acid will undergo deamination. This deamination occurs at a high rate because of the high activity of the deaminating ferments in the muscle. The rate is identical to the one observed in iodoacetate-poisoned muscle, as well as in muscle paste containing iodoacetic acid, fluoride, or just water. In a few minutes, all adenylic acid is being transformed to inosinic acid. Inhibiting glycolysis with fluoride or iodoacetate inhibits ATP synthesis, and AMP is deaminated.

Physiologically, the process could be explained as follows. During the cycle of anaerobic recovery processes, the first step of this process is that the structurally bound ATP is converted to adenylic acid; the products of this split, together with other members of the later reactions, are able to reform ATP. These other members consist, presumably, of reactions whereby phosphates are transferred from organic compounds to those substances necessary for biosynthesis (i.e., from phosphocreatine to adenylic acid, from an intermediary product of sugar utilization to creatine). The sequence of the anaerobic recovery processes is dependent on the previous oxidative recovery; in order for sugar to be metabolized, the coenzyme ATP must be present. If the anaerobic recovery starts to falter, the deamination of adenylic acid prevents formation of the coenzyme. The anaerobic reaction sequence ceases for the time it takes to replenish the glycolytic substrate, as well as the mother substance of the coferment, during oxybiontic recovery.

III

The relation between the existence of ATP and sugar utilization led to the conclusion that a process that is connected with ATP synthesis must exist. In phosphate–

muscle paste, no ammonia is formed; the addition of fluoride or iodoacetic acid, which alters sugar utilization, causes ammonia formation. If it is possible that the addition of substances that occur as intermediates in the sugar utilization suppresses ammonia formation in the phosphate paste in the presence of the above poisonous substances (e.g., if pyruvic acid or phosphoglyceric acid would reverse fluoride inhibition), certain conclusions could be drawn as to the role of these intermediate products. We investigated this question. The results of these experiments are evident; false results have been precluded since both the amount of ammonia formed and the ATP content of the muscle paste were determined separately.

1. In phosphate paste containing fluoride (N/400 to N/60 NaF) the addition of pyruvic acid and/or phosphoglyceric acid* causes cessation of ammonia formation, while the addition of lactic acid, glycerolphosphoric acid, or Harden–Young diester* did not affect the ammonia formation.

2. In phosphate paste containing iodoacetic acid, only phosphoglyceric acid is able to inhibit ammonia formation, all other compounds being ineffective.

As an example of the magnitude of these effects, the following experiment was carried out: paste containing fluoride but no pyruvic acid after 10 minutes incubation at 13°C contains 7.48 mg percent NH_3–N and 1.38 mg percent ATP–N. In the presence of pyruvic acid in the same paste (M/50 Na–pyruvate), 1.6 mg percent NH_3–N and 7.02 mg percent ATP–N was found after 10 minutes of incubation.

These experiments lead to the conclusion that the resynthesis of phosphocreatine and ATP is not dependent on the glycolysis process as a whole, but only on part of it. They also indicate that this relationship cannot be an "energetic coupling," but rather a phosphate transfer from molecule to molecule as Lohmann[9] discovered in the case of dephosphorylation of adenylic acid by phosphocreatine.

The observation that only phosphoglyceric acid was able to inhibit ammonia formation in the presence of iodoacetate in the muscle–phosphate paste gives this compound a special role in ATP synthesis.

Regarding the mechanism by which phosphoglyceric acid and pyruvic acid undergo changes, the following could be said. In fluoride paste, phosphoglyceric acid and pyruvic acid are effective, whereby the latter is the stronger one. Experiments carried out by Embden, Deuticke, and Kraft,[11] as well as Meyerhof and Kiessling,[12] concerning the intermediary process of glycolysis in muscle demonstrate that the conversion of phosphoglyceric acid to pyruvic acid is interrupted by fluoride poisoning. The reversion of ammonia formation by pyruvic acid could be related to the resynthesis of ATP as a final process in the formation of lactic acid from pyruvic acid. The reversion by phosphoglyceric acid, however, cannot go via pyruvic acid. Experiments in which phosphoglyceric acid inhibits ammonia formation in phosphate–fluoride paste revealed no methylglyoxal or lactic acid formation.

In iodoacetate–phosphate paste, only phosphoglyceric acid (not pyruvic acid) inhibits ammonia formation. The inhibition of sugar utilization by iodoacetic acid is

---

*We are extremely grateful to C. Neuberg for the gift of a substantial amount of this substance.

thought to be the interruption of the dismutation between pyruvic acid and the glycerolphosphate ester. We conclude that the connection to ATP synthesis (or to phosphocreatine) occurs at a step in the glucose utilization which can only be reached by pyruvic acid and phosphoglyceric acid in the fluoride paste and only by phosphoglyceric acid in the iodoacetic acid paste. We have ascertained that no lactic acid or methylglyoxal is formed in iodoacetic acid paste when phosphoglyceric acid is added.

The substances responsible for the transformation of phosphate via creatine to adenylic acid have to be between phosphoglyceric acid and pyruvic acid. Neuberg[13] demonstrated that more steps exist between these substances when he found diphosphoglyceric acid and its decomposition to pyruvic acid. The first steps of sugar utilization are not involved in the resynthesis of ATP, since the Harden–Young ester is ineffective and is converted to dihydroxyacetone phosphate[14] in the presence of fluoride and iodoacetic acid. It would be easy to demonstrate equations for the phosphate transfer from phosphoglyceric acid or diphosphoglyceric acid to creatine; however, this should wait until the energetics have been determined.

References

1. J. K. Parnas and W. Mozolowski, *Biochem. Z.*, **184**, 399 (1927).
2. W. Mozolowski and B. Sobczuk, *Biochem. Z.*, **265**, 41 (1933).
3. T. Mann, *Biochem. Z.*, **266**, 162 (1933).
4. H. K. Barrenscheen and W. Filz, *Biochem. Z.*, **253**, 422 (1932); **250**, 281 (1932).
5. G. Schmidt, *Z. Physiol. Chem.*, **179**, 243 (1928).
6. S. Chrzaszczewski and W. Mozolowski, *Biochem. Z.*, **194**, 233 (1928).
7. W. Mozolowski, T. Mann, and C. Lutwak, *Biochem. Z.*, **231**, 290 (1931).
8. G. Embden, *Klin. Wochschr.*, **9**, 1337 (1930).
9. C. Lohmann, *Naturwiss.*, **22**, 409 (1934).
10. J. K. Parnas, *Ann. Rev. Biochem.*, **1**, 443 (1932).
11. G. Embden, J. Deuticke, and H. Krafft, *Klin. Wochschr.*, **12**, 337, 373 (1934).
12. O. Meyerhof and W. Kiessling, *Biochem. Z.*, **267**, 313 (1934).
13. C. Neuber, W. Schuchardt, and A. Vercellone, *Biochem. Z.*, **271**, 221 (1934).
14. O. Meyerhof and K. Lohmann, *Biochem. Z.*, **271**, 89 (1934).

Editor's Comments on Papers 15 and 16

15 Warburg and Christian: About a New Oxidative Ferment and Its Absorption Spectrum
Biochem. Z., **254,** 349, 444–454 (1932)

16 Warburg, Christian, and Griese: The Hydrogen-transferring Coferment, Its Constitution and Mechanism
Biochem. Z., **282,** 157–164 (1935)

The research group with Otto Warburg became particularly well known due to their outstanding work in the field of aerobic respiration. The discovery of an oxidative enzyme, the "yellow enzyme" or "Zwischenferment" that we now call glucose 6-phosphate dehydrogenase (Paper 15; Warburg and Christian, 1933), together with the second cofactor, nicotinamide adenine dinucleotide phosphate (NADP) (Paper 16), and the identification of its end product, 6-phosphogluconic acid, led to the conclusion that yeasts possess a second pathway of carbohydrate utilization. It was recognized (Warburg and Christian, 1936, 1937) that NADP is absolutely necessary for the oxidation of glucose 6-phosphate to 6-phosphogluconate, and further, with different proteins (Warburg and Christian, 1936; Dickens, 1936; Lipmann, 1936), to ribose 5-phosphate (Dickens, 1938) before pyruvic acid is formed.

Most, if not all, of these experiments were carried out with either growing cells or crude and purified extracts. The individual substances were characterized either by specific spot testing (see Feigl, 1966) or by paper chromatography (see Block et al., 1958). All these methods had their limitations. The use of growing cells allowed the study of the metabolism of a particular compound, but the products of these reactions were utilized during growth, making it difficult to observe more than the end product of a long sequence of reactions. Thus most studies into metabolic reactions, their equilibria and reversibility, as well as inhibition and activation of the enzymes involved, were conducted mainly with the "resting cell technique" (Quastel, 1928). The discovery of dehydrogenation reactions was a result of these investigations (Quastel and Whetham, 1925; Quastel and Wooldridge, 1928).

15

About a New Oxidative Ferment and Its Absorption Spectrum

O. WARBURG and W. CHRISTIAN

*Translated expressly for this Benchmark
volume by H. W. Doelle from "Über ein
neues Oxydationsferment und sein
Absorptionsspektrum,"* Biochem. Z.,
254, *349, 444–454 (1932), with permission from Springer-Verlag*

Last year we described a water-soluble ferment–coferment system[1] that transfers molecular oxygen to hexosemonophosphate and is not inhibited by CO or HCN. Similar processes have been observed in *Chlorella*,[2] in yeast juice,[3] and in anaerobic bacteria.[4] There must be, therefore, oxidative ferments in nature that are different from the oxygen-transferring phäohemin of aerobic cells.

Such a ferment, which we found in bottom yeast,[5] will be described. It does not dialyze through cellophane; it becomes inactive if heated to 60°C in an aqueous solution; these aqueous solutions of the ferment are yellowish red. If the ferment is reduced, this color disappears. Shaking with oxygen reoxidizes the ferment and the solution again becomes colored. If one calls the reduced form of the ferment "leuco form" (since it does not absorb in the visible spectrum as the oxidized form does), the oxygen transfer reaction of the ferment is based on the change between the leuco and the colored form.

The leuco form of the ferment is oxidized to the colored form not only by molecular oxygen but also by methylene blue, which increases the reaction rate. Because of this characteristic, the ferment can be titrated by methylene blue, and it is possible to determine the absolute concentration of the active groups of the ferment. With the concentration known, it is then possible to obtain the absolute absorption spectrum by measuring light absorption at various wavelengths.

The carbon monoxide- and HCN-insensitive respiration of the Lebedew juice from yeast is an oxygen transfer carried out by the new ferment. We are of the opinion that the ferment transfers "heme oxygen" in the cell, not molecular oxygen.

---

[1]O. Warburg and W. Christian, *Biochem. Z.*, **242**, 206 (1931).
[2]O. Warburg, *Biochem. Z.*, **100**, 230 (1919).
[3]O. Warburg, *Biochem. Z.*, **231**, 493 (1931).
[4]O. Meyerhof and P. Finkle, *Chem. Zelle*, **12**, 157 (1925).
[5]A. Bertho and H. Glück, *Ann.*, **414**, 159 (1932).

Oxidation and Reduction of the Ferment

The substrate in our experiments was Robison's hexosemonophosphate. If the ferment transfers oxygen to this acid, the oxidation of the leuco form by molecular oxygen would be a direct chemical reaction. The reaction of the colored form is a catalytic process. A second ferment and a coferment are necessary for the hexosemonophosphate to reduce the colored form of the oxygen-transferring form to its leuco form. We call hexosemonophosphate, second ferment, and coferment the "reducing system." Solutions of the second ferment and the coferment are almost colorless, and thus far we have no reason to believe that either of the two absorb in visible light.

Content

* * * * * * *

III. The Oxygen-Transferring Ferment

To 1200 ml of fresh Lebedew juice from bottom yeast was added 480 ml of lead acetate (Liquor Plumbi subacetici DAB 6) and 20 drops of octanol. The mixture was vigorously shaken. The mixture was left 12 hr in a cold room and then centrifuged to obtain a precipitation that was as complete as possible. To the supernatant, which contained the ferment, was added 240 ml M/2 phosphate solution (85 parts secondary and 15 parts primary M/2 phosphate). The precipitated lead phosphate was centrifuged and discarded. The supernatant, containing the ferment, was concentrated to 240 ml under vacuum and 40°C. Frothing was prevented by the repeated addition of octanol. The concentrated liquid was clarified by centrifugation, and the supernatant was transferred into dialysis tubes and dialyzed at 0°C for 17 hr against

131

running distilled water. After clarification by centrifugation, the solution was further concentrated to 70 ml under vacuum at 40°C, centrifuged, incubated for 1 hr at 38°C and, finally, centrifuged at high speed.

The ferment solution is a clear, yellowish-red fluid that becomes inactive[6] if it is heated for 10 min at 60°C but can be stored in the refrigerator for weeks without activity loss.

If one studies a 2-cm-thick ferment solution under a spectroscope, one is able to observe that the light is completely absorbed from 520 nm toward the blue. The α-band of the hemochromogen of the Lebedew juice is visible at 550 nm as are the β- and β'-bands at 520 and 530 nm, respectively. Spectroscopic measurements (Section VII) demonstrated that the ferment solution contains $6 \times 10^{-5}\,M$/liter yellow-red ferment and $1 \times 10^{-5}\,M$/liter hemochromogen. The iron of the hemochromogen is in the reduced form in the solution and will not be oxidized if shaken with oxygen. It probably takes no part in the oxygen transfer reaction.

$$* \quad * \quad * \quad * \quad * \quad * \quad *$$

V. Oxygen Pressure and the Color of the Ferment Solution

As was mentioned in the introduction, the leuco form is oxidized to the colored form of the ferment not only by molecular oxygen, but also by methylene blue. It can be concluded, therefore, that the yellow-red ferment is not an "oxygen addition product" of the oxyhemoglobin type, but ferment and leuco ferment must exist in a relation similar to that of methylene blue and its leuco form. Common to both is the fact that the color does not change if the solution is freed of oxygen or saturated with different partial pressures of oxygen.

If the ferment transfers oxygen, however, the solutions are deeper in color at higher oxygen pressures (within certain limits). This phenomenon can be explained by the kinetic theory of the stationary conditions.

If C is the total concentration of the ferment, c_{ox} and c_{red} the concentrations of the oxidized and reduced form of the ferment, c_s the concentration of the reducing systems, and c_{O_2} the concentration of oxygen,

$$-\frac{dc_{ox}}{dt} = k_1 c_{ox} c_s - k_2 c_{red} c_{O_2} \tag{1}$$

where k_1 and k_2 are the rate constants of the oxidation and reduction.

In the stationary condition of oxygen transfer

$$0 = k_1 c_{ox} c_s - k_2 c_{red} c_{O_2} \tag{2}$$

---

[6] J. Banga and A. Szent-Gyorgyi observed a yellow pigment in heart muscle juice that can be reduced with hydrosulfite and reoxidized with air [*Biochem. Z.*, **246**, 203 (1932)]. It is possible that this pigment is a decomposition product of the ferment.

If one considers $c_\mathrm{red} = C - c_\mathrm{ox}$,

$$\frac{c_\mathrm{ox}}{C} = \frac{k_2 c_{O_2}}{k_2 c_{O_2} + k_1 c_s} \tag{3}$$

The "color index," c_ox/C, is that fraction of ferment that is present in the oxidized form under stationary conditions of oxygen transfer. The right side of equation (3) demonstrates the way in which this fraction is dependent upon the concentration of oxygen and the reducing systems. In general, c_ox/C is smaller than 1. If the oxygen pressure increases under constant c_s, c_ox/C increases and becomes equal to 1 as soon as $k_2 c_{O_2}$ has increased in comparison to $k_1 c_s$. In this case the ferment is completely oxidized.

A simple relationship exists between reaction rate of oxygen transfer and depth of color. If we use the expression α for the right side of equation (3),

$$c_\mathrm{ox} = C \times \alpha \tag{4}$$

whereby α is a function of the oxygen pressure at constant c_s.

The reaction rate of oxygen transfer under stationary conditions is, according to equation (1),

$$v = k_1 c_\mathrm{ox} c_s$$

Substituting c_ox with equation (4), we obtain

$$v = k_1 \times c_s \times C \times \alpha \tag{5}$$

For the relationship of the reaction rates during variations in the oxygen pressures,

$$\frac{v_1}{v_2} = \frac{\alpha_1}{\alpha_2} \tag{6}$$

which means that with the oxygen pressure at constant C and c_s, the reaction rates of the oxygen transfer are in direct relation to the color intensity.

We have tried to examine equation (6) quantitatively. A solution containing the oxygen-transferring ferment and the reducing system was saturated with oxygen at different partial pressures. The oxidation rate v was determined manometrically and the color depth α by light absorption. Since it was difficult to obtain an equilibrium in the solutions in the absorption containers at low partial pressures of oxygen during the measurement of color depth, the results were not satisfactory and we had to rely on guessing the color depth during shaking. In the manometric experiments equilibrium was easy to obtain. It can be demonstrated that changes in the oxidation rate and color depth are parallel during varying oxygen pressures. If one saturates parts of the same solution with oxygen at different pressures, the color deepens as the oxidation rates increase.

The following example should explain the conditions that apply for such experiments:

Two ml of ferment of the reducing system, 1.8 ml of coferment, 0.45 ml of 0.3 M hexosemonophosphate, and 3 ml of oxygen-transferring enzyme were mixed. Three ml of this mixture was added to a conical flask and shaken with different partial pressures of oxygen at a rate such that an increase in the shaking rate did not result in any further oxygen uptake. At this time the reacting solutions had obtained absorption equilibrium with the respective oxygen pressures, which existed in the gas phase. The results are shown in the following table:

Main compartment: Gas component:	3 ml mixture 5% O_2 (in argon)	3 ml mixture 100% O_2
ml O_2 uptake after 10 min	16	68
ml O_2 uptake after 20 min	27	129
ml O_2 uptake after 30 min	39	188
Color observed during shaking	Light	Dark

At 20°C; KOH in center well.

IV. Absorption Spectrum of the Oxygen-Transferring Ferment

The solution containing the oxygen-transferring enzyme, which was obtained as described in Section III, also contains a hemochromogen in a significant concentration. The absorption spectrum of the solution, therefore, represents not only the spectrum of the ferment, but the spectrum of a color mixture containing the yellow-red color and the hemochromogen.

In order to measure the spectrum of the ferment, one utilizes the fact that the spectrum of the hemochromogen remains, even after reduction. If one mixes the ferment solution with the reducing system and measures the light absorption both at oxygen saturation and in the absence of oxygen, two different spectra are obtained. The spectrum in the absence of oxygen is that of the hemochromogen, while the spectrum at oxygen saturation consists of the color mixture (hemochromogen + yellow-red color). The difference of the absorption coefficients $\alpha_{ox} - \alpha_{red}$ yields the absorption spectrum of the oxidized form of the ferment.

Two cells (Fig. 1) were filled with the following clarified mixture, obtained by centrifugation at 0°C: 3.8 ml of the solution containing the ferment of the reducing system, 7.6 ml of the coferment solution, 1.4 ml of 0.3 M K-hexosemonophosphate, and 12.0 ml of the oxygen-transferring ferment solution.

Cell 1 is filled with oxygen, cell 2 is closed airtight by a capillary and is ready to be measured as soon as the light absorption does not change in the blue-green (at 460 nm) (e.g., as soon as the yellow-red pigment is completely reduced).

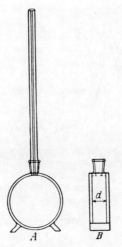

Fig. 1. Absorption vessel made of parallel quartz plates with a capillary for an airtight seal.

Table I. Measurements of the light absorption of the oxidized and reduced ferment solution

Wavelength, nm	Oxidized (hemochromogen + yellow-red pigment)		Reduced (hemochromogen)	
	i_0/i	$\ln i_0/i$	i_0/i	$\ln i_0/i$
400	7.88	2.07	5.49	1.70
410	13.0	2.56	8.73	2.17
415	16.1	2.78	10.9	2.39
420	13.9	2.63	9.13	2.21
430	4.9	1.59	3.26	1.18
440	3.78	1.33	2.23	0.80
450	3.49	1.25	1.80	0.59
460	3.43	1.23	1.73	0.55
470	3.40	1.22	1.63	0.49
480	2.93	1.08	1.54	0.43
490	2.64	0.97	1.46	0.38
500	2.07	0.73	1.41	0.34
510	2.32	0.84	1.56	0.445
520	2.07	0.73	1.65	0.50
530	1.75	0.56	1.46	0.38
540	1.48	0.39	1.34	0.29
550	1.68	0.52	1.64	0.50
560	1.28	0.25	1.21	0.19
570	1.17	0.16	1.15	0.14
580	1.15	0.14	1.10	0.095
590	1.10	0.096	1.08	0.077
600	1.07	0.068	1.04	0.040

Cell thickness is 1.07 cm; i_0/i is the ratio of light intensities at the end of the absorption.

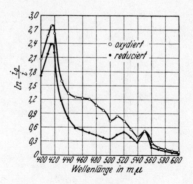

Fig. 2. Absorption spectrum of the oxidized and reduced ferment solution.

The results of the measurements are presented in Table I and in Fig. 2. The spectrum of the reduced solution is a typical hemochromogen spectrum with an α-band (550 nm), β-band (520 nm), and γ-main band (415 nm). From the spectrum of the oxidized solution it can be seen that the oxidation in the whole spectrum gives increased light absorption that is strongest in the blue-green and exhibits the largest differences at the ordinate.

Another experiment contained the following mixture: 8 ml of a solution containing the ferment of the reducing system, 16 ml of a coferment solution, 3 ml of 0.3 M K-hexosemonophosphate, and 24 ml of a solution containing the oxygen-transferring ferment.

The mixture was centrifuged first at room temperature and later at 0°C to obtain an absolutely clear solution and then filled into the cells as described earlier. Instead of reading the absorption separately, the oxidized solution was measured directly against the reduced one. If, at the same wavelength, the light intensity behind the oxidized solution is i_2 and behind the reduced solution is i_1, then $\ln i_1/i_2$ is proportional to the absorption coefficient of the oxidized form of the ferment.

Table II represents the results of the measurement, and Fig. 3 gives the absorption coefficient as function of the wavelength. The maximum of the absorption is at 470 nm with an indication of a minor band at 440 nm.

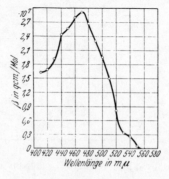

Fig. 3. Absorption spectrum of the oxidized form of the hydrogen-transferring ferment.

136

If one determines the absolute concentration of the ferment (as will be described in Section VII), the relative absorption coefficient can be recalculated to its absolute values. The latter values are given in the last column in Table II. They are, of course, dependent on the accuracy of the concentration measurement and can, thus, be ½ or double the value. The probable value of the absolute absorption coefficient for the spectral region of strongest absorption (470 nm) is 3×10^7 cm^2/M; the coefficient is not smaller than 1.5×10^7 and not larger than 6×10^7 cm^2/M.

Table II. Measurements of the absorption spectra of the oxygen transfer ferment

Wavelength, nm	i_1/i_2	ln i_1/i_2	$= 1/d \times 1/c \times $ ln i_1/i_2, cm^2/$M \times 10^7$
410	1.71	0.536	1.61
420	1.75	0.559	1.68
430	1.90	0.642	1.92
440	2.24	0.806	2.42
450	2.35	0.854	2.56
460	2.54	0.932	2.80
470	2.64	0.971	2.92
480	2.44	0.892	2.68
490	2.15	0.765	2.30
500	1.94	0.662	1.96
510	1.65	0.501	1.50
520	1.31	0.27	0.81
530	1.13	0.122	0.33
540	1.09	0.086	0.26
550	1.015	0.015	0.045
560	1	—	—
570	1	—	—
580	1	—	—
590	1	—	—
600	1	—	—

Cell thickness d = 1.07 cm. Possible concentration of the ferment c = 3.1×10^{-8} moles/ml.

The spectrum in Fig. 3 has been obtained with the assumption that the reduced form of the ferment does not absorb significantly in the visible region. As far as the hemochromogen is concerned, it could interfere if it has an oxidized and reduced form. This, however, is not the case, since the α-band of its oxidized and reduced form is identical (Fig. 2). If the hemochromogen is oxidized by oxygen, the α-band should disappear under oxygen saturation.

* * * * * * *

VIII. Rate Calculation of the Oxygen Transfer from Optical Measurements

The last section described a method that allows the calculation of the rate at which the oxidized form is reduced by the reducing system. [*Ed. Note:* That section has not been reproduced.] If c is the concentration of the oxidized ferment, the following relation exists at a constant concentration of the reducing system:

$$-\frac{dc}{dt} = k \times c$$

If a solution consisting of ferment and reducing system is shaken with oxygen, c is based at the constant value c_0. If the oxygen pressure is large enough, c_0 is equal to the total concentration of the ferment in the solution.

For the example given in the previous section,

$c = 3.1 \times 10^{-5}$ mole/liter $= 3.1 \times 10^{-8}$ mole/ml
k at 25°C $= 0.0175$ sec^{-1} $= 1.05$ min^{-1}

Does one assume that the reoxidation of the leuco form is the primary reaction, as in the case of the reoxidation of the leuco form of methylene blue?

1 leuco ferment + 1 O_2 = primary product of oxidation, the oxygen utilization per minute and ml of solution:

$$-\frac{dc}{dt} = k \times c_0 = 1.05 \times 3.01 \times 10^{-8} \text{ mole/min} = 0.73 \text{ mm}^3/\text{min}$$

We found an initial rate of 0.63 mm^3/min if the solution in which k and c_0 had been calculated was shaken at 25°C with 100 percent oxygen.

It should be noted that the conditions (low temperature and low concentration of the reducing system) were chosen in order to keep k small. If one adds small amounts of the ferment to large amounts of reducing system, as was done in the manometric experiment in Section IV, the value for k will be 60-fold. In this case, k cannot be determined by the optical method.

IX. Physiological Theory

In aerobic cells there exists not only molecular oxygen, but also the Fe^{3+} of the hemin as the oxidative substance whereby the latter reacts faster with the leuco form of the yellow-red pigment. In this case, a direct reaction does not exist between molecular oxygen and the leuco form of the yellow-red pigment:

$O_2 \rightarrow Fe^{2+}-\text{hemin} \rightarrow Fe^{3+}-\text{hemin} \rightarrow \text{leuco form of pigment} \rightarrow \text{pigment} \rightarrow \text{reducing system}$ (1)

If one inactivates the hemin with HCN, the following oxidative pathway occurs:

$O_2 \rightarrow \text{leuco form of pigment} \rightarrow \text{pigment} \rightarrow \text{reducing system}$ (2)

In general, the oxidation rates decrease if pathway (1) is replaced by pathway (2).

Only in the case of very small concentrations of the reducing system does the direct reaction between oxygen and the leuco form of the yellow-red pigment lead to a similar rate between oxidation paths (1) and (2). This may be explained as the way that the respiration of sugar-free *Chlorella,* which is small, cannot be inhibited by HCN, while the respiration of the sugar-containing *Chlorella,* which is large, can be inhibited by HCN.

In sugar-containing baker's yeast, the concentration of the reducing system is so large that a direct reaction between oxygen and the leuco form of the yellow-red pigment is not large enough; respiration is inhibited if one blocks the hemin with CO or HCN. If, however, the yeast is extracted according to the method developed by v. Lebedew, the hemin remains as residue, while the yellow-red pigment and the reducing system go into solution and one obtains a small respiration, which cannot be inhibited by CO and HCN.

We also want to remark that the reaction

$$Fe^{3+}-hemin \longrightarrow leucoform\ of\ pigment$$

is not the only reaction where the Fe^{3+} is reduced. Although the primary reaction of aerobic respiration is always the oxidation of Fe^{2+}–hemin, there may exist many ferments that would be able to reduce the Fe^{3+}–hemin.

139

16

The Hydrogen-Transferring Coferment, Its Constitution and Mechanism

O. WARBURG, W. CHRISTIAN, and A. GRIESE

*Translated expressly for this Benchmark
volume by H. W. Doelle from "Wasser-
stoffübertragendes Coferment, seine
Zusammensetzung und Wirkungsweise,"*
Biochem. Z., **282**, *157–164 (1935),
with permission from Springer-Verlag*

The coferment from red blood cells,[1] which we call hydrogen-transferring coferment, was purified until its catalytic activity did not increase further. Our purified coferment is easily soluble in water, does not crystallize, contains 12.9 percent nitrogen and 12.3 percent phosphorus, and produces, after hydrolysis, phosphoric acid, pentose, adenine, and a pyridine base that is the amide of nicotinic acid:

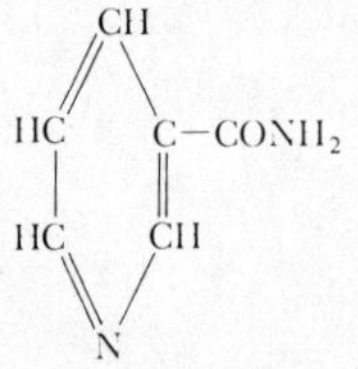

If one assumes that the coferment consists of 1 molecule of adenine, 1 molecule of nicotinamide, 3 molecules of phosphoric acid, and 2 molecules of pentose, one obtains the formula $C_{21}H_{28}N_7P_3O_{17}$. This agrees with the chemical analysis. The molecular weight would be 743, whereas measurements give 870.

* * * * * * *

Relation to Cozymase

The hydrogen-transferring coferment is not able to replace the cozymase of Harden's fermentation experiments,[2] and cozymase is not able to replace the

---

[1] O. Warburg and W. Christian, *Biochem. Z.*, **242**, 206 (1931); **254**, 438 (1932); **266**, 377 (1933); **274**, 112 (1934); **275**, 212 (1934); **275**, 464 (1935); **279**, 143 (1935); in the latter article, 25 percent should read 15 percent nicotinamide.

[2] O. Warburg and W. Christian, *Biochem. Z.*, **274**, 112 (1934).

hydrogen-transferring coferment in the oxidative process.[3] The hydrogen-transferring coferment and cozymase, therefore, have to be different substances.

A comparison of the chemical characteristics of cozymase, which were described by v. Euler and K. Myrbäck,[4] with those of the hydrogen-transferring coferment leads unmistakably to the conclusion that both substances are very closely related chemically. A number of years ago, v. Euler and K. Myrbäck showed that hydrolysis results in the products adenine, phosphoric acid, and pentose.

Zwischenferment [*Ed. Note:* Glucose 6-phosphate dehydrogenase]

Just as cozymase can react as a fermentative enzyme only in coordination with a special protein, the "zymase," the hydrogen-transferring coferment can react catalytically only together with special proteins, which we call "Zwischenferment."

* * * * * * *

I. About the Substrate and the Endproduct of the Oxidation in the Fermentation System

In all experiments with the fermentation system (yellow ferment + zwischenferment + coferment), the Robison ester hexosemonophosphate was the substrate. Hexosediphosphate and the Neuberg ester cannot be used as substrate, since they do not react significantly.

The Robison ester was purified as the calcium salt[5] ($C_6H_{11}PCaO_6 + H_2O$; molecular weight 316). During aldose determination according to the method of M. MacLeod and R. Robison,[6] 3.54 mg of calcium salt ($= 11 \times 10^{-3}$ mmole) required 3.10 ml of N/200 iodine solution ($= 15.5 \times 10^{-3}$ mmole). Since 1 molecule of free aldose uses 2 molecules of iodine, the aldose value of our substance was

$$\frac{15.5 \times 10^{-3}}{2.11 \times 10^{-3}} \times 100 = 96\%$$

Furthermore, since the aldose value of pure aldose monophosphoric acid according to R. Robison is smaller than 100 percent, our substance consisted mainly of aldose monophosphoric acid.

In order to transfer the calcium salt into the potassium salt, 4 g of calcium salt were ground in 40 ml of H_2O and 2.33 g of potassium oxalate ($K_2C_2O_4 + H_2O$; molecular weight 184). After 30 minutes, the solution was centrifuged and the phosphorus in the supernatant was determined colorimetrically.

---

[3]v. Euler and E. Adler, *Hoppe-Seyler*, **235**, 164 (1935).
[4]K. Myrbäck, *Co-zymase. Ergebnisse der Enzymforschung*, **2**, 139, Leipzig (1933).
[5]O. Warburg and W. Christian, *Biochem. Z.*, **254**, 438 (1932).
[6]M. MacLeod and R. Robison, *Biochem. J.*, **23**, 517 (1929).

Total Oxygen Consumption and Hydrogen Peroxide Formation

In order to obtain a complete oxidation of the hexose monophosphate in the fermentative system, we added to the main compartment of a cylindrical measuring container [*Ed. Note:* Warburg vessel] less hexosemonophosphate and more co-ferment (as during the determination of the coferment) to obtain the endpoint quickly; small amounts of zwischenferment were also added in order to have the least amount of hydrogen peroxide catalytically destroyed. Even the most pure zwischen-ferment preparation from Negelein contained traces of catalase.[7]

The cylindrical measuring flasks have two sidearms. One of the sidearms con-tained the yellow ferment, the other, the blood catalase (2 drops of a 1/100 dilution of red blood cells from rats). The gas phase contained oxygen, and the temperature was 38°C.

First the yellow ferment was added to the main compartment and shaken until oxygen consumption stopped. Then the catalase was added to the main compartment and shaken until no oxygen was being formed.

The results are presented in Table I. At the end of the oxidation, the solution contained 0.77 molecules of H_2O_2 per molecule of oxidized hexosemonophosphate. The oxygen consumption after the catalytic decomposition of H_2O_2 was 0.5 molecule per molecule of oxidized hexosemonophosphate. The loss of H_2O_2 could be due to catalase action of the zwischenferment preparation or to the side reaction

leuco ferment + H_2O_2 = yellow ferment + H_2O

Phosphohexonic Acid

It was assumed that after the consumption of the oxygen, phosphohexonic acid, an acid that R. Robison and E. J. King[8] obtained by oxidizing the Robison ester with bromide, was formed as a result of the oxidation of hexosemonophosphate.

In order to isolate phosphohexonic acid, the following experiment was set up: 50 ml of 0.4% NaOH; 5 ml of K-hexosemonophosphate containing 44 mg of phosphorus; 5 ml of a solution containing pure,[9] prepared yellow ferment from H. Theorell, which contained 30×10^{-8} mole of ferment; 10 ml of Zwischenferment solution, which contained 2 mg of dry substance; and 2.5 mg of coferment.

A mixture of a 5 percent CO_2–oxygen gas was forced through the solution for 3 hr at 38°C. The solution had an acetaldehyde odor. The protein was precipitated

---

[7]Crude zwischenferment solution from yeast contains considerable amounts of catalase. This was the reason A. Bertho and B. v. Zychilinski [*Liebig's Ann.*, **512**, 81 (1934)] could not find the hydrogen peroxide formed during the oxidation of the ferment system.
[8]R. Robison and E. J. King, *Biochem. J.*, **25**, 323 (1931); also M. MacLeod and R. Robison, *Biochem. J.*, **27**, 286 (1933).
[9]The use of crude yellow ferment would lead to the formation of "Hefegummi" [*Ed. Note:* "yeast rubber"; carbohydrate polymers] during the precipitation of the barium· salt.

Table I

	Vessel 1	Vessel 2
Main compartment	0.04 mg Zwischenferment 1.35 mg hexosemonophos- phate (K-salt) = 0.16 mg P 0.01 mg coferment, 2.3 ml H_2O	As vessel 1 but 5-fold coferment
Sidearm 1	10^{-8} mole yellow ferment in 0.25 ml H_2O	As vessel 1
Sidearm 2	0.1 ml catalase solution	
After addition of yellow ferment in 80 min	−101 cmm O_2, then constant	−101 cmm O_2, then constant
After addition of catalase in 10 min	+44 cmm O_2, then constant	+45 cmm O_2, then constant
Oxygen consumption after H_2O_2 decomposition	−101 + 44 = −57 cmm	−101 + 45 = −56 cmm O_2
$\dfrac{\text{Moles } O_2 \text{ consumed}}{\text{Moles substrate oxidized}}$	0.49	
$\dfrac{\text{Moles } H_2O_2 \text{ formed}}{\text{Moles substrate oxidized}}$	0.77	

At 38°C, Gas phase oxygen; 0.2 ml of 5 percent KOH in center well.

with the addition of 18 ml of 50 percent trichloroacetic acid, and after 1 hr of refrigeration, it was centrifuged. The addition of 3 ml of 1 M barium acetate and 4 ml of 13 N NaOH (phenolphthalein pink) caused a small precipitation that was centrifuged, but the residue was not investigated further. The addition of an equal volume of alcohol precipitated phosphohexonic acid as its neutral barium salt. The precipitate was washed with a little 50 percent alcohol and dissolved in 15 ml of water; N bromine water was added until congo red gave an acidic reaction. The acidic barium salt of the phosphohexonic acid was precipitated using a 5-fold volume alcohol; it weighed 320 mg. After 6 hr drying in high vacuum at 60°C, W. Lüttgens found:

$C_6H_{11}PBaO_{11}$ (mol. wt. 411)	C	H	P	Ba
Calculated	17.5	2.68	7.54	33.3
Found	17.8	2.71	7.23	31.9

The aldose determination, according to the method of M. MacLeod and R. Robison, did not use any iodine.

Eighty mg of the barium salt was treated with 2.61 ml of H_2O and 0.39 ml of

N N_2SO_4. The resulting barium sulfate was centrifuged, and the supernatant, which contained 2 mg of phosphorus per ml (in a 1-dm tube) turned the light $+0.01°$ at the wavelength 546 nm and $+0.28°$ after 2 hr of incubation at 70°C. Thus

$$[\alpha] \, \frac{\text{lactone}}{\text{546 nm}} = 15.6$$

When we oxidized the hexosemonophosphoric acid with bromine, according to the method of R. Robison and E. J. King, to produce phosphohexonic acid, we found

$$[\alpha] \, \frac{\text{lactone}}{\text{546 nm}} = 17.4$$

Fermentation of Phosphohexonic Acid

The addition of phosphohexonic acid, which had been obtained by the oxidation of the ferment system or bromine from hexosemonophosphoric acid, to Lebedew juice causes its fermentation. The rate of CO_2 development is smaller than during fermentation of hexosemonophosphoric acid or glucose, but is of the same order of magnitude. The final values for the CO_2 obtainable from phosphohexonic acid, hexosemonophosphate, and glucose are approximately equal.

This unexpected behavior of phosphohexonic acid in Lebedew juice is explained by the assumption that phosphohexonic acid is first reduced to hexosemonophosphate. In this case phosphohexonic acid would represent the oxidized form of a catalyst whose reduced form is hexosemonophosphate.

To measure the fermentation, we transferred into the main compartment of the cylindrical flask 2 ml of Lebedew juice (from yeast of the Schultheiss–Patzenhofer Brewery) and into the sidearms, 1/100 mmole of the appropriate acid. After the fermentation of the juice had ceased, we added the acids to the main compartment. The results are shown in Table II.

Table II

	(1)	(2)	(3)	(4)	(5)
Main compartment	2 ml Lebedew juice		(pH approx. 5.6)		
Sidearms	1/100 mmole glucose	hexosemonophosphate (1.8 mg)	1/100 mmole phospho- hexonic acid obtained by		0.2 ml H_2O
	0.31 mg P		bromide ferment 0.31 mg P		
	cmm O_2	cmm O_2	cmm O_2	cmm O_2	cmm O_2
After addition					
in 20 min	+294	+246	+124	+152	0
in 60 min	+326	+298	+305	+340	0
in 90 min	+326	+298	+305	+350	0

At 20°C; gas phase, air.

Editor's Comments on Paper 17

17   **Wood, Werkman, Hemingway, and Nier:** Heavy Carbon As a Tracer in Bacterial Fixation of Carbon Dioxide
J. Biol. Chem., **135**, 789–790 (1940)

Renewed interest in the elucidation of metabolic pathways was stimulated by the development of an entirely new research method. The application of "heavy" elements in form of ^{13}C and radioisotopes such as ^{14}C (see Carson, 1948; Calvin et al., 1949) certainly enabled research workers to follow the metabolic path of the carbon skeleton. The use of ^{13}C (Hevesy, 1938) in biochemical research was first introduced by Wood and coworkers (Paper 17) in their investigations into the bacterial fixation of carbon dioxide.

Using this new isotopic technique, Cori and Lipmann (1952) clarified the primary oxidation product of the glucose 6-phosphate oxidation as phosphogluconolactone, which is quickly converted to phosphogluconic acid. Horecker and his group (Horecker and Smyrniotis, 1952) confirmed Dickens's (1938) suggestion that ribose 5-phosphate is the product of phosphogluconic acid oxidation with the help of ^{14}C. The discovery of the cleavage of pentose phosphate to triosephosphate (Marmur and Schlenk, 1951) established the reaction sequence of oxidative glucose 6-phosphate metabolism, with pyruvic acid and carbon dioxide as intermediate and end product, respectively. The individual reaction sequence can be found in the excellent review by Gunsalus et al. (1955).

17

Reprinted from *J. Biol. Chem.*, **135**, 789–790 (1940)

LETTERS TO THE EDITORS

HEAVY CARBON AS A TRACER IN BACTERIAL FIXATION OF CARBON DIOXIDE*

Sirs:

Wood and Werkman[1] postulated that succinic acid is formed by combination of CO_2 and a 3-carbon compound. The validity of this suggestion has now been examined, with C_{13} as a tracer with suspensions of bacteria in C_{13} $NaHCO_3$ solutions. The C_{13} in the products has been determined with a mass spectrograph.

The natural molecular percentage ratio $C_{13}:C_{12}$ is approximately 1.10. Succinic acid is the only product from galactose which contained a concentration of C_{13} substantially differing from that of galactose. Evidently C_{13} CO_2 was fixed in succinic

	Initial NaHCO₃	Final NaHCO₃	Products*			
			Alcohols	Volatile acids	Succinic acid	CO₂
E. coli, mM per l..........	110.0	143.8	51.4†	20.6,‡ 1.12§	52.5	33.8
Galactose, % $C_{13}:C_{12}$......	4.36	2.80	1.07	1.08	1.49	
E. coli, mM per l..........	149.1	167.8	0.0	87.2,‡ 70.2§	34.3	18.7
Pyruvate, % $C_{13}:C_{12}$......	2.65	2.36		1.08, 1.53	1.27	
P. pentosaceum, mM per l..	108.1	80.1	6.2‖	6.1,‡ 90.6¶	21.7	−28.0
Glycerol, % $C_{13}:C_{12}$.......	2.62	2.15	1.19	1.25	1.30	

* 8.63 mM of lactic acid and 1.08 mM of H_2 also were formed in the pyruvate fermentation; 12.00 mM of H_2 in the galactose fermentation.

† Ethyl, ‡ acetic, § formic, ‖ propyl, ¶ propionic.

acid. Pyruvate gave similar results. Formic acid contained fixed CO_2. The quantitative distribution of C_{13} in products of *Propionibacterium pentosaceum* shows general distribution.

* The isotope separation and analysis were supported by a grant to the University of Minnesota for the use of isotopes in biological research by the Rockefeller Foundation.

[1] Wood, H. G., and Werkman, C. H., *Biochem. J.*, **34**, 129 (1940).

Probably CO_2 is fixed by 3-C and 1-C addition, the 4-C compound being converted to propionic acid and propyl alcohol containing fixed CO_2. The observed dilution of C_{13} in the final $NaHCO_3$ indicates that formation of CO_2 occurred from carbon originally from glycerol.

The succinate was converted into malate and fumarate; a heart muscle preparation was used. A portion was then oxidized with permanganate.[2] Malate yields 2 molecules of CO_2 and 1 of acetaldehyde; fumarate yields CO_2 and only a trace of acetaldehyde. A second portion was converted into oxaloacetate with *Micrococcus lysodeikticus.* 1 CO_2 was liberated from each oxaloacetate, with citric acid and aniline.[3] Both methods demonstrate that substantially all the fixed CO_2 is in the carboxyl groups of succinic acid and that the methylene carbons have only the natural complement of C_{13}.

Escherichia coli and *Propionibacterium pentosaceum* fix CO_2 with formation of succinic acid. A possible mechanism is as follows: $CO_2 + CH_3COCOOH = COOH \cdot CH_2 \cdot CO \cdot COOH$, $COOH \cdot CH_2COCOOH + 4H = COOHCH_2 \cdot CH_2COOH + H_2O$.

Bacteriology Section   H. G. WOOD
 Agricultural Experiment Station   C. H. WERKMAN
 Iowa State College
 Ames

Departments of Physiological Chemistry and Physics   ALLEN HEMINGWAY
 University of Minnesota   A. O. NIER
 Minneapolis

Received for publication, July 19, 1940

[2] Friedemann, T. E., and Kendall, A. I., *J. Biol. Chem.,* **82,** 23 (1929).
[3] Ostern, P., *Z. physiol. Chem.,* **218,** 160 (1933).

Editor's Comments on Paper 18

18 **Entner and Doudoroff:** Glucose and Gluconic Acid Oxidation of *Pseudomonas saccharophila*
J. Biol. Chem., **196**, 853–862 (1952)

In their studies with *Pseudomonas saccharophila*, N. Entner and M. Doudoroff observed (Paper 18) that the C_1-labeled glucose was recovered almost quantitatively as carbon dioxide and that the utilization of glucose by this organism involves a split into two three-carbon fragments before oxidative assimilation takes place. Although the latter finding would agree with the classical EMP scheme, the former agrees with the HMP mechanism. Thus a third pathway that branches from glucose 6-phosphate and bears the name of both research workers (Entner–Doudoroff pathway or ED pathway) was discovered. This pathway is unique to microorganisms and has not been detected in animal tissues. The final evidence was provided by Wood and his research group (Wood and Schwerdt, 1953, 1954; Kovachevich and Wood, 1955), who isolated and characterized the corresponding enzymes, 6-phosphogluconic dehydrase and 2-keto-3-deoxy-6-phosphogluconate aldolase. The discovery by Entner and Doudoroff in 1952 brought the number of pathways for glucose utilization to three, all of which are interconnected as is demonstrated in Figure 1, and all of which produce the important intermediate pyruvic acid.

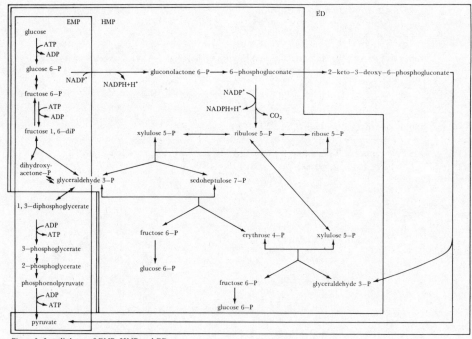

Figure 1. Interlinkage of EMP, HMP and ED
pathways of glucose metabolism

18

Reprinted from *J. Biol. Chem.*, **196**, 853–862 (1952)

GLUCOSE AND GLUCONIC ACID OXIDATION OF PSEUDOMONAS SACCHAROPHILA*

By NATHAN ENTNER and MICHAEL DOUDOROFF

(*From the Department of Bacteriology, University of California, Berkeley, California*)

(Received for publication, December 31, 1951)

There has been increasing evidence recently that the so called "hexose-monophosphate shunt," involving a direct oxidative attack on the C_6 skeleton of glucose, is of fundamental significance in the metabolism of certain microorganisms and perhaps in most biological systems. This oxidative mechanism has been observed in various bacteria (1–9), animal tissues (10–12), molds (13), and even in yeast Lebedev juice (14).

All of the mechanisms of glucose metabolism reported to date, other than the classical Embden-Meyerhof scheme, have in common the fact that CO_2 is produced largely from the 1st carbon atom of glucose. In the Embden-Meyerhof scheme, on the other hand, the carboxyl groups of pyruvic acid, which are an important source of CO_2, are derived from the 3rd and 4th carbon atoms of glucose.

In an experiment with a resting cell suspension of *Pseudomonas saccharophila*, in which C_1-labeled glucose was decomposed aerobically, it was found that the labeled carbon was almost quantitatively recovered as CO_2. Previous experiments suggested that a mechanism other than a primary decarboxylation of a C_6 skeleton to yield a pentose might be operative. It had been shown that (1) intact cells of *P. saccharophila* assimilate almost two-thirds of the carbon of glucose, pyruvate, or lactate, (2) the α- and β-carbons of pyruvate or lactate are assimilated, while the carboxyl group appears almost entirely as CO_2, and (3), when assimilation is inhibited with dinitrophenol (DNP), pyruvic acid accumulates in the oxidation of glucose. These observations suggested that, just as in the classical glycolytic scheme, the utilization of glucose by this organism involves a split into two 3-carbon fragments before oxidative assimilation takes place.

The studies to be reported indicate that such a split of the glucose skeleton does indeed occur, 2 molecules of pyruvic acid being formed from a molecule of glucose. The carboxyl group of 1 of the pyruvic acid molecules is derived from the 1st carbon atom of glucose. The key step in this scheme appears to be the cleavage of 6-phosphogluconic acid or an isomer of this compound to yield pyruvic acid and triosephosphate.

* Part of this work was performed under a contract between the Office of Naval Research and the University of California.

Methods

Cells were grown on a liquid mineral medium as previously described (15), with glucose or sodium gluconate as the sole carbon source.   Resting cell suspensions were prepared by centrifuging liquid cultures inoculated 24 hours previously, washing, and resuspending in $M/30$ phosphate buffer at pH 6.8.   Enzyme preparations were obtained by grinding washed, centrifuged cells with levigated alumina powder according to the method of McIlwain (16) and gradually adding 5 parts of $M/30$ buffer solution of pH 7, either tris(hydroxymethyl)aminomethane or phosphate.   During this operation the containers and solutions were all kept at 0°.   After centrifugation of the alumina-ground cell suspension in a Servall centrifuge at 12,000 r.p.m. for 30 minutes, a clear viscous solution high in protein content was obtained.   This was used immediately or stored at $-20°$ until needed.

Oxygen consumption and CO_2 evolution were determined with the Warburg respirometer.

Pyruvic acid was determined by decarboxylation with ceric sulfate (17) or colorimetrically (18) as carbonate-extractable 2,4-dinitrophenylhydrazone.

Methylglyoxal was determined colorimetrically by preparing the bis-2,4-dinitrophenylhydrazone (or osazone) and developing the color with 5 per cent alcoholic NaOH.   In mixtures of pyruvic acid and methylglyoxal the color contributed by the pyruvate hydrazone was eliminated by washing the bishydrazone with acidic alcohol or by applying simultaneous equations for the color absorption at 440 mμ and 570 mμ on the Beckman spectrophotometer.

Total triose was measured as methylglyoxal after distillation of the sample from 10 per cent H_2SO_4.

Glucose was determined manometrically by oxidation with notatin, the glucose oxidase of *Penicillium notatum* (19).   This method was also used to prepare radioactive gluconate from labeled glucose.

All phosphate determinations were carried out according to the method of Fiske and Subbarow (20).   Triosephosphate was measured as phosphate liberated in N KOH after 20 minutes incubation at room temperature. Dihydroxyacetone phosphate and glyceraldehyde phosphate were differentiated by determining alkali-labile phosphate before and after I_2 oxidation in dilute Na_2CO_3.   To obtain demonstrable amounts it was necessary to trap the triosephosphate with hydrazine sulfate according to the method of Meyerhof and Junowicz-Kocholaty (21).   Adenosinetriphosphate (ATP) was measured as 7 minute-hydrolyzable phosphate.

Radioactivity was determined by drying the sample in question on copper disks and counting in a Geiger-Müller, model 1000B, counting chamber. Counts were made on the hydrazone or bishydrazone of pyruvate or methylglyoxal, respectively, in order to obtain the activity of the parent compound. The activity of the carboxyl group of pyruvate was obtained by collecting the CO_2 liberated from the action of ceric sulfate or yeast carboxylase in CO_2-free KOH, followed by treating according to methods previously described (15).

Oxygen consumption by enzyme preparations was mediated by the use of methylene blue as hydrogen carrier (1:20,000), while experiments conducted under anaerobic conditions were carried out in evacuated Thunberg tubes.

EXPERIMENTAL

Glucose and Gluconate Utilization by P. saccharophila Poisoned with DNP and with Arsenite

Intact cells of *P. saccharophila* were grown, harvested, and studied with the Warburg respirometer as previously described (15). They were allowed to oxidize glucose labeled in the C_1 position[1] with C^{14} in the presence of 0.00025 M DNP and of 0.002 M arsenite respectively. Under proper conditions in the presence of these poisons, pyruvic acid was found to accumulate in the medium, almost in theoretical yield of 2 moles per mole of glucose used (see Table I).

The pyruvic acid was identified[2] and assayed for C^{14} as the 2,4-dinitrophenylhydrazone, and the activity of the carboxyl group was determined by decarboxylation with ceric sulfate and with yeast carboxylase. In all cases the specific activity of pyruvate was found to be very close to half the specific activity of glucose on the molar basis. All of the C^{14} content of pyruvate could be accounted for by the C^{14} content of the carboxyl group. Similar results were obtained with C_1-labeled gluconate[3] as substrate when cells grown with gluconate as substrate were used (see Table I). It therefore appears that 2 molecules of pyruvic acid are formed from glucose or from gluconic acid, the carboxyl group of one of which comes from the 1st carbon atom of the substrate.

Exchange of Carboxyl Groups with CO₂ or Formate

It seemed possible that the C_6 compound might be first degraded to a C_5 compound by the loss of the 1st carbon atom as CO_2 or formic acid, and

---

[1] The C_1-labeled glucose was prepared by Dr. J. C. Sowden and was generously supplied by Dr. W. Z. Hassid of the Division of Plant Biochemistry, University of California, and by Dr. I. C. Gunsalus of the University of Illinois.

[2] Melting point of 2,4-dinitrophenylhydrazone of the reaction product, 214–216°; of 2,4-dinitrophenylhydrazone of pyruvate, 215–216°; mixed melting point, 214–216°; all melting points uncorrected.

[3] The labeled gluconic acid was prepared from C_1-labeled glucose by oxidation with notatin.

that the C_5 compound could give rise to 2 pyruvic acid molecules by a C_2–C_3 split and the subsequent addition of the C_1 fragment to the C_2 fragment. This would imply an equilibration of the carboxyl group of pyruvate formed in the reaction with either CO_2 or formic acid. Experimental evidence does not support the above hypothesis. No exchange

TABLE I

Utilization of C_1-Labeled Glucose and Gluconic Acid by Intact Cells of P. saccharophila in Presence of DNP and Arsenite

The reactions were carried out for from 2 to 3 hours at 30° in the Warburg respirometer. To each vessel were added 2 ml. of cell suspension (D 0.450 with 600 mμ filter on the Klett colorimeter), 0.6 to 0.7 ml. of inhibitors in appropriate concentration, and 0.2 ml. of C_1-labeled glucose or gluconate (0.05 M) from the side arm. When the reaction was complete, the contents of each vessel were removed and centrifuged, and the supernatant or KOH from the center well analyzed by the methods described.

Amounts expressed in micromoles per ml. of reaction mixture; specific activities as counts per micromole per minute.

Substrate Inhibitor	Glucose Dinitrophenol (0.00025 M)	Glucose Arsenite (0.002 M)	Gluconate Arsenite (0.002 M)	Glucose Iodoacetate (0.002 M)
Substrate utilized	1.1	3.49	3.56	2.85
Pyruvic acid produced	1.9	5.82	5.59	2.0
Methylglyoxal produced	*	*	*	2.2
O_2 used	4.0	3.52	2.31	2.7
CO_2 produced	2.9	0.88	1.80	0.8
Specific activity of				
Glucose or gluconate	364	1000	1000	541
Pyruvate	186	515	502	560
Methylglyoxal	*	*	*	4
COOH group of pyruvate	182	530	550	473
Respiratory CO_2	42	350	360	168

* Not determined.

between labeled formate and the carboxyl group of pyruvate could be detected during the oxidation of glucose.

An exchange between labeled CO_2 and the carboxyl group of pyruvate was observed both during the active formation of pyruvate from glucose and after the exhaustion of glucose. However, these exchanges were not great, especially in the presence of DNP (see Table II). It is also significant that in the presence of this poison the specific activity of the respiratory CO_2 produced during glucose oxidation was much lower than the specific activity of the carboxyl group of pyruvate. It is apparent from Table I that in all of the experiments some pyruvate is oxidized to yield CO_2.

Glucose and Gluconate Utilization by P. saccharophila Poisoned with Iodoacetate

Further insight into the mechanism of the glucose oxidation by *P. saccharophila* was gained by using cells poisoned with 0.002 M monoiodo-

TABLE II

Exchange of Carboxyl Group of Pyruvate with CO_2 by Intact Poisoned Cells

Experiments 1 and 5 with labeled glucose in the absence of CO_2. Experiments 2, 4, and 6 with labeled glucose or pyruvate and with inactive CO_2 in the gas phase. Experiments 3 and 7 with inactive glucose and labeled CO_2.

In presence of 0.002 M arsenite				
	Experiment 1	Experiment 2	Experiment 3	Experiment 4
Glucose (initial), μM per vessel	10	10	10	None
CO_2 (initial), % in gas phase	None	10	3.5	10
Pyruvate (initial), μM per vessel	"	None	None	17.8
" (final), " " "	17.8	18.6	18.8	18.8
Specific activity (counts per μM per min.) of				
Glucose (initial)	1180	1180	0	
CO_2 (initial)		0	20,700	0
COOH of pyruvic acid (initial)				609
COOH of pyruvic acid (final)	609	550	1,920	517

In presence of 0.00025 M DNP			
	Experiment 5	Experiment 6	Experiment 7
Glucose (initial), μM per vessel	Not determined		
CO_2 (initial), % in gas phase	None	10	3.5
Pyruvate (final), μM per vessel	12.3	15.5	11.2
Specific activity (counts per μM per min.) of			
Glucose (initial)	1180	1180	0
CO_2 (initial)		0	20,700
COOH of pyruvic acid (final)	603	573	473

acetate (see Table I). Under these circumstances the reaction proceeds with an oxygen uptake of approximately 0.5 mole per mole of glucose, as indicated by a sudden sharp break in the rate of oxygen uptake. The principal accumulated products in the medium were found to be pyruvate and methylglyoxal. These were identified by their respective hydrazone and bishydrazone.[4] 1 mole of glucose yielded approximately 1 mole each

[4] Melting point of 2,4-dinitrophenylhydrazone of the reaction product, 214-216°; of 2,4-dinitrophenylhydrazone of pyruvate, 215-216°; mixed melting point, 214-216°;

of pyruvic acid and methylglyoxal. Small quantities of as yet unidentified products (probably triose) also appeared to be present. By again employing C_1-labeled glucose, the portion of the hexose skeleton from which each of the two C_3 fragments is derived was determined. The pyruvic acid was found to have the same specific activity as the glucose, all of the C^{14} being in the carboxyl group. The methylglyoxal, on the other hand, was completely inactive.

When gluconate was provided as substrate to gluconate-adapted cells poisoned with iodoacetate, the same two products were obtained and identified.

Experiments with Enzyme Preparations from Glucose-Grown Cells

The occurrence of the pathway for glucose oxidation thus far indicated in experiments with intact cells was substantiated by experiments with enzymes obtained by grinding the cells with levigated alumina.

Initial Phosphorylation (Hexokinase)—The necessity for an initial phosphorylation soon became apparent when it was found that the enzyme preparations could reduce methylene blue in evacuated Thunberg tubes upon the addition of glucose-6-phosphate but not of glucose. A hexokinase reaction was demonstrated by the disappearance of 7 minute-hydrolyzable phosphate when the enzyme preparation was incubated with glucose and ATP. The product of the reaction between ATP and glucose was tentatively identified as glucose-6-phosphate. Fructose-6-phosphate was also formed, indicating the presence of phosphohexoisomerase. An assay for fructose-6-phosphate, coupled with a study of the rate of hydrolysis of the barium-soluble fraction of the mixture of phosphoric esters, indicated that the mixture contained 23.5 per cent fructose-6-phosphate and 76.5 per cent glucose-6-phosphate. This corresponds closely to the previously known ratio of the two compounds under equilibrium conditions.

Oxidation of Glucose-6-phosphate—An appreciable rate of oxygen uptake could be obtained with glucose-6-phosphate as substrate, provided methylene blue was employed as a hydrogen carrier. Glucose, on the other hand, did not increase the oxygen uptake above the endogenous rate. Thus, with 2.5 ml. of reaction mixture, containing 2.0 ml. of enzyme preparation, 0.1 ml. of 0.1 per cent methylene blue, and 0.1 γ each of diphosphopyridine nucleotide and triphosphopyridine nucleotide, after aerobic incubation for 180 minutes at 30°, 1.6 μM of oxygen were taken up in the absence of substrate, 1.65 μM in the presence of 20 μM of glucose, and 4.1 μM in the presence of 20 μM of glucose-6-phosphate. With the last substrate only 1.2 μM of CO_2 were produced. In the presence of arsenite pyruvic acid was found

of bishydrazone of the reaction product, 305–307°; of bishydrazone of methylglyoxal, 305–307°; mixed melting point, 305–307° (all uncorrected).

to accumulate, thus revealing the presence of the entire complement of enzymes necessary for the production of pyruvate from glucose-6-phosphate.

Utilization of 6-Phosphogluconate—To show that 6-phosphogluconate could be attacked at a rate commensurate with the utilization of glucose-6-phosphate, the rate of production of pyruvate from these substrates was measured. In the presence of methylene blue and 0.002 M arsenite, pyruvate was formed at almost identical rates from either substrate. In an experiment in which the enzyme preparation was shaken under aerobic conditions at 30° with glucose-6-phosphate and with 6-phosphogluconate, 8 μM of each per ml., respectively, in the presence of 0.004 per cent methylene blue, 0.002 M arsenite, and 0.04 γ each of diphosphopyridine nucleotide and triphosphopyridine nucleotide, 1.8 μM of pyruvic acid were produced per ml. per hour from the former substrate and 1.94 μM from the latter.

Anaerobic Split of 6-Phosphogluconate to Pyruvic Acid and Triosephosphate—It is apparent from previous experiments that the conversion of 6-phosphogluconate to two C_3 compounds should not require the presence of oxygen. Under anaerobic conditions 6-phosphogluconate could readily be observed to undergo a split to approximately equal amounts of pyruvic acid and a 3-carbon compound on the oxidation level of a triose. That this compound is not methylglyoxal was clear from the fact that practically no bishydrazone was formed upon the addition of 2,4-dinitrophenylhydrazine to the reaction mixture. Upon distillation from 10 per cent H_2SO_4, however, methylglyoxal was found abundantly in the distillate, demonstrating the presence of a triose.

Since methylglyoxal was not formed directly in the reaction, analyses were carried out both for triosephosphate and free triose as products of cleavage of 6-phosphogluconate. However, due to a rapid phosphatase reaction, triosephosphate (as alkali-hydrolyzable phosphate) could be demonstrated only in minute amounts. The use of fluoride as a phosphatase inhibitor or of cyanide as a "trapping agent" proved to be ineffective, since these poisons apparently prevent the cleavage of 6-phosphogluconic acid. On the other hand, when 0.05 M hydrazine sulfate was added to the reaction mixture and the hydrazine subsequently removed with benzaldehyde, considerable alkali-hydrolyzable phosphate was found to accumulate. If the reaction was allowed to proceed for a short time (10 minutes) in the presence of hydrazine, all of the triose could be accounted for as the phosphorylated compound. The disappearance of the bulk of the alkali-hydrolyzable phosphate after iodine oxidation indicates that the compound in question is glyceraldehyde phosphate.

When 2 ml. of enzyme preparation were allowed to react for 10 minutes in a 30° water bath in the presence of 20 μM of 6-phosphogluconate and 0.05 M neutralized hydrazine sulfate, an analysis of the products showed the accumulation of 1.12 μM per ml. of pyruvic acid, 1.20 μM per ml. of alkali-hydrolyzable phosphate, and 1.10 μM per ml. of total triose, indicating that all of the latter compound exists in the phosphorylated form. After iodine oxidation according to the method of Meyerhof and Junowicz-Kocholaty (21), there was a disappearance of the alkali-hydrolyzable phosphate to the same extent that iodine oxidation caused the disappearance of alkali-labile phosphate from known solutions of glyceraldehyde phosphate (about 80 per cent under the conditions that were employed).

Pyruvate Production from Phosphoglyceric Acid and Glyceraldehyde Phosphate—Pyruvate formation could be observed quite readily when phosphoglyceric acid was incubated anaerobically with the enzyme preparation, although measurable amounts of phosphoenol pyruvate could not be demonstrated. The aerobic formation of pyruvate from glyceraldehyde phosphate, however, proceeded rather poorly, owing probably to the very strong phosphatase activity of the enzyme preparation with this compound. No pyruvate was formed by the enzyme preparations from non-phosphorylated glyceric acid or glyceraldehyde.[5]

DISCUSSION

The above experiments show that glucose and gluconic acid can be metabolized by *P. saccharophila* through the cleavage of a 6-carbon compound on the oxidative level of gluconic acid to yield 1 molecule of pyruvic acid and 1 of glyceraldehyde phosphate. The utilization of glucose appears to involve the phosphorylation of this compound to glucose-6-phosphate and its oxidation to 6-phosphogluconic acid. The latter compound is then split in such a way as to give rise to pyruvic acid, the carboxyl group of which is derived from the C_1 position, and to glyceraldehyde phosphate. It seems likely that a rearrangement of the phosphogluconic acid molecule takes place prior to the split. An intermediate which would fulfil the requirements would be 2-keto-3-desoxy-6-phosphogluconic acid, the carboxylated analogue of desoxyribose-5-phosphate. The cleavage of such a compound would be analogous to that reported by Racker (22), in which desoxyribose-5-phosphate gives rise to acetaldehyde and glyceraldehyde phosphate. Such a compound has not yet been found in the reaction mixtures or prepared synthetically.

It has further been shown that phosphoglyceraldehyde (though poorly) as well as phosphoglyceric acid gives rise to pyruvic acid under appropriate conditions in the presence of enzyme preparations, while glyceraldehyde

---

[5] Glyceric acid and phosphoglyceric acid were generously supplied by Dr. H. A. Barker of the Division of Plant Biochemistry, University of California, glyceraldehyde (DL mixture) by Dr. H. O. L. Fischer of the Department of Biochemistry, University of California, and the glyceraldehyde phosphate (DL mixture) by Dr. E. Baer of the University of Toronto.

and glyceric acid are not attacked. This suggests the operation of the classical mechanism for the oxidation of trioses (23–26). The effect of iodoacetate on intact cells supports this view.

The massive conversion *in vivo* of triosephosphate to methylglyoxal in the presence of iodoacetate appears to be a new phenomenon, which again revives the question of the possible biological rôle of this compound, which was suggested in early experiments of Neuberg and Kobel (27). Though one must be aware of the possibility of a spontaneous conversion of triose to methylglyoxal, this does not appear to be the case in view of the almost quantitative accumulation of the latter compound and the failure to obtain an observable reduction of Fehling's solution in the cold.

The further oxidation of the pyruvate formed from glucose by intact cells to yield CO_2 and cell material appears to follow the pattern previously postulated on the basis of a comparison of the oxidative assimilation with different substrates and of the interpretation of experiments with labeled compounds (28, 29, 15). The carboxyl group of the pyruvic acid appears as CO_2, while most of the rest of the carbon atoms are assimilated. This explains the almost quantitative recovery of the 1st carbon atom of glucose as respiratory CO_2, and the assimilation of two-thirds of the glucose molecule. It is, at present, impossible to say whether the phosphopyruvic acid which is probably formed is oxidized directly or first dephosphorylated.

The above reactions involved in the degradation of glucose may be summarized in sequence as follows:

(1) Glucose $\xrightarrow{\text{ATP}}$ glucose-6-phosphate

(2) Glucose-6-phosphate $\xrightarrow{\frac{1}{2}O_2}$ 6-phosphogluconic acid

(3) 6-Phosphogluconic acid $\rightarrow$ (?) $\rightarrow$ pyruvic acid + 3-phosphoglyceraldehyde

(4) 3-Phosphoglyceraldehyde $\xrightarrow[\text{(intact cells)}]{\frac{1}{2}O_2}$ 3-phosphoglyceric acid

(4, *a*) 3-Phosphoglyceraldehyde $\xrightarrow[\text{(enzyme preparation)}]{-\text{phosphate}}$ triose (glyceraldehyde?)

(4, *b*) 3-Phosphoglyceraldehyde $\xrightarrow[\text{(intact cells, IAc)}]{-\text{phosphate, } -H_2O}$ methylglyoxal

(5) 3-Phosphoglyceric acid $\xrightarrow{-\text{phosphate, } -H_2O}$ pyruvic acid

(6) 2 pyruvic acid $\xrightarrow[\text{(intact cells)}]{O_2}$ $2CO_2 + 4(CH_2O)$(cell material)

The authors wish to thank Dr. P. K. Stumpf, Dr. H. A. Barker, Dr. H. O. L. Fischer, and Mr. E. Putman for their generous advice and for some of the chemicals used in the experiments.

SUMMARY

1. In studies with intact cells and crude enzyme preparations of *Pseudomonas saccharophila*, it has been shown that glucose and gluconic acid can be utilized in such a way as to yield 2 pyruvic acid molecules, the carboxyl group of one of which is derived from C_1 of glucose.

2. The utilization of glucose appears to involve its phosphorylation to glucose-6-phosphate, the oxidation of this compound to 6-phosphogluconic acid, and the subsequent cleavage to yield pyruvic acid from the first 3 carbon atoms and glyceraldehyde phosphate from the last 3.

3. Glyceraldehyde phosphate can then be converted to pyruvic acid by intact cells poisoned with dinitrophenol or arsenite, to free triose by enzyme preparations, or to methylglyoxal by intact cells poisoned with iodoacetate.

4. The previous observations on the oxidative assimilation with glucose and the appearance of the C_1 of glucose as respiratory CO_2 are in complete agreement with the proposed scheme of glucose degradation.

BIBLIOGRAPHY

1. Cohen, S. S., and Raff, F., *J. Biol. Chem.*, **188,** 501 (1951).
2. Scott, D. B. M., and Cohen, S. S., *J. Biol. Chem.*, **188,** 509 (1951).
3. Cohen, S. S., *J. Biol. Chem.*, **189,** 617 (1951).
4. Cohen, S. S., *Bact. Rev.*, **15,** 131 (1951).
5. Stokes, F. N., and Campbell, J. J. R., *Arch. Biochem.*, **30,** 121 (1951).
6. Entner, N., and Stanier, R. Y., *J. Bact.*, **62,** 181 (1951).
7. Rappoport, D. A., Barker, H. A., and Hassid, W. Z., *Arch. Biochem. and Biophys.*, **31,** 326 (1951).
8. Lampen, J. O., Gest, H., and Sowden, J. C., *J. Bact.*, **61,** 97 (1951).
9. Gibbs, M., and DeMoss, R. D., *Federation Proc.*, **10,** 189 (1951).
10. Dickens, F., *Nature*, **138,** 1057 (1936).
11. Dickens, F., *Biochem. J.*, **32,** 1628, 1645 (1938).
12. Dickens, F., and Glock, G. E., *Nature*, **166,** 33 (1950).
13. Foster, J. W., Chemical activities of fungi, New York, chapter 15 (1949).
14. Horecker, B. L., and Smyrniotis, P. Z., *Federation Proc.*, **10,** 199 (1951).
15. Wiame, J. M., and Doudoroff, M., *J. Bact.*, **62,** 187 (1951).
16. McIlwain, H., *J. Gen. Microbiol.*, **2,** 288 (1948).
17. Krebs, H. A., and Johnson, W. A., *Biochem. J.*, **31,** 645 (1937).
18. Friedemann, T. E., and Haugen, G. E., *J. Biol. Chem.*, **147,** 415 (1943).
19. Birkinshaw, J. H., and Raistrick, H., *J. Biol. Chem.*, **148,** 459 (1943).
20. Fiske, C. H., and Subbarow, Y., *J. Biol. Chem.*, **66,** 375 (1925).
21. Meyerhof, O., and Junowicz-Kocholaty, R., *J. Biol. Chem.*, **149,** 71 (1943).
22. Racker, E., *Nature*, **167,** 408 (1951).
23. Meyerhof, O., and Lohmann, K., *Biochem. Z.*, **271,** 102 (1934); **273,** 60 (1934).
24. Warburg, O., and Christian, W., *Biochem. Z.*, **286,** 81 (1936).
25. Meyerhof, O., Ohlmeyer, P., and Mohle, W., *Biochem. Z.*, **297,** 113 (1938).
26. Negelein, E., and Brömel, H., *Biochem. Z.*, **301,** 135 (1939).
27. Neuberg, C., and Kobel, M., *Biochem. Z.*, **203,** 463 (1928).
28. Doudoroff, M., *Enzymologia*, **9,** 59 (1940).
29. Doudoroff, M., Kaplan, N., and Hassid, W. Z., *J. Biol. Chem.*, **148,** 67 (1943).

Editor's Comments on Paper 19

19   **Krebs and Johnson:** The Role of Citric Acid in Intermediate Metabolism in Animal Tissues
    Enzymologia, **4**, 148–156 (1937)

Parallel to the pathway investigations, interest in the energetics of these pathways was stimulated (Dische, 1936–1937). It was Hans Krebs and his renowned research team who made the breakthrough in the oxidative breakdown of carbohydrates. In their epoch-making publication (Paper 19), Krebs and Johnson reported that citric acid promotes oxidation in muscle in the presence of carbohydrates and 2-oxoglutarate and succinate were obtained as products of this oxidation. A further observation noted that citric acid was produced upon addition of oxalacetate to muscle. From these observations Krebs concluded that the necesary C_2 compound for this condensation must come from the carbohydrate metabolism. Thus the "citric acid cycle," "tricarboxylic acid cycle," or "Krebs cycle," was discovered. With this cycle it was now possible to explain why the main end product of oxidative carbohydrate utilization was carbon dioxide (Krebs, 1943).

At the same time it was also recognized that the fundamental branching-off point for anaerobic and aerobic carbohydrate utilization must be at the pyruvate level (Lipmann, 1937, 1954).

19

Reprinted from *Enzymologia*, **4**, 148–156 (1937)

The role of citric acid in intermediate metabolism in animal tissues

BY

H. A. KREBS AND W. A. JOHNSON

(From the Departm. of Pharmacol., Univ. of Sheffield)

(29.VI.37)

During the last decade much progress has been made in the analysis of the anaerobic fermentation of carbohydrate, but very little is so far known about the intermediate stages of the oxidative breakdown of carbohydrate. A number of reactions are known in which derivatives of carbohydrate take part and which are probably steps in the breakdown of carbohydrate; we know furthermore, from the work of Szent-Györgyi [20] that succinic acid, fumaric acid and oxaloacetic acid play some role in the oxidation of carbohydrate, but the details of this role are still obscure.

In the present paper experiments are reported which throw new light on the problem of the intermediate stages of oxidation of carbohydrate; in conjunction with the work of Szent-Györgyi [20], Stare and Baumann [19] and Martius and Knoop [13, 14] the new experiments allow us to outline the principal steps of the oxidation of sugar in animal tissues.

I. Methods.

1. Tissue. Pigeon breast muscle was used for the majority of the experiments described in this paper. The tissue was minced in a LATAPIE mincer immediately after killing and usually suspended in 3—7 volumes of 0,1 M sodium phosphate buffer (ph = 7,4). On further dilution of the suspension the rate of metabolism decreased.

2. Quantitative determination of citric acid. The method of PUCHER, SHERMAN and VICKERY [17] was used; citric acid is oxidised to pentabromoacetone which is subsequently converted by means of sodium sulphide to a coloured material suitable for colorimetric determination. As pointed out by PUCHER c.s. the method is suitable for the determination of quantities between 0,1 and 1 mg. It is fairly specific; there are only a few other substances which yield also a yellow coloured material, and the only substance which interfered in our experiments was oxaloacetic acid. In pure solution 0,5 millimol oxaloacetate yielded $1,98 \cdot 10^{-3}$ millimol ,,citric acid''. The yield of ,,citric acid'' is increased by 50 % if pyruvic acid is present at the same time and this suggests that bromine, like hydrogen peroxide (MARTIUS and KNOOP [13]) brings about a synthesis of citric acid from oxaloacetic and pyruvic acid. This interfering reaction can be removed if oxaloacetic acid is decomposed by heating the solution for one hour in neutral or weakly acid medium after deproteinisation. Although oxaloacetate is not completely decomposed if heated in pure solution the destruction is practically complete in the deproteinised tissue extract. This effect may be explained by the observations of POLLAK [16] and LJUNGGREN [10] which demonstrate a catalytic influence of amino compounds on the decompositions of β-ketonic acids.

3. Quantitative determination of succinic acid. The method used was a modification of SZENT-GYÖRGYI's [20] manometric method. The details will be described in full elsewhere.

4. Quantitative determination of α-ketoglutaric acid. The α-ketoglutaric acid was quantitatively determined by estimation of the amount of succinic acid formed on oxidation. In an aliquot sample the preformed succinic acid is determined and the figure obtained is substracted from the sample treated with the oxidising agent. Suitable oxidising agents are cold permanganate or ceric sulphate in acid medium. Under our conditions both reagents gave identical results. The ceric sulphate method is better if significant amounts of α-hydroxyglutaric acid or glutamic acid are present, since these two substances react more readily with permanganate than with ceric sulphate to yield succinic acid. Citric acid, iso-citric acid and cis-aconitic acid do not yield succinic acid if treated with permanganate or ceric sulphate.

5. Quantitative determination of succinic acid in the presence of malonic and α-ketoglutaric acid. Malonic acid interferes with the manometric determination of succinic acid and has therefore to be removed first. The removal is brought about by a principle suggested by

WEIL-MALHERBE [22]). To the neutral solution containing the three substances are added 1 ccm 2 M sodium sulphite and 2 ccm 3 M tartaric acid and the solution is then extracted continuously with ether in a KUTSCHER-STEUDEL [9]) extractor. Under our conditions extraction of succinic acid was complete in 30 minutes, whilst α-ketoglutaric acid remains quantitatively in the aqueous phase. The ethereal extract which also contains malonic acid is freed from ether, dissolved in water and treated with permanganate in acid solution in order to destroy the malonic acid and is then extracted with ether again. This second ethereal extract contains the succinic acid ready for the manometric determination.

   6. Metabolic Quotients. According to the usual convention the quantities of metabolites are expressed in μl even if they are not gases; 1 millimol citric acid, for instance, is considered equivalent to $22400\,\mu l$. The rate of metabolic reaction is expressed by the quotient $\dfrac{\text{substrate metabolised}}{\text{mg dry tissue} \times \text{hour}}$ In the case of muscle the dry weight was considered to be 20 % of the wet weight.

II. Catalytic effect of citrate on respiration.

   If muscle tissue is minced and suspended in 6 volumes of phosphate buffer a high rate of respiration is observed initially, but after 20—40 minutes the rate begins to fall off. If citrate is added the rate of respiration is often increased and the falling off of respiration is always much retarded. This effect is brought about by small quantities of citrate, and comparing the extra respiration with the citrate added we find that the extra oxygen uptake is by far greater than can be accounted for by the complete oxidation of citrate. An example is the following experiment:

TABLE I.

Effect of citrate on respiration of minced pigeon breast muscle.
(Manometric experiment)

Time (min.)	$\mu l\ O_2$ absorbed by 460 mg muscle (wet weight) suspended in 3 ccm phosphate saline	
	No substrate added	0,15 ccm 0,02 M sodium citrate added
30	645	682
60	1055	1520
90	1132	1938
150	1187	2080

   In this experiment the citrate caused an increased respiration of $893\,\mu l$, whilst $302\,\mu l\ O_2$ are calculated for the complete oxidation of the citrate added.

   The magnitude of the effect of citrate shows considerable variations from experiment to experiment; the effect appears to be dependent on the amounts of citrate and other substrates preformed in the tissue. The effect is more pronounced if glycogen, or hexosediphosphate, or α-glycerophosphate are added to the muscle, and we presume therefore that the substrate the oxidation of which is catalysed by citrate, is a carbohydrate or a related substance.

   An example in which citrate promotes catalytically the oxidation of α-glycerophosphate is given in Table II. There is only a small effect of citrate in this experiment if added alone to the suspension, but a very considerable effect is observed if α-glycerophosphate is present.

   SZENT-GYÖRGYI [20]) and STARE and BAUMANN [19]) have shown that fumarate, oxaloacetate, and succinate have a similar catalytic effect under the same experimental conditions, a fact of great importance to which we shall refer later.

   The problem of the mechanism of this citrate catalysis can be approached in various ways.

TABLE II.

Effect of citrate on the respiration of pigeon breast muscle in the presence of α-glycerophosphate.

(40°; 140 min.; 460 mg muscle (wet weight) in 3 ccm phosphate saline per flask; manometric experiment)

Substrates added	μl O$_2$ absorbed
—	342
0,15 ccm 0,02 M citrate	431
0,3 ccm 0,2 M glycerophosphate	757
0,3 ccm 0,2 M glycerophosphate + 0,15 ccm 0,02 M citrate	1385

We have chosen the investigation of the intermediate stages of the breakdown of citrate in the tissues. If all the stages are known the mechanism of the catalytic effect will be clear.

III.   Rate of disappearance of citric acid in muscle.

Since citric acid reacts catalytically in the tissue it is probable that it is removed by a primary reaction but regenerated by a subsequent reaction. In the balance sheet no citrate disappears and no intermediate products accumulate. The first object of the study of intermediates is therefore to find conditions under which citrate disappears in the balance sheet. We find that some poisons bring about this effect, for instance arsenite (Table III) or malonate. If one of these two substances is present, very large amounts of citric acid disappear provided that oxygen is available. Obviously the poisons leave the breakdown of citric acid unaffected whilst they check the synthesis of citric acid.

TABLE III.

Disappearance of citric acid in pigeon breast muscle in the presence of arsenite (3.10^{-3} mol.).

(3 ccm muscle suspension containing 750 mg wet muscle were shaken for 40 min. at 40°)

μl citrate added	μl citrate found after 40 min.	μl citrate used	Q$_{citrate}$
1120	30	1090	—10,9
2240	972	1268	—12,7
4480	2790	1690	—16,9

IV.   Conversion of citric acid into α-ketoglutaric acid.

The oxidation of citric acid in the presence of arsenite or malonate is not complete. Only one or two molecules of oxygen are absorbed for each molecule of citric acid removed and the solution must therefore contain intermediate products of oxidation of citric acid.

Although it has long been known that citric acid is readily metabolised (see ÖSTBERG [15]), SHERMAN c.s. [18])), the pathway of the breakdown remained obscure until early 1937, when

MARTIUS and KNOOP [13, 14]) working with citrico dehydrogenase from liver discovered that the oxidation of citric acid by methylene blue yields α-ketoglutaric acid. We are able to confirm MARTIUS and KNOOP's results with other tissues and with molecular oxygen as the oxidising agent.

In previous work it had been shown that arsenite is a specific inhibitor for the oxidation of α-ketonic acid in animal tissues. It had been possible, for example, to stop the oxidation of glutamic acid [6]) and of proline [23]) at the stage of α-ketoglutaric acid. We find now that large quantities of α-ketoglutaric acid are present in those suspensions in which citric acid was oxidised in the presence of arsenite.

For example: 46 grammes (wet weight) of minced muscle was suspended in 145 ccm phosphate buffer and shaken in an atmosphere of oxygen for one hour in three large flasks of the shape described previously ([5]) with 11,5 ccm 1 M citrate and 6 ccm 0,1 M arsenite. After one hour 40 ccm of trichloro-acetic acid (30 %) was added and 190 ccm filtrate was treated with 1 gramme 2,4 dinitrophenyl-hydrazine dissolved in 100 ccm 2 N HCl. A precipitate was formed immediately. It was collected after two hours on a sintered glass filter, and thoroughly washed with 0,1 N hydrochloric acid and water. The precipitate weighed 1,199 grammes and proved to be practically pure 2,4-dinitrophenyl-hydrazone of α-ketoglutaric acid (M.P. 217° C). On recrystallisation from aqueous alcohol a substance was obtained which gave the correct melting and mixed melting points (222° C). The calculated total yield of dinitrophenylhydrazone is $1{,}199 \frac{249}{190} = 1{,}57$ grammes, or 4,82 millimol.

The quantitative analysis of the deproteinised filtrate with the manometric method gave no succinic acid, but 0,0612 millimol α-ketoglutaric acid per 3 ccm filtrate or 5,07 millimol in the total volume. Both methods, isolation and manometric method, thus agree very well, the former as expected giving a slightly lower figure.

The determination of citric acid in another aliquot of the filtrate showed that 4,64 mg of citric acid were left per ccm liquid, or 6,02 millimol in the total volume. The amount of citric acid added was 11,5 millimol so that the amount metabolised was 5,48 millimol. The yield of α-ketoglutaric acid as will be seen from Table 4 is thus as complete as could be expected in the circumstances.

TABLE IV.

Citric acid metabolised	5,48	millimol	
α-Ketoglutaric acid formed (manometrically)	5,07	,,	(yield 93 %)
α-Ketoglutaric acid formed (as hydrazone) .	4,82	,,	(yield 88 %)

V. Conversion of citric acid into succinic acid.

In the presence of malonate the oxidation of citrate is checked at the stage of succinic acid as shown by the following experiment: 7,5 grammes (wet weight) minced pigeon muscle were suspended in 22,5 ccm phosphate buffer (0,1 M; ph = 7,4) and 3 ccm 0,2 M sodium citrate and 1 ccm 1 M malonate were added. The suspension was shaken for 40 min. in an atmosphere of oxygen, and then deproteinised by adding 34 ccm water, 2 ccm 50 % sulphuric acid and 2 ccm 15 % sodium tungstate. In the filtrate succinic and α-ketoglutaric acids were determined manometrically. 3 ccm contained 472 μl succinic acid and 80 μl α-ketoglutaric acid; α-keto-glutaric acid was also identified by the isolation of the 2,4-dinitrophenylhydrazone.

VI. Synthesis of citric acid in the presence of oxaloacetic acid.

The new results of the citric acid breakdown, in conjunction with previous work on the oxidation of succinic acid in tissues may be summarised by the following series:

citric acid → α-ketoglutaric acid → succinic acid → fumaric acid → l-malic acid → oxaloacetic acid → pyruvic acid.

If it is true that the oxidation of citric acid is a stage in the catalytic action of citric acid then it follows that citric acid must be regenerated eventually from one of the products of oxidation. We are thus led to examine whether citric acid can be resyn-thesised from any of the intermediates of the citric acid breakdown.

Systematic experiments show that indeed large quantities of citric acid are formed if oxaloacetic acid is added to muscle anaerobically, whilst all the other intermediates, including pyruvic acid yield no citric acid under the same conditions. It is because the synthesis of citric acid from oxaloacetic acid does not require molecular oxygen and because citric acid is stable in the tissue anaerobically that it is possible to demonstrate the synthesis of citric acid in a simple experiment.

Minced pigeon breast muscle was suspended as usual in 3 volumes phosphate buffer and 3 ccm suspension were measured into a conical manometric flask the sidearm of which contained 0,3 ccm 1 M oxaloacetate. In the centre chamber a stick of yellow phosphorus was placed and the gas space was filled with nitrogen. After the removal of oxygen the oxaloacetate was added to the tissue and the flask was shaken in the water bath for 20 mins. During this period about $1000 \mu l$ CO_2 were evolved. After the incubation, the suspension was quantitatively transferred into 25 ccm 6 % trichloracetic acid and the volume was made up to 50 ccm. Citric acid was determined in the filtrate and 0,0131 millimol (293 μl) citric acid were found. Qcitrate is thus $\dfrac{293 \times 3}{150} = 5,86$. No citrate was present in the controls.

This experiment shows that muscle is capable of forming large quantities of citric acid if oxaloacetic acid is present and the question arises from which substance the two additional carbon atoms of the citric acid molecule are derived. Addition of various possible precursors such as acetate, or pyruvate, or of α-glycerophosphate had no effect on the rate of citric acid synthesis, but this negative result is no proof against the participation in the synthesis of one of these substances. Pyruvic acid and acetic acid arise rapidly from oxaloacetic acid and it may be that the tissue is already saturated with these substances if oxaloacetic acid alone has been added.

The fact that the catalytic effect of citrate is more pronounced if glycogen, or hexose-monophosphate, or α-glycerophosphate are present suggests that the substance condensing with oxaloacetate is derived from carbohydrate. We may term it provisionally as ,,triose'', leaving it open whether triose reacts as such or as a derivative for example as a phosphate ester, or pyruvic acid or acetic acid.

A synthesis of citric acid from a C_4-dicarboxylic acid and a second substance has often been discussed, especially with reference to the citric acid fermentation of moulds (see [1, 24]), though it has not been shown before to occur in animal tissues.

MARTIUS and KNOOP [12] showed recently that citric acid is formed in vitro if oxaloacetate and pyruvate are treated with hydrogen peroxide in alkaline medium. This model reaction is an interesting analogy and it suggests that the synthesis of citric acid may be a comparatively simple reaction *).

VII. Role of citric acid in the intermediate metabolism.

1. Citric acid cycle. The relevent facts concerning the intermediate metabolism of citric acid may now be summarised as follows:

1. Citrate promotes catalytically the oxidations in muscle tissue, especially if carbohydrates have been added to the tissue.

2. Similar catalytic effects are shown by succinate, fumarate, malate, oxalo-acetate (SZENT-GYÖRGYI [20], STARE and BAUMANN [19]).

3. The oxidation of citrate in muscle passes through the following stages: citric acid → α-ketoglutaric acid → succinic acid → fumaric acid → l-malic acid → oxaloacetic acid.

4. Oxaloacetic acid reacts with an unknown substance to form citric acid.

-----

*) See also the work of CLAISEN and HORI [3].

These facts suggest that citric acid acts as a catalyst in the oxidation of carbohydrate in the following manner:

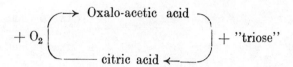

$$+ O_2 \quad \longrightarrow \text{Oxalo-acetic acid} \quad + \text{"triose"}$$
$$\text{citric acid} \longleftarrow$$

According to this scheme oxaloacetic acid condenses with „triose" to form citric acid, and by oxidation of citric acid oxaloacetic acid is regenerated. The net effect of the „citric acid cycle" is the complete oxidation of „triose".

The synthesis of citric acid from oxaloacetic acid as well as the oxidation of citric acid to oxaloacetic has been experimentally verified. The only hypothetical point in the scheme is the term „triose", though we may consider it as certain that the substance condensing with oxaloacetic acid is related to carbohydrate.

The proposed scheme outlines a pathway for the oxidation of carbohydrate. Many details must necessarily be left open at the present time, but a few points will be discussed in the following sections.

2. Origin of the C_4-dicarboxylic acid. According to the scheme succinic acid or a related compound is necessary as „carrier" for the oxidation of carbohydrate and the question of the origin of succinic acid arises. We have shown previously ([8]) that succinic acid can be synthesised by animal tissues in small amounts if pyruvic acid is available. The physiological significance of the synthesis is now clear: it provides the carrier required for the oxidation of carbohydrate.

3. Further intermediate stages. (a) iso-Citric acid. WAGNER-JAUREGG and RAUEN [22]) and MARTIUS and KNOOP [13,14]) have suggested that iso-citric acid is an intermediate in the oxidation of citric acid. We find that iso-citric acid is indeed readily oxidised in muscle, the rates of oxidation of citric acid and iso-citric acids being about the same.

(b) cis-Aconitic acid. cis-aconitic acid, discovered by MALACHOWSKI and MASLOWSKI[11]), was first discussed as an intermediate by MARTIUS and KNOOP [13]) and MARTIUS[14]) showed that it yields readily citric acid with liver. We have examined the behaviour of cis-aconitic acid in muscle and other tissues and find that it is oxidised as readily as citric acid. The conversion of cis-aconitic acid into citric acid is also brought about by tissue extracts. One milligramme muscle tissue (dry weight) converts up to 0,1 mg cis-aconitic acid into citric acid per hour (40°; ph = 7,4).

MARTIUS and KNOOP [13,14]) assume that the reaction cis-aconitic $\rightleftarrows$ citric acid is reversible and believe that it plays a role in the breakdown of citric acid. It cannot yet be said, however, whether the reaction is an intermediate step in the breakdown or in the synthesis of citric acid.

(c) Oxalo-succinic acid. The oxidation of iso-citric acid would be expected to yield in the first stage oxalo-succinic acid (MARTIUS and KNOOP). This β-ketonic acid is only known in the form of its esters, since the free acid is unstable in a pure state. In acid solution it is readily decarboxylated and yields α-ketoglutaric acid (BLAISE and GAULT [2])).

(d) Detailed citric acid cycle. The information available at present about the intermediate steps of the cycle may be summarised thus:

154

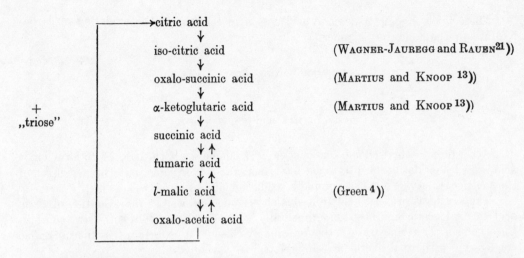

+
„triose"

citric acid
↓
iso-citric acid   (WAGNER-JAUREGG and RAUEN[21])
↓
oxalo-succinic acid   (MARTIUS and KNOOP [13])
↓
α-ketoglutaric acid   (MARTIUS and KNOOP [13])
↓
succinic acid
↓↑
fumaric acid
↓↑
l-malic acid   (Green [4])
↓↑
oxalo-acetic acid

4. Reversible steps. Succinic acid arises according to our scheme by oxidative reactions from oxaloacetic acid, via citric and α-ketoglutaric acids. Anaerobic experiments, however, show succinic acid can also be formed by reduction from oxaloacetic acid (see also SZENT-GYÖRGYI). The reactions succinic acid → fumaric acid → l-malic acid → oxaloacetic acid are thus reversible under suitable conditions.

The outstanding problem in this connection is the question of the oxidative equivalent of the reduction. At least a partial answer may be given. The synthesis of citric acid as shown in section VI takes place anaerobically, although it is an oxidative process. A reductive process equivalent to the oxidation must therefore occur at the same time. The reduction of oxaloacetic acid to succinic acid is the only reduction of sufficient magnitude (see the next section) known so far to occur simultaneously with the citric acid synthesis and we assume therefore it is the equivalent for the synthesis of citric acid.

5. Effect of malonate. It follows from the preceding paragraph that succinic acid can arise from oxaloacetic acid in two different ways (a) oxidatively via citric and α-ketoglutaric acids (b) reductively via l-malic and fumaric acids. That two different ways and therefore two different enzymic systems bring about the conversion of oxaloacetic into succinic acid can be demonstrated with the aid of malonate. Malonate inhibits specifically the reaction succinic acid ⇄ fumaric acid. Aerobically it will therefore increase the yield of succinic acid from oxaloacetic acid since it prevents its secondary breakdown. Anaerobically, on the other hand, it will inhibit the formation of succinic acid, since in this case the succinic dehydrogenase is concerned with the formation of the succinic acid. The following experiment shows that the results are as expected.

TABLE V.

Effect of malonate on the aerobic and anaerobic conversion of oxaloacetic into succinic acid.

(0,75 grammes wet muscle in 3 ccm phosphate buffer; 40° C; ph = 7,4)

Experimental conditions (final concentration of the substrates)	μl succinic acid formed in 40 min.
1. O_2; 0,1 M oxaloacetate;	1086
2. O_2; 0,1 M oxaloacetate; 0,06 M malonate	1410
3. N_2; 0,1 M oxaloacetate;	1270
4. N_2; 0,1 M oxaloacetate; 0,06 M malonate	834

166

6. Citric acid cycle in other tissues. We have tested the principal points of the citric acid cycle in various other animal tissues and find that brain, testis, liver and kidney of the rat are capable of oxidising citric acid as well as synthesising it from oxaloacetic acid. Of these four tissues testis shows the highest rate of synthesis and this is of interest in view of the work of THUNBERG's school on the occurrence of citric acid in spermatic fluid. 1 mg (dry weight) rat testis forms anaerobically up to 0,02 mg citric acid per hour if oxaloacetic acid is present.

Whilst the citric acid cycle thus seems to occur generally in animal tissues, it does not exist in yeast or in *B. coli*, for yeast and *B. coli* do not oxidise citric acid at an appreciable rate.

7. Quantitative significance of the citric acid cycle. Though the citric acid cycle may not be the only pathway through which carbohydrate is oxidised in animal tissues the quantitative data of the oxidation and resynthesis of citric acid indicate that it is the preferential pathway. The quantitative significance of the cycle depends on the rate of the slowest partial step, that is for our experimental conditions the synthesis of citric acid from oxaloacetic acid. According to the scheme one molecule of citric acid is synthesised in the course of the oxidation of one molecule of „triose", and since the oxidation of triose requires 3 molecules O_2, the rate of citric acid synthesis should be one third of the rate of O_2 consumption if carbohydrate is oxidised through the citric acid cycle. We find for our conditions:

Rate of respiration (Q_{O_2}) = —20

Rate of citric acid synthesis ($Q_{citrate}$) = + 5,8

The observed rate of the citric acid synthesis is thus a little under the expected figure (—6,6), but it is very probable that the conditions suitable for the demonstration of the synthesis (absence of oxygen) are not the optimal conditions for the intermediate formation of citric acid, and that the rate of citric acid synthesis is higher under more physiological conditions. This is suggested by the experiments on the aerobic formation of succinic acid from oxaloacetic acid (Table IV). $Q_{succinate}$, in the presence of malonate and oxaloacetate is +14,1, and if citrate is an intermediate stage the rate of citrate formation must be at least the same. But even the observed minimum figures of the rate of the synthesis justify the assumption that the citric acid cycle is the chief pathway of the oxidation of carbohydrate in pigeon muscle.

8. The work of SZENT-GYÖRGYI. SZENT-GYÖRGYI[20] who first pointed out the importance of the C_4-dicarboxylic acids in cellular respiration, came to the conclusion that respiration, in muscle, is oxidation of triose by oxaloacetic acid. In the light of our new experiments it becomes clear that SZENT-GYÖRGYI's view contained a correct conception, though the manner in which oxaloacetic acid reacts is somewhat different from what SZENT-GYÖRGYI visualised. The experimental results of SZENT-GYÖRGYI can be well explained by the citric acid cycle; we do not intend, however, to discuss this in full in this paper.

Summary.

1. Citric acid catalytically promotes oxidations in muscle, especially in the presence of carbohydrate.

2. The rate of the oxidative removal of citric acid from muscle was measured. The maximum figure for $Q_{citrate}$ observed was — 16,9.

3. α-Ketoglutaric acid and succinic acid were found as products of the oxidation of citric acid. These experiments confirm MARTIUS and KNOOP's results obtained with liver citric dehydrogenase.

4. Oxaloacetic acid, if added to muscle, condenses with an unknown substance to form citric acid. The unknown substance is in all probability a derivative of carbohydrate.

156

5. The catalytic effect of citrate as well as the similar effects of succinate, fumarate, malate and oxaloacetate described by Szent-Györgyi and by Stare and Baumann are explained by the series of reactions summarized in section VII 3 d.

6. The quantitative data suggest that the „citric acid cycle" is the preferential pathway through which carbohydrate is oxidised in animal tissues.

———————

We wish to thank the Medical Research Council and the Rockefeller Foundation for grants and Professor E. J. Wayne for his help and advice.

1) Bernhauer, Ergebn. Enzymf. **3**, 185 (1934). — 2) Blaise, Gault, C. R. **147**, 198 (1908). — 3) Claisen, Hori, Ber. Chem. Ges. **24**, 120 (1891). — 4) Green, Biochem. Jl. **30**, 2095 (1936). — 5) Krebs, Zs. phys. Chem. **217**, 191 (1933). — 6) Krebs, Zs. phys. Chem. **218**, 151 (1933). — 7) Krebs, Biochem. Jl. **29**, 1620 (1935). — 8) Krebs, Johnson, Biochem. Jl. **31**, 645 (1937). — 9) Kutscher, Steudel, Zs. phys. Chem. **39**, 474 (1903). — 10) Ljunggren, Katalytisk Kolsyreavspjälkning ur Ketokarbonsyror, Lund 1925. — 11) Malachowski, Maslowski, Ber. Chem. Ges. **61**, 2524 (1928). — 12) Martius, Knoop, Zs. phys. Chem. **242**, I (1936). — 13) Martius, Knoop, Zs. phys. Chem. **246**, 1 (1937). — 14) Martius, Zs. phys. Chem. **247**, 104 (1937). — 15) Östberg, Skand. Arch. Phys. **62**, 81 (1931). — 16) Pollak, Hofmeisters Beitr. **10**, 232 (1907). — 17)Pucher, Sherman, Vickery, Jl. of Biol. Chem. **113**, 235 (1936). — 18) Sherman, Mendel, Vickery, Jl. of Biol. Chem. **113**, 247, 265 (1936). — 19) Stare, Baumann, Proc. Roy. Soc. **B 121**, 338 (1936). — 20) Szent-Györgyi c.s., Bioch. Zs. **162**, 399 (1925); Z. phys. Chem. **224**, 1 (1934), **236**, 1 (1935), **244**, 105 (1936) **247**, I (1937). — 21) Wagner-Jauregg, Rauen, Zs. phys. Chem. **237**, 227 (1935). — 22) Weil-Malherbe, Biochem. Jl. **31**, 299 (1937). — 23) Weil-Malherbe, Krebs, Biochem. Jl. **29**, 2077 (1935). — 24) Wieland, Sonderhoff, Ann. Chem. Pharm. Liebig **503**, 61 (1933).

Editor's Comments on Paper 20

20 **Lohmann and Schuster:** Investigations into the Cocarboxylase
Biochem. Z., **294**, 193–197, 201 (1937)

Soon after Peters (1936) had discovered a connection between thiamine (vitamin B$_1$) and pyruvic acid oxidation, Lohmann and Schuster (Paper 20) established the first mechanism of pyruvic acid metabolism. Both workers found that the cocarboxylase (thiamine pyrophosphate) found to be present in dried yeast (Auhagen, 1933) was the prosthetic group of yeast carboxylase, which is responsible for the decarboxylation of pyruvic acid to acetaldehyde and carbon dioxide.

Lipmann and his research group devoted their activity to pyruvic acid oxidation. Using *Lactobacillus delbruckii*, Lipmann (1939) observed that this oxidation was different from the one suggested by Lohmann and Schuster (Paper 20), as it was completely dependent upon the presence of inorganic phosphate, and that the acetate formation resulted in the net production of ATP. Lipmann thus concluded that "acetate-phosphate" must be the link between pyruvate and acetate (Lipmann, 1940, 1941, 1944). This was soon established as "active acetate," e.g., an acetyl-transferring compound (Lipmann, 1945).

This acetyl phosphate was also found to be an intermediate in the anaerobic utilization of pyruvate to carbon dioxide and to acetic, formic, lactic, and succinic acids by *Escherichia coli* (Kalnitzky and Werkman, 1942, 1943). This "hydroclastic" split, whereby pyruvic acid is split into formic and acetic acids, was shown to be a reversible phosphoroclastic split (Utter and Werkman, 1943; Utter et al., 1944; Lipmann and Tuttle, 1944; Utter et al., 1945).

20

Investigations into the Cocarboxylase

K. LOHMANN AND P. SCHUSTER

*Translated expressly for this Benchmark
volume by H. W. Doelle from "Untersuchungen über die Cocarboxylase,"
Biochem. Z., 294, 193–197, 201
(1937), with permission from
Springer-Verlag*

IV. Chemical Studies

Qualitative analysis revealed the presence of C, H, N, S, P, and Cl. Difficulties were experienced with the quantitative N and S analyses. N was measured according to Dumas and S according to Pregl and in a microcombustion tube according to Carius. Both methods gave equally good results for S, which revealed, together with the N values obtained, a ratio of 4:1. Finally we determined N according to Kjeldahl after digestion with 2 ml of concentrated H_2SO_4, $CuSO_4$ + K_2SO_4, and the addition of 30 mg of glucose. We determined S as $BaSO_4$ after oxidation with excess aqueous $KMnO_4$ solution, which was heated 10 minutes in the water bath; reduction of the Mn oxides in acidic solution with H_2O_2; hot precipitation with $BaCl_2$ that was filtrated by suction; addition of 2 ml of N HCl; and heating to dryness over a water bath. The residue was taken up in water with the addition of a drop of $2 N$ HCl and filtered, and the precipitate was washed.

The molecular weight of the cocarboxylase–HCl has not yet been determined. From the above chemical analysis we calculated it to be 479.9, assuming the presence of 1 atom of S.

Analysis: $C_{12}H_{21}O_8N_4P_2SCl$. 5.078 mg = 5.745 mg of CO_2; 2.055 mg of H_2O - 4.15 mg = 3.48 ml of $N/100$ HCl = 0.487 mg of N (Kjeldahl) - P (colorimetrically), inorganic P_2O_5, zero; 15-min hydrolysis 6.51%; total P 13.00% - 10.05 mg = 4.94 mg of $BaSO_4$ - 8.52 mg = 2.55 mg of AgCl (direct precipitation with $AgNO_3$) - 4.997 mg = 1.43 mg of AgCl (micro-Carius).

	C, %	H, %	N, %	P, %	S, %	Cl, %
Calculated	30.08	4.42	11.71	12.96	6.69	7.40
Found	30.85	4.53	11.72	13.00	6.78	7.41

The binding of the sulfur: The cocarboxylase produces a positive "plumbit" as the vitamin B_1 and a negative sulfhydryl reaction, as well as a very faint "Fichtenspan" reaction.

The binding of chlorine: Chlorine is present in the aqueous solution in its ionic form.

The binding of phosphorus: Phosphorus is present as a phosphoric ester. One molecule is released by hydrolysis after 15 min of treatment with N HCl at 100°C, whereas the second is very difficult to hydrolyze.

Thus the formula for cocarboxylase could be written as

$$C_{12}H_{16}N_4SO \times HCl \times 2H_3PO_4 \, (-2H_2O) + 1H_2O$$

Alkaline kidney phosphatase (dialyzed kidney extract 1:1) hydrolyzes (preferably) the easy hydrolyzable phosphate and the second one very slowly. The loss of cocarboxylase activity parallels the hydrolyzed phosphate; similar results in the case of fractionated hydrolysis in $N/10$ HCl (see Table 1).

Table 1. Inactivation of cocarboxylase after enzymatic and chemical hydrolysis of the easily hydrolyzable P

	Time, min	Easily hydrolyzable P split, %	Activity loss, %
Phosphatase treatment	15	27	26
	60	63	55
Hydrolysis in $N/10$ HCl	60	77	71

During enzymatic separation with acidic phosphatases (prostataphosphatase, gratefully obtained from Dr. Kutscher[1]), both phosphate molecules were split at equal rates, which were much slower than in the case of glycerolphosphoric acid (pH 5.0). After complete separation of the P (a number of days at 37°C with toluene) the protein was precipitated with mercuric chloride–HCl; the filtrate, after removal of mercury and good aeration, was precipitated with $HAuCl_4$, and the crystalline gold salt decomposed without further purification by H_2S. Crystals were formed from the concentrated solution in ethanol–ether that (after recrystallization in F. and mixture-F.) were identical to the aneurin–HCl (micro-F. 249°C; mixture-F. 250°C; identical to the pikronolate).

The basic substance of the cocarboxylase is thus identical with vitamin B_1. The cocarboxylase is a double-phosphorylated aneurin (vitamin B_1).

During the oxidation of cocarboxylase with alkaline ferricyanide, a blue fluorescent compound develops, as is the case with aneurin[2] (in acidic solution, the compound is fluorescent green). This oxidation occurs in an alkaline bicarbonate

[1]W. Kutscher and A. Worner, *Biochem. Z.*, **239**, 109 (1936).
[2]R. A. Peters, *Nature*, **135**, 107 (1935); G. Barger, F. Bergel, and A. R. Todd, *Ber. Deut. Chem. Ges.*, **68**, 2257 (1935).

solution; the oxidation rate increases with increasing $[OH^-]$. Vitamin B_1 reacts very similarly and can also be oxidized in alkaline bicarbonate solution, despite literature reports to the contrary. In an alkaline bicarbonate solution, the oxidation of the cocarboxylase can be directed in such a way that exactly 2 atoms of H are oxidized. The oxidation product cannot yet be obtained in crystalline form.

During Williams' sulfite treatment,[3] a phosphorus-free pyrimidine (as sulfonic acid) and a double phosphorylated thiazol was obtained, of which one phosphoric acid can be split easily after hydrolysis for 15 min with N HCl at 100°C; the other is difficult to hydrolyze, as was the case with cocarboxylase.

Experiment: 130 mg of cocarboxylase–HCl is dissolved in 2.0 ml of water and neutralized with 0.3 ml of N NaOH to pH 5.0; 200 mg of sodium bisulfite is added. After 3 days at room temperature, during which a white crystallate soon develops, the solution was concentrated in a vacuum desiccator to 0.5 ml and filtered. The crystals were washed with 3 drops of water. The weight of the crystals was 53.4 mg (calculated: 54.3 mg). The substance was recrystallized with hot water. Result: 47 mg of $C_6H_9O_3N_3S$ (mol. wt. 203.2).

Analysis: 5.170 mg = 6.670 mg of CO_2 and 2.135 mg of H_2O - 2.324 mg = 0.410 ml of N_2 (754/20°) - 3.587 mg = 3.953 mg of $BaSO_4$.

Calculated: C, 35.44%; H, 4.46%; N, 20.68%; S, 15.78%.

Found: C, 35.19%; H, 4.62%; N, 20.39%; S, 15.14%.

The compound does not melt at 360°C. It is quite possible that it is the same 2-methyl-4-amino-5-sulfonic acid-methyl pyrimidine, which was obtainable after the same treatment of aneurine.

* * * * * * *

All results obtained indicate the occurrence of an unsymmetrical pyrophosphate ester for the binding of both phosphoric ester molecules. Evidence for this assumption was obtained by alkaline titration and the separation of inorganic pyrophosphate.

Titration: 65.6 mg of cocarboxylase–HCl was dissolved in 2 ml of water and titrated with $N/10$ NaOH against methyl orange and afterward against phenolphthalein as an indicator. The 65.6 mg corresponded to 0.137 mmole of cocarboxylase, which used 0.141 mmole of alkaline (= 1.03 equivalents) against methyl orange and, further, 2.8 mmoles of alkaline (= 2.04 equivalents) against phenolphthalein. In the cocarboxylase–HCl molecule we have, therefore, a strong acid group with a dissociation constant of about pH 3.5 and two weaker acid groups with constants between pH 3.5 and 8.5. The molecule itself has three strong acid groups (Cl^- and two primary hydroxyl groups of phosphoric acid) and two weaker ones if one assumes the existence of a diphosphoric ester (one weak one if one assumes a pyrophosphoric acid ester). Vitamin B_1–$(HCl)_2$ possesses one weak acid group with the dissociation constant pK_B 5 according to the titration curves of Williams.[4] This result is

[3]R. R. Williams, R. R. Waterman, J. C. Keresztesy, and E. R. Buchman, *J. Amer. Chem. Soc.*, **57**, 536 (1935).

[4]R. R. Williams and A. E. Ruehle, *Amer. J. Chem. Soc.*, **57**, 1856 (1935).

based on the fact that one HCl molecule is being neutralized with the quarternary N because of salt formation; the other is weakened because of the amino group at the pyrimidine ring. The same is the case with the cocarboxylase–HCl, where, of the three strong acid groups, one is completely neutralized and the second is so weakened that it reacts as a weak acid group. Since there is only one further weak acid group, an unsymmetrical pyrophosphate ester must exist. The following scheme demonstrates the loss of a weak acid group as a result of binding as an unsymmetrical pyrophosphoric acid ester. The index 0 means neutralized acid; the index 1, strong acid; and index 2, weak acid:

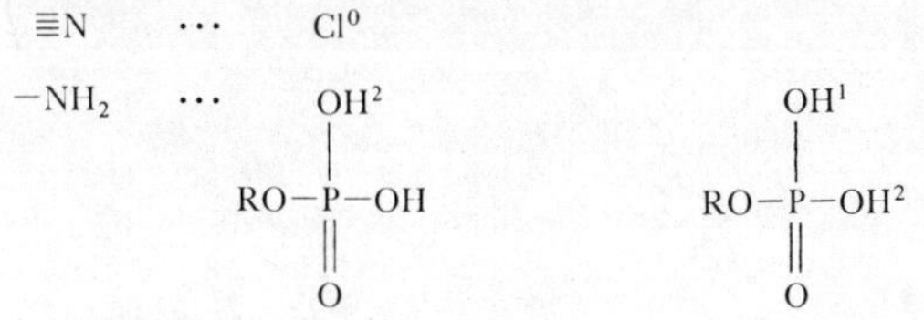

$$
\begin{array}{lll}
\equiv\!N & \cdots & Cl^0 \\[4pt]
-NH_2 & \cdots & OH^2 \qquad\qquad\qquad OH^1 \\
& & \quad| \qquad\qquad\qquad\qquad | \\
& & RO-P-OH \qquad\quad RO-P-OH^2 \\
& & \quad\| \qquad\qquad\qquad\qquad \| \\
& & \quad O \qquad\qquad\qquad\qquad O
\end{array}
$$

Acid groups of a diphosphoric acid ester

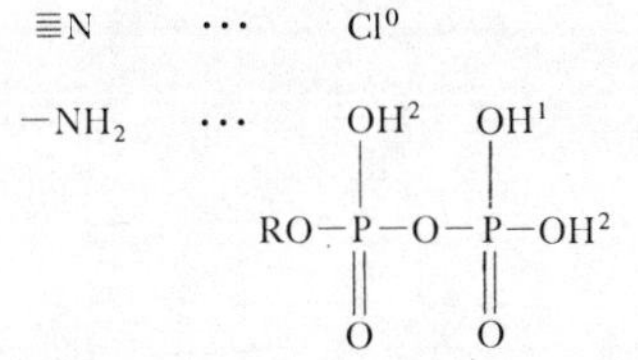

$$
\begin{array}{lll}
\equiv\!N & \cdots & Cl^0 \\[4pt]
-NH_2 & \cdots & OH^2 \quad OH^1 \\
& & \quad| \qquad | \\
& & RO-P-O-P-OH^2 \\
& & \quad\| \qquad \| \\
& & \quad O \qquad O
\end{array}
$$

Acid group of an unsymmetrical pyrophosphoric acid ester

Separation of pyrophosphate. After 3 to 4 hr boiling of cocarboxylase in $2\,N$ NaOH over a boiling water bath (~ 0.5 percent solution), not only the easily removable inorganic phosphate is being released, but the difficultly hydrolyzable phosphate is almost completely converted into easily hydrolyzable phosphate. The percentage of P obtained was as follows:

	Before saponification	After saponification
Inorganic phosphate	0	20
After 7 min hydrolysis in N HCl	47	94
After 15 min hydrolysis in N HCl	50	96

The separation of inorganic phosphate during saponification correlates with the amount obtainable in splitting inorganic pyrophosphate under identical conditions.

* * * * * * *

173

Constitution of Cocarboxylase

Since sulfite treatment resulted in a diphosphorylated thiazol and a phosphate-free pyrimidine, and the results of the titration and alkaline saponification indicate the presence of an asymmetrical pyrophosphate acid, the cocarboxylase should have the following constitution:

Cocarboxylase (diphosphoaneurin)

Editor's Comments on Paper 21

21 Baddiley, Thain, Novelli, and Lipmann: Structure of Coenzyme A
Nature, **171**, 76 (1953)

During the work on cell-free acetylation (Lipmann, 1945), the action of a new co-enzyme was observed. It was identified as a pantothenic acid derivative (Lipmann et al., 1947) for which the term "coenzyme A" (CoA) was introduced (Novelli and Lip-mann, 1947). Again it was Lipmann and his coworkers who established the final structure of this coenzyme (Paper 21; Baddiley, 1955). The implication of this discovery does not need further explanation. Earlier reports that pantothenic acid stimulates fermentation and, particularly, respiration of yeast with sucrose as substrate (Pratt and Williams, 1939; Dorfmann et al., 1942) hinted at a connection between this vita-min and the citric acid cycle (Teague and Williams, 1942; Hills, 1943). It was soon realized that pyruvic acid oxidation via the Krebs cycle must involve a common acetyl derivative (Wood, 1946) as well as coenzyme A for the catalytic reaction (Novelli and Lipmann, 1947; 1950; Stern and Ochoa, 1949). The functioning of two enzymes was suggested (Stern et al., 1950), one that activates acetyl phosphate and a second which causes the active acetate to combine with oxalacetate to produce citric acid.

21

Reprinted from *Nature*, **171**, 76 (1953)

LETTERS TO THE EDITORS

The Editors do not hold themselves responsible for opinions expressed by their correspondents. No notice is taken of anonymous communications

Structure of Coenzyme A

CHEMICAL[1] and enzymic[2] studies from these two laboratories suggested that coenzyme A is best represented by formula (I) (cf. ref. 3). While the synthesis of various fragments of the molecule[4] has lent considerable support to this structure, the enzymic and chemical evidence did not agree on one point. This concerned the nature of a substance obtained by the action of nucleotide pyrophosphatase on the coenzyme and which stimulated the growth of *Acetobacter suboxydans*[5]. Although not isolated in a chemically pure state, it was thought to be a simple phosphate of pantothenic acid[6]. None of the synthetic pantothenic acid phosphates showed activity towards this organism ; consequently, it was suggested[1] that this 'Acetobacter-stimulatory factor' might be pantetheine-4'phosphate (II). An unambiguous synthesis of (II) is described here.

D : L - Pantetheine - $O^{2'}$: S dibenzyl ether was prepared from pantothenic acid - 2'benzyl ether by reaction with ethyl chloroformate and then 2-benzyl-thioethylamine. Phosphorylation with dibenzyl chlorophosphonate and removal of the four benzyl groups with sodium in liquid ammonia gave D : L-pantetheine-4'phosphate.

A more reliable method of assay for the 'Acetobacter-stimulatory factor' consists in its resynthesis to coenzyme A by a partially purified enzyme system isolated from pigeon liver[7]. This system does not respond to pantetheine or to pantothenic acid phosphates. Synthetic D : L - pantetheine - 4'phosphate, when examined in this system, showed an activity equivalent to 265 units of coenzyme A per milligram,

which represents a 47 per cent conversion into coenzyme A. This is in excellent agreement with the expected 50 per cent conversion for the optically inactive substance.

Pure D(+)-pantetheine-4'phosphate, $[\alpha]_D^{18}$ 10·8°, was synthesized by direct phosphorylation of pantetheine with dibenzyl chlorophosphonate followed by removal of benzyl groups with sodium in liquid ammonia. This method, although ambiguous, is very convenient in operation, and the product showed a coenzyme A activity in the above test of 450 units/ mgm., which represents an 82 per cent conversion.

This synthesis establishes beyond doubt the structure of the pantetheine phosphate part of the coenzyme molecule, and it is hoped to extend these studies to the synthesis of pyrophosphates more closely related to coenzyme A.

Full details of this work will be published separately elsewhere.

J. BADDILEY
E. M. THAIN
Lister Institute of Preventive Medicine,
London, S.W.1.

G. D. NOVELLI
F. LIPMANN
Biochemical Research Laboratory,
Massachusetts General Hospital,
and the Dept. of Biochemical Chemistry,
Harvard Medical School, Boston, Mass.
Dec. 12.

[1] Baddiley, J., and Thain, E. M., *J. Chem. Soc.*, 2253 (1951) ; 3783 (1952).
[2] Gregory, J. D., Novelli, G. D., and Lipmann, F., *J. Amer. Chem. Soc.*, **74**, 854 (1952).
[3] Wang, T. P., Schuster, L., and Kaplan, N. O., *J. Amer. Chem. Soc.*, **74**, 3204 (1952).
[4] Baddiley, J., and Thain, E. M., *J. Chem. Soc.*, 246, 3421 (1951).
[5] King, T. E., Locher, L. M., and Cheldelin, V. H., *Arch. Biochem.*, **17**, 483 (1948).
[6] Novelli, G. D., "Phosphorus Metabolism", **1**, 414 (Baltimore, 1951).
[7] Levintow, L., and Novelli, G. D., abstract of paper presented at the Atlantic City Meeting of the American Chemical Society, p. 33 c (1952).

$$PO_3H_2$$
$$\overline{\quad O \quad}$$

CH.CH.CH.CH.CH$_2$.O.P.O.P.O.CH$_2$.CMe$_2$.CH.CO.NH.CH$_2$.CH$_2$.CO.NH.CH$_2$.CH$_2$.SH

with OH groups; O O O and O O above; OH OH and OH markings

(I)

H$_2$O$_3$PO.CH$_2$.CMe$_2$.CH.CO.NH.CH$_2$.CH$_2$.CO.NH.CH$_2$.CH$_2$.SH

OH

(II)

Editor's Comments on Paper 22

22 **Stadtman, Novelli, and Lipmann:** Coenzyme A Function in and Acetyl Transfer by the Phosphotransacetylase System
J. Biol. Chem., **191**, 365–367, 370, 374–376 (1951)

It was again the research group directed by F. Lipmann that discovered in the enzyme phosphotransacetylase (Paper 22) the link between acetylphosphate and coenzyme A that established acetylphosphate as the source of acetyl groups. This enzyme was first purified from *Clostridium kluyveri* (Stadtman, 1952). The final proof of the participation of this enzyme in the aerobic breakdown of pyruvic acid came when Stadtman (1952) showed that phosphotransacetylase catalyzes a net synthesis of acetyl CoA and isolated this compound by paper chromatography. At the same time he identified acetyl CoA as a thioester of coenzyme A and acetic acid.

The final link from pyruvate to citric acid was established by Ochoa and coworkers (Korkes et al., 1950, 1951; Ochoa et al., 1951; Stern et al., 1951; Stern and Ochoa, 1952), who studied the enzymatic synthesis of citric acid. They observed the condensing enzyme catalyzing a reversible reaction between acetyl CoA and oxalacetate to yield CoA and citrate and reported that the free-energy change of −12,000 cal suggested a role of acetyl CoA as an energy-rich compound equivalent to ATP (see Lynen, 1953).

22

Reprinted from *J. Biol. Chem.*, **191**, 365–367, 370, 374–376 (1951)

COENZYME A FUNCTION IN AND ACETYL TRANSFER BY THE PHOSPHOTRANSACETYLASE SYSTEM*

By E. R. STADTMAN,† G. DAVID NOVELLI, AND FRITZ LIPMANN

(*From the Biochemical Research Laboratory, Massachusetts General Hospital, and the Department of Biological Chemistry, Harvard Medical School, Boston, Massachusetts*)

(Received for publication, February 27, 1951)

Lipmann and Tuttle (1) discovered that certain bacterial extracts catalyze a rapid interchange of inorganic and acetyl-bound phosphate. They suggested that this exchange might be due in part to a reversibility of the phosphoroclastic decomposition of pyruvate; however, the observation that the exchange was surprisingly unaffected by addition of acetyl acceptors like formate led them to suspect that unknown factors may be also involved.

More recently, Stadtman and Barker (2) reinvestigated the phosphate exchange reaction in cell-free extracts of *Clostridium kluyveri*. They found that substitution of arsenate for phosphate in these extracts resulted in a very rapid and complete hydrolysis of acetyl phosphate. The marked similarity between these reactions and the reactions catalyzed by the bacterial transglucosidase system, previously described by Doudoroff *et al.* (3, 4), led to the proposal that the phosphate exchange and arsenolysis reactions of acetyl phosphate were catalyzed by an acetyl-transferring enzyme (Stadtman and Barker (2); Lipmann (5)).

Concurrently, acetyl phosphate, until recently refractive with regard to acetyl donor function, was found to serve as a C_2 precursor in the synthesis of butyrate and hexanoate by extracts of *C. kluyveri* (6), and, in particular, it showed a surprising activity in the coenzyme A (CoA)-linked citric acid synthesis by extracts of *Escherichia coli* (7).

These observations became of even greater interest when it was found that microbial extracts could activate acetyl phosphate to serve as an acetyl donor for various CoA-dependent acetylation reactions catalyzed by animal enzyme preparations (8–10). Attempts to identify this "activator" function of microbial extracts led to the proposition that the phosphate exchange and arsenolysis system may be responsible for the acetyl transfer from acetyl phosphate. This possibility prompted us to embark

* Aided by grants from the Commonwealth Fund, the National Cancer Institute, the United States Public Health Service, and an institutional grant of the American Cancer Society to the Massachusetts General Hospital.

† Postdoctorate Research Fellow of the Atomic Energy Commission. Present address, National Heart Institute, National Institutes of Health, Bethesda 14, Maryland.

on a more detailed study of the mechanisms of phosphate exchange and arsenolysis. Particularly, viewed in conjunction with the recently reported observations on an acetyl donor function of the pyruvate-formate exchange system (11, 12), these studies appear to open new approaches to the problem of acetyl transfer.

Materials and Methods

Microbial Preparations—In the majority of experiments reported in this paper, extracts of *C. kluyveri* were applied. Lyophilized extracts of these organisms were prepared as previously described (13). Generally 1 to 2.5 per cent solutions of the lyophilisate were used. In a few experiments, extracts of *E. coli* were used. This preparation is described further in the text.

Acetyl Phosphate—Lithium monoacetyl phosphate was prepared by the method of Lipmann and Tuttle (14) or by reaction of isopropenyl acetate with phosphoric acid (15). For the estimation of acetyl phosphate, the hydroxamic acid method was used (16). For radioactivity studies, the inorganic and acetyl phosphate fractions were separated by differential calcium precipitation as described by Lipmann and Tuttle (17).

Radioactivity Determination—To determine P^{32}, 0.05 to 0.1 ml. of the solution to be tested was uniformly distributed on a copper disk, dried, and the radioactivity measured with a Tracerlab autoscaler having a thin windowed Geiger tube.

Protein Determination—The protein content of the bacterial extracts was estimated by turbidity measurements of trichloroacetic acid precipitates. The bacterial extract, containing 0.1 to 2.0 mg. of protein, was made up with water to a volume of 2 ml., and 3 ml. of 5 per cent trichloroacetic acid solution were added. The resulting suspension was allowed to stand for 30 seconds and the turbidity was measured in a Klett-Summerson colorimeter, with a No. 54 filter. Crystalline egg albumin was used as standard. The turbidity is a linear function of the amount over a range of 0.1 to 5 mg.

CoA Determination—The coenzyme content was determined by the enzymatic acetylation method of Kaplan and Lipmann (18). CoA determinations were also carried out by use of the arsenolysis method. As will be discussed below, arsenolysis of acetyl phosphate is, over a wide range, linearly proportional to CoA concentrations and may be used very conveniently for assay purposes.

Arsenolysis of Acetyl Phosphate—The arsenolysis was generally measured under the following standardized conditions: the enzyme was incubated with a mixture of lithium acetyl phosphate, 0.025 M; cysteine, 0.01 M; tris(hydroxymethyl) aminomethane buffer (pH 8.0) (19), 01. M; potassium arsenate,[1] 0.05 M; CoA, if added; total volume, 1.0 ml., 28°. After several 10 minute intervals, 0.2 ml. aliquots of the mixture were analyzed for acetyl phosphate. For controls, two similar mixtures, one without arsenate and one without CoA, were used. Under such conditions, as was found previously (2), the rate of arsenolysis is constant until 85 to 90 per cent of the acetyl phosphate is decomposed.

* * * * * * *

Proportionality of Coenzyme Concentration with Activity—In Table IV, experiments are reproduced in which an ammonium sulfate fraction was used as the enzyme. Two results of interest appear from these data. Experiment 1 shows straight proportionality between coenzyme concentration and activity up to 20 units per ml. Even with considerably higher concentrations of CoA, the concentration-activity curve does not bend. This makes the system very well suited for CoA assay. In contrast to the liver system (18), in which CoA is synthesized from various fragments (21, 22), this assay has the further advantage of responding exclusively to intact CoA. In Experiment 2, CoA preparations of different purity are

TABLE IV

Proportionality of Arsenolysis with CoA Concentration

Experiment No.	CoA sample[*]	CoA added	Units per ml.	Δ, μM acetyl P in 15 min.
		mg. per ml.		
1	0	0	0	0.6
	S-519-C (55 units per mg.)	0.036	2	2.6
	"	0.091	5	5.7
	"	0.18	10	10.3
	"	0.36	20	20.6
2	A$_2$512 (67 units per mg.)	0.15	10	11.3
	W (4.5 units per mg.)	2.22	10	10.3

Conditions, 0.05 M potassium arsenate; 0.1 M tris(hydroxymethyl)aminomethane (pH 8.0); 22 μM acetyl P; 0.01 M cysteine; 0.002 M MgCl$_2$; 0.5 mg. of enzyme (from Lot L); ammonium sulfate fraction, between 70 and 90 per cent saturation. Final volume 1 ml.

[*] Preparations obtained from hog liver; Sample W represents a rather early fraction, while the other two preparations are more highly purified.

compared at equal potency. The correspondence of activity and potency is independent of purity, and confirms CoA as the true activator of this system.

* * * * * * *

The failure of animal enzyme preparations to utilize synthetic acetyl phosphate as an acetyl donor can now be attributed to absence of a phosphotransacetylase. This confirms earlier unpublished experiments by Lipmann and Tuttle, who found, with tissue homogenates, no exchange between acetyl-bound and inorganic phosphate. A survey of several groups of microorganisms has shown that the phosphotransacetylase is present in many bacteria: *Proteus morganii, Lactobacillus delbrueckii, Clostridium tetanamorphum, Clostridium butylicum, E. coli.* The enzyme can so far not be detected in yeast.

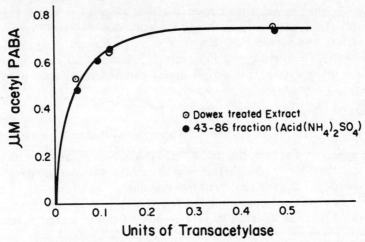

Fig. 1. The effect of the concentration of transacetylase on acetylation of PABA by pigeon liver enzyme. Conditions as given in Table VI, except that two bacterial enzyme preparations were used. ⊙, Dowex-treated bacterial extract (Lot N); ●, acid ammonium sulfate fraction precipitating at 43 to 86 per cent saturation.

DISCUSSION

In view of the general rôle of CoA in acetyl transfer reactions, the intermediate formation of acetyl∼CoA had been an attractive proposition. The evidence presented here and earlier experience appear to bear out the assumption that there exists an acetyl∼CoA with an energy-rich link between the acetyl group and the coenzyme, either free or protein-bound. In the first part of this paper, it was shown that the transacetylase reaction, as represented by phosphate exchange or arsenolysis of acetyl phosphate, is CoA-dependent. The exchange reaction is therefore formulated as follows:

Acetyl∼phosphate + CoA-Protein I $\rightleftharpoons$ acetyl∼CoA-Protein I + phosphate (1)

The donor function of this system for acetyl acceptor systems, furthermore, suggests the transfer of acetyl~CoA from transacetylase Protein I to an acceptor; for instance, enzyme Protein II, specific for aromatic amines.   This may be formulated as follows:

Acetyl~CoA-Protein I + amine-Protein II →

$$\text{acetyl amine} + \text{Protein I} + \text{Protein II} + \text{CoA} \quad (2)$$

The easiest interpretation. is to assume that acetyl~CoA dissociates from Protein I and CoA assumes an acetyl carrier function.   This aspect, however, remains to be further substantiated.

Previous experiments have shown already that a variety of donor as well as acceptor systems may react together to perform acetyl transfer reactions.   Chou *et al.* isolated the ATP-acetate donor system from pigeon liver extract and recombined it with a variety of acceptor systems (8). And recently, Chantrenne and Lipmann (11) showed that *E. coli* extracts contain a donor system that derives acetyl groups directly from pyruvate by way of a formate exchange system.

Pyruvate (= acetyl formate) + CoA-Protein III ⇌

$$\text{acetyl~CoA-Protein III} + \text{formate} \quad (3)$$

The similarity between Reactions 1 and 3 has been pointed out already (11), and the terms "phosphotransacetylase" and "formotransacetylase" are proposed for the respective enzyme systems.

From data obtained during the last few years (7, 10, 26), the conclusion is ventured that the so called "active acetate," fed into a great variety of synthetic channels, is acetyl~CoA, which may be derived by a variety of enzyme reactions from a variety of acetyl-donating molecules.   In turn, acetyl~CoA may donate its acetyl residue to a variety of acceptor systems.

SUMMARY

Coenzyme A is required for the catalysis of interchange of acetyl-bound and inorganic phosphate and for the arsenolysis of acetyl phosphate by a phosphotransacetylation enzyme present in extracts of *Clostridium kluyveri* and other bacteria.   The rate of arsenolysis is directly proportional to coenzyme A concentration.   The phosphotransacetylase has been partially purified by ammonium sulfate fractionation.

Phosphotransacetylase-coenzyme A + acetyl phosphate was shown to donate acetyl groups for acetylation of aromatic amines to a specific pigeon liver acceptor fraction.   The acetyl transfer function of coenzyme A is discussed in the light of these experiments.

Methods are described for the removal of coenzyme A from bacterial extracts by treatment with an ion exchange resin or charcoal.

BIBLIOGRAPHY

1. Lipmann, F., and Tuttle, L. C., *J. Biol. Chem.*, **158,** 505 (1945).
2. Stadtman, E. R., and Barker, H. A., *J. Biol. Chem.*, **184,** 769 (1950).
3. Doudoroff, M., Barker, H. A., and Hassid, W. Z., *J. Biol. Chem.*, **168,** 725 (1947).
4. Doudoroff, M., Barker, H. A., and Hassid, W. Z., *J. Biol. Chem.*, **170,** 147 (1947).
5. Lipmann, F., *Harvey Lectures*, **44,** 99 (1950).
6. Stadtman, E. R., and Barker, H. A., *J. Biol. Chem.*, **180,** 1117 (1949).
7. Novelli, G. D., and Lipmann, F., *J. Biol. Chem.*, **182,** 213 (1950).
8. Chou, T. C., Novelli, G. D., Stadtman, E. R., and Lipmann, F., *Federation Proc.*, **9,** 160 (1950).
9. Stadtman, E. R., *Federation Proc.*, **9,** 233 (1950).
10. Stern, J. R., Shapiro, B., and Ochoa, S., *Nature*, **166,** 403 (1950).
11. Chantrenne, H., and Lipmann, F., *J. Biol. Chem.*, **187,** 757 (1950).
12. Strecker, H. J., Wood, H. G., and Krampitz, L. O., *J. Biol. Chem.*, **182,** 525 (1950).
13. Stadtman, E. R., and Barker, H. A., *J. Biol. Chem.*, **180,** 1085 (1949).
14. Lipmann, F., and Tuttle, L. C., *Arch. Biochem.*, **13,** 373 (1947).
15. Stadtman, E. R., and Lipmann, F., *J. Biol. Chem.*, **185,** 549 (1950).
16. Lipmann, F., and Tuttle, L. C., *J. Biol. Chem.*, **158,** 505 (1945).
17. Lipmann, F., and Tuttle, L. C., *J. Biol. Chem.*, **153,** 571 (1944).
18. Kaplan, N. O., and Lipmann, F., *J. Biol. Chem.*, **174,** 37 (1948).
19. Gomori, G., *Proc. Soc. Exp. Biol. and Med.*, **62,** 1251 (1946).
20. DeVries, W. H., Govier, W. M., Evans, J. S., Gregory, J. D., Novelli, G. D., Soodak, M., and Lipmann, F., *J. Am. Chem. Soc.*, **72,** 4838 (1950).
21. Novelli, G. D., Kaplan, N. O., and Lipmann, F., *Federation Proc.*, **9,** 209 (1950).
22. Novelli, G. D., Gregory, J. D., Flynn, R. M., and Schmetz, F. J., Jr., *Federation Proc.*, **10,** 229 (1951).
23. Bratton, A. C., and Marshall, E. K., Jr., *J. Biol. Chem.*, **128,** 537 (1939).
24. Kaplan, N. O., and Lipmann, F., *J. Biol. Chem.*, **176,** 459 (1948).
25. Kaplan, N. O., and Soodak, M., *Federation Proc.*, **8,** 211 (1949).
26. Soodak, M., and Lipmann, F., *J. Biol. Chem.*, **175,** 999 (1948).

Editor's Comments on Paper 23

23 Lynen and Ochoa: Enzymes of Fatty Acid Metabolism
Biochim. Biophys. Acta, **12**, 299–314 (1953)

Acetyl CoA, however, not only plays an important part in the metabolism of pyruvic acid, but it was also found to be an important intermediate in fatty acid metabolism and synthesis. Although it was shown earlier (Lehninger, 1944, 1945, 1946; Grafflin and Green, 1948; Drysdale and Lardy, 1953) that the two-carbon units removed successively from fatty acid chains during oxidation are identical to the two-carbon units derived from the decarboxylation of pyruvate, it was Lynen and Ochoa (Paper 23), who established the S-acyl derivatives of coenzyme A as the most important intermediates in fatty acid metabolism. The results of Lynen and Ochoa established the close link between the catabolism of carbohydrates and fatty acids and the fatty acid biosynthesis.

23

Reprinted from *Biochim. Biophys. Acta*, **12**, 299–314 (1953)

ENZYMES OF FATTY ACID METABOLISM*

by

FEODOR LYNEN

Biochemische Abteilung, Chemisches Universitäts-Laboratorium, München (Deutschland)

AND

SEVERO OCHOA

Department of Pharmacology, New York University College of Medicine, New York, N.Y. (U.S.A.)

Work of recent years (for reviews see [3, 5, 30]) has thrown much light on the mechanism of the β-oxidation of fatty acids formulated by KNOOP in 1904[32]. Through the use of isotopic tracer techniques[74, 53, 75] and of cell-free tissue preparations capable of oxidizing fatty acids[50, 43, 37–40, 20, 15, 16] it was established that the two-carbon units removed successively from fatty acid chains during β-oxidation are identical to the two-carbon units derived from carbohydrate through the oxidative decarboxylation of pyruvic acid[39]. Further, these units can either condense with one another—or with longer fatty acid chains—to bring about fatty acid synthesis, or can undergo oxidation via the citric acid cycle[74, 53, 6, 39, 40, 20]. Work with extracts of *Clostridium kluyveri* demonstrated that fatty acid synthesis occurs by a reversal of β-oxidation[61–63, 28]. Evidence was also obtained that in the process of synthesis, in both bacteria[4, 66] and animal tissues[1, 78, 52], the methyl end of "acetic acid" units is added to the carboxyl end of a fatty acid chain.

Further progress was hampered by the failure to detect intermediates during fatty acid oxidation or synthesis although from the early work of DAKIN[14] the corresponding α,β-unsaturated, β-hydroxy- and β-keto derivatives would be expected to be involved. Such a view would be in agreement with the observations that, at least in some tissues, the above compounds are oxidized at about the same rate as the corresponding fatty acids[31, 20].

The finding that fatty acids are not oxidized unless they undergo a preliminary activation and the fact that this activation is dependent on the generation of energy-rich phosphate[50, 43, 37, 38, 42, 20, 33, 61, 62, 63, 29, 15, 16] suggested that the actual intermediates might not occur as the free acids[28]. The identification of the two-carbon unit as S-acetyl coenzyme A**[46, 47, 65, 51, 71, 34, 59, 45] shed new light on the problem and strongly suggested

* The experimental work reported in this paper was aided by grants from the Deutsche Forschungsgemeinschaft and the Firma C. H. Boehringer Sohn, Ingelheim (University of Munich), and the United States Public Health Service, the American Cancer Society (recommended by the Commitee on Growth of the National Research Council), and by a contract (N6onr279, T.O. 6) between the Office of Naval Research and New York University College of Medicine. The authors are indebted to the Rockefeller Foundation for travelling fellowships which facilitated collaboration between their two laboratories.
** The following abbreviations are used: Coenzyme A (reduced), CoA, CoÄ-SH or CoA-SH; S-acyl coenzyme A derivatives, S-Acyl CoA, acyl-S-CoÄ, acyl-S-CoA, or simply acyl CoA; adenosine triphosphate, ATP; adenosine-5'-phosphate, AMP; pyrophosphate, PP; oxidized and reduced diphosphorpyridine nucleotide, DPN+ and DPNH; oxidized and reduced flavin adenine dinucleotide, FAD and FADH$_2$.

that the active intermediates might be the CoA derivatives of the fatty acids[47, 3, 30]. This belief was reinforced by the observation that S-acetyl CoA or the S-acyl derivatives of higher fatty acids can be generated enzymically through a reaction of the fatty acid with acyl phosphates in the presence of CoA[59, 60] or with CoA and ATP[11, 44, 15, 36, 49, 72, 23, 16, 41, 67]. Finally, work on the enzymic breakdown and synthesis of acetoacetate and other β-keto fatty acids[7, 76, 9, 24, 75, 58, 70, 64, 3, 21, 68, 22] opened the way for an understanding of the mechanism whereby fatty acid chains are shortened or elongated, by the removal or addition of acetyl CoA, during fatty acid oxidation or synthesis.

By employing synthetic S-acyl analogues of the fatty acid derivatives of CoA[48, 55] or the CoA fatty acid derivatives themselves[48, 69, 67] more recently made available by chemical or enzymatic synthesis, it has been possible to characterize and isolate from animal tissues some of the enzymes of fatty acid metabolism and obtain a clearer picture of the process as a whole. The development of rapid and sensitive optical methods of assay, whose introduction in enzymology we owe to OTTO WARBURG, has greatly facilitated the task of purifying the individual enzymes and studying their mechanism of action. The work described in this paper owes much to WARBURG's pioneering contributions which opened up new avenues of approach to dynamic biochemistry.

Fatty acid cycle

The results of the work summarized above and of the more recent work to be discussed in this paper show that fatty acid oxidation and synthesis proceed through the reactions illustrated in Fig. 1.

Fatty acid synthesis is accomplished through repetition of a cycle of four consecutive reactions: (a) condensation of two molecules of acetyl CoA to form acetoacetyl CoA and CoA–SH, (b) reduction of acetoacetyl CoA to β-hydroxybutyryl CoA, (c) dehydration of β-hydroxybutyryl CoA to crotonyl CoA, and (d) reduction of crotonyl CoA to butyryl CoA. A new cycle is started by the reaction of butyryl CoA with another molecule of acetyl CoA, to form β-ketocaproyl CoA + CoA–SH, and so forth. The cycle is repeated eight times until stearyl CoA is formed. All four reactions of the fatty acid cycle are reversible and fatty acid oxidation, once the fatty acid is

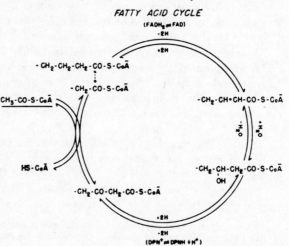

Fig. 1. Fatty acid cycle

activated through conversion to the corresponding acyl CoA derivative, proceeds by a reversal of the above sequence. The acetyl CoA split off at the end of each sequence is either oxidized via the citric acid cycle, by reacting with oxalacetate to form citrate and CoA–SH[51, 71], or is converted to acetoacetyl CoA + CoA–SH. In liver, acetoacetyl CoA is hydrolysed by a specific deacylase with formation of CoA–SH and acetoacetate[69a, 11a]. The presence of this enzyme would seem to account for the formation of free aceto-

References p. 313/314.

acetate in this organ. In either case CoA–SH is made available for activation of further fatty acid molecules.

The equilibrium of reaction (a) is predominantly in favor of the thioclastic splitting of the β-ketoacyl CoA derivatives. For this reason the name β-ketothiolase, or simply thiolase, has been proposed for this class of enzymes[48]. The equilibrium of reaction (b) favors reduction of the β-keto derivative, hence the name β-ketoreductase has been proposed for this group of enzymes[48]. The name crotonase has been suggested[67] for the enzyme or enzymes catalyzing reaction (c) and, finally, the name ethylene reductase has been used[55] to designate the enzyme or enzymes catalyzing reaction (d).

There are two main mechanisms for activation of fatty acids, *i.e.*, for the synthesis of their S-acyl CoA derivatives: (a) by a reaction with CoA–SH and ATP which, as we shall see later, results in the reversible formation of the corresponding acyl CoA, AMP and PP, and (b) by transfer of CoA from certain acyl CoA compounds such as acetyl CoA or succinyl CoA. Animal tissues, such as liver, heart, and kidney, utilize mainly the first mechanism while *C. kluyveri* utilizes the second. Extracts of this organism catalyze the reversible transfer of CoA from acetyl CoA to such fatty acids as propionate or butyrate[60]. Because of the presence of phosphotransacetylase[59], in the presence of CoA such extracts can utilize acetyl phosphate for activation.

A transferring enzyme of rather limited specificity is present in heart and probably in skeletal muscle and kidney but appears to be absent from liver. This enzyme catalyzes the reversible transfer of CoA from succinyl CoA to acetoacetate[21,68,69,22]. Through the formation of acetoacetyl CoA the enzyme activates acetoacetate, produced in the liver and carried by the blood stream to the peripheral tissues, for oxidation in these tissues via the tricarboxylic acid cycle (see reference no. 8). The latter in turn generates the necessary succinyl CoA through the oxidation of α-ketoglutarate which, as shown by recent work[26,54,27], reacts with CoA–SH and DPN$^+$ to form succinyl CoA, CO_2, and DPNH.

S-acyl fatty acid derivatives

Synthetic S-acetoacetyl and S-crotonyl derivatives of N-acetyl thioethanolamine[48a] have been found to act as substrates of β-ketoreductase and ethylene reductase respectively[48,55]. These structural analogues of the natural S-acyl CoA derivatives have therefore provided suitable substrates for the isolation of the two enzymes. Further, the two model compounds have characteristic absorption spectra. This made it possible not only to predict the optical properties of the corresponding natural substrates, *i.e.*, S-acetoacetyl and S-crotonyl CoA, but also to develop convenient optical methods for the assay of several enzymes. Thus, the analogues have greatly facilitated the study of individual steps of fatty acid metabolism.

S-acetoacetyl-N-acetyl thioethanolamine was obtained as a colourless crystalline compound (m.p., 60°) through reaction of N-acetyl thioethanolamine with diketene. As a solid, the compound is in the keto form but it undergoes rapid enolization in solution as can be shown with the ferric chloride reaction and by the change in its absorption spectrum. At equilibrium the percentage of enol is higher in solutions of the thioester

$$CH_3-\overset{O}{\underset{|}{C}}-CH_2-\overset{O}{\underset{|}{C}}-S-CH_2-CH_2-NH-CO-CH_3 \rightleftharpoons CH_3-\overset{OH}{\underset{|}{C}}=CH-\overset{O}{\underset{|}{C}}-S-CH_2-CH_2-NH-CO-CH_3$$

than in those of acetoacetic ethyl ester, a fact which was first observed by BAKER AND REID with acetoacetic thioethyl ester[2].

References p. 313/314.

The absorption spectrum of S-acetoacetyl-N-acetyl thioethanolamine is shown in Fig. 2. At pH 6.2 the compound has a band with a maximum at 233 mμ; this absorption

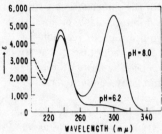

peak is characteristic of the thioester bond[57,60]. At pH 8.0 an additional band appears with a maximum at 303 mμ. This band is to be attributed to the formation of an enolate ion and, as shown in Fig. 3, depends on the pH. The increasing absorption parallels the increasing dissociation as the pH is raised. The pK' of the compound was found to be 8.54.

S-crotonyl-N-acetyl thioethanolamine was obtained in

$$CH_3—CH=CH—\overset{O}{\overset{\|}{C}}—S—CH_2—CH_2—NH—CO—CH_3$$

Fig. 2. Ultraviolet absorption spectrum of S-acetoacetyl-N-acetyl thioethanolamine.

crystalline form (m.p., 61.5–62°) through reaction of crotonyl chloride with the lead salt of N-acetyl thioethanolamine[55]. Its absorption spectrum is shown, along with that of free crotonate, in Fig. 4. It is evident that with the binding of the unsaturated acid to sulfur there is a shift toward longer wavelengths of the absorption due to the double bond. Free crotonate has a maximum (not shown on the figure) at 204 mμ while the thioester has a maximum at 224 mμ. The thioester has an additional band at 263 mμ which is possible due

to the $—\overset{O}{\overset{\|}{C}}—S—$group. The shift of the two absorption maxima toward longer wavelengths may be a reflection of the resonance between the double bond and the thio-ester linkage, a fact which is of great importance for the chemical reactivity of the former.

A number of S-acyl CoA derivatives of fatty acids have now become available through chemical or enzymic

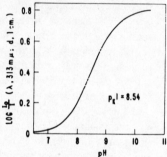

Fig. 3. pH Dependence of light absorption of S-acetoacetyl-N-acetyl thioethanolamine at 313 mμ. $c = 5 \cdot 10^{-5}$ M; $d = 1.0$ cm.

synthesis. Solutions of acetoacetyl CoA can be readily prepared by the enzymic transfer of CoA from succinyl CoA to acetoacetate. This reaction has made possible the isolation of acetoacetyl CoA[69] and its routine preparation for the assay of β-ketothiolase. Succinyl CoA itself can be prepared enzymically with α-ketoglutaric dehydrogenase[54,27] or by means of the reaction between succinate, CoA, and ATP, of KAUFMAN et al.[26,27]. However, the compound can be obtained much more readily by the synthetic procedure of SIMON AND SHEMIN[56] with CoA–SH and succinic anhydride. The method of SIMON AND SHEMIN has further been applied to the preparation of other S-acyl CoA derivatives such as acetyl, propionyl, butyryl, and crotonyl CoA. S-acyl fatty acid derivatives have also been prepared by

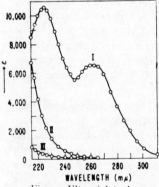

Fig. 4. Ultraviolet absorption spectra of S-crotonyl-N-acetyl thioethanolamine (I), crotonate (II), and N-acetyl thioethanolamine (III), at pH 7.0.

means of the enzymic reaction of fatty acids with CoA–SH and ATP[21a] and, in the case of the acetyl and propionyl derivatives, through the phosphotransacetylase catalyzed reaction between CoA–SH and the corresponding acyl phosphates[59]. Finally, S-acetoacetyl and S-β-hydroxybutyryl

References p. 313/314.

CoA have recently become available through chemical synthesis. T. WIELAND[77] has succeeded in synthesizing these compounds by reaction of CoA–SH with the thio-esters of acetoacetic or β-hydroxybutyric acid and thiophenol. S-acetoacetyl CoA has also been prepared through the interaction of CoA–SH with diketene[14a].

The absorption spectra of acetoacetyl CoA and crotonyl CoA are essentially the same as those of their thioethanolamine analogues. The main difference is that, in contrast to N-acetyl thioethanolamine, CoA absorbs in the 260 mμ region because of its adenine group. This does not interfere with the enol band of acetoacetyl thioesters but interferes to some extent with the 263 mμ band of the crotonyl derivatives. However, the extinction coefficient of the latter compounds at this wavelength is very high and the interference of the adenine moiety of crotonyl CoA can be eliminated by addition of adenine nucleotide, for example adenylic acid, to the blank cell.

In contrast to the optical behavior of the acetoacetyl and crotonyl CoA derivatives, β-hydroxyacyl and saturated acyl CoA compounds show only the thioester band at 233 mμ in addition to the adenine band. It is therefore possible in enzymic experiments, to follow the appearance and disappearance of β-ketoacyl or dehydroacyl CoA compounds if β-hydroxyacyl or acyl CoA compounds are involved in the reaction. At pH 8.0 the enol absorption of acetoacetyl thioesters is markedly increased by magnesium ions[67a], probably through formation of a chelate structure. This increase in absorption can conveniently be made use of to increase the sensitivity of the optical enzyme tests.

ENZYMES OF FATTY ACID METABOLISM

Activating enzymes. As already stated the main mechanism for the activation of fatty acids in animal tissues is through a reaction of the fatty acid with CoA–SH, in the presence of ATP, to yield the corresponding S-acyl CoA, AMP, and PP. This reaction requires the presence of Mg ions. The first reaction of this type to be studied in detail was the activation of acetate by an enzyme present in liver, yeast, and other tissues[11]. The mechanism of the over-all reaction was established by LIPMANN *et al.*[44] with partially purified enzyme preparations from liver and yeast (Reaction 1). Similar results were obtained by HILZ AND LYNEN (unpublished experiments) with a highly purified enzyme

$$CH_3-COOH + HS-Co\bar{A} + ATP \rightleftharpoons CH_3-\overset{\overset{\text{O}}{\|}}{C}-S-Co\bar{A} + AMP + PP \qquad (1)$$

from yeast and by GREEN and collaborators[21, 23] with purified enzymes from heart muscle and liver. The acetate enzyme is active also with propionate.

Recent experiments[25] suggest that the over-all reaction occurs in three steps as indicated below:

(a) ATP + enzyme $\rightleftharpoons$ AMP-enzyme + PP
(b) AMP-enzyme + CoA $\rightleftharpoons$ CoA-enzyme + AMP
(c) CoA-enzyme + acetate $\rightleftharpoons$ acetyl-CoA + enzyme

The occurrence of reaction (a) is supported by the incorporation of labelled PP into ATP in the presence of a partially purified enzyme from yeast. This exchange is dependent upon the presence of Mg^{+2}. Reaction (c) is supported by the incorporation of isotopic acetate into acetyl CoA in the presence of the enzyme.

An enzyme catalyzing the activation of fatty acids from C_4 to C_{12} was isolated from ox liver in D. E. GREEN's laboratory[72]. The enzyme catalyzes Reaction 2. The same

References p. 313/314.

enzyme preparation was active on α,β-unsaturated and β-hydroxy derivatives. The formation of crotonyl- and β-hydroxybutyryl CoA by liver enzymes under similar

$$-CH_2-CH_2-COOH+HS-Co\bar{A}+ATP \rightleftharpoons -CH_2-CH_2-\overset{O}{\overset{\|}{C}}-S-Co\bar{A}+AMP+PP \quad (2)$$

conditions has also been observed in other laboratories[41,67]. The activation of higher fatty acids, presumably C_{14} to $_{18}$, by ATP and HS-CoA is catalyzed by yet another enzyme discovered by KORNBERG AND PRICER[36,35] in liver. KORNBERG's enzyme catalyzes the formation of S-stearyl CoA, AMP, and PP from stearic acid, HS-CoA and ATP.

CoA transferases. In *Cl. kluyveri* extracts activation of fatty acids appears to occur predominantly by transfer of CoA from acetyl-S-CoA. The first enzyme of the CoA transferase type was discovered by STADTMAN in extracts of *Cl. kluyveri* and named CoA transphorase[60]. The enzyme catalyzes the reversible transfer of CoA from acetyl-CoA to propionate (Reaction 3).

$$CH_3-\overset{O}{\overset{\|}{C}}-S-Co\bar{A}+CH_3-CH_2-COOH \rightleftharpoons CH_3-COOH+CH_3-CH_2-\overset{O}{\overset{\|}{C}}-S-Co\bar{A} \quad (3)$$

Cl. kluyveri extracts also catalyze the transfer of CoA from acetyl CoA to butyrate, vinyl acetate, and lactate[60a]. This enzyme (enzymes) is (are) similar to the succinyl-CoA-acetoacetate transferase of heart muscle but with different substrate specificity.

The reversible transfer of CoA from succinyl CoA to acetoacetate was discovered independently by GREEN and co workers[21,22] and by STERN *et al.*[68,69]. The enzyme which, as already mentioned, is present in heart and probably in skeletal muscle and kidney but not in liver, catalyzes Reaction 4. In the early stages of purification[69] the

$$HOOC-CH_2-CH_2-\overset{O}{\overset{\|}{C}}-S-Co\bar{A}+CH_3-CO-CH_2-COOH \rightleftharpoons$$
$$HOOC-CH_2-CH_2-COOH+CH_3-CO-CH_2-\overset{O}{\overset{\|}{C}}-S-Co\bar{A} \quad (4)$$

enzyme assay was based on the rate of citric acid synthesis from succinyl CoA and acetoacetate in the presence of oxalacetate, an excess of thiolase, and crystalline citrate condensing enzyme, as indicated by the reactions below:

Succinyl—S—Co$\bar{A}$ + acetoacetate $\rightleftharpoons$ succinate + acetoacetyl—S—Co$\bar{A}$ (transferase)
Acetoacetyl—S—Co$\bar{A}$ + HS—Co$\bar{A}$ $\rightleftharpoons$ 2 acetyl—S—Co$\bar{A}$ (thiolase)
2 Acetyl—S—Co$\bar{A}$ + 2 oxalacetate + 2 H$_2$O $\rightleftharpoons$ 2 citrate + 2 HS—Co$\bar{A}$ (citrate condensing enzyme)

Sum: Succinyl—S—Co$\bar{A}$ + acetoacetate + HS—Co$\bar{A}$ + 2 oxalacetate + 2 H$_2$O $\rightleftharpoons$ Succinate + 2 citrate + 2 HS—Co$\bar{A}$

A heated ammonium sulfate fraction from ox liver, free of transferase, was used as the source of thiolase. After removal of thiolase, the transferase assay was based on the increase in optical density at pH 8.1 and wavelength 305 mμ due to the formation of acetoacetyl-S-CoA. Although magnesium ions are not required for the reaction, as mentioned previously, Mg^{+2} markedly augments the light absorption and was added to the reaction mixture in order to increase the sensitivity of the assay.

The enzyme has been isolated from pig heart and purified about 700-fold over the initial phosphate extract[67a]. The purification involved ammonium sulfate and acetone fractionation, removal of inactive proteins by heat and by adsorption on Ca phosphate

References p. 313/314.

gel, fractionation with ethanol in the presence of Zn ions, and refractionation with ammonium sulfate.

Fig. 5 shows the appearance of the enol band of S-acetoacetyl thioesters when succinyl CoA is incubated with acetoacetate and transferase at pH 8.1, indicating the formation of S-acetoacetyl CoA. Within the range 290 to 330 mμ this band corresponds closely with the corresponding band of S-acetoacetyl-N-acetyl thioethanolamine. It may also be seen that most of the absorption in this region disappears after the further addition of CoA–SH and thiolase since the equilibrium position of the thiolase reaction favors the formation of acetyl CoA. The forward course and the reversal of the transferase

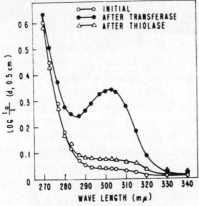

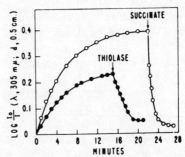

Fig. 5. Spectral changes accompanying the enzymatic synthesis and breakdown of S-acetoacetyl CoA at pH 8.1 Volume, 1.5 ml; $d = 0.5$ cm; temp. 25°.—O—O— S-Succinyl CoA ($\sim 0.1 \mu M$). —●—●— After establishment of equilibrium on addition of acetoacetate (50 μM) and transferase (60 μg of protein). —△—△— After further addition of CoA–SH (0.15 μM) and thiolase (90 μg of protein). Acetoacetate and CoA–SH added to both blank and experimental cells. MgCl$_2$ (8.0 μM) present in reaction mixture.

Fig. 6. Optical demonstration of transferase and thiolase activities. Volume, 1.5 ml; $d = 0.5$ cm; pH, 8.1; temp., 25°. Upper curve: Transferase (17 μg of protein) added at zero time to a mixture of succinyl CoA ($\sim 0.11 \mu M$) and acetoacetate (50 μM); succinate (40 μM) added at the arrow. Lower curve: Transferase (17 μg of protein) added at zero time to a mixture of succinyl CoA ($\sim 0.06 \mu M$) and acetoacetate (50 μM); CoA–SH (0.15 μM) and thiolase (2.7 μg of protein) added at the arrow. Other details as in Fig. 5.

reaction as followed at 305 mμ are shown in Fig. 6. The upper curve shows the increase in absorption at 305 mμ on adding transferase to a mixture of succinyl CoA and acetoacetate and the reversal of the reaction by succinate after equilibrium was established. The equilibrium constant of the transferase reaction (K_{eq} = (Succinate) (acetoacetyl-S-CoA)/Succinyl-S-CoA) (acetoacetate)) is about 10^{-2} at pH 8.1.

The acetoacetyl CoA formed by the reaction between succinyl CoA and acetoacetate, in the presence of transferase, was isolated as a crude alcohol-insoluble barium salt and further purified by paper chromatography[69]. In ethanol-acetate its R_F is 0.52 at 24°, while that of acetoacetate is 0.75. Like acetyl CoA[46, 47], acetoacetyl CoA gives a positive sulfhydryl reaction with nitroprusside only after alkaline hydrolysis.

Some insight into the mechanism of action of the transferase has been gained by experiments with methylene labelled ^{14}C-succinate[19a]. When ^{14}C-succinate and succinyl-CoA are incubated with transferase a rapid exchange of free- and thioester-bound succinate occurs. This suggests the possibility that succinyl CoA, or acetoacetyl CoA, reacts with the enzyme to form a CoA-enzyme compound which retains the energy of the

References p. 313/314.

thioester bond and can transfer CoA to the free acid, acetoacetic or succinic. The reaction could be visualized as involving a carboxyl group of the enzyme as indicated below:

$$HOOC\text{---}CH_2\text{---}CH_2\overset{O}{\overset{\|}{\text{---}C}}\text{---}S\text{---}Co\bar{A} + Enzyme\text{---}COOH \rightleftharpoons$$

$$HOOC\text{---}CH_2\text{---}CH_2\text{---}COOH + Enzyme\overset{O}{\overset{\|}{\text{---}C}}\text{---}S\text{---}Co\bar{A}$$

$$Enzyme\overset{O}{\overset{\|}{\text{---}C}}\text{---}S\text{---}Co\bar{A} + CH_3\text{---}CO\text{---}CH_2\text{---}COOH \rightleftharpoons$$

$$Enzyme\text{---}COOH + CH_3\text{---}CO\text{---}CH_2\overset{O}{\overset{\|}{\text{---}C}}\text{---}S\text{---}Co\bar{A}$$

The best preparations of transferase so far obtained are free of thiolase and, under the conditions of the optical assay, catalyze the formation of 250 moles of acetoacetyl-CoA per minute per 100,000 g of enzyme at 25°. As assayed optically, the purified transferase catalyzes the transfer of CoA from succinyl CoA to acetoacetate, β-ketovalerate, β-keto*iso*caproate, and β-ketocaproate in order of decreasing activity. β-ketooctanoate is inactive. The enzyme catalyzes the transfer of CoA from acetoacetyl CoA to succinate but not to β hydroxybyturate, crotonate, butyrate or octanoate.

β-keto thiolase. The enzyme catalyzing Reaction 5 has been partially purified from sheep liver[48] and more extensively from pig heart[50a]. The enzyme has also been referred to as the acetoacetate condensing enzyme[69]. In the lower curve of Fig. 6, addition of CoA-SH and thiolase to a mixture of succinyl CoA and acetoacetate previously incubated with transferase is shown to cause a decrease in optical density at 305 mμ due to cleavage of the acetoacetyl CoA formed by the CoA transfer reaction. The assay used for the purification of the pig heart enzyme was based on the decrease in optical density at

$$CH_3\text{---}CO\text{---}CH_2\overset{O}{\overset{\|}{\text{---}C}}\text{---}S\text{---}CoA + HS\text{---}CoA \rightleftharpoons 2CH_3\overset{O}{\overset{\|}{\text{---}C}}\text{---}S\text{---}CoA \qquad (5)$$

pH 8.1 and wavelength 305 mμ with acetoacetyl CoA and CoA–SH as substrates in the presence of Mg^{+2}. Solutions of acetoacetyl CoA were prepared every few days by incubating synthetic succinyl CoA and acetoacetate with purified CoA-transferase. When the reaction reached equilibrium, the pH of the mixture was brought to 5.5 with acetic acid, the solution was heated to 75° for 2 minutes to destroy the transferase, cooled, centrifuged and the supernatant adjusted to pH 8.0. Acetoacetyl CoA was stable for several days if stored at −18° when not in use.

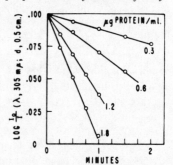

The enzyme has been purified about 300 fold over the initial phosphate extract through steps involving ammonium sulfate and acetone fractionation, removal of inactive proteins at pH 5.3, refractionation with ammonium sulfate, and low temperature ethanol fractionation in the presence of Zn ions. The time course of the reaction in the optical test with varying concentrations of purified pig heart enzyme is shown in Fig. 7.

Fig. 7. Optical thiolase test. Tris (hydroxymethyl) amino - methane-HCl buffer pH 8.1, 200 μM; MgCl$_2$, 8.0 μM; reduced glutathione, 10.0 μM; CoA-SH, 0.15 μM; S-acetoacetylCoA, ∼0.03 μM. Volume, 1.5 ml; d = 0.5 cm; temp., 25°.

The thioclastic cleavage of acetoacetyl CoA to acetyl CoA results not only in a decrease of light absorption at 305 mμ but also in a concomitant increase in the absorption in the 240 mμ region

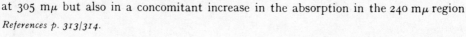

References p. 313/314.

due to the formation of a second thioester bond, since two molecules of acetyl CoA are formed per molecule of acetoacetyl CoA disappearing. In the presence of CoA-SH, oxalacetate, thiolase, and citrate condensing enzyme, acetoacetyl CoA yields two molecules of citrate per molecule of sulfhydryl (*i.e.*, per molecule of CoA–SH) appearing[69], according to the following reactions:

Acetoacetyl—S—CoA + HS—CoA ⇌ 2 acetyl—S—CoA (thiolase)

2 Acetyl—S—CoA + 2 oxalacetate + 2 H_2O ⇌ 2 citrate + 2 HS—CoA (citrate condensing enzyme)

Sum · Acetoacetyl—S—CoA + HS—CoA + 2 oxalacetate + 2 H_2O ⇌ 2 citrate + 2 HS—CoA

The equilibrium position of the thiolase reaction is very far toward cleavage[48, 68, 69]. For this reason it was not feasible to use this reaction for the isolation of acetoacetyl CoA. Determinations of the equilibrium constant $(K'_{eq} = (\text{Acetyl-S-CoA})^2/(\text{Acetoacetyl CoA})(\text{CoA-SH}))$ by means of the optical method gave an approximate value of $5 \cdot 10^4$ at pH 8.1, and $1 \cdot 10^4$ at pH 9.0.

The reversibility of the reaction can be demonstrated by the optical method as previously reported[48]. The synthesis of acetoacetyl CoA from acetyl CoA can be followed directly at alkaline pH (∼ 9.0) as a small increase in the optical density at 305 mμ in the presence of large amounts of acetyl CoA[48a], or indirectly through coupling with the β-keto reductase to effect the oxidation of reduced DPN[48].

The purified heart enzyme is highly specific for acetoacetyl CoA. β-Ketovaleryl CoA reacts at 20% of the rate of acetoacetyl CoA, and β-ketocaproyl- and *iso*caproyl-CoA react practically not at all. This is in contrast to the broader specificity of crude enzyme fractions[68] and indicates that there must be other thiolases, acting on S-β-ketoacyl CoA derivatives of higher chain length.

Under the conditions of the optical test, the best preparations of the heart enzyme so far obtained catalyze the cleavage of 3000 to 4000 moles of acetoacetyl CoA per minute per 100,000 g of enzyme at 25°. When coupled with β-keto reductase about 30 times more acetoacetate condensing enzyme must be used in the back reaction to reach the rates obtained in the direction of acetoacetyl CoA cleavage.

β-Ketothiolase has been found to be inhibited by sulfhydryl reagents such as iodoacetic acid or arsenoxide[48a]. This indicates that the enzyme is an "SH enzyme" and suggests the following mechanism of action:

(a) R—CH$_2$—CO—CH$_2$—$\overset{\overset{\text{O}}{\|}}{\text{C}}$—S—CoA + HS-Enzyme ⇌ R—CH$_2$—$\overset{\overset{\text{O}}{\|}}{\text{C}}$—S-Enzyme + CH$_3$—$\overset{\overset{\text{O}}{\|}}{\text{C}}$—S—CoA

(b) R—CH$_2$—$\overset{\overset{\text{O}}{\|}}{\text{C}}$—S-Enzyme + HS—CoA ⇌ R—CH$_2$—$\overset{\overset{\text{O}}{\|}}{\text{C}}$—S—CoA + HS-Enzyme

Such a mechanism is further supported by experiments[45a] with CoA labelled with ^{35}S. On incubation of propionyl-S-CoA with ^{35}S-H-CoA, in the presence of purified heart thiolase, radioactive propionyl-S-CoA is formed indicating the occurrence of the following reaction:

Propionyl S—CoA + HS-enzyme ⇌ Propionyl-S-enzyme + HS—CoA

The above mechanism provides an explanation for the unequal isotope distribution in acetoacetate observed during oxidation of isotopic fatty acids in liver[10, 13, 12, 19, 18]. For example, octanoic acid labelled with ^{14}C in the carboxyl group can yield acetoacetate in which the ratio of the radioactivity in the carbonyl and carboxyl carbons is less than unity. Some acetoacetate labelled exclusively in the carboxyl group must arise when

References p. 313/314.

non-labelled acetoacetyl-S-CoA from the last four carbons of the fatty acid chain reacts with thiolase to give non-labelled acetyl-S-enzyme and this in turn reacts with labelled

acetyl-S-CoA from the pool to yield CH_3—CO—CH_2—$\overset{\overset{\displaystyle O}{\|}}{C}{}^*$—S—CoA. This is shown schematically in Fig. 8 for the case of caproic acid.

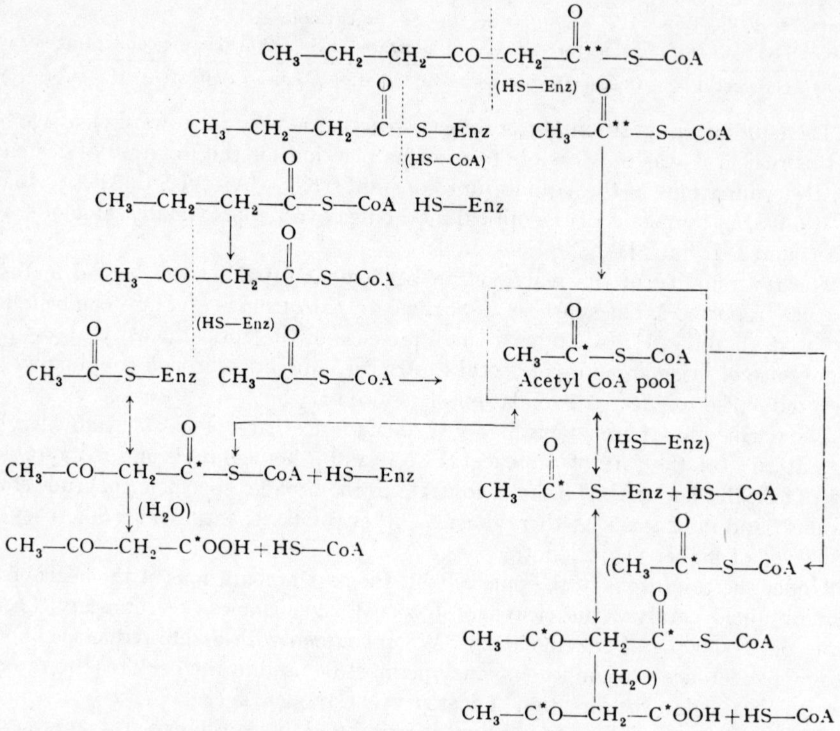

$$CH_3-CH_2-CH_2-CO\text{--}CH_2-\overset{\overset{O}{\|}}{C}{}^{**}-S-CoA$$

(HS—Enz)

$$CH_3-CH_2-CH_2-\overset{\overset{O}{\|}}{C}\text{--}S-Enz \qquad CH_3-\overset{\overset{O}{\|}}{C}{}^{**}-S-CoA$$

(HS—CoA)

$$CH_3-CH_2-CH_2-\overset{\overset{O}{\|}}{C}-S-CoA \quad HS-Enz$$

$$CH_3-CO\text{--}CH_2-\overset{\overset{O}{\|}}{C}-S-CoA$$

(HS—Enz)

$$CH_3-\overset{\overset{O}{\|}}{C}-S-Enz \quad CH_3-\overset{\overset{O}{\|}}{C}-S-CoA \longrightarrow$$

$$\boxed{\begin{array}{c} O \\ \| \\ CH_3-C{}^*-S-CoA \\ \text{Acetyl CoA pool} \end{array}}$$

$$CH_3-CO\text{--}CH_2-\overset{\overset{O}{\|}}{C}{}^*-S-CoA+HS-Enz$$

(H_2O)

$$CH_3-CO\text{--}CH_2-C{}^*OOH+HS-CoA$$

(HS—Enz)

$$CH_3-\overset{\overset{O}{\|}}{C}{}^*-S-Enz+HS-CoA$$

$$(CH_3-\overset{\overset{O}{\|}}{C}{}^*-S-CoA$$

$$CH_3-C{}^*O-CH_2-\overset{\overset{O}{\|}}{C}{}^*-S-CoA$$

(H_2O)

$$CH_3-C{}^*O-CH_2-C{}^*OOH+HS-CoA$$

Fig. 8. Asymmetric labelling of acetoacetate from carboxyl-labelled caproic acid.

β-keto-reductase. This enzyme catalyzes Reaction 6. The finding that

$$CH_3-CO-CH_2-\overset{\overset{O}{\|}}{C}-S-Co\bar{A}+DPNH+H^+ \rightleftharpoons CH_3-CHOH-CH_2-\overset{\overset{O}{\|}}{C}-S-Co\bar{A}+DPN^+ \quad (6)$$

the acetoacetyl-S-CoA analogue, S-acetoacetyl-N-acetyl thioethanolamine, was readily reduced by DPNH in the presence of enzyme solutions from various sources afforded a convenient assay for this enzyme. Employing this assay the enzyme was purified some 300-fold from sheep liver extracts by a procedure involving three steps: precipitation with ethanol, denaturation of inactive protein at 55°, and fractionation with ammonium sulfate[48]. The time course of the reaction in the optical test with varying concentrations of the purified enzyme is shown in Fig. 9.

The reaction is readily reversible but, at pH 7.35 with equimolecular amounts of DPNH and the acetoacetyl thioethanolamine derivative, it proceeds in the direction of reduction of the latter to the extent of 95 %. The equilibrium constant of the reaction $(K'_{eq} = \text{(S-β-hydroxybutyryl compound) (DPN}^+)/\text{(S-acetoacetyl compound) (DPNH))}$

References p. 313/314.

194

has been found[48a] to be $5.2 \cdot 10^2$ at pH 7.0. The enzyme does not react with free acetoacetate or with ethyl acetoacetate; it also fails to react with S-acetoacetyl glutathione. With acetoacetyl-S-CoA the reaction is much faster than with the thioethanolamine derivative. This is undoubtedly due to the much higher affinity of the enzyme for the natural compound. In fact, in kinetic studies with S-acetoacetyl-N-acetyl thioethanolamine it was not possible to reach saturation of the enzyme with the analogue[48a].

In the presence of thiolase, β-keto reductase, and DPNH, the latter is oxidized on addition of acetyl-S-CoA; DPN⁺, β-hydroxybutyryl-S-CoA and HS-CoA are the reaction products[48]. This occurs according to the reactions below:

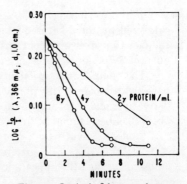

Fig. 9. Optical β-keto reductase test. Pyrophosphate buffer pH 7.4, 50 μM; DPNH, 0.13 μM; S-acetoacetyl-N-acetyl thioethanolamine, 5.0 μM. Volume, 2.0 ml; $d = 1.0$ cm; temp. 25°.

$$2CH_3 - \overset{O}{\overset{\|}{C}} - S - Co\bar{A} \rightleftharpoons HS - Co\bar{A} + CH_3 - CO - CH_2 - \overset{O}{\overset{\|}{O}} - S - Co\bar{A} \quad \text{(thiolase)}$$

$$CH_3 - CO - CH_2 - \overset{O}{\overset{\|}{C}} - S - Co\bar{A} + DPNH + H^+ \rightleftharpoons CH_3 - CHOH - CH_2 - \overset{O}{\overset{\|}{C}} - S - Co\bar{A} + DPN^+ \quad \text{(reductase)}$$

$$Sum: 2CH_3 - \overset{O}{\overset{\|}{C}} - S - Co\bar{A} + DPNH + H^- \rightleftharpoons CH_3 - CHOH - CH_2 - \overset{O}{\overset{\|}{C}} - S - Co\bar{A} + HS - Co\bar{A} + DPN^-$$

The formation of HS-CoA can be followed through the appearance of sulfhydryl groups. β-hydroxybutyryl-S-CoA was extracted from the acidified reaction mixture with *p*-cresol and converted into the corresponding hydroxamic acid by reaction with hydroxylamine. The β-hydroxybutyrohydroxamic acid was identified by paper chromatography (R_F in aqueous butanol, 0.29). On incubation of the natural β-hydroxybutyryl-S-CoA with DPN⁺ and purified β-ketoreductase at pH 9.05, the reduction of DPN⁺, followed at 340 mμ, is accompanied by the formation of acetoacetyl-S-CoA as shown by the increase in optical density at 303 mμ.

As previously mentioned both β-hydroxybutyryl- and acetoacetyl-S-CoA have recently become available synthetically. The course of the β-ketoreductase reaction with these two compounds[48a] is shown in Fig. 10.

LEHNINGER AND GREVILLE[41] have recently reported the interesting observation that liver contains two different β-ketoreductases. One of them catalyzes the reversible oxidation of free *l*-hydroxybutyrate by DPN⁺, the other catalyzes the reversible oxidation

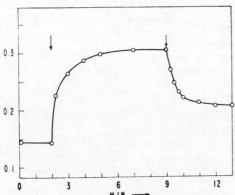

Fig. 10. Optical experiments with β-keto reductase. Pyrophosphate buffer pH 6.58, 100 μM; DPN⁺, 5.0 μM; S-β-hydroxybutyryl CoA, 2.0 μM. Volume, 2.0 ml; λ, 366 mμ; $d = 1.0$ cm; temp. 21°. β-keto reductase (1.5 mg of protein) added at the first arrow. S-acetoacetyl CoA (0.43 μM) added at the second arrow.

References p. 313/314.

of d-β-hydroxybutyryl-S-CoA by DPN$^+$. The latter reaction, which is undoubtedly catalyzed by the β-ketoreductase here described, was demonstrated by making use of the fact that liver also contains enzymes catalyzing the formation of d- or l-β-hydroxybutyryl-S-CoA in the presence of ATP, CoA-SH, and d- or l-β-hydroxybutyrate.

The chain-length specificity of the β-ketoreductase is still unknown and it is not possible to decide at this time whether more than one enzyme is concerned with the CoA derivatives of β-keto and β-hydroxy acids from C_4 to C_{18}. The purified reductase described above has been found to act rapidly on S-β-ketocaproyl-N-acetyl thioethanolamine[48a].

Crotonase. Synthetic S-crotonyl CoA is converted to S-acetoacetyl CoA, in the presence of DPN, by crude enzyme preparations from heart or liver[67]. The reaction can be followed through the appearance of the absorption band of DPNH at 340 mμ or that of acetoacetyl-S-CoA at 305 mμ. Also, on addition of HS-CoA, citrate condensing enzyme, and oxalacetate, crotonyl-S-CoA acts as an acetyl donor for citrate synthesis; the required thiolase was present in the crude enzyme preparation used. These observations, together with the fact that reduced leucosafranine is oxidized by synthetic β-hydroxybutyryl-S-CoA in the presence of partially purified preparations of ethylene reductase[55] indicate the occurrence of an enzyme catalyzing the reversible Reaction 7 below. The name crotonase has been suggested for this enzyme[67]. The enzyme has no action on free

$$CH_3-CH=CH-\overset{\overset{\displaystyle O}{\|}}{C}-S-CoA + H_2O \rightleftharpoons CH_3-CHOH-CH_2-\overset{\overset{\displaystyle O}{\|}}{C}-S-CoA \qquad (7)$$

crotonate or on the S-crotonyl derivatives of N-acetyl thioethanolamine, glutathione or thioglycolic acid.

As already mentioned the spectrum of S-crotonyl CoA is similar to that of S-crotonyl-N-acetyl thioethanolamine. This is readily apparent when the contribution of the adenine moiety of the CoA derivative is eliminated by reading S-crotonyl CoA against a solution containing an identical amount of the compound but previously subjected to alkaline hydrolysis. The difference spectrum so obtained[52a], illustrated in Fig. 11, shows absorption maxima at 224 and 263 mμ like S-crotonyl-N-acetyl thioethanolamine. The crotonyl CoA was obtained through reaction of CoA-SH with crotonic anhydride following the method of SIMON AND SHEMIN[56].

The decrease in light absorption at 263 mμ when crotonase acts on crotonyl CoA affords a simple method of assay for this enzyme. The purification of the enzyme from ox liver has recently been undertaken. Through steps involving denaturation of inactive proteins by acidification and heat, followed by acetone, ammonium sulfate and low temperature ethanol fractionation, preparations of the enzyme have been obtained representing about 100-fold purification over the original extract[52a]. The preparations are free of fumarase showing that fumarase and crotonase are distinct enzymes. Crotonase has a remarkably high activity as may be seen in Fig. 12. which shows the time course of the reaction in the optical test with varying amounts of the enzyme. The equilibrium

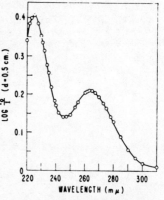

Fig. 11. Difference ultraviolet absorption spectrum of S-crotonyl CoA before and after alkaline hydrolysis of the thioester bond. $c \simeq 6 \cdot 10^{-5}$ M in each cell; $d = 0.5$ cm; pH, 7.5. Crotonyl CoA in blank cell previously hydrolyzed with alkali.

References p. 313/314.

constant of the reaction has not yet been determined but it appears to favor the S-β-hydroxyacyl derivatives. Nothing can as yet be said as to the chain-length specificity of crotonase and consequently the occurrence of several enzymes of this type is not excluded.

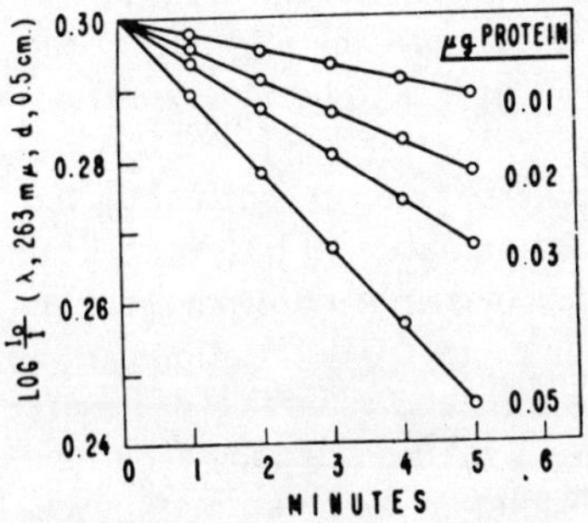

Crotonase would also appear to convert S-vinylacetyl CoA to the β-hydroxybutyryl derivative[21a]. If so, an equilibrium would be established between the S-acyl CoA derivatives of crotonic, vinylacetic, and β-hydroxybutyric acid. This might explain the observation that vinylacetate can be either oxidized or reduced by extracts of *C. kluyveri*[28,62]. The failure of crotonate to replace vinylacetate in this system[62] may have been due to failure of the bacterial extracts to activate crotonate.

Ethylene reductase. Ethylene reductase was detected in liver extracts[55] by a method similar to that employed by FISCHER AND EYSENBACH to study fumarate reductase[17]. Leucosafranine is oxidized by S-crotonyl-N-acetyl thioethanolamine, but not by free crotonate, in the presence of an enzyme from liver.

Fig. 12. Optical crotonase test. Tris (hydroxymethyl) aminomethane-HCl-buffer pH 7.5, 100 μM; egg albumin, 0.1 mg; ethylenediamine tetraacetate, 1.5 μM; S-crotonyl CoA, $\sim$ 0.5 μM. 2.0 μM of AMP in blank cell. Volume, 1.5 ml; $d = 0.5$ cm; temp., 25°.

The reaction is shown in Fig. 13. Here again a natural compound, in this case crotonyl-S-CoA, could be replaced by its readily synthesized thioethanolamine analogue. The

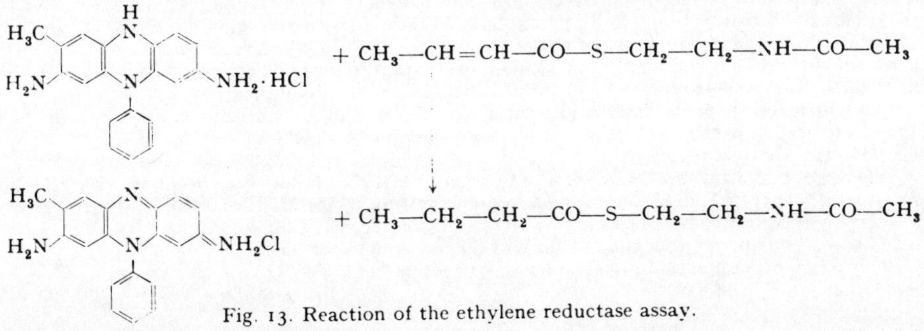

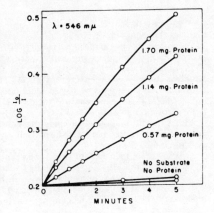

H₃C—CH=CH—CO—S—CH₂—CH₂—NH—CO—CH₃

CH₃—CH₂—CH₂—CO—S—CH₂—CH₂—NH—CO—CH₃

Fig. 13. Reaction of the ethylene reductase assay.

enzyme assay, in which the appearance of colour from the leucodye is followed, is illustrated in Fig. 14. By the use of this assay ethylene reductase was purified about 80-fold from sheep liver extracts through steps involving acetone fractionation, adsorption and elution from calcium phosphate gel, and ammonium sulfate fractionation. Solutions of the purified enzyme are yellow in colour. A colourless, almost inactive

Fig. 14. Optical ethylene reductase test. Phosphate buffer pH 7.1, 140 μM; leucosafranine T, 0.5 μM; S-crotonyl-N-acetyl thioethanolamine, 2.6 μM. Volume, 2.1 ml; $d = 0.5$ cm; temp. 17°.

References p. 313/314.

protein can be precipitated from these solutions with ammonium sulfate at pH 3.6 as in the method of WARBURG AND CHRISTIAN[73] for the resolution of the flavoprotein D-amino acid oxidase. The activity of the protein can be restored by the addition of flavin adenine dinucleotide which has been found to be the prosthetic group of the enzyme. Thus, like fumarate reductase, ethylene reductase appears to be a flavoprotein. DPNH or TPNH cannot substitute for the leucodye.

In line with the above observations GREEN and co-workers[20a] have recently reported on the isolation of flavoproteins from ox liver catalyzing the oxidation of butyryl-S CoA and some higher acyl-S-CoA derivatives in the presence of triphenyltetrazolium as hydrogen acceptor. The prosthetic group appears also to be FAD.

There is thus little doubt that the enzymes of the ethylene reductase class are flavoproteins. The nature of the electron transport system in the cell mediating the transfer of hydrogen from the reduced flavoprotein to molecular oxygen is still unknown. During fatty acid synthesis, hydrogens made available through oxidation of carbohydrate as reduced pyridine nucleotides must be transferred to the ethylene reductase flavoproteins to effect the reduction of the α,β-unsaturated S-acyl-CoA fatty acid derivatives. How such interaction takes place is also unknown.

SUMMARY

The intermediates in the biological breakdown and synthesis of fatty acids are S-acyl derivatives of coenzyme A.

Fatty acid synthesis is accomplished through repetition of a cycle of four consecutive reactions: a. Condensation of two molecules of acetyl CoA to form acetoacetyl CoA and coenzyme A (CoA–SH); b. reduction of acetoacetyl CoA to β-hydroxybutyryl CoA; c. dehydration of β-hydroxybutyryl CoA to crotonyl CoA, and d. reduction of crotonyl CoA to butyryl CoA. A new cycle is started by the reaction of butyryl CoA with another molecule of acetyl CoA, to form β-keto-caproyl CoA + CoA–SH, and so forth. The cycle is repeated eight times until stearyl CoA is formed.

All four reactions of the fatty acid cycle are reversible and fatty acid oxidation, once the fatty acid is activated through conversion to the corresponding S-acyl CoA derivative, proceeds by a reversal of the above sequence.

There are two main mechanisms for activation of fatty acids: (a) By a reaction with ATP and CoA to form S-acyl CoA, adenosine monophosphate and pyrophosphate, and (b) by transfer of CoA from certain acyl CoA compounds such as acetyl CoA or succinyl CoA.

The isolation and identification of some of the key enzymes of fatty acid metabolism is outlined and their mechanism of action discussed.

RÉSUMÉ

Les intermédiaires dans la dégradation et la synthèse biologique des acides gras sont des dérivés S-acylés du coenzyme A.

La synthèse des acides gras est le résultat de la répétition d'un cycle de 4 reactions consécutives: (a) condensation de deux molécules d'acétyl CoA conduisant à l'acétoacétyl CoA et au coenzyme A (CoA–SH), (b) réduction de l'acétoacétyl CoA en β-hydroxybutyryl CoA, (c) déshydratation du β-hydroxybutyryl CoA en crotonyl CoA, et (d) réduction du crotonyl CoA en butyryl CoA. Un nouveau cycle recommence par la réaction du butyryl CoA avec une autre molécule d'acétyl CoA, qui donne le β-cétocaproyl CoA + CoA–SH, et ainsi de suite. Le cycle se répète huit fois jusqu'à la formation du stéaryl CoA.

Les quatre réactions du cycle des acides gras sont réversibles et l'oxydation d'un acide gras, après son activation par transformation en dérivé S-acylé du CoA, suit le chemin inverse de la synthèse.

Il y a deux mécanismes principaux d'activation des acides gras: (a) par une réaction avec ATP et CoA qui donne du S-acyl CoA, de l'adénosine monophosphate et du pyrophosphate et (b) par transfert du CoA de certains acyl CoA, tels que l'acétyl CoA et le succinyl CoA.

L'isolement et l'identification de quelques-uns des enzymes essentiels au métabolisme des acides gras sont esquissés et leur mécanisme d'action discuté.

References p. *313/314.*

ZUSAMMENFASSUNG

Die Zwischenprodukte bei dem biologischen Abbau und bei der Synthese der Fettsäuren sind S-Acylderivate des Coenzyms A.

Die Fettsäuresynthese wird erreicht durch die Wiederholung eines Kreislaufs von 4 aufeinander-folgenden Reaktionen: a. Der Kondensation von 2 Molekülen Acetyl-CoA zu Acetoacetyl-CoA und Coenzym A (CoA–SH), b. der Reduktion des Acetoacetyl-CoA zu β-Hydroxybutyryl-CoA, c. der Dehydratisierung des β-Hydroxybutyryl-CoA zu Crotonyl-CoA und d. der Reduktion des Crotonyl-CoA zu Butyryl-CoA. Ein neuer Kreislauf wird begonnen mit der Reaktion des Butyryl-CoA mit einem anderen Molekül Acetyl-CoA unter Bildung von β-Ketocaproyl-CoA und CoA–SH, usw. Dieser Kreislauf wird 8 mal wiederholt bis Stearyl-CoA gebildet ist.

Alle 4 Reaktionen des Fettsäurekreislaufs sind reversibel und die Fettsäureoxydation verläuft über die umgekehrten Stufen der obigen Folge, wenn einmal die Fettsäure durch Überführung in das entsprechende S-Acyl-CoA aktiviert ist. Es gibt 2 Hauptmechanismen für die Aktivierung der Fettsäuren: a. Eine Reaktion mit ATP und CoA unter Bildung von S-Acyl-CoA, Adenosin mono-phosphat und Pyrophosphat, und b. eine Überführung des CoA von gewissen Acyl-CoA-verbindungen wie Acetyl-CoA oder Succinyl-CoA.

Die Isolierung und Identifizierung einiger Schlüsselenzyme des Fettsäurestoffwechsels wird umrissen und der Wirkungsmechanismus besprochen.

REFERENCES

[1] H. S. ANKER, *J. Biol. Chem.*, 194 (1952) 177.
[2] R. B. BAKER AND E. E. REID, *J. Am. Chem. Soc.*, 51 (1929) 1567.
[3] H. A. BARKER, in W. D. MCELROY AND B. GLASS, *Phosphorus Metabolism*, Vol. I, p. 204, Johns Hopkins Press, Baltimore (1951).
[4] H. A. BARKER, M. D. KAMEN AND B. T. BORNSTEIN, *Proc. Natl. Acad. Sci.*, 31 (1945) 373.
[5] K. BLOCH, *Ann. Rev. Biochem.*, 21 (1952) 273.
[6] R. O. BRADY AND S. GURIN, *J. Biol. Chem.*, 186 (1950) 461.
[7] F. L. BREUSCH, *Science*, 97 (1943) 490; *Enzymologia*, 11 (1944) 169.
[8] F. L. BREUSCH, in *Symposium sur le Cycle Tricarboxylique*, IIe Congrés International de Biochmie p. 35. Paris (1952).
[9] F. L. BREUSCH AND H. KESKIN, *Enzymologia*, 11 (1944) 243.
[10] J. M. BUCHANAN, W. SAKAMI AND S. GURIN, *J. Biol. Chem.*, 169 (1947) 411.
[11] T. C. CHOU AND F. LIPMANN, *J. Biol. Chem.*, 196 (1952) 89.
[12] D. I. CRANDALL, R. O. BRADY AND S. GURIN, *J. Biol. Chem.*, 181 (1949) 845.
[13] D. I. CRANDALL AND S. GURIN, *J. Biol. Chem.*, 181 (1949) 829.
[14] H. D. DAKIN, *J. Biol. Chem.*, 6 (1909) 203, 221.
[14a] K. DECKER AND F. LYNEN, unpublished.
[15] G. R. DRYSDALE AND H. A. LARDY, in W. D. MCELROY AND B. GLASS, *Phosphorus Metabolism*, Vol. II, p. 281. Johns Hopkins Press, Baltimore (1952).
[16] G. R. DRYSDALE AND H. A. LARDY, *J. Biol. Chem.*, 202 (1953) 119.
[17] F. G. FISCHER AND H. EYSENBACH, *Ann. Chem.*, 530 (1937) 99.
[18] R. P. GEYER, M. CUNNINGHAM AND J. PENDERGAST, *J. Biol. Chem.*, 185 (1950) 461; 188 (1950) 185.
[19] R. P. GEYER, L. W. MATTHEWS AND F. J. STARE, *J. Biol. Chem.*, 180 (1950) 1037.
[19a] C. GILVARG, unpublished.
[20] A. L. GRAFFLIN AND D. E. GREEN, *J. Biol. Chem.*, 176 (1948) 95.
[20a] D. E. GREEN, reported at meeting of Federation of Biological Societies, Chicago, April 1953.
[21] D. E. GREEN, *Science*, 115 (1952) 661.
[21a] D. E. GREEN, personal communication.
[22] D. E. GREEN, D. S. GOLDMAN, S. MII AND H. BEINERT, *J. Biol. Chem.*, 202 (1953) 137.
[23] M. P. HELE, *Federation Proc.*, 12 (1953) 216.
[24] F. E. HUNTER AND L. F. LELOIR, *J. Biol. Chem.*, 159 (1945) 295.
[25] M. E. JONES, F. LIPMANN, H. HILZ AND F. LYNEN, *J. Am. Chem. Soc.*, 75 (1953) 3285.
[26] S. KAUFMAN, in W. D. MCELROY AND B. GLASS, *Phosphorus Metabolism*, Vol. I, p. 370. Johns Hopkins Press, Baltimore (1951).
[27] S. KAUFMAN, C. GILVARG, O. CORI AND S. OCHOA, *J. Biol. Chem.* 203 (1953) 869.
[28] E. P. KENNEDY AND H. A. BARKER, *J. Biol. Chem.*, 191 (1951) 419.
[29] E. P. KENNEDY AND A. L. LEHNINGER, *J. Biol. Chem.*, 190 (1951) 361.
[30] E. P. KENNEDY AND A. L. LEHNINGER, in W. D. MCELROY AND B. GLASS, *Phosphorus Metabolism* Vol. II, p. 253. Johns Hopkins Press, Baltimore (1952).
[31] A. KLEINZELLER, *Biochem. J.*, 37 (1943) 678.
[32] F. KNOOP, *Beitr. Chem. Physiol. Pathol.*, 6 (1904) 150.

[33] W. E. KNOX, B. N. NOYCE AND V. H. AUERBACH, *J. Biol. Chem.*, 176 (1948) 117.
[34] S. KORKES, A. DEL CAMPILLO, I. C. GUNSALUS, AND 'S. OCHOA, *J. Biol. Chem.* 193 (1951) 721.
[35] A. KORNBERG, in W. D. MCELROY AND B. GLASS, *Phosphorus Metabolism*, Vol. II, p. 245. Johns Hopkins Press, Baltimore (1952).
[36] A. KORNBERG AND W. E. PRICER Jr., *J. Am. Chem. Soc.*, 74 (1952) 1617.
[37] A. L. LEHNINGER, *J. Biol. Chem.*, 154 (1944) 309; 157 (1944) 363.
[38] A. L. LEHNINGER, *J. Biol. Chem.*, 161 (1945) 437.
[39] A. L. LEHNINGER, *J. Biol. Chem.*, 161 (1945) 413; 164 (1946) 291.
[40] A. L. LEHNINGER, *J. Biol. Chem.*, 165 (1946) 131.
[41] A. L. LEHNINGER AND G. D. GREVILLE, *J. Am. Chem. Soc.*, 75 (1953) 1515.
[42] A. L. LEHNINGER AND E. P. KENNEDY, *J. Biol. Chem.*, 173 (1948) 753.
[43] L. F. LELOIR AND J. M. MUÑOZ, *J. Biol. Chem.*, 153 (1944) 53.
[44] F. LIPMANN, M. E. JONES, S. BLACK AND R. M. FLYNN, *J. Am. Chem. Soc.*, 74 (1952) 2384.
[45] J. W. LITTLEFIELD AND D. R. SANADI, *J. Biol. Chem.*, 199 (1952) 65.
[45a] F. LYNEN, unpublished experiments.
[46] F. LYNEN AND E. REICHERT, *Angew. Chem.*, 63 (1951) 47, 490.
[47] F. LYNEN, E. REICHERT AND L. RUEFF, *Ann. Chem.*, 574 (1951) 1.
[48] F. LYNEN, L. WESSELY, O. WIELAND AND L. RUEFF, *Angew. Chem.*, 64 (1952) 687.
[48a] F. LYNEN, G. VOGELMANN, L. WESSELY, O. WIELAND AND W. SEUBERT, unpublished.
[49] H. A. MAHLER, in W. D. MCELROY AND B. GLASS, *Phosphorus Metabolism*, Vol. II, p. 286. Johns Hopkins Press, Baltimore (1952).
[50] J. M. MUÑOZ AND L. F. LELOIR, *J. Biol. Chem.*, 147 (1943) 355.
[50a] S. OCHOA, J. HARTING AND M. C. SCHNEIDER, unpublished.
[51] S. OCHOA, J. R. STERN AND M. C. SCHNEIDER, *J. Biol. Chem.*, 193 (1951) 691.
[52] G. POPJÁK, G. D. HUNTER AND T. H. FRENCH, *Biochem. J.*, 54 (1953) 238.
[52a] I. RAW AND J. R. STERN, unpublished.
[53] D. RITTENBERG AND K. BLOCH, *J. Biol. Chem.*, 160 (1945) 417.
[54] D. R. SANADI AND J. W. LITTLEFIELD, *J. Biol. Chem.*, 201 (1953) 103.
[55] W. SEUBERT AND F. LYNEN, *J. Am. Chem. Soc.*, 75 (1953) 2787.
[56] E. J. SIMON AND D. SHEMIN, *J. Am. Chem. Soc.*, 75 (1953) 2520.
[57] B. SJÖBERG, *Z. physik. Chem.*, 52 B (1942) 209.
[58] M. SOODAK AND F. LIPMANN, *J. Biol. Chem.*, 175 (1948) 999.
[59] E. R. STADTMAN, *J. Biol. Chem.*, 196 (1952) 527, 535.
[60] E. R. STADTMAN, *Federation Proc.*, 11 (1952) 291; *Abstracts 122nd Meeting Am. Chem. Soc.*, 32 C (1952).
[60a] E. R. STADTMAN, personal communication.
[61] E. R. STADTMAN AND H. A. BARKER, *J. Biol. Chem.*, 180 (1949) 1085, 1095, 1117, 1169.
[62] E. R. STADTMAN AND H. A. BARKER, *J. Biol. Chem.*, 181 (1949) 221.
[63] E. R. STADTMAN AND H. A. BARKER, *J. Biol. Chem.*, 184 (1950) 769.
[64] E. R. STADTMAN, M. DOUDOROFF AND F. LIPMANN, *J. Biol. Chem.* 191 (1951) 377.
[65] E. R. STADTMAN, G. D. NOVELLI AND F. LIPMANN, *J. Biol. Chem.*, 191 (1951) 365.
[66] E. R. STADTMAN, T. C. STADTMAN AND H. A. BARKER, *J. Biol. Chem.*, 178 (1949) 677.
[67] J. R. STERN AND A. DEL CAMPILLO, *J. Am. Chem. Soc.*, 75 (1953) 2277.
[67a] J. R. STERN AND A. DEL CAMPILLO, unpublished.
[68] J. R. STERN, M. J. COON AND A. DEL CAMPILLO, *Nature*, 171 (1953) 28.
[69] J. R. STERN, M. J. COON AND A. DEL CAMPILLO, *J. Am. Chem. Soc.*, 75 (1953) 1517.
[69a] J. R. STERN, M. J. COON AND A. DEL CAMPILLO, unpublished observations.
[70] J. R. STERN AND S. OCHOA, *J. Biol. Chem.*, 191 (1951) 161.
[71] J. R. STERN, B. SHAPIRO, E. R. STADTMAN AND S. OCHOA, *J. Biol. Chem.*, 193 (1951) 703.
[72] S. WAKIL AND H. R. MAHLER, *Federation Proc.*, 12 (1953) 285.
[73] O. WARBURG AND W. CHRISTIAN, *Biochem. Z.*, 298 (1938) 150.
[74] S. WEINHOUSE, G. MEDES AND N. F. FLOYD, *J. Biol. Chem.* 155 (1944) 143.
[75] S. WEINHOUSE, G. MEDES AND N. F. FLOYD, *J. Biol. Chem.*, 166 (1946) 691.
[76] H. WIELAND AND C. ROSENTHAL, *Ann. Chem.*, 554 (1943) 241.
[77] T. WIELAND AND L. RUEFF, *Angew. Chem.*, 65 (1953) 186.
[78] I. ZABIN, *J. Biol. Chem.*, 189 (1951) 355.

Received June 22nd, 1953

Editor's Comments on Paper 24

24 **Kornberg and Krebs:** Synthesis of Cell Constituents from C_2-Units by a Modified Tricarboxylic Acid Cycle
Nature, **179**, 988–991 (1957)

A second epoch-making contribution came from the research group of H. A. Krebs, the discoverer of the tricarboxylic acid cycle. Soon after they had established the tricarboxylic acid cycle and its role in terminal respiration, the found that the cycle must also be involved in the synthesis of amino acids or other carbon compounds (Krebs et al., 1952). Using [^{14}C]-acetate as the carbon source, most of the research activity was directed at the acids of the Krebs cycle as well as amino acids (Goldschmidt et al., 1956). If an organism continuously withdraws acids from the Krebs cycle for its amino acid biosynthesis, it must have some way of replenishing them in order to provide oxalacetate, which is necessary for citrate formation and the normal functioning of the tricarboxylic acid cycle. The discovery of the formation of glyoxylic acid (Campbell et al., 1953) and the enzymes isocitritase (Saz, 1954; Smith and Gunsalus, 1955; Olson, 1954) and malate synthetase (Wong and Ajl, 1957) led Kornberg and Krebs to their second epoch-making discovery (Paper 24), the establishment of the "glyoxylate cycle" or "dicarboxylic acid cycle" (see also Kornberg and Elsden, 1961). The presence of this cycle was soon confirmed in fungi (Kornberg and Collins, 1958; Collins and Kornberg, 1960), *Pseudomonas* (Kornberg, 1957, 1958; Kornberg et al., 1958; Kornberg and Quayle, 1958; Kornberg and Madsen, 1957; 1958), *Escherichia coli* (Kornberg et al., 1959, 1960), and yeast (Barnett and Kornberg, 1960).

With the elucidation of the major pathways of carbohydrate metabolism and the two cycles for respiration and synthesis, the basic routes of catabolism had been established (see Horecker, 1961–1962). The period of research now gave way to investigations on the molecular level.

24

Reprinted from *Nature*, **179**, 988–991 (1957)

SYNTHESIS OF CELL CONSTITUENTS FROM C₂-UNITS BY A MODIFIED TRICARBOXYLIC ACID CYCLE

By Dr. H. L. KORNBERG and Prof. H. A. KREBS, F.R.S.

Medical Research Council Cell Metabolism Research Unit, Department of Biochemistry,
University of Oxford

MAJOR advances have recently been made towards the closure of one of the outstanding gaps in the knowledge of intermediary metabolism. This gap concerns the metabolic processes by which two-carbon compounds, such as acetate or ethanol, can be converted to cell constituents in those organisms which can meet all their carbon requirements from these compounds. Bacteria of the genus *Pseudomonas*, many strains of *Escherichia coli* and many moulds belong to this group. The occurrence of a cyclic process, representing a modification of the tricarboxylic acid cycle, has been newly established in these organisms.

Experiments on Acetate-grown Cells of *Pseudomonas*

To find the first, or an early, metabolic product of acetate, acetate labelled with carbon-14 was added to cells of *Pseudomonas KB* 1 [1] growing on ammonium acetate as sole carbon source, and the radioactive compounds formed after very short periods of incubation were located by autoradiography and analysed [2]. In the hands of Calvin and his collaborators, this procedure had led to the identification of phosphoglyceric acid as the first organic compound containing fixed carbon dioxide in photosynthesizing cells [3]. However, analogous experiments with acetate on whole cells of *Pseudomonas* [2,4] remained inconclusive. This organism oxidizes acetate by the reactions of the tricarboxylic acid cycle [1,2], and the intermediates of this cycle therefore became rapidly labelled. Even after only 3 sec., citrate, malate, fumarate and succinate, and some amino-acids directly derived from the cycle (glutamate and aspartate), contained radioactive carbon. It did not prove possible in these experiments to limit the radioactivity to virtually one compound, as in the case of photosynthesis. The distribution of the radioactivity among the labelled compounds formed from labelled acetate, and the change of labelling with time, suggested that acetate entered the tricarboxylic acid cycle at two points, to form citrate at one and a C₄-dicarboxylic acid at another [2]. Subsequent work on extracts [5,6] confirmed this conclusion.

Malate Synthetase

A decisive step was the observation made on extracts of *Pseudomonas* that the removal of acetate can be promoted in two ways. The first, established in 1951 by Ochoa, Stern and Schneider [7], consists of the addition of oxaloacetate, in the presence of coenzyme A and adenosine triphosphate. The reactions occurring under these conditions are the well-established stages of the tricarboxylic acid cycle leading to citrate :

Acetate + coenzyme A + ATP →
    acetyl coenzyme A (+ AMP + PP) [*]
Acetyl coenzyme A + oxaloacetate →
    citrate (+ coenzyme A) [*]

The second way of promoting acetate utilization consists of the addition of glyoxylate, in the presence of coenzyme A and adenosine triphosphate. The metabolic process responsible for this removal of acetate proved to be identical with the malate synthetase reaction discovered by Wong and Ajl [8] in extracts of *E. coli* :

Acetate + coenzyme A + ATP + glyoxylate →
    malate (+ coenzyme A + AMP + PP) [*]

The action of malate synthetase is closely analogous to that of the citrate-forming condensing enzyme [7]. In both cases, the methyl group of acetyl coenzyme A condenses with a —CO.COOH grouping.

Isocitritase

Pseudomonas was already known to possess an enzyme which can supply glyoxylate. This is the 'isocitritase' which splits *iso*citrate to glyoxylate and succinate [9-12] :

<pre>
COOH   COOH
| |
CH.CH(OH).COOH   CH₂   O
| → | +   ‖
CH₂   CH₂   HC.COOH
| |
COOH   COOH
</pre>
Isocitric acid   Succinic acid   Glyoxylic acid

This enzyme, which belongs to the class of aldolases, has also been found in *Penicillium chrysogenum* [13] and *E. coli* [14]. The reaction is reversible. Saz and Hillary [14] suggested that its function might be to provide glyoxylate for the biosynthesis of glycine and, in reverse, to provide a cyclic mechanism for the oxidation of compounds more highly oxidized than acetate, such as glycine and glycollate. It has also been suggested [14] that the glyoxylate may be oxidized to carbon dioxide and water, possibly via formate, and that this therefore represents an alternative mechanism for the complete oxidation of acetate.

The 'Glyoxylate Bypass'

The following results [5,6] show that the glyoxylate, formed by the action of *iso*citritase, can react with acetyl coenzyme A to form malate :

(a) Cell-free extracts of *Pseudomonas*, in the presence of glutathione, adenosine triphosphate and coenzyme A, catalyse the condensation of labelled

---

[*] These compounds (in brackets) have not been identified in the present work, but are presumed to arise, by analogy with previous work

acetate and glyoxylate to form malate as the only labelled compound.

(*b*) When *iso*citrate is used instead of glyoxylate in the above system, malate is again the only labelled compound formed in short-term experiments.

(*c*) Incubation of extracts with *iso*citrate leads to the production of equal amounts of glyoxylate and succinate. In the presence of acetate, coenzyme *A* and adenosine triphosphate, the glyoxylate disappears and malate is formed. The amounts of *iso*citrate utilized are approximately equal to the amount of succinate, and the amounts of malate + glyoxylate, formed.

(*d*) No malate is formed when boiled cell extracts are used for the above experiments, nor when acetate, coenzyme *A* or adenosine triphosphate is omitted.

It is evident that the combined action of *iso*citritase and malate synthetase can replace the steps of the tricarboxylic acid cycle leading from *iso*citrate to malate. In the tricarboxylic acid cycle, these steps are oxidative :

$$Isocitrate + 1\tfrac{1}{2}\,O_2 \rightarrow malate + 2\,CO_2$$

whereas the combined action of *iso*citritase and malate synthetase is an anaerobic process :

$$Isocitrate + acetate \rightarrow succinate + malate$$

The existence of this 'glyoxylate bypass'[5] implies that there are two variants of the tricarboxylic acid cycle in *Pseudomonas*. One is the well-established terminal pathway of acetate oxidation (Fig. 1). The effect of one turn of this cycle is the complete oxidation of acetate :

$$CH_3COOH + 2\,O_2 \rightarrow 2\,CO_2 + 2\,H_2O$$

The second variant employs most of the reactions of the tricarboxylic acid cycle but substitutes the 'glyoxylate bypass' for the degradative reactions between *iso*citrate and malate. The net effect of one turn of this cycle, henceforth referred to as the 'glyoxylate cycle' (Fig. 2), is the synthesis of one molecule of succinate from two molecules of acetate :

$$2\,CH_3COOH + \tfrac{1}{2}\,O_2 \rightarrow HOOC.CH_2.CH_2.COOH + H_2O$$

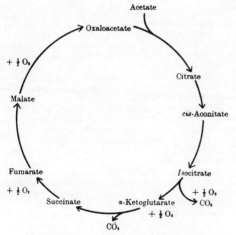

Fig. 1. The main stages of the tricarboxylic acid cycle
Acetate reacts in the form of acetyl coenzyme *A*. The net effect of one turn is : acetate + 2 O₂ → 2 CO₂

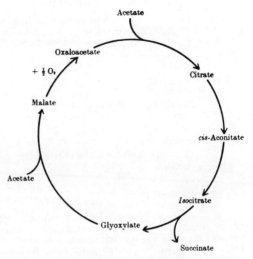

Fig. 2. The main stages of the 'glyoxylate cycle', which is a variant of the tricarboxylic acid cycle
Acetate reacts in the form of acetyl coenzyme *A*. The net effect of one turn of the cycle is 2 acetate + ½O₂ → succinate. If the succinate formed is further metabolized, the cycle, together with the subsequent reactions of succinate, can lead to the synthesis of other metabolites

The occurrence of a reaction leading from two molecules of acetate to one molecule of succinate was first postulated by Thunberg[15] in 1920, and later by Knoop[16]. These authors assumed a rather direct condensation of two molecules of acetate ('Thunberg condensation') ; but it is now apparent that the same effect can be achieved by an entirely different mechanism, involving as intermediate stages the reactions of the glyoxylate cycle :

Acetate + oxaloacetate	→ citrate
Citrate	→ *iso*citrate
*Iso*citrate	→ succinate + glyoxylate
Acetate + glyoxylate	→ malate
Malate + ½ O₂	→ oxaloacetate

Sum : 2 acetate + ½ O₂   → succinate.

Biological Role of the Glyoxylate Cycle

The glyoxylate cycle accounts for the net synthesis of C_4-dicarboxylic acids from acetate when this is the sole source of carbon, and it therefore provides the oxaloacetate required for the continued operation of the tricarboxylic acid cycle. It is also a key step in the synthesis of many cell constituents. Extracts of *Pseudomonas*, in the presence of pyridine nucleotides, can convert malate to phosphopyruvate, which can yield hexoses by the reversal of the reactions of glycolysis[17,18]. Hexoses in turn can supply pentoses through the pentose phosphate cycle, as well as the carbon skeletons of several amino-acids. The intermediates of the tricarboxylic acid cycle together with acetyl coenzyme *A* are already known to supply the carbon skeletons of most amino-acids. Such intermediates, drained from the tricarboxylic acid cycle, can be readily regenerated from acetate by the glyoxylate cycle.

Conversion of Fat to Carbohydrate

In what has already been discussed, it is implied that the glyoxylate cycle could also account for the conversion of fat to carbohydrate, the stages being :

fatty acid
↓
acetyl coenzyme A
↓ (glyoxylate cycle)
succinate
↓
oxaloacetate
↓ (Utter–Kurahashi reaction, ref. 18)
phosphopyruvate
↓
carbohydrate

It is uncertain to what extent a net conversion of fat to carbohydrate takes place in higher animals, but this conversion is known to occur in seedlings rich in oil, such as those of the castor bean (*Ricinus*). Cell-free extracts of castor bean seedlings contain *isocitritase* and malate synthetase, and are able to catalyse the formation of malate from acetate and *isocitrate* via the glyoxylate bypass[19]. In conjunction with the reactions whereby fatty acids give rise to acetyl coenzyme A, and those whereby malate produces phosphopyruvate[18], the bypass thus provides a route for the net conversion of fat to carbohydrate.

Tissues of higher animals are known to be capable of incorporating labelled acetate (and therefore the carbons of fatty acids) into carbohydrates ; but this does not imply a net conversion of fat to carbohydrate. When labelled acetate enters the tricarboxylic acid cycle, the citrate formed is labelled in such a manner as to lead, on completion of one turn of the cycle, to the formation of C_4-dicarboxylic acids still retaining all the isotope of the added acetate : the two molecules of carbon dioxide evolved are not directly derived from the added acetate. Hence, although the entry of two carbon atoms (as acetate) has been followed by the liberation of two carbon atoms (as carbon dioxide), and no net synthesis has occurred, the C_4-dicarboxylic acids of the tricarboxylic acid cycle have nevertheless become labelled. Since these acids can readily give rise to phosphopyruvate[17], isotope will also appear in carbohydrates, but will not be accompanied by any net formation of carbohydrate. The glyoxylate cycle, by supplying extra C_4-dicarboxylic acids from acetate, could, however, account for a net synthesis of carbohydrate from acetate and hence from fat. It remains to be investigated whether higher animals can under special conditions—such as when fat is the main source of energy—convert fat into carbohydrate, and whether this involves the glyoxylate cycle.

Synthesis of Citric and Fumaric Acid in Moulds

The conversion of sugars to citric acid by *Aspergillus niger* is taken to involve a fission of C_6-sugars to triose phosphates, oxidation to pyruvate, the fixation of carbon dioxide to form oxaloacetate, and a condensation of this with a molecule of acetyl coenzyme A derived from another molecule of pyruvate (see Chain[20]).

This pathway cannot account for the synthesis of citric acid from acetate or from other two-carbon compounds. The occurrence of *isocitritase* in at least one mould[13] suggests that the accumulation of citric acid involves the glyoxylate cycle, the intermediate stages being :

Acetate + *isocitrate*	→ succinate + malate
Malate + $\frac{1}{2}$ O_2	→ oxaloacetate
Succinate + O_2	→ oxaloacetate
2 Acetate + 2 oxaloacetate	→ 2 citrate
Citrate	→ *isocitrate*

Sum : 3 Acetate + $1\frac{1}{2}$ O_2 → citrate

Citrate, besides being the end-product of acetate utilization under these conditions, also acts in the manner of a catalyst, in that it initiates the sequence of reactions and is regenerated by them.

Foster and his co-workers[21,22] concluded from isotopic data that the synthesis of fumaric acid from acetate or ethanol in the mould *Rhizopus nigricans* involved a 'dicarboxylic acid cycle', in which the two methyl groups of acetate or ethanol, via the Thunberg condensation, give rise to the two methylene carbons of the C_4-compound. The experimental results are, however, in even better agreement with the assumption that fumarate is formed by the reactions of the glyoxylate cycle, the steps being :

Isocitrate	→ succinate + glyoxylate
Acetate + glyoxylate	→ malate
Malate + $\frac{1}{2}$ O_2	→ oxaloacetate
Acetate + oxaloacetate	→ citrate
Citrate	→ *isocitrate*
Succinate + $\frac{1}{2}$ O_2	→ fumarate

Sum : 2 Acetate + O_2 → fumarate

The accumulation of fumarate in this organism could be ascribed to the absence or low activity of fumarase. As in the case of the citric acid-forming moulds, citrate and *isocitrate* act like catalysts.

Conclusion

Recent work, carried out in several laboratories, has established the occurrence of a metabolic cycle in micro-organisms which can derive all their carbon requirements from two-carbon compounds. The cycle (see Fig. 2) represents a variant of the tricarboxylic acid cycle. The stages between *isocitrate* and malate are replaced by reactions in which glyoxylate is a key metabolite. The cycle is therefore referred to as the 'glyoxylate cycle'.

The main discoveries which led to the elaboration of the cycle were : (1) the finding that *isocitrate*, apart from undergoing dehydrogenation, is split enzymically to form succinate and glyoxylate[9–14,23] ; (2) the recognition by Wong and Ajl[8] of an enzyme system bringing about the synthesis of malate from glyoxylate and acetyl coenzyme A ; (3) the demonstration of the ready occurrence of the combined action of the two enzyme systems in cell-free extracts[5,6,19].

The overall effect of one turn of the glyoxylate cycle is the formation, from two molecules of acetate, of one molecule of C_4-dicarboxylic acid. This, together with acetate, can serve as a precursor of many cell constituents. The cycle is therefore a stage in the synthesis of cell material from acetate. It can also account for the net formation from acetate of citric, fumaric and other organic acids in moulds[20].

The key reactions of the glyoxylate cycle have further been demonstrated in *Ricinus* seedlings[19]. In these seedlings, it can account for the conversion of fat to carbohydrate.

[1] Kogut, M., and Podoski, E. P., *Biochem. J.*, **55**, 800 (1953).

[2] Kornberg, H. L., *Biochem. J.* (in the press).

[3] Calvin, M., "The Harvey Lectures", **46**, 218 (1950–1951). (C. C. Thomas Publ. Co., Springfield, Ill.)

[4] Kornberg, H. L., *Biochim. Biophys. Acta*, **22**, 208 (1956).

[5] Kornberg, H. L., and Madsen, N. B., *Biochim. Biophys. Acta* (in the press).

[6] Kornberg, H. L., and Madsen, N. B., *Biochem. J.* (in the press).

[7] Ochoa, S., Stern, J. R., and Schneider, M. C., *J. Biol. Chem.*, **193**, 691 (1951).

[8] Wong, D. T. O., and Ajl, S. J., *J. Amer. Chem. Soc.*, **78**, 3230 (1956).

[9] Saz, H. J., *Biochem. J.*, **58**, xx (1954).

[10] Smith, R. A., and Gunsalus, I. C., *J. Amer. Chem. Soc.*, **76**, 5002 (1954).

[11] Smith, R. A., and Gunsalus, I. C., *Nature*, **175**, 774 (1955).

[12] Saz, H. J., and Hillary, E. P., *Biochem. J.*, **62**, 563 (1956).

[13] Olson, J. A., *Nature*, **174**, 695 (1954).

[14] Wong, D. T. O., and Ajl, S. J., *Nature*, **176**, 970 (1955).

[15] Thunberg, T., *Skand. Arch. Physiol.*, **40**, 1 (1920).

[16] Knoop, F., *Klin. Wochschr.*, **2**, 60 (1923).

[17] Krebs, H. A., *Bull. Johns Hopkins Hosp.*, **95**, 19 (1954). Bartley, W., *Biochem. J.*, **56**, 387 (1954). Bartley, W., and Avi-Dor, Y., *Biochem. J.*, **59**, 194 (1955).

[18] Utter, M. F., and Kurahashi, K., *J. Biol. Chem.*, **188**, 847 (1953).

[19] Kornberg, H. L., and Beevers, H., *Nature* (in the press).

[20] Chain, E. B., Proc. 3rd Int. Congr. of Biochemistry, Brussels 1955, p. 523 (Academic Press, Inc., New York, 1956).

[21] Foster, J. W., Carson, S. F., Anthony, D. S., Davis, J. B., Jefferson, W. E., and Long, M. V., *Proc. U.S. Nat. Acad. Sci.*, **35**, 663 (1949).

[22] Foster, J. W., and Carson, S. F., *Proc. U.S. Nat. Acad. Sci.*, **36**, 219 (1950).

[23] Campbell, J. J. R., Smith, R. A., and Eagles, B. A., *Biochim. Biophys. Acta*, **11**, 544 (1953).

III
Metabolism of Inorganic Compounds

Editor's Comments on Paper 25

25 **Schloesing and Müntz:** On Nitrification by Organized Ferments
Compt. Rend. Acad. Sci., Paris, **84**, 301–303 (1877)

The first report that microorganisms might be involved in the mineralization of soil, converting ammonia to nitrate, was given by Schloesing and Müntz (Paper 25) in 1877 and the following years (1878, 1879). The first publication was chosen to indicate the beginning of soil microbiology.

Warrington verified these experiments and started to investigate the nutritional requirements (1878) of these microorganisms. He obtained cultures that converted ammonia to nitrite (1879) and cultures that converted nitrite to nitrate but were unable to oxidize ammonia (1883). He did not, however, succeed in obtaining pure cultures.

25

On Nitrification by Organized Ferments

J. J. T. SCHLOESING and A. MÜNTZ

*Translated expressly for this Benchmark
volume by G. Gordon of the University
of Queensland, Australia, from "Sur la
nitrification par les ferments organisés,"*
Compt. Rend. Acad. Sci., Paris, **84**,
301–303 (1877)

It is generally accepted that nitrates formed in the soil arise from the combustion of ammonia and nitrogenous materials, but the mechanism of this combustion is far from known. Is nitrification the result of a purely chemical reaction between gaseous oxygen and nitrogenous compounds? Is it carried out by the intermediary functioning of organisms? Or is it brought about by both processes at the same time? These questions have been asked since Monsieur Pasteur showed that certain organisms, such as the mycoderma of wine and vinegar, have the ability to transfer atmospheric oxygen to the most diverse organic substances, and thus are most active in the destruction of nonliving organic matter. Furthermore, Monsieur Pasteur has proven that, while organic substances are less alterable than compounds that nitrify in soil, they display a unique resistance to oxygen when they are kept sterile. On comparing these two concepts, it is supposed that some organized agents are less active in the case of rapid combustion and nitrification under aerobic conditions, but they do have the ability to destroy nitrogenous materials by oxidation and to nitrify. Delving deeply into these ideas, Monsieur Pasteur has declared since 1862 that the study of nitrification was a revival of new information on the functions of combustive organisms. The experiment that we are going to relate confirms the theory of L. Pasteur without emphasizing his precision.

During a recent enquiry into irrigation by drainage water, one of us wished to know if the presence of humic water in a soil was necessary for purification of this water (in other words, the total combustion of the undissolved materials). To determine this, a large, 1-m-long, glass tube was filled with 5 kg of quartz sand (red calcined material) and mixed with 100 g of powdered limestone. The sand was moistened each day with a constant amount of drainage water, calculated so that the liquid took a week to descend the tube. During the first 20 days there was no appearance of nitrification, and the amount of ammonia in the filtrate remained invariable. Then nitrate appeared, the quantity of which increased very quickly. It was soon established that the effluent drainage water from the apparatus contained no trace of ammonia.

If, as in this experiment, the organic materials and ammonia have been destroyed by oxidation caused by oxygen acting directly without intermediary steps, it can be asked why it takes 20 days before combustion begins. This delay is better understood by hypothesizing the presence of organized ferments that act evidently only after accidental inoculation and development of their germs.

Beginning in July, the experiment lasted for 4 months, after which we diffused chloroform vapor into the tube. One of us has shown that this compound suspends all activity of organized ferments without inhibiting the soluble ferments in any way. Thus, if the observed nitrification was produced by organisms, chloroform must halt it by paralyzing its agents. If, however, nitrification was a simple chemical reaction, chloroform would not modify it at all. We then placed on our sand a vessel full of chloroform from which vapor was diffused into the tube by a stream of forced air. We have said that the daily addition of drainage water takes a week to run through the sand, and in that time we were not able to observe the disappearance of nitrate. After 10 days the sand had been washed by displacement; last month's liquid no longer contained any nitrate, and all the ammonia remained in the drainage water. Upon evaporation the liquid left a residue that was perceptibly colored and odorous, as if the drainage water had been filtered but not purified.

Having maintained the chloroform vapor in our tube for 2 weeks (from November 27 to December 12), we removed the vessel that produced it. For the next 2 weeks, the liquid issuing from the tube continued to have an odor characteristic of chloroform, which disappeared toward the end of December. Nevertheless, during January, the tube remained at an average temperature of 15 degrees, but no nitrate was produced. Without doubt our nitrifying organisms were dead, and the drainage water did not contain any replacement, perhaps because it was already in an advanced state of putrefaction. On February 1, we attempted an incubation of these germs. A sample of surface soil in the process of nitrifying must contain many of them, so we made a suspension in water of 10 g of earth well known to us for its nitrifying ability, and poured the cloudy water over the surface of our sand. Nitrate was evident on the exact day we looked for it, February 9. Its proportion has increased since then, so we think that before long the conditions that existed prior to the application of chloroform will be reestablished.

It now remains for us to discover and isolate the nitrifying organisms. We have the firm hope of accomplishing this while following the path so clearly traced by Monsieur Pasteur for the research of this group.

As for the purification of drainage waters, our experiment demonstrated that an absolutely sterile sandy soil, containing limestone as a base for nitric acid, became an excellent purifier. In an arable soil, the combustive and nitrifying agents are already present, and the purification of drainage waters proceeds from the first day of irrigation. In an absolutely sterile soil, purification is retarded until these agents have developed sufficiently. From the point of view of purification, this is very probably the main difference between these two types of soil.

Editor's Comments on Paper 26

26 Winogradsky: On the Organisms of Nitrification
Compt. Rend. Acad. Sci., Paris, **110**,1013–1016 (1890)

There is no doubt that Sergei Winogradsky was one of the outstanding microbiologists of the past century. Winogradsky succeeded in the isolation of the cultures similar to those of Warrington and studied their physiology (Paper 26). He quickly realized that more than one species must be involved in the process of ammonia oxidation. He therefore called his culture a "physiological type." These investigations also led Winogradsky to define the nature of chemolithotrophic life, which was the main reason for selecting this paper from his publications on this subject (1890).

26

On the Organisms of Nitrification

S. WINOGRADSKY

*Translated expressly for this Benchmark
volume by G. Gordon of the University of
Queensland, Australia, from "Sur les
organismes de la nitrification,"* Compt.
Rend. Acad. Sci., Paris, **110**,
1013–1016 (1890)

Before resuming research on nitrification that I have pursued for a year, I would like to recall the starting point of my preceding work.

The studies included two groups of organisms, both included in my paper, which oxidize inorganic substances and which I have called sulfobacteria and ferrobacteria.[1]

The first group are found in natural waters containing hydrogen sulfide and do not live in media lacking this constituent. This gas is avidly absorbed and oxidized by the cells, which become filled with sulfur, which is in turn destroyed by oxidation and excreted into the surrounding medium as sulfuric acid. The second group oxidize ferrous iron salts, and its survival is closely bound to the presence of these compounds in the nutritive medium.

My effort to discover the physiological significance of these phenomena has led me to the belief that, during the growth of these organisms, such inorganic compounds take the place of fermentative material, which is organic material for a great many microbes. As a logical result (confirmed by experimentation), these beings have a group of physiological qualities that can be summarized as follows: all the energy necessary for their vital functions is formed by combustion of mineral compounds, consumption of organic matter during growth is extremely low, and carbon compounds that cannot nourish organisms lacking chlorophyll serve as a source of carbon.

The remarkable work by Messieurs Schloesing and Müntz was first to shed light on the role of lower organisms in nitrification. Although a high probability of the existence of a special nitrifying agent was suggested, they have not reported an iolation from soil, this natural medium so rich in diverse microbes. It is the isolation and culture in the pure state of the nitrifying ferment that is today both the primary aim of much microbiological experiment and the rather large obstacle on which a

---

[1]"On the sulfobacteria" (*Botan. Zeitung*, 1887); "On the ferrobacteria" (*Ibid.*, 1888); "Contribution to the physiological and morphological study of bacteria," 1st fasc., Leipzig, 1888; "Physiological studies on the sulfobacteria" (*Ann. Inst. Pasteur*, Vol. III, No. 2).

number of knowledgable men have foundered. To the present time, the conclusions of Messieurs Schloesing and Müntz relative to the existence of a special nitric ferment has not been confirmed by bacteriologists and botanists.[2]

First it was necessary to solve this problem. I am convinced that the failure of my predecessors was due to the use of gelatinous media for the isolation and culture of the microbes. Nitrifying organisms refuse to grow, with the result that passage of a mixture of microbes obtained from totally nitrified soil through this medium kills all those that are active and enriches all those that are ineffective. A continued study of culture conditions favorable for the first group and unfavorable for the second has led me, not without difficulty, to eliminate the foreign species one by one and to obtain many pure cultures of the nitrifying species. Under normal conditions of experimental microbiology, this study was as rigorous as could be desired by adopting the recent experiments of Monsieur Schloesing on nitrification in soil as a standard for comparison.

The study of the physiological properties of these organisms, which are more suitable for experimentation than the more delicate organisms of my previous work, has not only justified my care but has led to the discovery of a new matter that I would like to report to the Academy.

Applying previously acquired information to this study of organisms capable of oxidizing mineral substances, I first cultivated the nitrification microbe in a medium comprising only that material which pure natural water would contain. As addition of hydrocarbon compounds appeared unfavorable for growth, I tried, in preference, a mineral solution completely lacking organic carbon as a culture. In this liquid, which gave the organism no carbon compounds other than carbon dioxide and carbonates, neither the abundance of multiplication nor the intensity of its action appeared to diminish for several months.

The conclusion was made that this organism assimilates the carbon of carbon dioxide. This is rendered irrefutable by the measurement of carbon dioxide in the cultures, which demonstrates that accumulation of organic carbon is constant.

The nitrification organism, which is colorless, is capable of complete synthesis of its substance from carbon dioxide and ammonia. It accomplished this synthesis independently of light, and without energy other than that liberated by oxidation of ammonia. This new mechanism is contradictory to fundamental physiological doctrine, according to which complete synthesis of organic material in nature takes place only in chlorophyllic plants by the action of light rays.

It is not very probable that the action of the nitrifying ferment follows a chlorophyllic action, for oxygen is never released. Another supposition, that an amide, perhaps urea, is the first step in the synthesis, is the only one to be plausible to me.[3]

This question, as well as those concerning the physiology and morphology of the nitrifying ferment, needs to be studied in more detail.

---

[2]See the history contained in my article "Studies on the organisms of nitrification" (*Ann. Inst. Pasteur*, Vol. IV, No. 4).
[3]An article discussing these questions in more detail will appear in the next issue of *Annales de l'Institut Pasteur*.

Editor's Comments on Paper 27

27 Winogradsky: About Sulfur Bacteria
   Botan. Zeitung, **45**, 489–507 (1887)

   Before he studied the nitrifying organisms, Winogradsky concerned himself with sulfur bacteria, especially *Beggiatoa.* He established (Paper 27, 1888, 1889) that *Beggiatoa* deposits sulfur in the protoplasm as a result of hydrogen sulfide oxidation, but he stated that this sulfur deposition depends on culture conditions (Paper 27) and therefore is no absolute consequence of sulfide oxidation. Thus all bacteria that oxidize hydrogen sulfide, sulfur, and thiosulfate were called sulfur bacteria, irrespective of sulfur deposition. Winogradsky was able to formulate these fundamental principles of sulfur oxidation despite the fact that he was not able to obtain a pure culture of *Beggiatoa.* It took a further decade before Keil (1912) succeeded in this task.

27

About Sulfur Bacteria

S. WINOGRADSKY

*Translated expressly for this Benchmark
volume by H. W. Doelle from "Über
Schwefelbakterien,"* Botan. Zeitung,
45, *489–507 (1887)*

The genus *Beggiatoa* comprises the most commonly known and widely distributed members of those organisms for which I suggest the common description "sulfur bacteria." These bacteria form a most peculiar physiological group because of the strange role sulfur plays in their life processes.

Since Cramer showed in 1870[1] that the dark, strongly light-reflecting particles in the *Beggiatoa* filaments consist of sulfur, these organisms have been objects of continuous research.

Cohn[2] (1875) confirmed Cramer's findings and found that a number of other bacteria (e.g., *Clathrocystis roseopersinina, Monas okenii, Monas vinosa, Monas warmingii Ophidomonas sanguinea*) also contained particles that are identical with those of *Beggiatoa*. Cohn investigated the growth conditions of these organisms and tried to explain the development of the sulfur deposits, which are regarded as extraordinary in the plant kingdom, in their cells. He observed, in particular, the fact that these organisms can live in water that contains the gas hydrogen sulfide to the saturation point; this is "an adaptation to living conditions that are deadly for all other plants and animals; these red organisms (*Monas okenii, vinosa, Clathrocystis*, and others mentioned earlier) appear to multiply only under these conditions."[3] In fact, one finds *Beggiatoa* and all the other sulfur-containing bacteria mainly in waters that contain dissolved hydrogen sulfide. The *Beggiatoa* are, it is known, characteristic inhabitants of sulfur springs; every one of these springs contains them and they show such good growth as can not be found elsewhere in nature. The white slimy mass that forms has been known for a long time and was thought of as being a lifeless organic substance, which precipitates from water (baregine, glairine). These observations gave Cohn the idea

---

[1]Ch. Müller, *Chem. Phys. Beschreibung der Thermen von Baden in der Schweiz* (1870).
[2]Cohn, *Beitr. Biol. Pflanzen*, Bd. I, Heft 3 (1875).
[3]*Loc. cit.*, S. 170.

that a connection must exist between the growth of the *Beggiatoa* and the presence of hydrogen sulfide in the water; he expressed the opinion that the life process of *Beggiatoa* and the other sulfur-containing organisms is the cause of sulfate reduction and the formation of sulfur metals or free hydrogen sulfide in sulfur springs and elsewhere in nature. Thus those organisms must be able to resist the poisonous influence of the hydrogen sulfide gas, and "must possess the ability to develop and multiply normally in oxygen-free water," since water containing hydrogen sulfide cannot contain oxygen.[4] During the process of sulfate reduction, sulfur is deposited as particles or crystals in these organisms. "The latter appears to suggest that the hydrogen sulfide is absorbed by these organisms and oxidized inside the cells."[5]

In regard to the last sentence I would like to note that it is not clear how this hydrogen sulfide oxidation works because of the existence of energetic reductions that Cohn has described; also, these organisms are living in water that does not contain free oxygen.

Although Cohn has never reported a direct experiment to prove his ideas about the sulfate-reducing activities of these organisms, he made a number of very interesting observations which support his ideas. The first of these dates back to 1863; he observed that *Beggiatoa* stored in a bottle of "Landecker" thermal water developed a strong hydrogen sulfide odor. A similar observation was made by Lothar Meyer[6] during the analysis of Landecker sulfur water. He found that the water containing the algae (*Beggiatoa*), if stored 4 months in a closed bottle, contained five times more free hydrogen sulfide than the fresh thermal water. Therefore, "it is possible that the hydrogen sulfide content of the springs is caused by these algae."[7]

Plauchud[8] tried to solve the question experimentally; after a number of experiments he came to the same conclusion as Cohn. To a fluid that contained $CaSO_4$ and small amounts of organic substance were added algae from sulfur springs (sulfuraires). Hydrogen sulfide formation was a constant result under these conditions; it ceased after heating to the boiling point, addition of chloroform, phenol, etc. The interrupted hydrogen sulfide formation resumed after the addition of small amounts of living "sulfuraires." These experiments showed without any doubt that the hydrogen sulfide formation was caused by the activity of living organisms; they produced, however, no conclusions about which organisms were involved, since no microscopical investigations had been carried out that would have produced evidence that under those conditions one of the sulfuraires (e.g., *Beggiatoa*) could grow well, whereas other bacteria were absent or developed only in minute quantities.

Etard and Olivier[9] cultivated *Beggiatoa* under different conditions. They observed that the *Beggiatoa* filaments lose their particles in a fluid that did not contain sulfate, but they reappeared after the addition of gypsum. These sulfur particles

---

[4]*Loc. cit.*, S. 177.
[5]*Loc. cit.*, S. 180.
[6]*J. Prakt. Chem.*, Bd. 91 (1864).
[7]*Loc. cit.*, S. 6.
[8]*Compt. rend.* (1878).
[9]*Compt. rend.* (1882).

"constituent un témoin des phénomènes de réductions s'accomplissant dans le proto-plasme de l'être vivant." Duclaux,[10] taking the experiments of the French authors as a base, regards it as possible that the sulfur springs organisms (sulfuraires) reduce sulfate and, especially, gypsum, resulting in the excretion of sulfur or hydrogen sulfide. The actual mechanism of these processes is unclear: does sulfate reduction always result in hydrogen sulfide, which is oxidized in contact with the oxygen of the air and causes the sulfur deposits in the cells, or is the sulfur formed directly from H_2SO_4 ("réduction à l'état de soufre d'une partie de l'acide sulphurique")? The second explanation by Duclaux is more likely, since the first one includes an oxidative process that cannot occur in the protoplasm[11] ("dont le protoplasme ne peut être le siège").

In restricting myself to this brief historical review of the most important work on these questions I would like to add that the opinion of Cohn has been included in some physiological and bacteriological textbooks.

I

I started my investigations in November 1885 in the Institute of Botany in Strass-burg. In the summer of 1886 I came to the following results:

1. *Beggiatoa* does not participate in sulfate reduction and hydrogen sulfide formation.

2. Sulfur is formed by oxidation of hydrogen sulfide and incorporated in the plasma of the *Beggiatoa* cells.

So far my results are in complete agreement with those of Hoppe-Seyler. Although the question of sulfate reduction and the mechanism of sulfur excretion in *Beggiatoa* could be regarded as having been solved by the work by Hoppe-Seyler, it may not be fruitless to add my own investigations, which have been carried out independently and by different methods.

* * * * * * *

Beggiatoa is widely distributed in nature. They appear in almost every swamp and pond and wherever dead plant parts decay. However, it is not always possible to find *Beggiatoa* in these places by direct microscopy, since they are present only in small numbers; one finds a filament here and there only by chance. I also found *Beggiatoa* in the pond of the botanical garden of Strassburg in these small numbers. In order to obtain enough material for my investigations, I took water from the pond, added mud and plant residues, and left it standing for a long time at room temperature.

I could not obtain any growth of *Beggiatoa*. They did not grow and all cultures were a failure. The growth of *Beggiatoa* appears to depend on certain conditions. One

---

[10]*Microbiologie*, S. 719 (1883).
[11]*Loc. cit.*, S. 720.

of the conditions necessary for the growth of *Beggiatoa* appears to be the presence of a minimum quantity of sulfate in the water. The ponds of Strassburg contain very small amounts of sulfate. Addition of decaying plant material did not cause the hydrogen sulfide odor to develop. The addition of small amounts of gypsum resulted in an immediate multiplication of *Beggiatoa*.

I now used the following procedure: I cut the rhizome of a freshly harvested water plant (*Butomus*) into small sections, put some in a deep vessel, and added spring water with some gypsum. I did not sterilize the vessel or the water. After covering the vessel with a glass plate I left it standing. I observed the same phenomena in all these cultures. After 3–4 days in the darkness of a warm room the water was barely turbid, and *Cladothrix* with green *Oscillaria* appeared at the surface, together with bacterial zooglea; after 5–6 days a weak odor of hydrogen sulfide can be recognized, which soon becomes stronger. Careful investigation of the contents of the vessel shows that no multiplication of *Beggiatoa* had taken place. At the surface one finds only dead *Cladothrix* filaments and the bacterial zooglea, while on the bottom the *Butomus* pieces are covered with a tremendous number of different bacteria. Once started, hydrogen sulfide formation continues for months, if one keeps the vessel in the dark; otherwise green *Oscillaria* and green bacterial zooglea develop, and the hydrogen sulfide odor gradually disappears. At the surface, a thick layer of sulfur develops. This excretion of hydrogen sulfide and sulfur at the surface continues until all the gypsum is decomposed. If one adds some gypsum, the process begins anew. If one investigates such a vessel from time to time, a significant growth of *Beggiatoa* can be observed after approximately 4 weeks. After 2 months almost all organisms have disappeared from the surface, and *Beggiatoa* has grown vigorously; they form fine white nets and clusters that are visible with the naked eye at the glass walls near the surface.

These experiments showed that *Beggiatoa* takes no part in the decomposition of gypsum, since they appear in significant amounts only long after the process has started. It is easy to prevent growth of *Beggiatoa* in such experiments by using boiled *Butomus* sections and gypsum. Hydrogen sulfide odor appears as usual, but no *Beggiatoa* does even after a long period of time, since spring water does not normally contain *Beggiatoa*.

A more vigorous hydrogen sulfide development can be obtained if macerated hay is added to gypsum-containing water. Hay is cut into small pieces, macerated in water for 10 days, and boiled in large quantities of water, which is repeatedly renewed. A handful is transferred into a deep vessel containing water and gypsum; a small amount (knife tip) of mud from swamps is added. The fluid develops a hydrogen sulfide odor which becomes very strong after 2–3 days. The fluid stays clear and is opalescent in the upper layers because of sulfur excretion. On the surface, bacterial zooglea develop and a thick layer of sulfur is formed. Microscopic investigations of the vessel contents reveal different forms of bacteria on the surface and at the bottom of the vessel; even here no *Beggiatoa* or sulfur bacteria develop during the first 15 days. From that point on they develop slowly and appear in large quantities after 4–6 weeks.

Cohn and Lothar Meyer have already observed that *Beggiatoa* develops hydrogen sulfide in a closed bottle. My observations confirm the hydrogen sulfide formation under these conditions. In May 1886 I filled five bottles three-fourths full of sulfur spring water from Langenbruck, added *Beggiatoa*-containing mud from the same spring, and left these securely closed at room temperature. I investigated the content of these bottles every 2–3 days. After 4–5 days I realized that the hydrogen sulfide odor had intensified. It became very strong and a thick sulfur layer developed at the surface. As far as *Beggiatoa* was concerned, the filaments became immobile after 3–4 days and many were completely disorganized. This dying out of the *Beggiatoa* continued and after 2 weeks not a trace could be found in the fluid. The hydrogen sulfide formation continued for months. Hydrogen sulfide could be formed partly by reduction of sulfate of the water during the decaying process of *Beggiatoa,* and partly from the sulfur particles of *Beggiatoa.* The latter is undoubtedly the case if *Beggiatoa* is cultivated in water that contains little or no amounts of sulfate, as is the case with the spring water or distilled water. Only the sulfur particles in the cells of *Beggiatoa* can serve as a source for hydrogen sulfide formation; these sulfur particles are transformed to hydrogen sulfide with the help of H^+, which is formed during the decaying process of the filaments.

The following experiments demonstrate this best: one takes some (5–6) *Beggiatoa* flakes, transfers these into a drop of spring water on a microscope slide, and covers it with a large coverslip so that the *Beggiatoa* flakes are in the center. If one does not handle these filaments very carefully during this procedure, they die very quickly because of their sensitive nature; the addition of distilled water speeds this process. The preparation is left in the normal humid chamber. After some time, a large number of bacteria appear between the swollen and disorganized filaments; at the same time, sulfur deposition starts at the periphery of the preparation and proceeds to such an extent that the drop and coverslip appear yellowish white. During this time the sulfur disappears from the decaying filaments in the center of the preparation. A test of the fluid under the coverslip for hydrogen sulfide with lead paper (filter paper dipped into a solution containing PbO and KOH and dried) showed conclusively that free hydrogen sulfide is present. It is quite obvious that the sulfur of the dead filaments in the center of the preparation is converted into hydrogen sulfide, which diffuses into the fluid and is oxidized by contact with air to sulfur at the periphery of the preparation. This process can take weeks and it is, therefore, possible to observe it step by step. In this way the hydrogen sulfide formation, which many research workers found in closed bottles containing *Beggiatoa,* can be explained. The decay of the dead filaments was regarded as part of the life process.

I come now to the investigations concerning the sulfur inclusions of the *Beggiatoa,* their formation, nature, etc. However, first I must explain in some detail the method that I used, since it deviates from the ones normally used. Usually one employs the pure culture method for investigations of the metabolism of lower organisms, their fermentative activities, etc. One grows the appropriate organism in a flask, protected from contamination, for a certain time and studies the chemical conversions that occur as a result of the life processes. A main factor is, of course, the purity of the culture; the organism under study must be able to grow in the experimental flask completely isolated from all other organisms. This condition is very difficult, if not impossible, to obtain with *Beggiatoa*. There is no method available for the complete isolation of *Beggiatoa*. The gelatine method, which serves so well in the isolation of bacteria, does not work, since *Beggiatoa* dies very quickly after gelatine solidifies. All my endeavors in attempting to isolate *Beggiatoa* and to obtain pure material were in vain. The *Beggiatoa* material, as pure as it often appeared to be, is always contaminated with bacteria, the reason for which appears to be that *Beggiatoa* in nature, excluding sulfur springs, only grow in the presence of these bacteria (e.g., because of the decompositions they carry out in the substrate). One can, therefore, never be confident that even the smallest inoculation of *Beggiatoa* does not contain these bacteria. Thus the abovementioned experiment of Plauchud (where hydrogen sulfide formation was stopped by heating and resumed after the addition of *Beggiatoa* filaments) can be explained by supposing that some bacteria enter the fluid with the inoculum and are able to begin the decaying process of the dead filaments of *Beggiatoa*.

Even if we succeeded in isolating a few *Beggiatoa* filaments, the living conditions of these plants, as we shall see later, are so strange that it would be very difficult to grow them under normal cultural conditions in a specified amount of fluid. This growth would be extremely slow compared to that of other bacteria, which makes a large-scale experiment almost impossible. I finally succeeded in finding culture conditions under which the attached bacteria did not develop. The possibility of such bacterial growth, however, is always there and it sometimes occurs. Therefore, it is very important to carry out continuous microscopic controls of the cultures.

Because of the reasons outlined above I decided to consider only those results which were obtained with microscopic cultures. I did not use any special apparatus for my microscopic cultures. I put a *Beggiatoa* flake into a drop of fluid on the microscope slide and covered it with a coverslip of 18 mm². In order to maintain a fluid level of specific depth, a few pieces of broken coverslip were put into the drop. Between observations, such cultures were kept in humid chambers. The fluid can be renewed as necessary. The liquid flow thus created causes a separation of the bacteria and infusoria from the *Beggiatoa* filaments, since the latter do not swim freely, but grow along the glass and cannot be washed off so easily. Even the strongest fluid flow cannot wash out the filaments; in other words, one can wash the culture as often as one wants. *Beggiatoa* grows beautifully under such conditions. Such a culture can serve for a long time; I kept some for 2 months, during which I occasionally had to remove some filaments.

In such cultures I was able to study, at my leisure, both the influence of environmental factors on the growth, nutrition, etc., of *Beggiatoa* on a single growth of filament and, with the help of microchemical reactions, some chemical transformations of the substrate.

I now return to the sulfur inclusions of the *Beggiatoa*. The *Beggiatoa* filaments found in nature exhibited large variations in their sulfur particles. The amount and distribution of these particles led scientists to use these as morphological characteristics for the identification of the respective *Beggiatoa* species; Cohn, Engler, and Winter used them as part of the *Beggiatoa* species characterization. Zopf believes that

220

the sulfur content depends upon the age of the filaments; young filaments should contain no or only a few sulfur particles. Olivier and Etard report that cultivation in sulfate-free liquids causes disappearance of sulfur particles; they reappear upon the addition of gypsum. They have, however, neither directly observed the disappearance and reappearance of the sulfur particles nor described the precise conditions under which either occurs.

My own investigations soon revealed that the sulfur content of the filaments is no morphological characteristic and does not depend upon the age of the filaments, only upon the culture conditions. Depending upon those conditions, the filaments can be filled with sulfur particles or contain no sulfur particles at all. They go readily from one stage to the other. If one puts a flake from sulfur-enriched filaments into a microscopic culture and cultivates it in spring water, one can easily observe the disappearance of the sulfur particles from the filaments. In order to observe this accurately, it is not even necessary to observe the same filament, since *Beggiatoa* taken from a mass culture usually exhibits the same particle content and loses these at the same rate. It is, therefore, sufficient just to note the number of particles in the filaments. I will give an example. Sulfur-enriched filaments were put into a microscopic culture in spring water. After 24 hr all filaments already contained much less sulfur; after 24 or 48 hr only a few filaments contained barely recognizable particles; most filaments exhibited no trace of sulfur. This phenomenon is very obvious and is impossible to overlook in a microscopic culture. I will return later to this phenomenon; I will show, then, how this disintegration works and what importance this process has for *Beggiatoa*. I have mentioned these observations only because I had the opportunity to obtain filaments free of sulfur particles and was thus able to study the conditions of sulfur deposition.

The following question should be answered by direct observation: Is the sulfur in the *Beggiatoa* cells formed by reduction from SO_4 or by oxidation from H_2S? To answer this question I cultivated the filaments either in spring water with H_2S or in the same water with calcium sulfate. To keep the filaments in a constant hydrogen sulfide-containing medium, the following single apparatus was used. A large bell jar (Glasglocke) was closed by a double-bored stopper with two glass tubes, one of which penetrated deep into the jar and dipped into a small dish with water containing approximately 1 g of calcium sulfide (Schwefelcalcium); the other is only a small tube, which could be blocked by attaching a piece of rubber tubing and a clamp or glass rod. The latter served as an air exit when acid was added through the large glass tubing. In the interior of the bell jar moist filter paper was attached to the glass walls, and the whole jar was made airtight on a glass plate with the help of some Vaseline. I put my microscopic cultures under the bell jar and added some drops of diluted HCl via the large glass tube into the dish containing calcium sulfide. Hydrogen sulfide developed, which gradually diffused into the drop of culture, where it was oxidized to sulfur. If one uses completely sulfur-free filaments, one finds numerous little particles in the filaments, which look like black spots under the largest magnification, after only 3–5 hr. After 24 hr the same filaments are completely filled with these sulfur particles. If one transfers the culture into a normal humid chamber, the sulfur disappears

221

from the filaments but reappears as soon as the culture is returned to the hydrogen sulfide–containing jar. This experiment can easily be repeated many times if one takes care to develop more hydrogen sulfide every 2–3 hr; a strong hydrogen sulfide formation should be avoided, since the filaments are easily damaged and may even die.

The rate and constancy by which *Beggiatoa* deposits sulfur in H_2S-containing culture medium shows that the sulfur formation occurs only from H_2S solution; it is impossible to assume that the process can occur through reduction of SO_4 followed by oxidation of hydrogen sulfide. Nevertheless, I also arranged a number of microscopic cultures in spring water with gypsum. Cultures in fluids that contain excess sulfate do not need special attention: the decay, which is caused by bacteria in the mud and dead *Beggiatoa* cells, results in hydrogen sulfide production. In pure cultures in a solution containing gypsum, the sulfur in the filaments disappears as fast as in the spring water without hydrogen sulfide. Of the five microscopic slide cultures in spring water that contains gypsum, four gave the abovementioned results. The fifth culture behaved entirely differently. During the whole observation time (40 days) the filaments were full of sulfur. I found the cause for this strange behavior to be the result of a mass of dead *Cladothrix* filaments which were introduced into the culture by accident; the decay of these caused a hydrogen sulfide formation from calcium sulfate. The presence of hydrogen sulfide in the drop of culture could be confirmed throughout the observation period by testing the solution with lead oxide paper, or by the smell of the solution. A similar convincing result was obtained from a third series of experiments. I cultivated *Beggiatoa* in "Langenbrucker" sulfur water,[12] in which they grow very well. This water contains large amounts of sulfates. Before use I left it standing in an open vessel until the hydrogen sulfide odor had completely disappeared. Then I

---

[12]Since I used this water frequently in my studies, I include the complete analysis, which was carried out by Bunsen. The cold alkaline–saline water of the "Waldquelle" [*Ed. Note:* forest spring] at Bad Langenbrucken contains per 1000 parts:

Calcium carbonate	3.4055
Magnesium carbonate	2.6503
Calcium sulfate, anhydrous	3.1478
Magnesium sulfate	5.0528
Sodium sulfate	2.1245
Potassium sulfate	0.2072
Calcium phosphate (three basic in carbonic acid)	0.2157
Potassium chloride	0.1358
Ferrous sulfide (dissolved in calcium sulfide)	0.0459
Aluminium oxide (Tonerde)	0.0414
Calcium sulfide	0.0569
Silica (Kieselerde)	0.1735
Carbon dioxide	2.3561
Hydrogen sulfide	0.0994
Traces of organic substances and calcium fluoride	

19.7128

arranged a series (eight) of completely identical microscopic slide cultures. Half of these I washed twice daily with the same water; to the other half I added a few drops of hydrogen sulfide water per 5 ml of the water. In the former cultures, the filaments soon lost all their sulfur and did not form more. In the other half of the cultures, the filaments were always full of sulfur. The difference between the black filaments filled with sulfur and the colorless filaments without sulfur was very obvious, despite the fact that both cultures were offered the same amount of sulfate. The only difference in the constitution of the fluid was the hydrogen sulfide in the cultures of the second half of the experiment.

All these experiments show conclusively that *Beggiatoa* forms its sulfur only from hydrogen sulfide.

Editor's Comments on Papers 28 and 29

28 **Beijerinck:** About *Spirillum desulfuricans* as Cause for Sulfate Reduction
   Zentr. Bakteriol., Abtlg. II, **1**, 104–114 (1895)

29 **Deherain:** The Reduction of Nitrate in Arable Soil
   Compt. Rend. Acad. Sci., Paris, **124**, 269–273 (1897)

During this period of great activity in microbiology, Beijerinck discovered yet another organism, which did not oxidize sulfur compounds but reduced them (Paper 28; see also Beijerinck, 1895). He isolated the sulfate reducer *Spirillum desulfuricans* (now *Desulfovibrio desulfuricans*).

This discovery was soon followed by that of denitrification (Paper 29), which established that both the sulfur and the nitrogen cycle occur in nature. These discoveries, together with the isolation of colorless organisms (*Thiobacillus*) that oxidize hydrogen sulfide or thiosulfate (Nathanson, 1902; Beijerinck, 1904), as well as the isolation and characterization of hydrogen bacteria (Kaserer, 1906) and methane bacteria (Söhngen, 1906), established a basic knowledge of the metabolism of inorganic compounds.

In addition to the extensive investigations into the respiratory activity of the nitrifiers by Meyerhof (1916), S. A. Waksman continued the study of sulfur oxidation (Lipmann et al., 1921; Waksman, 1922) and isolated *Thiobacillus thiooxidans* (Waksman and Joffee, 1921, 1922). They found that this organism oxidizes elementary sulfur to sulfuric acid and derives its carbon from the carbon dioxide of the atmosphere. Furthermore, Waksman and Starkey (1923) also established the relationship between the amount of sulfur present and the velocity of oxidation.

Although Winogradsky had already indicated in 1890 that a certain unity concept exists among the complex group of chemolithotrophic microorganisms, the first and concise demonstration of the biochemical unity concept can be found in the excellent review by Baas-Becking and Parks (1927).

28

About *Spirillum desulfuricans* as Cause for Sulfate Reduction

W. M. BEIJERINCK

*Translated expressly for this Benchmark volume by H. W. Doelle from "Über Spirillum desulfuricans als Ursache von Sulfatreduktion," Zentr. Bakteriol., Abtlg. II, **1**, 104–114 (1895)*

Since the ferment occurs in my original cultures only in minute amounts compared with the usual species, a method had to be found to accumulate sulfate bacteria. This was made possible using what I call separation flasks, which are shown in Figs. 1 and 2.[1] The purpose of this flask is to separate the anaerobes from the main cell mass constituting aerobes of an ordinary culture, which was grown under limited air supply. This is done on the assumption that bacteria usually possess a higher specific weight than the nutritional medium, and since nonmotile[2] forms have no possibility of floating upward they sediment out.[3] The flask is a modification of the fermentation flask, which is unique in possessing a glass tubing that has an open connection at the highest point of the gas tubing. This can be obtained in two ways. In Fig. 1 this tube is outside the flask and leads to a capillary that, because of complete filling of the gas tube and outside tube, permits a flow only at excess pressure and, at the same time, prevents the addition of oxygen.

The flask can be used only if no gas development occurs in the culture, since, otherwise, the natural separation of bacteria with different gas requirements is lost.

If, in this flask, one incubates on an appropriate nutrition medium, a mixture of bacteria containing aerobes and obligate and facultative anaerobes, the following distribution can be obtained: the aerobes collect in the spherical part and at the bottom of the flask. The separation is very sharp. Investigations of the culture fluid above this line in the gas tube show only a few aerobes. If aerobes are cultivated

---

[1]The flasks were given to me by Dr. Rohrbeck from Berlin.
[2]Whether motile or not is unimportant.
[3]Bacteria exist that are able to grow in broth of the same specific weight; e.g., the lactic acid ferment can be cultivated in wort of 10° Balling. They are distributed, of course, throughout the liquid, even in the gas tube. The lactic acid bacteria, however, are facultative anaerobes. In my opinion, aerobic forms accumulate even in wort of 20° Balling below a distinct line on the bottom of the glass tube.

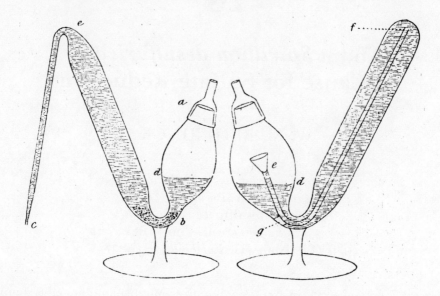

Fig. 1. Flask for the rough separation of anaerobes and aerobes. During sulfate reduction, ferrous sulfide formation appears first in precipitate *b*. A drop of sulfide ferment can be obtained from the tip of capillary *c* if the flask is tilted; *db* consists mainly of aerobic bacteria; *a* is a glass lid.

Fig. 2. Another form of separation flask. A small glass tube *g*, in which one end is open and the other is in the form of a funnel, is melted into an ordinary fermentation flask. If the broth is inoculated with a mixture of anaerobes and aerobes between *e* and *d*, i.e., outside the open glass tube, the anaerobes will collect mainly inside the tube and can be withdrawn at *e* for further inoculations. The inner tube can be closed off at *e* with a drop of paraffin.

alone in a fermentation flask, the culture fluid in the gas tube stays completely clear, whereas that in the globe and the lower parts of the flask are very turbid. Fluorescent bacteria (e.g., *B. fluorescens nonliquefaciens*) in meat bouillon give excellent and picturesque results.[4]

The facultative anaerobes either are uniformly distributed throughout the culture fluid or accumulate in the spherical part because of their weight. However, they are present in large numbers in the gas tube.

The obligate anaerobes are uniformly distributed throughout the culture fluid; thus their relative number, particularly in relation to the aerobes, is significantly larger in the gas tube.

Experience revealed that after a strong reduction, many more sulfide *Spirillum* can be obtained from the capillary than from any other method.

The second form of the separation flask is presented in Fig. 2. The tube for

---

[4]See also Th. Smith, "Das Gärungskölbchen in der Bakteriologie," *Zentral. Bakteriol.*, Bd. VII, 503 (1890); Bd. XIV, 864 (1893).

leading off the anaerobes is inside the flask. This tube ends either open at the top of the gas tube or in a small funnel inside the spherical portion. In either case it is easy to take material from the flask with a platinum needle for further experiments.

At the beginning of an experiment, the flask is filled with a sterilized and air-free nutrient solution to a level so that the little funnel is outside the fluid. Inoculation follows in the usual way, making certain that nothing goes into the funnel. This inoculation should be carried out with a large amount of material immediately after cooling to avoid the addition of air. During cooling only the spherical part of the flask is held under the water tap, to avoid any transfer of oxygen-containing air into the upper part of the gas tube, which can occur as the result of the drop of cold fluid into the warmer. With some experience it is possible to inoculate the spherical part at 25°C although the fluid in the gas tube is still at 66°C. These remarks are also applicable to the flask shown in Fig. 1. If one fears that humidity will cause water to condense at the rim of the funnel and infect the inner tube by dropping into it, one could block the inner tube with paraffin. This paraffin layer can later easily be penetrated by a platinum wire while obtaining inoculation material of facultative and obligate anaerobes. For the following experiments, the inoculum used was either mud from a creek or sediment from a previous reduction; the accumulation of the sulfide ferment can be observed in the inner tube.

This culturing method made further progress through the observation that the presence of common little water spirilla enhanced growth of the ferment. As I cultured various types of *Spirillum tenue* Cohn for a longer period of time, this characteristic was explored further.

Spirillum tenue grows on common nutrient agar slowly but without difficulty. The soil should be weakly alkaline and contain neutral salts of organic acids. The presence of peptone is advantageous. Of my three varieties, two do not liquify gelatine; the third does to a small extent. Beautiful cultures develop in meat bouillon with spirilla having 20 and more coils. The formation of calcium carbonate in solid and liquid substrates is characteristic of the spirilla.

The fluids generally used for filling the separation flasks are the same as given for the raw [*Ed. Note:* original?] culture. However, I also used different mixtures. During simultaneous inoculation of *Spirillum tenue*, I found that the concentration of organic material in the sulfate solution can be much higher than without the organisms. However, sugars must be kept out to avoid fermentation and acid formation.

The liquids were, in all cases, freed of oxygen by boiling and after the flasks were filled, they, too, were heated.

For example, I filled a flask with the following solution: water from a creek containing ¼ percent malate, ¼ percent peptone siccum, and 1/10 percent Mohr salt [*Ed. Note:* ferrous ammonium sulfate], which was made alkaline with sodium carbonate.

After 24 hr at 28°C, the flask, which was inoculated with creek water and *Spirillum tenue*, exhibited iron sulfide formation.

For another experiment, the flask was filled with creek water containing ¼ percent asparagine, 1/5 percent $MgSO_4$, 1/5 percent K-phosphate, 1/10 percent ferrolactate, and 1 percent sodium carbonate. Inoculation was carried out as before. Although *Spirillum tenue* does not grow well in this mixture, bacterial development was good, and after 48 hr at 30°C, strong H_2S and ammonium sulfide formation occurred. Even a pure ½ percent peptone solution with 1/10 percent Mohr salt and a bit of sodium carbonate produced growth. It could be shown that, in general, the reduction was stronger as the content of organic compounds capable of being reduced increased. However, since the organic compounds first have to undergo decomposition by other bacteria, it can take some time before the reduction is visible. The highest concentrations I studied were in a solution containing 1 percent sodium malate, ½ percent asparagine, ¼ percent K-phosphate, ¼ percent NaCl, ¼ percent sodium carbonate, and 1/10 percent Mohr salt in creek water. After 3 days at 28°C, FeS was produced. I wish to emphasize that the mixed infection with *Spirillum tenue* enhances but is not essential for these experiments.

Using this nutritional liquid, a flocculent precipitate, in which the sulfide ferment accumulates with the production of black spots, appears in bend *b* of the flask. This black color later spreads throughout the glass tube and the black flakes settle on the vertical glass wall. Since these flakes develop into long vertical streaks obviously as the result of the gravity of the sulfide ferment, one could assume that these bacteria are nonmotile under optimal conditions. The experiments indicate that, in general, even motile bacteria normally do not move; they do so only if it is absolutely necessary.

The isolation from these reduction flasks containing the sulfide ferment is relatively easy with gelatine and agar.

The agar culture was obtained as follows: A very clear, twice-filtered, aqueous agar solution was washed for a longer period of time with distilled water to remove all

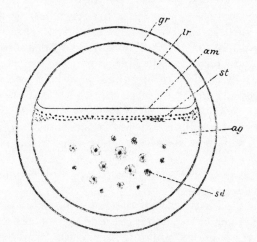

Fig. 3. Mixed culture of *Spirillum tenue* (*st*) and *S. desulfuricans* (*sd*) in agar (*ag*) between two glass plates separated by a glass ring (*gr*). The empty compartment is only partly filled as *lr* is air and *am* the agar level. The layer of *Spirillum tenue* colonies lies a specific distance from the agar level and thus has formed under reduced oxygen tension. The colonies of *Spirillum desulfuricans* and the surrounding area are black because of the ferrous sulfide deposit.

soluble material; distilled water was frequently poured and removed from the solid agar in the boiling flask. The agar was melted and boiled and then a very small amount of nutrient solution (which contained sodium malate, asparagine, and potassium phosphate) was added, and was again boiled to remove all oxygen. During the cooling of the agar, one drop of a clear solution of Mohr salt, together with traces of sodium carbonate, was added to prevent the appearance of turbidity. After a small drop from the capillary of the reduction flask was added and mixed vigorously, the agar was poured into test tubes, flat glass dishes, or glass containers and immediately cooled with water. The glass dishes were 1 millimeter deep and 1 decimeter wide, closed by a polished glass plate. The container (Fig. 3) consists of the well-known wide glass rings, fitted with ground-glass plates of equal diameter, which create a space equal to the thickness and diameter of the glass rings. Even this experimental method does not completely exclude the oxygen and, therefore, it would not be possible to cultivate the sulfide ferment. However, there are a great number of bacteria that take up the oxygen residues in the inoculum, create a completely oxygen-free medium, and thus make it possible for the sulfide ferment to grow and to form colonies after 2–3 days. If the contaminants are spirilla, the colonies will grow slowly and the reduction goes slowly until all sulfate is reduced and the iron is precipitated as iron sulfide. If other bacteria are involved as contaminants, the results are variable and often not explainable. Often the reduction starts vigorously, ceases after 2–3 days, and does not restart. The colonies are so small that it is better to repeat the experiment. It is advisable to use only well-developed colonies for further cultivation, since the number of bacteria is small even in those and barely exceeds 1000. The colonies obtained by this method appear large, which is mainly because of the iron sulfide coat; if one dissolves this coat in acid, the colonies disappear and become invisible to the naked eye. The growth of the colonies can be enhanced if the agar plate containing the colonies is dipped (wholly or partly) into a nutrient solution that favors sulfate reduction. If the fluid is renewed several times, growth can continue for some time. Thin agar plates can be rolled together and transferred into a stoppered, wide-neck flask. One transfers agar layers between glass plates into glass boxes that can be filled up with the culture fluid and closed airtight with ground-glass plates. However, even this trick does not exclude the development of small bacteria, and I had considerable difficulty maintaining sterility during the transfer of colonies. The difficulty of isolation depends on the last manipulation, and isolated cultures are very hard to use in further experiments, since it is difficult to obtain a completely oxygen-free culture area without the help of living organisms. Our lack of knowledge in regard to the bacteria of peptone decomposition, the most interesting species of which are also anaerobes, demonstrates that I am not the only one experiencing these difficulties.[5]

---

[5]I like to note that there exist two classes of anaerobic bacteria. One class, which is represented by the butyl ferment, is able to absorb the last traces of oxygen from the nutrient medium, whereupon the morphologically characteristic "oxygen form" appears [*Die Butylalkoholgärung*, p. 27, Amsterdam (1893)]. The second class, which includes the sulfide ferment, does not possess such an oxygen form and requires complete removal of oxygen to develop.

In any case I only spent as much time with pure cultures as was necessary to secure morphological characteristics and to observe the fact that sulfate reduction of the ferment is possible without the help of other bacteria.

Let us look at the characteristics of the colonies. It does not matter whether they are grown in agar or gelatine, since no different forms were observed, and the gelatine was not liquefied.

In the absence of iron salts the very small colonies have no special characteristics, and pigment formation is completely absent.[6]

In the presence of iron salts, the colonies are quite visible (Fig. 3). It should be noted, however, that the characteristics caused by the sulfur–iron are characteristic for the sulfide ferment only under the conditions that no other sulfur source is available as sulfate; they can also be found in the case of bacteria that form H_2S by different systems. The latter, of course, do not possess the morphology of spirilla; thus a microscopic diagnosis is always possible. The spirillum form is, however, not always distinct in the sulfide ferment.

The reduced colonies can appear in two forms, either with a diffuse, gradually disappearing sulfur–iron sphere or as intense black points without a sphere. The cause of this difference is unknown to me; only those colonies with a sphere were able to continue reduction. The appearance of motile organisms in the second form is not a distinction between life or death. Since I did not succeed in observing a constant morphological difference between bacteria of both colony forms, I have no reason to believe that they are different bacterial species. It should be noted, however, that colonies possessing the sphere developed only similar forms.

The sphere around the colonies consists, as stated earlier, of iron sulfide (Fig. 4). It exists as a uniform precipitate, gradually losing the coloring of the agar or gelatine, and as a little globular, rarely irregular, lumpy precipitate. The small globules are nearly equal in size and can be mistaken as micrococci. Since they are completely soluble in HCl, there is no reason to believe that they consist of an organic skeleton (since they develop with the much larger calcium carbonate sparites if sodium carbonate and calcium chloride react in the presence of protein or gelatine). The globules are situated in the colonies, distributed between the bacteria in small numbers.

The experiments described thus far always assumed that water spirilla are present in excess in the separation flask, apart from the reduction ferment. This was achieved by the addition of *Spirillum tenue* to the inoculum with the sulfide ferment. With the addition of peptone or acidic organic salts with Mohr salt as S source and indicator, *Spirillum tenue* reproduces so vigorously that all other bacteria are completely suppressed. As a consequence, only *Spirillum tenue* and the sulfide ferment develop a certain number of colonies between the glass plates; foreign bacterial colonies, especially the aerobes, are almost completely eliminated.

I wish to draw attention to a peculiarity in the growth of *Spirillum tenue* that is of importance in regard to the relation of the microorganisms to free oxygen. This peculiarity is the unique distribution of *Spirillum* colonies in the substrate; the colonies

---

[6]Zelinsky's *Bacterium hydrosulfureum ponticum* liquefies gelatine and produces a brown pigment.

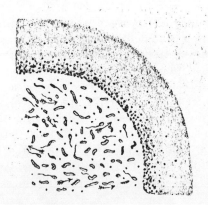

Fig. 4. Colony of *Spirillum desulfuricans* enlarged from Fig. 3. It shows the numerous ferrous sulfide precipitates in the agar and colonies. The *Spirillum* cells are partly dead and black. Mobility is indicated by arrows.

accumulate at a certain distance from the meniscus and only there do they appear in visible size (*st*, Fig. 3). Above and below this zone they cannot be localized. The colonies apparently develop in an area of the nutrient medium where a certain low oxygen tension exists. On another occasion I was able to determine three types according to their mobility: the aerobic, the spirilla, and the anaerobic type, depending upon whether they accumulate on places of high, medium, or low oxygen tension. We see now that these three mobility types find their analog in growth conditions. The basic explanation is probably that growth and mobility obtain an optical density maximum at identical oxygen tension. The question now arises as to whether *Spirillum tenue* exhibits a medium or a maximal CO_2 release at a medium tension. The latter possibility is probably the case, since oxygen supply completely inhibits CO_2 release in obligate aerobes.

Let us return to the sulfide ferment. The colonies in agar or gelatine are constituted of short spirilla with few coils that are approximately 4μ long and 1μ thick; only a few reach greater length or remain shorter. The number of coils is ½–1 and rarely can one find more than 1 coil. Most of them are slowly mobile, as long as no oxygen is excluded. If this gas is allowed to enter the preparation, the more mobile organisms withdraw toward the limited-oxygen region in the middle of the preparation; the less mobile ones remain immobile. It is the same behavior as I found earlier[7] with the influence of oxygen on the mobility of the anaerobic butyl ferment. In those colonies that developed in the presence of iron salts, the black micrococcus-type iron sulfide precipitate is distributed among the bacteria (Fig. 4). Dead spirilla attract iron sulfide precipitation, obtain an intensive black color, and swell tremendously, exposing the spirillum structure.[8]

---

[7]*Zentral. Bakteriol.*, Bd. XIV, 841 (1893).

[8]During my experiments I once observed a significant number of spirillum species that deposited sulfur–iron globules inside the cell in mobile and living conditions. R. Koch also appears to have found such a species and named it *Spirillum leucomelaenum* [*Mitt. Gesundh.*, Bd. I, 48 (1881)]. (Koch said "after Perty"; however, I looked in "Kleinste Lebensformen" and was not able to find this name.)

On many of the sulfide species I was able to observe without difficulty a terminal flagellum or a terminal cluster of flagella. The size of the ferment in liquid is normally smaller than in the colonies on solid medium, although the spirilla form is always visible. I believe therefore, that I can give our ferment the name *Spirillum desulfuricans*.

When I try to introduce the sulfide ferment here as a member of the genus *Spirillum*, I have to emphasize that such an introduction can only be a provisional one, since it is certain that the presently known *Spirillum* species differ among themselves. One example is their behavior toward free oxygen. Three sharply separable types can be observed through their colony growth in solid media, as well as through the mobility of their "respiration form." We find the aerobic type in *Spirillum tyrogenum* (also in the case of cholera), the *Spirillum tenue* type and the anaerobic type in *Spirillum desulfuricans*.

It is possible that these physiological differences come from distant systematic relationships that will allow our artificial genus *Spirillum* to be separated into three natural genera. To do this, however, we need a better view of the bacterial system as a whole.

Having obtained *Spirillum desulfuricans* in a pure culture, the difficulties of making further studies are certainly not all overcome. To the contrary, they are much greater than in the raw material. The main problem is that of oxygen removal, and everyone who is confronted with this problem knows the tedious repetition and radical treatments necessary if one wants to exclude the influence of aerobic micro-organisms. The use of ferric sulfate instead of Mohr salt may be one suggestion; however, this is only a last resort. Although I studied the sulfide ferment for over 2 years, such problems have so far prevented me from gaining a more complete knowledge of the biology of this ferment. The time factor is critical if one considers that it takes 3–4 weeks to obtain the result of each reduction experiment and that most experiments with pure cultures are failures. The following questions have, for example, not been answered as yet: Is the sulfide ferment able to reduce other compounds in the same way as it does sulfate (e.g., ferri salts, nitrate, etc.)? Are those sulfide ferments that occur in clay along the coastline and cause extensive sulfide formation identical with *Spirillum desulfuricans*? What is the influence of the salt content on the ferment? Does the sulfide ferment in our creeks and ponds, as well as that in the soil, belong to one and the same species? The important questions of the depth to which the sulfide ferment occurs in soil and the indications of where sulfate reduction has been completed in the appropriate soils also remain unsolved.

29

The Reduction of Nitrate in Arable Soil

P. P. DEHERAIN

*Translated expressly for this Benchmark
volume by G. Gordon of the University of
Queensland, Australia, from "La réduction des nitrates dans la terre arable,"*
Compt. Rend. Acad. Sci., Paris, **124**,
269–273 (1897)

In 1873 our colleague, Monsieur Schloesing, discovered that soil closed in a flask loses nitrogen from the nitrates it contains to the free state.

Later, in 1882, Messieurs Gayon and Dupetit on the one hand, and Monsieur Maquenne and myself on the other, attributed this reduction to the activity of anaerobic ferments. Several years ago Monsieur Breal discovered a denitrifying ferment, or strain, that was active even in contact with air.

Quite recently a German agronomist, Monsieur Wagner, again found in farm animal feces the ferment (or a similar species, discovered by Monsieur Breal), whose presence is believed to constitute a serious danger to farm cultivation.

In order to avoid adding these denitrifying ferments to the soil, it was proposed to destroy them by treating the fertilizing manure with sulfuric acid before spreading it. It appeared to me that the question merited a serious examination and that, before advising farmers to spend considerable sums on acidifying their manure, it was expedient to see if the danger was as pressing as had been believed.

My first consideration was to verify the existence of denitrifying ferments in straw and in solid animal waste. I succeeded easily in observing the disappearance of nitrates from dilute solutions of saltpeter [*Ed. Note:* HNO_3] and traces of potassium phosphate exposed to free air and primed with some straw, fresh manure, or horse manure and maintained in an oven at 30°C. Upon evaporating the previously inoculated solutions, potassium bicarbonate and a very small quantity of organic nitrogenous material was found.

I then looked for the carbonated organic material which was acknowledged as the best nutrient for denitrifying bacteria, I soon recognized that they prospered in liquids containing nitrate, phosphate, and starch. When 200 mg of saltpeter, 250 mg of starch, and 10 mg of potassium nitrate was added to 100 ml of distilled water inoculated with an active liquid, the nitrate disappeared completely after 48 hr at 30°C.

The very small quantity of organic nitrogenous material remainng in solution convinced me that the nitrogen must be released into the free state. Therefore, a flask was filled with liquid containing starch, a known weight of saltpeter, and potassium nitrate and closed with a stopper carrying a tube in which the liquid flows back, finally collecting the gas over mercury. Almost the exact quantity of nitrogen introduced was found in the gaseous state; of 100 ml of gas evolved, 12 ml were found as nitrous oxide. Monsieur Maquenne and I, in previous research on the reduction of nitrates in arable soil, recognized the presence of this gas.[1]

This reduction in a closed vessel is sufficiently rapid as to be evident in a short period of time: a round flask containing 1 liter of liquid, 2.5 g of starch, 2 g of saltpeter, and 0.1 g of potassium nitrate, inoculated with several cubic centimeters of an active culture, forming several cubic centimeters of a mixture of nitrogen, nitrous oxide, and carbon dioxide in an hour.

Free nitrogen is liberated from nitrates and reduction is most rapid in a sealed vessel. The denitrifying bacteria probably utilize only the oxygen from nitrates, and by passing a stream of air across the solution, the reduction could be retarded or even completely prevented. A slow stream of air does not affect activity, but when the passage of the air is accelerated, reduction slows down. Nevertheless, if the starch is carefully replaced, it takes no more than 8 days for the reduction to be complete.

Since denitrifying bacteria are found on straw and in animal wastes, it is probable that they would be encountered in cultivated soils to which farm manure is so frequently applied. In effect, nitrate reduction is obtained by inoculation of solutions of saltpeter and starch with soil. However, the activity of these denitrifying bacteria is not sufficient to impede aerated soil that is moistened, maintained at a suitable temperature, and charged with considerable quantities of nitrate; if the development of denitrifying organisms is favored by the addition of starch to the soil, the nitrates will be diminished.

Their reduction is verified by incorporating into soil excremental materials that are naturally charged with denitrifying bacteria. To succeed in the destruction of nitrates in soil by this addition it is necessary to introduce enormous quantities of these excremental materials. By employing analogous proportions to those used by German agronomists (namely, by mixing between 200 and 400 g of horse manure to 2 kg of soil), nitrate reduction is assisted, and it is this which has led some writers to recommend the treatment of manure with sulfuric acid.

Before accepting this conclusion, it is useful to note that the proportions of soil and manure used in the preceding experiments are entirely out of all proportion not only with usage but also with the possibilities of cultivation. In effect, applying 200 g of manure to 2 kg of soil would be to apply one-tenth of its weight. In other words, it would be necessary to apply to 1 hectare, which weighs 4000 tons, 400 tons of manure, which is not feasible. A very good fertilizing farm manure comprises more than 200 times the weight of soil. Eighty tons of manure would be applied to 4000 tons per

---

[1]*Ann. Agron.*, Vol. IX, 5.

hectare. But, if additional soil is used in the experiment (that is, 500 g of soil and 10 g of manure), the nitrates not only fail to disappear, they increase.

From time immemorial, farmers have employed farm manure with great profit. It is indeed extraordinary to suppose that the application of this manure, "far from favoring the formation in soil of nitrate, the most precious nitrogenous fertilizer," brings about its destruction. Our correspondent, Monsieur Pagnoul, has recently found large proportions of nitrate in soil enriched with farm manure. Also, some years ago, numerous comparative analyses of drainage water from manured soils and those left without fertilizer showed that a considerable quantity of nitrogen from manure appeared to be in the form of nitrate. However, all nitrogen introduced is not recovered as nitrate. But if this nitrogen has vanished to the gaseous state by the destruction of a product from nitrate, the soils enriched by farm manure would be conserved over the years as durably fertile. This nitrogen is not dissipated; it remains incorporated in the soil in the form of humus. It is precisely because manure possesses an action of great duration that nitrification of these nitrogenous materials proceeds slowly, and it constitutes the most valuable of all fertilizers.

Today we know how to strengthen its action with sodium nitrate; there is no need to fear that the denitrifying bacteria of manure will act in a disastrous way on the added nitrate, for there is no reason to scatter these two fertilizers at the same moment. All competent farmers distribute manure in autumn and nitrate in spring. The advantage of mixing these manures is already recognized, and their use becomes more general each year. Although manure and nitrate are incorporated into the soil at the same time, after several weeks more nitrate can be found in this soil than was put into it, provided that the farm manure has been applied in moderate doses, similar to those that are used daily.

I now believe that to advise farmers to treat manure with sulfuric acid before spreading it would involve them in an expenditure that is not only excessive but also useless and disastrous. Useless because denitrifying bacteria only exercise their action as long as they grow to enormous masses but are never used. Disastrous because, instead of applying a fertilizer advantageously to all soils, only a mixture of straw, potassium sulfate, and ammonium sulfate would be directed to the fields. But, as is known, the latter fertilizer is suitable only for heavy soils. It is without perceptible effect in many light soils and becomes dangerous in limestone soils.

I have been zealously aided in this work, carried out mostly at l'Ecole de Grignon by Monsieur Marcille, chemist at the Agronomic Station, and I am happy to thank him for his skillful collaboration.[2]

_____

[2]Details of these experiments will appear *in extenso* in the February 1897 issue of *Annales Agronomiques*.

Editor's Comments on Paper 30

30 Milhaud, Aubert, and Millet: Chemoautotrophic Carbon Metabolism. Cycle for Carbon Dioxide Assimilation
Compt. Rend. Acad. Sci., Paris, **243**, 102–105 (1956)

Research into the biochemistry of ammonia, nitrite, and sulfur oxidation came to a standstill until Calvin and his research group discovered the autotrophic CO_2-fixation mechanism (Bassham et al., 1954). Although Santer and Vishniac (1955) and Trudinger (1955, 1956) suspected the same mechanism to operate in *Thiobacillus thioparus, T. denitrificans,* and hydrogen bacteria, it was Milhaud and coworkers (Paper 30) who showed that the pattern of radioactivity after fixation of $^{14}CO_2$ was similar to the distribution found in photosynthetic organisms, which was confirmed later by Suzuki and Werkman (1958).

30

Chemoautotrophic Carbon Metabolism: Cycle for Carbon Dioxide Assimilation

G. MILHAUD, J.-P. AUBERT, and J. MILLET

*Translated expressly for this Benchmark volume by G. Gordon of the University of Queensland, Australia, from "Métabolisme du carbone dans la chimiautotrophie. Cycle d'assimilation de l'anhydride carbonique," Compt. Rend. Acad. Sci., Paris, **243**, 102–105 (1956), with permission from the Académie des Sciences*

The scheme of autotrophic carbon dioxide fixation is identical to that of chlorophyllic assimilation, as shown by the distribution of radioactivity in carbon atoms of compounds formed by *Thiobacillus denitrificans* after a short exposure to $^{14}CO_2$. The cyclic nature of the scheme is also established.

We have previously shown[1] that 3-phosphoglyceric acid is the first stable product of autotrophic carbon dioxide assimilation and have established the simultaneous presence of ribulose-diphosphate, sedoheptulose-phosphate, and fructose 6-phosphate.

In order to deduce the mechanism of CO_2 incorporation, we analyzed the radioactivity in each of the carbon atoms of 3-phosphoglyceric acid, fructose 6-phosphate, sedoheptulose-phosphate, and ribulose-diphosphate. Furthermore, we have studied the effect of CO_2 concentration and of reducing power on the relative distribution of these different intermediates.

Methods

Methods of culture for *Thiobacillus denitrificans*, incubation in the presence of CO_2, and isolation of intermediates have previously been described.[1,2]

Glyceric acid was degraded according to the method using periodic acid.[2] Radioactivity in fructose was determined by a combination of periodic acid oxidation,[3] oxidation of its phenylosazone to periodate,[4] and alcoholic fermentation. Ribulose and sedoheptulose, and their phenylosazones, were oxidized by periodic acid. These two oxidations are sufficient for analysis of ribulose. For sedoheptulose, carbon-4 is obtained by oxidation to sedoheptulosane by periodic acid.[5] The resultant dialdehyde

237

is oxidized to the diacid by bromine,[5] the calcium salt of which is pyrolyzed at 500°C, which allows the analysis of carbon-5 radioactivity.

Results

A. Distribution of Radioactivity

The table compares the various analyses obtained with incubation in $^{14}CO_2$ for 10 seconds. The results are total incorporation of radioactivity expressed as a percentage.

3-Phosphoglyceric acid		Fructose 6-P		Sedoheptulose-P		Ribulose-di-P	
C_1	94	C_1	1	C_1	0	C_1	10
C_2	4	C_2	1	C_2	0	C_2	10
C_3	2	C_3	49	C_3	32	C_3	80
		C_4	47	C_4	29	C_4	0
		C_5	1	C_5	39	C_5	0
		C_6	1	C_6	0		
				C_7	0		

B. Effect of Carbon Dioxide Concentration

We rapidly changed the CO_2 concentration by centrifuging the bacteria previously exposed to $^{14}CO_2$ and resuspending them in normal growth medium lacking CO_2. The kinetic analyses of radioactivity incorporated into 3-P-glyceric acid and ribulose-di-P is compared in Fig. 1.

C. Effect of Reducing Power

In the same way we were able to decrease reducing power by centrifuging the bacteria and then resuspending them in normal growth medium containing $^{14}CO_2$ but lacking thiosulfate and nitrate. The kinetic analysis of radioactivity incorporated into 3-P-glyceric acid (APG) and ribulose-di-P (RDP) is compared in Fig. 2.

Discussion

The labeling of these phosphorylated substances is sufficiently different after 10 seconds of exposure to $^{14}CO_2$ to allow the suggestion of a pathway for the forma-

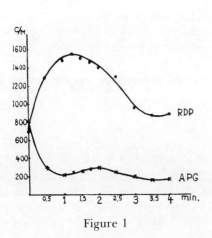

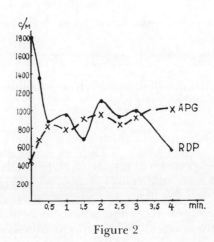

Figure 1   Figure 2

tion of these compounds. The labeling of 3-P-glyceric acid at the lone carboxyl group is in concordance with the hypothesis of a hydroclastic carboxylation of ribulose-di-P catalyzed by carboxydismutase.[6]

Fructose-6-P, carbon-3 and carbon-4 of which contain nearly all the radioactivity of the compound, could be formed by condensation of C_3-fragments provided by 3-P-glyceric acid.

Furthermore, transketolase[7,8] catalyzes the following reactions:

(I) Fructose-6-P + glyceraldehyde-3-P $\rightleftharpoons$ erythrose-4-P + ribulose-5-P
(II) Sedoheptulose-7-P + glyceraldehyde-3-P $\rightleftharpoons$ ribose-5-P + ribulose-5-P
And transaldolase[9] catalyzes
(III) Fructose-6-P + erythrose-4-P $\rightleftharpoons$ sedoheptulose-7-P + glyceraldehyde-3-P

Starting with fructose-6-P of the type

$$C-C-C^*-C^*-C-C-P$$

and glyceraldehyde-3-P of the type

$$C^*-C-C-P$$

labeling in the various compounds was distributed in the following fashion according to the following equations:

(I) $C-C-C^*-C^*-C-C-P + C^*-C-C-P \rightleftharpoons C^*-C^*-C-C-P + C-C-C^*-C-C-P$

(III) $C-C-C^*-C^*-C-C-P + C^*-C^*-C-C-P \rightleftharpoons C-C-C^*-C^*-C^*-C-C-P + C^*-C-C-P$

(II) $C-C-C^*-C^*-C^*-C-C-P + C^*-C-C-P \rightleftharpoons C^*-C^*-C^*-C-C-P + C-C-C^*-C-C-P$

So the sedoheptulose-7-P formed according to (III) will be of the type

$$C—C—C^*—C^*—C^*—C—C—P$$

and that the ribulose-di-P from ribulose-5-P, formed according to equations (I) and (II), will be of the type

$$P—C^*—C^*—C^{***}——C—C—P$$

The experimental results agree perfectly with this method of marking.

Finally, the results compared in Fig. 1 show that when CO_2 is removed, 3-P-glyceric acid diminishes while ribulose-di-P accumulates. Figure 2 shows that suppression of reducing power immediately corresponds to an accumulation of 3-P-glyceric acid and a drop in ribulose-di-P. This demonstrates the presence of a cycle relying on ribulose-di-P and 3-P-glyceric acid.

Conclusion

All these results agree with the following cycle:

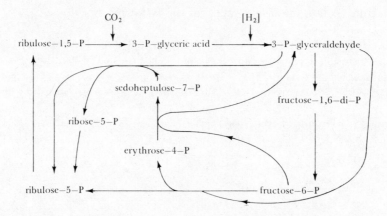

This scheme, originally proposed by Calvin[10] to explain the mechanism of CO_2 assimilation during photosynthesis, is now more widely applicable since it also explains CO_2 assimilation during chemautotrophic growth.

References

1. J. P. Aubert, G. Milhaud, and J. Millet, *Compt. Rend.*, **242**, 2059 (1956).
2. J. A. Bassham, A. A. Benson, and M. Calvin, *J. Biol. Chem.*, **185**, 781 (1950).
3. Y. Khouvine and G. Arragon, *Bull. Soc. Chim.*, **8**, 676 (1941).
4. Y. J. Topper and A. B. Hastings, *J. Biol. Chem.*, **179**, 1255 (1949).
5. W. T. Haskins, R. M. Hann, and C. S. Hudson, *J. Amer. Chem. Soc.*, **74**, 2198 (1952).
6. J. R. Quayle, R. C. Fuller, A. A. Benson, and M. Calvin, *J. Amer. Chem Soc.*, **76**, 3610 (1954).
7. B. L. Horecker and P. Z. Smyrniotis, *Methods in Enzymology*, Vol. 1, p. 371. Academic Press, New York (1955).
8. G. de la Haba and E. Racker, *Methods in Enzymology*, Vol. 1, p. 375. Academic Press, New York (1955).
9. B. L. Horecker and P. Z. Smyrniotis, *Methods in Enzymology*, Vol. 1, p. 381. Academic Press, New York (1955).
10. *Conferences et Rapports du III^c Congres International Biochemie*, p. 211. Vaillant-Carmande, Liege (1956).

Editor's Comments on Papers 31 and 32

31 **Postgate:** The Reduction of Sulphur Compounds by *Desulphovibrio desulphuricans*
    J. Gen. Microbiol., **5**, 725–738 (1951)

32 **Schlegel and Lafferty:** Growth of "Knallgas" Bacteria (*Hydrogenomonas*) Using Direct Electrolysis of the Culture Medium
    Nature, **205**, 308–309 (1965)

About the same time that Calvin and others were working on the problem of carbon dioxide fixation, the problem of denitrification (Allen and van Niel, 1952) and sulfate reduction (Butlin et al., 1949) was taken up again. Postgate and his research group were responsible not only for the advances in cultivating microorganisms (Postgate, 1951, 1953; Grossman and Postgate, 1953) but also for the further exploration into their biochemistry (Paper 31). In a similar way, Schlegel and his coworkers were responsible for the reinvestigation of the metabolism of hydrogen bacteria (Paper 32). The initial problems of cultivation having been solved, interest in the metabolic events of inorganic compounds was revived, and the publications since this time are numerous, as can be seen from the many reviews appearing in rapid sequence (Quastel and Scholefield, 1951; Schlegel, 1954, 1960, 1966; Butlin and Postgate, 1956; McElroy and Glass, 1956; Vishniac and Santer, 1957; Nason and Takahashi, 1958; Postgate, 1959, 1965; Lees, 1960; Gregory and Robbins, 1960; Taniguchi, 1961; Nason, 1962; Peck, 1962; Vishniac and Trudinger, 1962; Campbell and Postgate, 1965; Trudinger, 1967; Aleem, 1970).

$$31$$

$$31$$

31

Reprinted from *J. Gen. Microbiol.*, **5**, 725–738 (1951)

The Reduction of Sulphur Compounds by *Desulphovibrio desulphuricans*

BY J. R. POSTGATE

Chemical Research Laboratory, Teddington, Middlesex

SUMMARY: *Desulphovibrio desulphuricans*, strain 'Hildenborough', was able to use sulphite, thiosulphate, tetrathionate, metabisulphite or dithionite in place of sulphate for growth. Resting cell suspensions reduced these ions using the theoretical amounts of hydrogen and forming the theoretical amount of sulphide, except in the case of dithionite, which probably decomposed spontaneously to sulphate and sulphur before being reduced.

The organism was unable to grow with or to reduce dithionate, perdisulphate, 'formaldehydesulphoxylate', sulphamate, benzenesulphonate, methanesulphonate, β-hydroxyethane-sulphonate, sodium ethylsulphate, dimethylsulphone or cystine. Elementary sulphur, if purified by re-distillation, was also not attacked. Five other strains of *D. desulphuricans*, four of them cultivated autotrophically, were also unable to grow with pure elementary sulphur.

Colloidal sulphur permitted slow growth, or slow hydrogen absorption when a resting cell suspension was used. This effect was not due to oxide impurities in the sulphur permitting growth, as an ultra-filtrate of colloidal sulphur had considerably less activity.

A study of the rates of H_2 uptake suggested that sulphur, thiosulphate and tetrathionate were not intermediates in normal sulphate reduction, but that sulphite was.

The sulphate-reducing bacteria were first described by Beijerinck (1895), and were subsequently investigated by many workers including van Delden (1903), Baars (1930), Starkey (1938), Butlin & Adams (1947), ZoBell & Rittenberg (1948) and Butlin, Adams & Thomas (1949 *b*). 'Growth' was usually estimated by the amount of black ferrous sulphide precipitate formed by reaction of the sulphide produced from the reduction of sulphate with the excess of ferrous salt added to the medium. Butlin, Adams & Thomas (1949 *b*) showed that this large amount of iron is unnecessary, though traces insufficient to form a visible precipitate of iron sulphide are needed for growth.

The media used for the cultivation of these organisms were based on the use of a carbon source such as lactic acid, glucose or, for growth in autotrophic conditions, bicarbonate. Except in the latter case the carbon source acted also as a hydrogen donor for sulphate reduction, and the ability of various organic compounds to act as hydrogen donors was studied by Baars (1930). Butlin & Adams (1947) showed that, in autotrophic media, mild steel could act as a hydrogen donor, due to the formation of an electrolytic film of hydrogen at its surface in contact with the medium. Stephenson & Stickland (1931) showed that a strain of this organism was able to utilize gaseous hydrogen, and that sulphate reduction proceeded quantitatively according to the equation:

$$SO_4'' + 4H_2 = S'' + 4H_2O.$$

243

Postgate (1949) reported similar results with washed cell suspensions which reduced sulphate, sulphite and thiosulphate. Baars (1930) found that sulphate-reducing bacteria would grow with sulphite, thiosulphate, 'hydrosulphite' (dithionite) or colloidal sulphur in place of sulphate, but not with 're-precipitated' sulphur. When studying marine halophilic strains ZoBell & Rittenberg (1948) added tetrathionate to this list.

Butlin, Adams & Thomas (1949b) showed that growth and sulphide formation occurred with sulphate, sulphite, thiosulphate, and, in contrast to Baars (1930), also with 're-precipitated' sulphur, in autotrophic as well as heterotrophic conditions.

Evaluation of growth by sulphide formation may be unsatisfactory, since sulphide formation can take place without cell division, and this technique has probably been used only because of its ease and convenience. In media based on lactic acid and salts, growth without added iron is not abundant, but it is improved by the addition of yeast extract (Butlin, Adams & Thomas, 1949b). Recently, a medium giving vigorous growth without precipitation of iron sulphide has been described (Postgate, 1951) and used to grow large amounts of cells for manometric studies (Postgate, 1949). Using a sulphate-free modification of this medium, one can observe the growth of the organisms directly and investigate the ability of various compounds to replace sulphate for growth. Some studies of this kind are reported below, together with a quantitative investigation of the reduction of certain sulphur compounds by resting cell suspensions.

METHODS

Organism. A strain of *D. desulphuricans* called 'Hildenborough' was used in this work except where otherwise stated. Its origin and the routine methods of maintenance were described by Postgate (1951). Washed inocula were used for all growth tests recorded here.

Media and Materials. To study the ability of substances to replace sulphate it was desirable to have a medium which permitted optimal growth in the presence of sulphate and none in its absence. Such a medium was not easily prepared because most peptone preparations contain sulphate. A medium was found, however, based on Difco 'Bacto-Tryptone' (Baird & Tatlock Ltd., London), which permitted only very limited growth in the absence of added sulphate, owing probably to its low content of inorganic sulphur ('Difco Manual', 1948). This medium contained 'Bacto-Tryptone', 5 g.; glucose, 10 g.; yeast extract (Difco), 4 g.; $MgCl_2.6H_2O$, 0·8 g., in 1 litre of distilled water; pH 7·2. This will be referred to as the *complex medium*.

For certain tests it was necessary that no growth at all should occur in the absence of added substrate, and for this purpose a modification of Starkey's medium (Starkey, 1938) was used, having the composition: KH_2PO_4, 0·5 g.; NH_4Cl, 1 g.; $CaCl_2.6H_2O$, 0·1 g.; $MgCl_2.6H_2O$, 1·1 g.; sodium lactate (British Drug Houses Ltd., 70 % w/w) 5·0 g., in 1 litre of distilled water; pH 7·5. This medium gave only limited growth in the presence of sulphate owing to the absence of complex organic supplements. It will be referred to as the *simple medium.*

Where possible, materials of 'Analar' grade were used, but in certain cases (mentioned in the text) such specimens were not available. Sodium tetrathionate was at first prepared from an ethanolic solution of iodine and sodium thiosulphate, using the method described by Partington (1946), and was reprecipitated twice with absolute ethanol before use. This procedure did not give a pure preparation, as is mentioned later. 'Analar' grade $Na_2SO_3.7H_2O$ was recrystallized.

Substances to be tested were usually sterilized by autoclaving for 10 min. at 10 lb./sq. in., but when the substances might be unstable to heat they were added without sterilization. Such cases are mentioned; at the end of the test the cultures were always examined for contaminants, but none were found.

Resting Cell Suspensions. Cell suspensions for use in the Warburg manometer were prepared by centrifuging a culture and resuspending the cells in aqueous NaCl (0·8 % w/v) so as to give a suspension containing between 2 and 3 mg. dry wt. of cells/ml. Traces of substrate carried through the washing procedure were eliminated by pre-incubating the suspension for about 20 min. in a stream of hydrogen before use. One ml. of this suspension was added to the manometer vessel with 1 ml. of KH_2PO_4 buffer (0·5 % w/v, pH 6·3) and the substrate (usually 2·5 μmol.) was added in 0·5 ml. of water to the side arm; 0·5 ml. of aqueous NaOH (15 % w/v) or cadmium chloride (10 % w/v) were contained in the centre cup together with filter paper or glass wool. The manometer vessels were incubated at 37°. Six determinations of the $-Q_{H_2}$ for sulphate with a certain suspension gave a mean value of 323 mm^3 H_2/mg. dry cells/hr. with a standard deviation of 29·25 mm^3/mg./hr.; five determinations of the hydrogen absorbed with *c.* 2·5 μmol. of Na_2SO_4 gave a mean absorption of 276·6 mm^3 H_2 with a standard deviation of 2·72 mm^3 H_2.

Sulphide Estimations. Attempts to estimate the sulphide formed in the manometer vessel by analysis of the NaOH-soaked paper in the centre cup were unsuccessful, but a method using cadmium chloride in place of NaOH, and glass wool in place of filter paper proved satisfactory and was used throughout this work.

The manometer vessels were set up with a pre-incubated cell suspension and phosphate buffer in the main compartment and substrate in the side-arm. A small plug of acid-cleaned glass wool was placed in the centre cup and 0·5 ml. of aqueous $CdCl_2$ (10 % w/v) was added. At the end of the experiment the plug was transferred with clean tweezers to a stoppered titration vessel containing 1 ml. of 0·1 N iodine and 4 ml. of 5 N-HCl, which was shaken and left for 5 min. The centre cup was then rinsed with the titration liquid, followed by distilled water, to remove the last traces of sulphide, and the washings were added to the titration vessel. The whole volume was back-titrated against 0·01 N sodium thiosulphate, using a drop of carbon tetrachloride as an internal indicator. This method gave satisfactory results down to about 0·3 μmol. of sulphide, provided the titration fluid was left until all

CdS had decomposed (5 min.), and provided the titration vessel was kept stoppered as much as possible to prevent back-oxidation of HI. The standard deviation calculated from 12 readings taken over some months was 0·1273 μmol. of sulphide. The use of $CdCl_2$ in place of NaOH in the manometer made no difference to the amount of gas absorbed with a given substrate, indicating that no CO_2 is formed during sulphate reduction and that no correction need be applied for this.

RESULTS

Growth Experiments

Without substrate. No growth occurred in sulphate-deficient simple medium, but some growth occurred in the sulphate-deficient complex medium. This 'blank' growth was probably due to sulphate and other reducible compounds present in the 'Bacto-Tryptone' and yeast extract; indeed, the former is known to contain 0·04 % of inorganic sulphur ('Difco Manual', 1948).

Sulphate. Sulphate is the natural hydrogen-acceptor for the growth of *D. desulphuricans.* In the sulphate-deficient complex medium the growth of the organism depended linearly on the sulphate concentration between about 0·5 and 10 μmol. sulphate/ml. Higher concentrations of sulphate depressed the growth rate to some extent, though the maximum stationary population was ultimately reached (Fig. 1). Optimal growth was given by 10 μmols sulphate/ml., and this concentration was therefore used for testing other compounds, except in the case of elementary sulphur (see below).

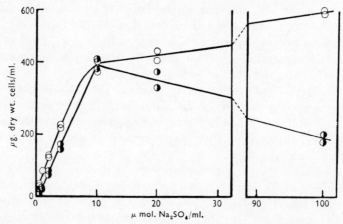

Fig. 1. Effect of sodium sulphate concentration on the growth of *D. desulphuricans* (Hildenborough) in a medium of glucose tryptone and yeast extract. ○ growth after 142 hr. incubation; ◑ growth after 92 hr. incubation.

Sulphite. Sodium sulphite could replace sulphate for the growth of *D. desulphuricans* in the sulphate-deficient complex medium (Table 1). It has been used in other media, at a concentration of 3 %, to purify crude cultures (Butlin, Adams & Thomas, 1949*b*) and has been observed to cause considerable elongation of the cells (Butlin, Adams & Thomas, 1949*a*).

Thiosulphate. Sodium thiosulphate could replace sodium sulphate for growth of the organism in the sulphate-deficient complex medium (Table 1).

Tetrathionate. Sodium tetrathionate could replace sodium sulphate for growth of the organism in sulphate-deficient complex medium, but growth took place more slowly (Table 1).

Table 1. *Growth of* D. desulphuricans (*Hildenborough*) *on a medium of glucose, peptone and yeast extract containing various substances in place of sulphate*

Test substance	Concentration M	24	48	72	96
		Growth after (hr.)			
Sulphate Na_2SO_4	10^{-2}	tr.	+	+++++	+++++
Sulphite Na_2SO_3	10^{-2}	tr.	+	+++++	+++++
Thiosulphate $Na_2S_2O_3$	10^{-2}	tr.	+	+++	+++++
Dithionate $Na_2S_2O_6$	10^{-2}	—	tr.	tr.	tr.
*Tetrathionate $Na_2S_4O_6$	10^{-2}	tr.	tr.	++	++++
*Dithionite $Na_2S_2O_4$	10^{-2}	—	tr.	+++	++++
Perdisulphate $(NH_4)_2S_2O_8$	10^{-2}	—	tr.	tr.	tr.
*Formaldehyde sulphoxylate $NaHSO_2 . HCHO$	10^{-2}	—	tr.	tr.	tr.
*Metabisulphite $K_2S_2O_5$	10^{-2}	tr.	tr.	++	+++
Benzenesulphonate $NaSO_3 . C_6H_5$	10^{-2}	—	tr.	tr.	tr.
Sulphur (B.D.H., re-ppt.) S	‡4×10^{-2}	—	tr.	+	+
*Sulphamate $NH_4 . SO_3NH_2$	10^{-2}	—	tr.	tr.	tr.
Methanesulphonate $NaO . SO_3 . CH_3$	10^{-2}	—	tr.	tr.	tr.
β-Hydroxyethanesulphonate $NaO . SO_2 . CH_2CH_2OH$	10^{-2}	—	tr.	tr.	tr.
†Sulphide Na_2S	10^{-2}	tr.	tr.	tr.	tr.
No addition	...	—	tr.	tr.	tr.
Sulphate Na_2SO_4	10^{-2}	—	tr.	+++++	++++
†Ethylsulphate $Na(C_2H_5)SO_4$	10^{-2}	—	—	—	tr.
Dimethylsulphone $(CH_3)_2SO_2$	10^{-2}	—	—	—	tr.
No addition	...	—	—	—	tr.

* Added without sterilization.   † Seitz filtered.   ‡ Added as suspension.

Dithionite. Sodium dithionite ('hydrosulphite' British Drug Houses Ltd.) replaced sulphate for the growth of the organism (Table 1), but it is likely that at the test pH value of 7·2, most of the S_2O_4'' ion had decomposed spontaneously. Solutions of the specimen used decomposed slowly in water with deposition of sulphur, and were therefore made up immediately before use and added without sterilization. Nevertheless, within 1 hr. a precipitate of sulphur was visible in the test medium, and it is likely that sodium dithionite supported growth because it decomposed spontaneously to sulphate.

Metabisulphite. It was thought desirable to test potassium metabisulphite since the S_2O_5 is known to exist as a separate ionic species in solution, though whether it was stable in the test conditions was not known. It replaced sulphate for growth of the organism (Table 1), but growth took place slowly and was less extensive.

Sulphur. 'Re-precipitated' sulphur (British Drug Houses Ltd.) supported only limited growth of the organism, though a suspension of 40 μg. atoms sulphur/ml. was used for testing in contrast to the 10 μmol./ml. solutions used of other substances (Table 1). This low activity might have two causes: (*a*) the low solubility of the substrate or (*b*) inactivity of the sulphur *per se* masked by the presence of active impurities. To test the second possibility a specimen of sulphur was distilled in an all-glass apparatus with a stream of oxygen-free nitrogen, ground in a flamed mortar and tested at once, without further sterilization. It did not support the growth of *D. desulphuricans*, and, since the preparation was perfectly satisfactory for the aerobic growth of *Thiobacillus thio-oxidans*, this failure was not due to a change in the allotropic state of the sulphur such as to render it biologically inactive.

Since the inactivity of purified sulphur contrasted with the reports of previous workers, it was studied in more detail. Cultures were set up with excess iron (FeCl$_2$, 0·5 mg./ml.), and also without, in sulphate-free simple medium and in sulphate-deficient complex medium. In the simple medium neither growth nor blackening occurred with the purified sulphur, and in the complex medium growth and blackening were equivalent to that obtained in the cultures without added substrate (Table 2). A test of the same kind using *D. desulphuricans* strain 'Teddington R' gave a similar result.

Table 2. *Growth and sulphide formation of* D. desulphuricans
(*Hildenborough*) *with sulphate and re-distilled sulphur* (1 *mg./ml.*)

With sulphate-deficient complex medium	Effect after (hr.)				
Addition	24	48	72	96	114
Sodium sulphate	—	+ +	+ + + +	+ + + + +	+ + + + +
Re-distilled sulphur	—	—	tr.	tr.	tr.
—	—	—	tr.	tr.	tr.
Sodium sulphate + FeCl$_2$	*	*	*	*	*
Re-distilled sulphur + FeCl$_2$	—	—	*	*	*
FeCl$_2$	—	—	*	*	*
With sulphate-deficient lactate medium					
Sodium sulphate	—	+	+ +	+ + +	+ + +
Re-distilled sulphur	—	—	—	—	—
—	—	—	—	—	—
Sodium sulphate + FeCl$_2$	*	*	*	*	*
Re-distilled sulphur + FeCl$_2$	—	—	—	—	—
FeCl$_2$	—	—	—	—	—

* Sulphide formation detected by precipitation of FeS from FeCl$_2$ (0·5 mg./ml.) added to the culture medium.

Four strains cultured in autotrophic medium (Butlin, Adams & Thomas, 1949*b*) were also tested for their ability to utilize freshly-distilled sulphur, using the sulphate-deficient simple medium in which lactic acid was replaced by sodium bicarbonate. They were all tested in the presence of FeCl$_2$ (0·5 mg./ml.) so that growth was indicated by blackening of the culture. Since it was not convenient to wash the inocula, the inoculum cells for the test were grown with 're-precipitated' sulphur in place of sulphate. In no case was growth or blackening detected in the presence of freshly-distilled sulphur. A specimen of re-distilled sulphur which had been left in air for about twenty days gave detectable blackening in autotrophic cultures.

It was possible that the sulphate-reducing bacteria were able to utilize sulphur only in the colloidal form—which was the form used by Baars (1930) —so a specimen of colloidal sulphur was obtained for testing in both simple and complex media. It supported the growth of both 'Hildenborough' and 'Teddington R' strains in these media. The specimen was known, however, to contain polythionic acid impurities equivalent to 0.0154% $H_2S_5O_6$, and the activity of the preparation may have been due to these. An ultra-filtrate of the sulphur sol was obtained by passing it through a 30–55 mμ. A.P.D. collodion membrame under 2 atm. N_2 pressure, and this also was able to support growth of the bacteria, though it was optically free from sulphur. These findings are illustrated in Table 3. In some experiments the ultra-filtrate supported distinctly less growth than the sol, but quantitative comparisons were most unreliable since the growth was judged by blackening due to FeS precipitation. Direct comparisons of the growth obtained with the sulphur sol and its ultra-filtrate could not be made owing to the opacity of the former.

Table 3. *Sulphide formation by* D. desulphuricans (*Teddington R*) *with colloidal sulphur and its ultra-filtrate*

With sulphate-deficient complex medium	Effect after (hr).			
Addition	24	48	72	96
Sodium sulphate+$FeCl_2$	*	*	*	*
Colloidal sulphur+$FeCl_2$	—	*	*	*
Ultra-filtrate+$FeCl_2$	—	*	*	*
With sulphate-deficient lactate medium				
Sodium sulphate+$FeCl_2$	—	*	*	*
Colloidal sulphur+$FeCl_2$	tr.	*	*	*
Ultra-filtrate+$FeCl_2$	tr.	*	*	*

Other compounds. The following compounds were tested and did not support growth, nor did they prevent the 'blank' growth that occurred in the complex medium: sodium dithionate (British Drug Houses Ltd., recryst. ×2), sodium formaldehyde sulphoxylate (British Drug Houses Ltd., the only available example of a compound containing the ion SO_2''), sodium benzene-sulphonate (British Drug Houses Ltd.), ammonium perdisulphate, ammonium sulphamate (Baird & Tatlock), sodium methanesulphonate (synthetic), sodium β-hydroxyethanesulphonate (synthetic), sodium ethylsulphate (synthetic) and dimethylsulphone (synthetic). For completeness, sodium sulphide was tested as a substrate for growth and was inactive, though its presence accelerated the 'blank growth', owing possibly to its strong reducing properties. Growth tests with these substances are recorded in Table 1.

Hydrogen uptake with cell suspension

Without substrate. Resting cell suspensions took up hydrogen slowly over a long period in the absence of reducible substrates; the $-Q_{H_2}$ was *c.* 15 mm³/mg./hr. (Fig. 3). In one experiment this 'blank' hydrogen uptake persisted for 48 hr., though the quotient was by then reduced.

Sulphide was not formed during the 'blank' hydrogen uptake, which, therefore, was unlikely to be due to the reduction of intracellular stores of sulphate-like material. Also, the rate of hydrogen absorption was unaffected by 10^{-3} M sodium selenate, which could have been sufficient to prevent the reduction of about 2×10^{-2} M sodium sulphate (Postgate, 1949).

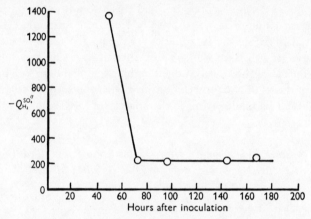

Fig. 2. Effect of the age of cultures of *D. desulphuricans* (Hildenborough) on the specific rate of sulphate reduction.

Sulphate. Resting cell suspensions in the Warburg manometer absorbed 4 mol. hydrogen/mol. sulphate, and 1 mol. sulphide was formed (Table 2, Fig. 3). This is consistent with the work of Stephenson & Stickland (1931). The specific rate of hydrogen absorption ($-Q_{H_2}^{SO_4''}$) depended on the concentration of cells present, between 0·218 and 2·18 mg. dry wt. cells/ml., and was independent of the sulphate concentration between 10^{-3} and 10^{-1} M-Na₂SO₄. Charcoal, which might have provided a greater surface for inter-action between the gas and liquid phases, did not affect the quotient, nor did ferrous ions, which remove sulphide from solution as ferrous sulphide.

The effect of age of the cells on the specific rate of hydrogen absorption is indicated in Fig. 2. Cells taken from a culture less than 48 hr. after inoculation showed an enhanced $-Q_{H_2}^{SO_4''}$; this corresponded to the period of active cell-division in the growth medium. In the stationary phase, however, the quotient remained constant for several days, so cultures in this phase of growth were used for general comparative work. The $-Q_{H_2}^{SO_4''}$ of such cells was in the region of 200 mm³/mg./hr. for *D. desulphuricans*, strain 'Hildenborough', though values between 150 and 350 mm³/mg./hr. have been obtained with this strain.

The greater specific rate of hydrogen absorption during growth suggests that sulphate reduction is the main energy-yielding reaction for cell mutiplication; Subba Rao & Sreenivasaya (1947) have shown that the rate of sulphate utilization by a halophil is greater during active cell-division, which is consistent with this view.

Although several substances, including lactic acid and glucose can be used as hydrogen-donors for cell growth in the absence of hydrogen, they were not utilized by resting cell suspensions when gaseous hydrogen was available. Glucose (1 %, w/v), peptone (1 %, w/v) and yeast extract (1 %, w/v) had no effect on the rate of sulphate reduction or on the amount of hydrogen absorbed/ion of sulphate. Sodium lactate (0·35 %, w/v) decreased the $-Q_{H_2}^{SO_4}$ slightly but did not affect the total amount of hydrogen taken up.

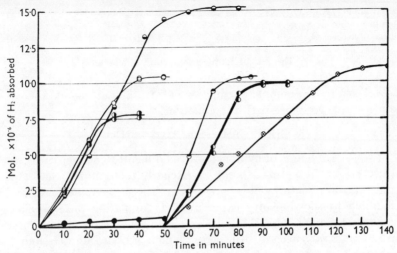

Fig. 3. Hydrogen adsorbed by resting cells of *D. desulphuricans* (Hildenborough) with various substrates.

The curves shown were taken from several experiments and their slopes are not directly comparable. $-Q_{H_2}$ values for the curve are given below. 2·5 μmol. of substrate were added in each test except in the case of sodium tetrathionate, when half this amount was used.

○ Sulphate, Na_2SO_4	210	◐ Dithionite, $Na_2S_2O_4$	220
◑ Sulphite, Na_2SO_3	210	◑ Thiosulphate, $Na_2S_2O_3$	164
◕ Metabisulphite, $K_2S_2O_5$	230	⊗ Tetrathionate, $Na_2S_4O_6$	60

● No added substrate 5·5.

Sulphite. Three mol. hydrogen were taken up/mol. Na_2SO_3 reduced (Fig. 3) and one mol. sulphide was formed (Table 2). For a given suspension, the $-Q_{H_2}^{SO_3}$ was greatest at pH 7·0, but it was only slightly lower at pH 6·3. The $-Q_{H_2}^{SO_3}$ was in general quantitatively similar to the $-Q_{H_2}^{SO_4}$ for the same strain, i.e. about 200 mm³/hr./mg., though on some occasions the sulphite quotient was found to be greater than the sulphate quotient.

Thiosulphate. Four mol. hydrogen were absorbed during the reduction of one mol. Na_2SO_3 (Fig. 3) and two mol. sulphide were formed (Table 4), corresponding to the equation:

$$S_2O_3'' + 4H_2 = S'' + H_2S + 3H_2O \ (or \ 2HS' + 3H_2O).$$

The optimal pH value for thiosulphate reduction was $7 \cdot 0 \pm 0 \cdot 2$, and the $-Q_{H_2}^{S_2O_3''}$ of a given suspension under optimal conditions averaged about 60 % of the $-Q_{H_2}^{SO_4''}$.

Table 4. *Sulphide formed and hydrogen absorbed by resting suspensions of* **D.** desulphuricans (*Hildenborough*) *with various substrates*

Substrate	Amount added (μmol.)	Hydrogen absorbed (μmol.)	Sulphide formed (μmol.)
Sulphate, Na_2SO_4	2·5	9·4 (10)	2·42 (2·5)
Sulphite, Na_2SO_3	2·5	7·3 (7·5)	2·40 (2·5)
Thiosulphate, $Na_2S_2O_3$	2·5	10·0 (10)	5·0 (5)
Tetrathionate, $Na_2S_4O_6$	1·25	11·2 (11·5)	4·82 (5)
Metabisulphite, $K_2S_2O_5$	1·5	8·9 (9)	3·0 (3)
Dithionite, $Na_2S_2O_4$	2·5	10·0 (10)	3·35 (2·5)

Theoretical figures are given in brackets.

Tetrathionate. The complete reduction of tetrathionate should theoretically take place in accordance with the equation:

$$S_4O_6'' + 9H_2 = S'' + 3H_2S + 6H_2O,$$

but the uptake of 9 mol. of hydrogen proved difficult to demonstrate. Indeed, an early report from this laboratory (Report, 1950) stated that 7 mol. of hydrogen/tetrathionate ion were absorbed. This discrepancy was probably attributable to the difficulty experienced in preparing pure specimens of sodium tetrathionate, for a 97 % pure specimen which was obtained later gave hydrogen uptakes in accord with theory: 9 mol. of hydrogen were found to be absorbed/ion of tetrathionate added, and 4 mol. of sulphide were formed (Table 4). Even with this relatively pure specimen of sodium tetrathionate, however, the total hydrogen uptakes varied more than usual and hydrogen uptakes less than theoretical were not uncommon; for example, six parallel tests with the 97 % pure specimen gave hydrogen uptakes of 8·9, 8·45, 8·1, 9·4, 8·5 and 9·0 mol. of hydrogen/tetrathionate ion. The reason for these deviations is not known. The optimal pH for the reduction of tetrathionate was pH 8·2 and the optimal $-Q_{H_2}^{S_4O_6''}$ amounted to only about 30 % of the $-Q_{H_2}^{SO_4''}$.

Dithionite. Four mol. hydrogen were taken up/ion of dithionite added, a result consistent with the view that the ion decomposes primarily to sulphate and sulphur, the first of which is reduced. However, sulphide-formation was consistently in excess of 1 mol. S''/ion S_2O_4'' required by the equation:

$$S_2O_4'' + 4H_2 = S'' + S + 4H_2O$$

though insufficient for the equation:

$$S_2O_4'' + 5H_2 = S'' + H_2S + 4H_2O$$

(see Table 4). Since freshly-prepared solutions of the specimen smelled of H_2S it is possible that the discrepancy was due to sulphide impurities. If this was the case, however, the values obtained for the hydrogen uptake must be regarded as excessive. The question was not studied further since dithionite is most unstable and very difficult to obtain pure.

Metabisulphite. Potassium metabisulphite was reduced straight-forwardly in the Warburg manometer with the uptake of 6 mol. H_2/ion S_2O_5'' and with the formation of 2 mol. sulphide (see Table 4):

$$S_2O_5'' + 6H_2 = 2HS' + 5H_2O.$$

Sulphur. No hydrogen uptake in excess of the blank was detected in the Warburg manometer using 're-precipitated' or re-distilled sulphur (10^{-5} g-atom/flask). Sulphur added as a colloidal sol containing polythionates ($0.0194\% H_2S_5O_6$) showed at first a slow hydrogen uptake ($-Q_{H_2}=20$ mm^3/mg./hr.) in excess of the blank and its ultra-filtrate ($-Q_{H_2}=7$ mm^3/mg./hr.). To see whether this was a genuine reduction of sulphur the flasks were shaken for 16 hr. in all, by which time the $-Q_{H_2}$ in all vessels was almost zero. The total amounts of hydrogen absorbed in the flasks containing sulphur corresponded to reduction of the sulphur present, and proportionate amounts of sulphide were found (Table 5). Traces of sulphide were also found in the flasks containing the ultra-filtrate of colloidal sulphur, and a small amount of hydrogen had been absorbed, but this can reasonably be ascribed to polythionate impurities known to be present in the sulphur sol.

Table 5. *Sulphide formed and hydrogen absorbed by resting suspensions of* D. desulphuricans (*Hildenborough*) *with colloidal sulphur and its ultra-filtrate*

Substrate	Amount added (μmol.)	Hydrogen absorbed (μmol.)	Sulphide formed (μmol.)
Sodium sulphate	2·5	10·1 (10)	2·54 (2·5)
Colloidal sulphur	4·66	5·30 (4·66)	5·05 (4·66)
Ultra-filtrate	*	0·62 (0)	0·203 (0)
No addition	—	0·40 (0)	0 (0)

Theoretical figures given in brackets.

* A volume of ultra-filtrate equivalent to 4·66 μmol. of sulphur in the unfiltered sol was added.

Other compounds. The following compounds were tested and were not reduced by resting cell suspensions: sodium dithionate, sodium formaldehyde sulphoxylate, ammonium perdisulphate, ammonium sulphamate, sodium methanesulphonate, sodium β-hydroxyethanesulphonate, sodium ethylsulphate, and dimethylsulphone. In view of the growth-promoting action of cysteine (Report, 1950; Postgate, 1951), cystine (British Drug Houses Ltd.) was tested in the Warburg manometer but was not reduced.

DISCUSSION

D. desulphuricans strain 'Hildenborough' was able to utilize sulphate, thiosulphate, sulphite and tetrathionate for growth and its resting metabolism.

It was also apparently able to use dithionite and metabisulphite, but it is likely that these compounds decompose spontaneously to sulphate and sulphite respectively before use. The organism was unable to utilize dimethyl-sulphone or several sulphur-containing oxy-acid ions, including two aliphatic and one aromatic sulphonates.

This and other strains of *D. desulphuricans* were unable to utilize elementary sulphur purified by re-distillation, and it is unlikely that this failure to grow was due to an allotropic change in the sulphur during purification since *Th. thio-oxidans* could use it for growth. Nor is it likely that an adaptive change in the bacteria is needed for sulphur utilization, since the four strains tested in autotrophic culture were first grown with impure sulphur—a condition likely to favour such an adaptation. No sign was obtained of growth-inhibitory impurities in the purified sulphur, since the 'blank' growth and hydrogen uptake was not prevented by these preparations. It is, therefore, likely that the activity of some sulphur preparations is due to the presence of oxidation products as impurities, and this view is favoured by the fact that a purified specimen of sulphur regained its activity after prolonged standing in air. In his original work on this subject Baars (1930) used colloidal sulphur prepared by the action of excess H_2S on SO_2, but this method also yields polythionates other than dithionate, which could have been responsible for the activity observed. Baars ensured the absence of sulphate and sulphite in his preparations, but did not check them for polythionates. In the present work, a sulphur sol prepared by a similar method was active, and since its ultra-filtrate was relatively inactive, the effect of the sol was probably not due to polythionates. In Baar's work, the yields of sulphide obtained from colloidal sulphur did not depend on the amounts of sulphur added, but in this work a direct quantitative relationship, between hydrogen absorbed, sulphide formed and colloidal sulphur added was found, which constitutes further evidence for the direct reduction of colloidal sulphur.

D. desulphuricans was able to use tetrathionate in place of sulphate, but unfortunately specimens of pure pentathionate and trithionate were not available for testing. The organism did not use dithionate, a result consistent with the theoretical view that this ion is not of the same structural type as the higher polythionates (Ephraim, 1934).

The mechanism of sulphate reduction. These studies raise some interesting points concerning the mechanism of the reduction of sulphate. The main substances found to be reducible were sulphate, sulphite, thiosulphate, tetra-thionate and colloidal sulphur, dithionite and metabisulphite being of secondary importance since they probably acted by spontaneous decomposition to one of the other ions. It is unlikely that sulphite, thiosulphate or tetrathionate underwent a preliminary decomposition to sulphate since the hydrogen uptakes and sulphide yields corresponded quantitatively to the reduction of the unchanged substrate: a preliminary decomposition would decrease the sulphide yield by formation of inactive sulphur, as may occur in the case of dithionite, and a preliminary oxidation to sulphate would cause considerably increased hydrogen uptakes to be found. Thus there is no doubt that these substances, as well as colloidal sulphur, are directly reduced by the organism, but it does not follow that they are necessarily intermediate in the normal reduction of sulphate. Since the sulphite ion requires three molecules of hydrogen for its reduction, as compared with four hydrogen molecules required by sulphate, the fact that the $-Q_{H_2}$ values were similar with these two compounds implies that the molar rate of sulphite utilization was greater than the molar rate of sulphate utilization by about 33 %. This suggests that sulphite is a normal intermediate in sulphate reduction, and this view is supported by the report (Postgate, 1949) that sulphite will overcome the inhibition of sulphate reduction by sodium selenate in a non-competitive manner. On the other hand, it is unlikely that thiosulphate and tetrathionate are intermediates in the normal reduction process since the specific rates at which these two compounds are reduced are less than those for sulphate and sulphite. These rates have been measured as the $-Q_{H_2}$ values for various substrates, and, whereas the $-Q_{H_2}^{SO_3''}$ and $-Q_{H_2}^{SO_4''}$ were usually similar for a given cell suspension, the $-Q_{H_2}^{S_2O_3''}$ was lower by about 40 % and the $-Q_{H_2}^{S_4O_6''}$ by about 60 %. Similarly, colloidal sulphur is probably not a normal intermediate since the $-Q_{H_2}^{S}$ amounted to only about 10 % of the $-Q_{H_2}^{SO_4''}$. The conclusion that thiosulphate and tetrathionate are not normal intermediates in sulphate-reduction is not surprising on theoretical grounds. Thiosulphate and tetrathionate are both less oxidized than sulphite, so they would presumably come at stages beyond sulphite in a scheme such as:

$$SO_4'' \longrightarrow SO_3'' \longrightarrow \text{——} \longrightarrow S''.$$

But the scheme as written above involves only divalent ions containing one sulphur atom, and for the appearance of ions containing more sulphur atoms a loss of electrons from the system must take place, e.g.:

$$2SO_3'' + 3H_2 = S_2O_3'' + 3H_2O + 2e'.$$

This is a formal oxidation, but is nevertheless not an impossible reaction, and one could picture a series of oxidative polymerizations occurring, coupled with reductions, which would lead to sulphide by way of polythio-ions. However, not only would electrons be continually lost in this process, but a logical result would be the formation of free sulphur or a very complex polythio-ion. Moreover, for the stages which can be represented as:

$$\text{polythio-ion } or \text{ sulphur} \longrightarrow \text{sulphide}$$

a considerable absorption of electrons by the system would be required as the converse of the oxidative polymerization stages.

Given suitable balance of the oxidative and reductive stages, hypotheses on these lines representing the mechanism of sulphate-reduction are not out of the question, but it is simpler to regard the normal process as:

$$SO_4'' \xrightarrow{\ H_2\ } SO_3'' \longrightarrow \left\{ \begin{array}{c} \text{unknown intermediates} \\ \text{containing 1 atom of} \\ \text{S per divalent ion} \end{array} \right\} \longrightarrow S''$$

and to regard the reduction of thiosulphate and tetrathionate as an independent process which would probably be written as:

$$S_4O_6'' \xrightarrow{H_2} S_2O_3'' \longrightarrow \left\{ \begin{array}{l} \text{further reductive} \\ \text{depolymerization} \end{array} \right\} \longrightarrow S''.$$

Even so, there is no evidence from the present work that thiosulphate is an intermediate in tetrathionate reduction, and it is possible that the two compounds are reduced by independent mechanisms.

The author wishes to thank Dr J. M. I. Jones of Crookes Laboratories Ltd. for gifts of standard sulphur sols, Mr W. H. Tomlinson of Oxford for a specimen of 97% sodium tetrathionate, Dr G. A. Maw for specimens of sodium methanesulphonate and β-hydroxyethanesulphonate and Mr H. D. Hollingworth for a specimen of dimethylsulphone. He is also indebted to Miss M. E. Adams for undertaking the work using strains of *D. desulphuricans* cultivated in autotrophic conditions; to Dr S. Jacobs for advice and assistance with the Elford ultrafilter, to Miss J. P. Cowne for preparing a specimen of sodium ethylsulphate and to Mr K. R. Butlin for his interest and advice. This paper is published by permission of the Director, Chemical Research Laboratory.

REFERENCES

Baars, E. K. (1930). *Over Sulphatreductie door Bacteriën*. Dissertation, W. D. Meinema, N.V., Delft, Holland.

Beijerinck, W. M. (1895). Über *Spirillum desulfuricans* als Ursache von Sulfatreduktion. *Zbl. Bakt.* (2 *Abt.*), 1, 1, 49, 104.

Butlin, K. R. & Adams, M. E. (1947). Autotrophic growth of sulphate-reducing bacteria. *Nature, Lond.*, 160, 154.

Butlin, K. R., Adams, M. E. & Thomas, M. (1949a). The morphology of sulphate-reducing bacteria. *J. gen. Microbiol.* 3, iii.

Butlin, K. R., Adams, M. E. & Thomas, M. (1949b). The isolation and cultivation of sulphate-reducing bacteria. *J. gen. Microbiol.* 3, 46.

Delden, A. van (1903). Beitrag zur Kenntnis der Sulphatreduktion durch Bakterien. *Zbl. Bakt.* (2 *Abt.*), 11, 31, 113.

Difco Manual (1948). 8th ed., Difco Laboratories, Detroit, Michigan.

Ephraim, F. (1934). *A Textbook of Inorganic Chemistry.* 2nd ed., London: Gurney & Jackson.

Partington, J. R. (1946). *General and Inorganic Chemistry.* London: MacMillan.

Postgate, J. R. (1949). Inhibition of sulphate-reduction by selenate. *Nature, Lond.*, 164, 670.

Postgate, J. R. (1951). On the nutrition of *D. desulphuricans. J. gen. Microbiol.* 5, 714.

Report (1950). *Chemistry Research*, 1949. H.M. Stationery Office, London.

Starkey, R. L. (1938). A study of spore formation and other morphological characteristics of *Vibrio desulphuricans. Arch. Mikrobiol.* 9, 268.

Stephenson, M. & Stickland, L. (1931). The reduction of sulphate to sulphide by molecular hydrogen. *Biochem. J.* 25, 215.

Subba Rao, M. S. & Sreenivasaya, M. (1947). Rate of reduction of sulphate by *Vibrio desulphuricans*, Konae. *Curr. Sci.* 9, 285.

ZoBell, C. E. & Rittenberg, S. C. (1948). Sulphate-reducing bacteria in marine sediments. *J. marine Res.* 7, 602.

(*Received 3 November* 1950)

32

Reprinted from *Nature,* **205**, 308–309 (1965)

Growth of 'Knallgas' Bacteria (*Hydrogenomonas*) using Direct Electrolysis of the Culture Medium

H. G. Schlegel and R. Lafferty

In view of the recent discussion pertaining to the use of the 'knallgas' bacteria for the regeneration of exhaled air[1–3], we should like to point out that it is possible to produce the oxygen–hydrogen mixture directly in the culture vessel by electrolysis of the mineral medium. Since the 'knallgas' bacteria of the *Pseudomonas* type (*Hydrogenomonas* strains *H* 16 and *H* 20) grow in chloride-free medium, oxygen and hydrogen can be produced in such a medium without interfering with side-effects using platinum electrodes with a relatively large surface area. Carbon dioxide is led directly into the culture vessel and removes excess oxygen. By using currents between 0·1 and 1·2 amp and at voltages not exceeding 5·3–5·5 V, good growth is achieved[1,4]. At low current-levels, growth is proportional to, and limited by, the hydrogen produced.

During growth, hydrogen, oxygen and carbon dioxide are consumed in the ratio of 8 : 3 : 1. Bacteria grown under these conditions can withstand a very high partial pressure of oxygen and contain very little reserve material (poly-β-

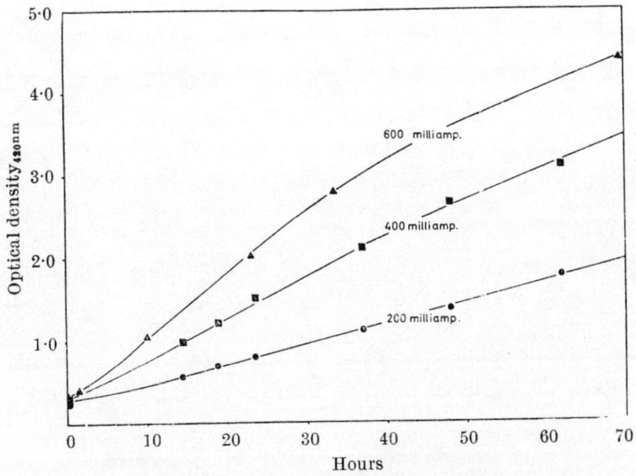

Fig. 1. Growth of *Hydrogenomonas* strain *H* 16 using electrolysis of culture medium for production of hydrogen and oxygen. Mineral medium (1 l.) was contained in a 2-l. culture vessel whose contents were magnetically stirred. Hydrogen and oxygen were produced using 2 platinum electrodes, each 16 cm², at currents of 200, 400 and 600 m.amp. Turbidity of the cell suspension properly diluted (ext. < 0·3) was measured at 420 nm with 1-cm cuvettes (Zeiss Elko III)

hydroxybutyric acid). Since hydrogen and oxygen are directly produced and consumed in the culture vessel, the electrolysis-culture method is simpler and less dangerous than other methods for the autotrophic growth of 'knallgas' bacteria. This method offers a number of distinct advantages for automatic continuous cultures.

This work was supported by funds from the Deutsche Forschungsgemeinschaft.

H. G. SCHLEGEL
R. LAFFERTY

Institut für Mikrobiologie,
Universität Göttingen,
Germany.

[1] Schlegel, H. G., *Raumfahrtforschung*, **8**, 65 (1964).
[2] Bongers, L. H., *Aerospace Med.*, **35**, 139 (1964).
[3] Chapman, D. D., Meyer, R., and Proctor, C. M., *Develop. Indust. Microbiol.*, **4**, 343 (1963).
[4] Schlegel, H. G., and Lafferty, R., *Zbl. Bakt.*, II Abt.,**118**, 483 (1964).

Printed in Great Britain by Fisher, Knight & Co., Ltd., St. Albans.

Editor's Comments on Paper 33

33 **Lipmann:** Biological Sulfate Activation and Transfer
   Science, **128,** 575–580 (1958)

The discovery of the first cytochrome (cyt. c_3) in any anaerobic microorganism (Postgate, 1956), as well as the establishment of adenosine 5-phosphosulfate (APS) as an intermediate in sulfate reduction (Paper 33) and thiosulfate oxidation (Peck, 1960), were milestones in the elucidation of the biochemistry of inorganic sulfur metabolism. The following paper was chosen because of its detailed description of the mechanism of group activation and its role in biosynthesis.

Biological Sulfate Activation and Transfer

Studies on a mechanism of group activation
and its role in biosynthesis are described.

Fritz Lipmann

Sulfate is bound, mostly in ester linkage, in a fairly large variety of compounds present rather commonly in living organisms. Of most importance among these compounds are the sulfated mucopolysaccharides, such as chondroitin sulfuric acid, the ground substance of cartilage, and the similar mucoitin-sulfuric acid in mucosous tissues. Heparin belongs in this group; it is outstanding for its high sulfate, partially bound here to the amino group of

the glucosamine moiety. Furthermore, a sulfurylated cerebroside is present in the brain and other tissues. On the other hand, conjugation with sulfate is a means of phenol detoxication in the animal body. This sulfate conjugation of the phenols, mainly in liver and the intestine, has been used for many years for the study of the mechanism of sulfate transfer.

With such a large number of metabolically-formed sulfurylated substances, it

appeared likely that there was a common metabolic carrier for activated sulfate which would serve as general sulfate donor in the enzymatic set-up of cells. This was all the more indicated when DeMeio (*1*), who pioneered in the field of sulfate activation, demonstrated that, in cell-free systems, ATP (*2*) could serve as the source of energy for sulfate activation. The kind of mechanism that occurs in sulfate activation was further clarified by Bernstein and McGilvery (*3*). All this work with the liver system indicated strongly that conjugation with phenol was a two-phasic process, the activation of sulfate being the primary, the transfer to phenol being a secondary and separate, step.

Since, therefore, in the process of activation the energy of a phosphoanhydride link of ATP

$$R \cdot O \cdot \overset{\overset{\displaystyle O}{\uparrow}}{\underset{\displaystyle O^-}{P}} \cdot O \cdot \overset{\overset{\displaystyle O}{\uparrow}}{\underset{\displaystyle O^-}{P}} \cdot O \cdot \overset{\overset{\displaystyle O}{\uparrow}}{\underset{\displaystyle O^-}{P}} \cdot O^- \quad (1)$$

apparently was transmitted to the sulfate, it seemed likely that the formation

Dr. Lipmann is a member of the staff of the Rockefeller Institute for Medical Research, New York, N.Y.

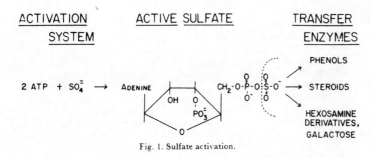

ACTIVATION SYSTEM   ACTIVE SULFATE   TRANSFER ENZYMES

2 ATP + SO$_4^=$ → ADENINE ... CH$_2$-O-P-O-S-O- →

→ PHENOLS

→ STEROIDS

→ HEXOSAMINE DERIVATIVES, GALACTOSE

Fig. 1. Sulfate activation.

of a *mixed* anhydride between sulfate and phosphate,

$$R \cdot O \cdot \overset{O}{\underset{O^-}{\overset{\uparrow}{P}}} \cdot O \cdot \overset{O}{\underset{O}{\overset{\uparrow}{S}}} \cdot O^- \qquad (2)$$

might represent this process of activation. However, no information about the chemistry of such a mixed anhydride was found in the literature. Pyrosulfates are well-known compounds,

$$^-O \cdot \overset{O}{\underset{O}{\overset{\uparrow}{S}}} \cdot O \cdot \overset{O}{\underset{O}{\overset{\uparrow}{S}}} \cdot O^- \qquad (3)$$

but they are very sensitive to water and are apparently about as unstable as organic acid anhydrides. For all these reasons, sulfate activation presented a rather special problem in group activation which seemed most attractive to me, and my co-workers and I decided, some three years ago, to try our hand at clearing up the chemistry of this intriguing reaction.

It will be helpful to start with the scheme in Fig. 1, which gives the essentials of the activation-transfer process as

Table 1. Active sulfate fraction, analytical data. Adenosine was determined by absorption at 260 mμ, ribose by the Orcinol procedure, and phosphate, by the method of Fiske and Subbarow. Total phosphate was determined by hydrolysis in $1N$ HCl acid. The 12- and 30-minute phosphate was determined by hydrolysis in $1N$ HCl at 100°C. Phosphate hydrolyzable by the 3'-nucleotidase was determined by the method of Kaplan (21).

Component	Amount
Adenosine	1
Ribose	0.95
Phosphate, total	1.98
Phosphate, 12-minute	0.53
Phosphate, 30-minute	1.04
Phosphate, 3'-nucleotidase	0.85
Sulfate, enzymatic	0.2–0.85

we were able to develop it. What I want to stress particularly is the strict separation between the activation process and the transfer reactions. The active sulfate is formed, as we now know and will explain in detail later, by a reaction between sulfate and two ATP's (4, 5), as a result of which adenosine-3'-phosphate-5'-phosphosulfate is formed. This appears to be the general sulfate donor in biological reactions, which, as suspected, carries sulfate in the form of a mixed anhydride. We have found this to be a sulfate donor in all cases studied so far —that is, in chondroitin sulfate and sulfatide synthesis, in steroid, and in phenol sulfurylation. Sulfate transfer from the activated sulfate to acceptors such as phenols, hydroxy steroids, and the hydroxy group of various compounds, and also probably amino groups, is catalyzed by enzymes which we call sulfokinases and which are more or less specific for the acceptor molecule.

This may serve as a general orientation. Now I want to discuss in detail, first, the isolation and identification of active sulfate and the enzymatic mechanism of its formation, carried out by Phillips W. Robbins (4–6). Then, second, I will discuss a number of sulfate acceptor reactions which have been and are being studied at the Rockefeller Institute for Medical Research by John D. Gregory, Yoshitsugu Nose, Furio D'Abramo, and Irving H. Goldberg.

Isolation and Identification of Active Sulfate

Helmuth Hilz, with whom this venture was started, found (7) that the reaction between ATP and sulfate appeared to yield pyrophosphate, and, using paper electrophoresis, he could show that the compound formed contained adenylic acid. This preliminary identification was carried out by the use of radioactive sulfate. In analogy to

other activation reactions, in particular to the recent studies on acetate activation, we tentatively thought of sulfate activation as a reaction between ATP and sulfate which, through a substitution of the terminal pyrophosphoryl group in ATP, led to the suspected anhydride between sulfate and substituted phosphate. However, some of the data did not fit with this interpretation, and at that stage we cautiously reported that our observations had yielded evidence for the formation of an adenyl sulfate derivative, of the exact structure of which we were not sure.

As is often the case in studies of an unknown "active" compound, especially a substance of which no chemical analog has been known before, we expected the compound to be very unstable. It had appeared, indeed, in these preliminary experiments that "active" sulfate was quite unstable to strong acid. To get a step further, it was necessary to clean up the enzymes and concentrate the sulfate activation system for use in medium-scale preparative runs (6); thus, Robbins succeeded in preparing 50-μmole samples of active sulfate from ATP and sulfate, and tried Dowex chromatography. Fortunately, it appeared that the phosphosulfate link was more stable to acid than had been expected; it is perfectly stable at neutral, or higher, pH, and it tolerated chromatography with rather concentrated formic acid in the cold. Active sulfate is strongly bound by Dowex-1, and it was possible to remove from the column all other adenine derivatives by treatment with $4N$ formic acid–0.3M ammonium formate. Then $5N$ formic acid–1M ammonium formate eluted the remaining active sulfate, and in this manner a rather homogenous fraction of active sulfate was obtained. During concentration of this fraction by lyophilization, however, part of the sul-

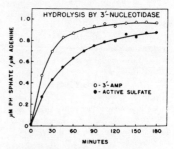

Fig. 2. Hydrolysis curve for active sulfate with 3'-nucleotidase compared to that for 3'-adenylic acid.

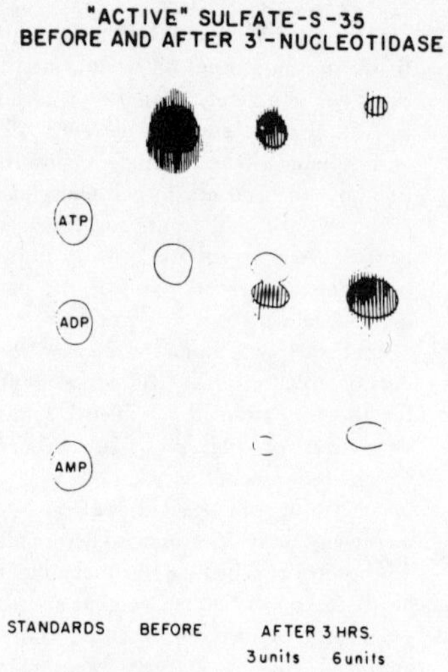

STANDARDS   BEFORE   AFTER 3 HRS.
                        3 units   6 units

Fig. 3. Radioautogram of paper electrogram in citrate buffer of pH 5.9. Encircled areas are ultraviolet quenching; shaded and black areas are radioautogram tracings (see Fig. 6 in 6).

fate was split off. The analysis of such a fraction is shown in Table 1.

It appeared from these data that the compound, to our surprise, contained two phosphates per adenine, and pentose. One phosphate was acid-stable, and the other one was unstable to heating with $1N$ HCl, but not as much so as would have been expected for a pyrophosphate link. The hydrolysis with acid rather suggested a 2'- or 3'-adenylic acid, particularly since the compound did not give the periodate reaction commonly obtained with adenosine-5'-phosphates. For further identification, Kaplan's 3'-nucleotidase was used. This enzyme liberated practically a full equivalent of phosphate from our "active" sulfate.

The active sulfate in all these cases was conveniently determined by enzymatic transfer to nitrophenol, the anion color of which disappears on conjugation.

As has been mentioned, during lyophilization part of the sulfate was split off, and this explains why the figures for sulfate in Table 1 vary between rather wide limits. Smaller batches, which could be lyophilized quickly, showed near equivalence between sulfate and adenosine. On the other hand, the sulfate-free residue gave ratios with regard to phosphate identical with those of active sulfate. In Fig. 2 the hydrolysis curve for active sulfate with 3'-nucleo-

tidase is compared with that for 3'-adenylic acid. Hydrolysis is slower for the active sulfate than for the monophosphate; in general, the 3'-adenylic acid is the substrate most rapidly hydrolyzed by this enzyme, while additional substitutes slow down reactivity.

The position of the sulfate in the molecule was largely identified by the use of radioactive sulfate. If a mixture of active sulfate and sulfate-free residue is exposed to the 3'-nucleotidase, the sulfate remains with adenylic acid, as is shown in the paper electrophoresis pattern of Fig. 3 by the overlap of ultraviolet quenching and radiotracing. If incubated with a sufficient amount of nucleotidase, the upper spot of PAPS disappears almost completely and a new spot appears instead, which could be identified as adenosine-5'-phosphosulfate (APS). On the other hand, a lower spot appears which is adenosine-5'-phosphate (AMP), derived by hydrolysis of PAP, the sulfate-free residue. The adenosine-5'-phosphosulfate could be identified by comparison with synthetic compound, prepared according to the method of Baddiley et al. (8). The structure and some of the properties of the active sulfate are explained in Fig. 4, where it may be seen that the phosphosulfate link is rather sensitive to hydrochloric acid; $0.1N$ HCl split the sulfate completely off in about half an hour at 37°C. These compounds have an ultraviolet absorption indistinguishable from that of adenylic acid. This excludes any possibility of sulfate being linked to the amino

group of adenine, since blocking of this amino group in all cases causes a shift of the ultraviolet absorption toward the visible.

For further identification, we argued that hydrolysis of the phosphosulfate link should liberate a secondary phosphate. This was shown to be the case by means of electrotitration between pH 5 and 8 before and after hydrolysis. All this evidence makes us feel sure that we are dealing with a compound of the constitution shown in the figures. This constitution has now been confirmed through synthesis by Baddiley et al. (9).

Two Enzymatic Steps in Biosynthesis of Active Sulfate

The unexpected appearance of two separately linked phosphates in the active sulfate, as now identified, indicated right away a two-phasic synthesis as likely. Initially, we had speculated (7) on the possibility of adenosine-5'-phosphosulfate being active sulfate, formed by pyrophosphate substitution on ATP. It now appeared that this reaction was the first step in the sequence shown in Fig. 5. This was completed by a second reaction, of phosphokinase type, whereby the terminal phosphate of a second ATP was transferred to the 3'-position of APS. The initial reaction is catalyzed by an enzyme which we call sulfurylase. It catalyses the attack of one of the oxygens of sulfate on the proximal phosphorus in adenosine-5'-triphosphate with

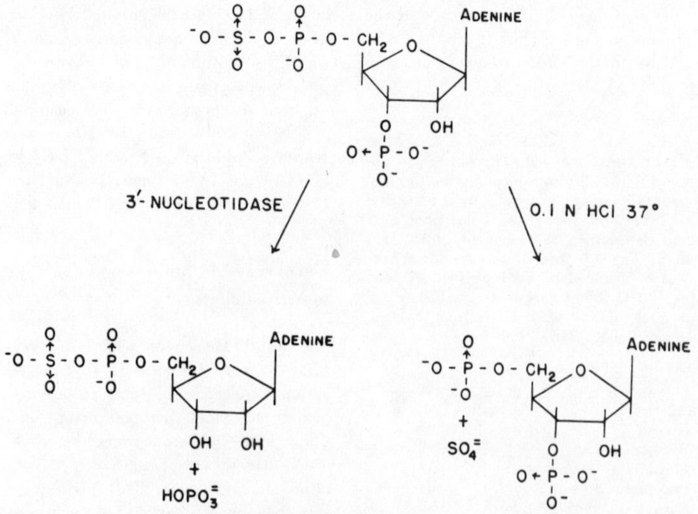

Fig. 4. Active sulfate and hydrolysis products.

the displacement of pyrophosphate by sulfate. The APS, thus formed initially, in *entirely inactive* as a sulfate donor in enzymatic reactions.

It is important to realize that the reaction as written is actually much more favored energetically in the backward direction; in other words, the sulfuryl potential in APS is considerably higher than the pyrophosphoryl potential in ATP. We believe that this energetic situation is the reason for the further phosphorylation. In this manner, the energy of a second energy-rich phosphate is used to force the reaction into the forward direction by a "masking" of the reaction product through 3'-phosphorylation. The over-all energy balance, even then, is not too favorable, and the rather energy-rich phosphosulfate bond becomes still further stabilized through removal of the initial reaction product, pyrophosphate, by the quite ubiquitous pyrophosphatase.

In proving this mechanism, the independent work of Bandurski et al. (10) has been rather important. These workers found that the sulfate activation sys-

tem in yeast could be separated into two inactive fractions, active only after recombination. When Bandurski's work came to our attention, we turned to the yeast system for elaboration of the mechanism, as it appeared preferable to the liver system we had used so far. Confirming Bandurski, we were able to separate from yeast two fractions, which were identified with (i) sulfurylase, and (ii) APS-kinase.

Sulfurylase was measured, as is indicated in Table 2, in the reverse direction by means of synthetic APS. Sulfurylase from yeast could be rather highly purified by electrophoresis on Geon 426, as is shown in Fig. 6. With this purified enzyme, equilibrium studies were made which showed that, as seen in Fig. 7, a small but definite amount of APS was formed in the forward direction. The equilibrium constant for the reaction

$$ATP + S \rightleftharpoons APS + PP$$

at pH 8 is approximately 10^{-8}, and therefore $\Delta F°$ equals 11,000 cal. But APS was found to have a high affinity to APS-kinase, giving, indeed, the highest re-

action rate at the lowest measurable concentration, $5.10^{-6}M$. The amounts formed enzymatically are, under "physiological" conditions, probably of similar magnitude, and therefore the little that is formed can thus immediately be phosphorylated by APS-phosphokinase and can thereby be eliminated from equilibrium. This drives the reaction in the direction of synthesis of PAPS, helped by pyrophosphatase, removing pyrophosphate, the other product of sulfurylase reaction. There are interesting general implications in this use of two or more energy-rich phosphates for the fixation of bonds of higher group potential, such as the phosphosulfate bond, the additional energy serving to pull an initially-formed, thermodynamically very unstable compound over the energy hump:

$$ATP + S \xleftarrow{\text{sulfurylase}} APS + PP \qquad \Delta F°, +11{,}000 \quad (4)$$

$$PP \xrightarrow{\text{PP-ase}} 2P \qquad \Delta F°, -5{,}000 \quad (5)$$

$$APS + ATP \xrightarrow{\text{APS-kinase}}$$
$$PAPS + ADP + H^+ \quad \Delta F°, -6{,}000 \quad (6)$$

$$2ATP + S \rightarrow PAPS + 2P + ADP$$
$$\text{over-all} \quad \Delta F°, \qquad 0 \quad (7)$$

The energy data are rough approximations, to give an impression of the over-all $\Delta F°$, which, taking into account the formation, at pH 8, of H$^+$ as calculated for hexokinase in (11), just about balances.

Transfer of Active Sulfate to Various Acceptors

With the solution of the problem of sulfate activation, the way had been opened to approach more intelligently the metabolic utilization of sulfate. This, in a sense, forced us to enter metabolic territory rather foreign to the experience of workers in our laboratory—some steroid metabolism but, more seriously, polysaccharide synthesis and lately some lipid chemistry. Generally, in these experiments, isolated PAPS was not used, but rather PAPS was fed in by way of an enriched enzymatic generating system from yeast (5) or liver (6). For confirmation, the various acceptor reactions were then checked with isolated PAPS.

Except in the case of phenol and steroid conjugation, we are still in the more exploratory phase, using almost exclusively S^{35} as a guide. We have made available cell-free preparations from embryonic cartilage for synthesis of chon-

Table 2. Separation of yeast enzymes. National Bakers yeast was used, and extracts were prepared essentially according to the method of Jones *et al.* (22). The formation of ATP from APS was measured by following pyrophosphate disappearance or by measuring ATP formation with hexokinase and glucose-6-phosphate dehydrogenase. Formation of PAPS was followed by transfer to nitrophenol or by PAP assay. The PAP assay depends on the catalytic activity of PAP in the transfer of sulfate from *p*-nitrophenol to phenol. The rate of nitrophenol formation is measured at 400 mμ in the Beckman DU spectrophotometer. The reaction between APS and P was routinely followed by measuring the disappearance of P with chromatographic checks on ADP formation.

Fraction	ATP-sulfurylase (APS + PP → ATP) – PP, (μmole/mg hr)	APS-kinase (APS + ATP → PAPS) PAPS, (μmole/mg hr)
Dialyzed extract, I	2.1	
NaCl precipitate, II	10.1	0.55
17–23 percent EtOH, III	22.1	3.5
pH 5.4 precipitate, IVa	85.0	0.6
Supernatant + 10 percent EtOH, IVb	0.5	4.1
40–50 percent (NH$_4$)$_2$SO$_4$, V	0	12.5

Table 3. Sulfate transfer from PAPS^{35} to chondroitin sulfate. The enzyme preparation, prepared from three chick embryos, as in the previous experiments, was extracted with 6.5 ml of saline-phosphate solution and centrifuged. The supernatant was mixed with 0.25 ml of PAPS^{35}, and 1 ml was immediately heated (zero time). Each tube contained 1 ml of enzyme in a 1.35-ml total and 15,000 counts. Precipitation was with sodium acetate and 3 vol of alcohol; there were 10 washings with 80 percent alcohol.

Incubation (37°C) (hr)	PAPS^{35}	ATP 1 μmole	UTP 1 μmole	Count/min	Δ	Incorporation (%)
0	+	–	–	80		
2	+	–	–	340	260	1.7
2	+	+	–	600	520	3.4
2	+	–	+	670	590	4
2	+	+	+	550	470	3

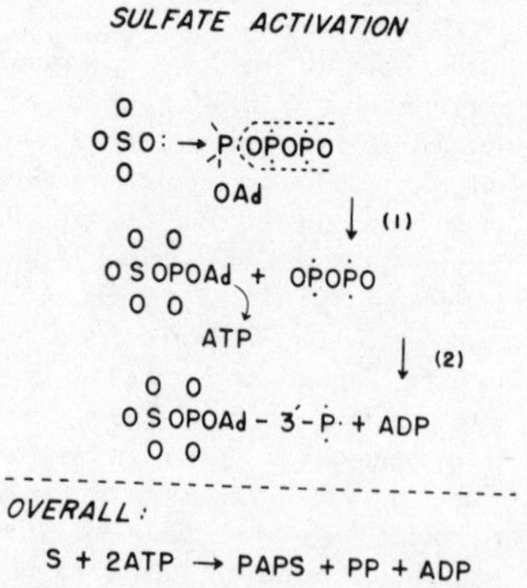

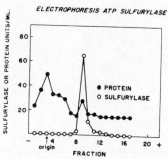

OVERALL :

S + 2ATP → PAPS + PP + ADP

Fig. 5. Reaction 1: the displacement by sulfate of pyrophosphate in ATP, yielding APS, is catalyzed by sulfurylase. Reaction 2: the phosphorylation of APS by the terminal phosphate of ATP is catalyzed by APS-phosphokinase.

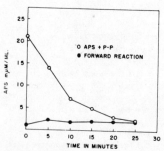

Fig. 6. Electrophoresis in a Geon 426 (Goodrich) bed (see Fig. 8).

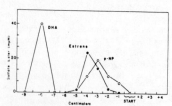

Fig. 7. Equilibrium experiment; ATP-sulfurylase.

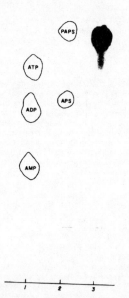

Fig. 8. Electrophoresis of rat enzymes in a Geon 426 (Goodrich) bed.

droitin sulfate, and from rat liver and brain for synthesis of sulfatide, but many needed details are still missing.

For orientation, I would like to refer once more to Fig. 1, in which it may be seen that, after resolving the left and middle part of the scheme, which concerns the generation of active sulfate, we now move into the nearly virgin territory of sulfate utilization outlined in the right-hand part of the figure.

Conjugation of Steroids and Phenols

This reaction has been studied by De-Meio (12), and by Roy in England (13), and we have used the latter's method for the estimation of sulfurylated steroids. Y. Nose, from the University of Kyoto, has worked in my laboratory on the separation of the enzymes responsible for the conjugation of phenols and polycyclic acceptors, using mainly electrophoresis of a prepurified liver preparation. It may be seen in Fig. 8 (14) that by this means three enzyme fractions were obtained, one for dihydroandrosterone and other 3′-β-OH steroids. Another enzyme conjugates with estrone and is different from ordinary phenol-sulfokinase. The last-named, however, seems to accept sulfate relatively unspecifically on a great variety of variously substituted phenols, as elaborated in greater detail by John D. Gregory (15). The dihydroandrosterone sulfokinase also reacts with isoandrosterone and with progesterone, all having a 3′-β-hydroxyl. It therefore appears to be a 3′-β-hydroxy-steroid sulfokinase.

It should be mentioned that in nitrophenyl sulfate, the sulfate group was shown by John Gregory (15) to be of a group potential only less than 2000 calories below that of PAPS; a PAP-mediated sulfate transfer from nitrophenol to phenol has been studied with phenol-sulfokinase. Nitrophenyl sulfate was also shown, by Egami and his collaborators (16), to act as sulfate donor in a sulfatase-catalyzed, PAP-independent reaction, which reminds one of the rather outstanding activity of nitrophenyl phosphate for donating phosphate unspecifically with phosphatase (17).

Synthesis of Chondroitin Sulfate

The structure of chondroitin sulfate is presented in Fig. 9, for orientation. After unsuccessfully trying various cartilage preparations, which had been shown by other workers to incorporate radioactive sulfate in chondroitin sulfate in in vivo or in slice experiments, we turned to embryonic cartilage from 15-day-old chick embryos, which yielded rather active nonparticulate extracts. Figure 10 shows that active sulfate was formed in such an extract, together with small amounts of the precursor APS; in this experiment, the charcoal absorbate of the incubate was eluted with pyridine and then put on the paper for electrophoresis.

Chondroitin sulfuric acid was isolated by the usual methods of precipitating

Chondroitin
sulfate A or C

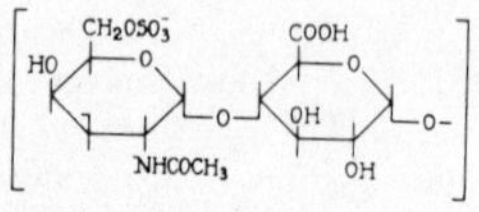

Fig. 9. Repeating unit of chondroitin sulfate.

Fig. 10. Radioautogram of paper electrogram from $SO_4^{35=}$ incubated cartilage extract. Cartilages from two embryos were homogenized in 3 ml of saline phosphate to which 12 μmole of Mg^{++}, 10 μmole of Na-ATP, 1.5 μmole of UTP, 2 μmole of glutamine, 2.7 ml of enzyme, and 2 ml of $SO_4^{35=}$ (100 μc, carrier-free) were added; the total volume was 5.3. The mixture was incubated for 2 hours at 37°C. Markers electrographed on the same paper strip are identified in radioautograms Nos. 1 and 2 by ultraviolet quenching, as indicated by encircling lines. Number 3 represents the radioautogram of paper electrogram in citrate buffer (pH 5.9) of the pyridine eluate from a charcoal adsorbate of incubate.

579

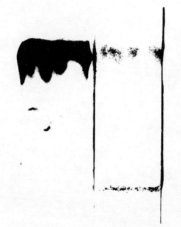

Fig. 11. Comparison between radioautogram and toluidine blue staining of the paper electrogram of chondroitin sulfuric acid obtained from extracts of chick embryo cartilage incubated with S³²-sulfate. The toluidine blue color (right) did not photograph as well as the radioautogram (left). Nevertheless, the analogous outline of the tracings made by the two methods appears clear.

from acetate-containing solution either with alcohol or with cetyltrimethylammonium salt. Radioactive sulfate and other compounds were removed by appropriate washing. Figure 11 shows that radioactivity overlapped exactly with the chondroitin sulfuric acid; a phosphate buffer medium was used for paper electrophoresis and toluidine blue, for the spotting of the chondroitin sulfate. Tables 3 and 4 (from *18*) show some preliminary studies on the mechanism of this reaction. It may be seen in Table 3 that the sulfate of PAPS³⁵ was transferred to chondroitin sulfate. An indication of a participation of uridylic acid

in the synthesis may be seen in the slightly better activation, in this case, when UTP was used instead of ATP. In other experiments, however, UTP was often inhibitory. Table 4 shows that with these extracts, ATP and magnesium were necessary for chondroitin sulfate synthesis from inorganic sulfate. This was also true if isolated PAPS was used, confirming the *de novo* synthesis of polysaccharide. Further evidence for *de novo* synthesis of chondroitin sulfate in these extracts was obtained by showing incorporation of radioactive acetate.

A great deal remains to be done. The polysaccharide field is a vast area of chemistry, and I have to confess that it is not our intention to become polysaccharide chemists. However, we will try to stay with this type of reaction for a little while, since it has been forced on us through our progress with sulfate activation. For similar reasons, we ventured also into the equally complex field of lipid synthesis. Irving Goldberg is studying in vitro incorporation of sulfate into lipid fractions. He has obtained preliminary evidence of a formation in liver extracts and brain homogenates of a sulfatide similar to Blix's cerebroside sulfate (*19*), shown in Fig. 12. This problem seemed attractive to me mainly because we might, from present experience, anticipate here a direct transfer of a galactose sulfate derivative to ceramide. This would present a simpler metabolic sequence than chondroitin sulfate synthesis, which is complicated by the polymerization problem. That, however, makes the latter all the more challenging.

Finally, I would like once more to underline the fact that we are dealing, in the area of sulfate transfer, with a process in which a central activated

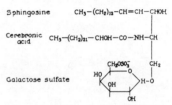

Fig. 12. The structure of cerebroside sulfate according to Blix (*19*).

molecule is first elaborated. This carries the sulfate in activated form, and from there, sulfate is picked up by quite a large number of separate acceptor enzymes which we call sulfokinases. This is a repetition of a rather general scheme in biosynthesis. It has been well defined in the case of acetyl activation and transfer (*20*) and, of course, with phosphate activation and transfer, and it seems to apply in many other cases of group transfer.

References and Notes

1. R. H. DeMeio, M. Wizerkaniuk, E. Fabriani, *J. Biol. Chem.* 203, 257 (1953).
2. The following abbreviations have been used in this article: ADP, adenosinediphosphate; AMP, adenosine monophosphate; APS, adenosine-5'-phosphosulfate; ATP, adenosine triphosphate; CoA, coenzyme A; P, inorganic phosphate; PAP, 3',5'-diphosphate; PAPS, adenosine-3'-phosphate-5'-phosphosulfate (active sulfate); PP, pyrophosphate; S, sulfate; UTP, uridine triphosphate.
3. S. Bernstein and R. W. McGilvery, *J. Biol. Chem.* 199, 745 (1952).
4. P. W. Robbins and F. Lipmann, *J. Am. Chem. Soc.* 78, 2652 (1956).
5. ——, *ibid.* 78, 6409 (1956).
6. ——, *J. Biol. Chem.* 229, 837 (1957).
7. H. Hilz and F. Lipmann, *Proc. Natl. Acad Sci. U.S.* 41, 880 (1955).
8. J. Baddiley, J. G. Buchanan, R. Letters, *J. Chem. Soc.* 1957, 1067 (1957).
9. ——, *Proc. Chem. Soc. (London)* 1957, 147 (1957).
10. L. G. Wilson and R. S. Bandurski, *Arch. Biochem. Biophys.* 62, 503 (1956); R. S. Bandurski, L. G. Wilson, C. L. Squires, *J. Am Chem. Soc.* 78, 6408 (1956).
11. E. A. Robbins and P. D. Boyer, *J. Biol Chem.* 224, 121 (1957).
12. R. H. DeMeio, M. Wizerkaniuk, I. Schreibman, *ibid.* 213, 439 (1955).
13. A. B. Roy, *Biochem. J.* 63, 294 (1956).
14. Y. Nose and F. Lipmann, in preparation.
15. J. D. Gregory and F. Lipmann, *J. Biol. Chem.* 229, 1081 (1957).
16. S. Suzuki, N. Takahashi, F. Egami, *Biochim. et Biophys. Acta* 24, 444 (1957).
17. B. Axelrod, *Advances in Enzymol.* 17, 159 (1956).
18. F. D'Abramo and F. Lipmann, *Biochim. et Biophys. Acta* 25, 211 (1957).
19. G. Blix, *Z. physiol. Chem. Hoppe-Seyler's* 219, 82 (1933).
20. F. Lipmann, *Science* 120, 855 (1954); ——, in *Metabolism of the Nervous System*, D. Richter, Ed. (Pergamon, London, 1957), p. 329.
21. T. P. Wang, L. Shuster, N. O. Kaplan, *J. Biol. Chem.* 206, 299 (1954). We are indebted to Dr. Kaplan for a sample of 3'-nucleotidase.
22. M. E. Jones *et al.*, *Biochim et Biophys. Acta* 12, 141 (1953).

Table 4. Incorporation of S³⁵O₄⁼ into chondroitin sulfate. Condyles from tibias and femurs of three chick embryos were broken up in deep-freeze-cooled mortar with quartz sand, with 6 ml of saline and 0.01M phosphate (pH 7.4), and centrifuged at 6000g (International centrifuge) for 10 minutes. The supernatant was mixed with 1.2 ml of carrier-free S³⁵O₄⁼ (60 μc). There was 1 ml of enzyme-S³⁵ mixture in each sample; final volume was 1.35 ml.

Sample No.	Incu-bation (37°C) (hr)	ATP 5 μmole	Mg 6 μmole	Gluta-mine 1 μmole	UTP 1 μmole	Counts/ min	%
1	0	–	–	–	–	60	
2	2	–	–	–	–	60	
3	2	–	–	–	–	405	
4	2	–	+	–	–	4760	0.6
5	2	–	+	+	–	5390	0.7
6	2	–	+	+	–	2007	0.28

IV
Aromatic Carbon Metabolism

Editor's Comments on Papers 34 and 35

34 Stanier: Simultaneous Adaptation: A New Technique for the Study of Metabolic Pathways
J. Bacteriol., **54**, 339–348 (1947)

35 Stanier and Hayaishi: The Bacterial Oxidation of Tryptophan: A Study in Comparative Biochemistry
Science, **114**, 326–330 (1951)

The beginning of research on aromatic carbon metabolism goes back to Kaserer (1906), who demonstrated for the first time the utilization of methane by mixed cultures of soil bacteria. These investigations were continued by Söhngen (1906), who noted the disappearance of methane with increased growth and carbon dioxide production, and who isolated *Bacillus methanicus* (*Methanomonas methanica*) from enrichment cultures. Söhngen (1913) also showed that paraffin was more readily attacked by 17 different species of soil bacteria than were petroleum ether, paraffin oil, and crude petroleum. Microbial assimilation of aromatic hydrocarbon was first reported by Störmer (1908), who isolated *Bacillus hexacarbovorum* and organisms capable of utilizing toluene and xylene.

The discovery and development of the method of simultaneous adaptation (Paper 34) made it possible to study the course of any microbial metabolic process that is under adaptive enzymatic control. One example of such studies has been selected (Paper 35) to demonstrate how different pathways may occur for the same substrate. The oxidation of tryptophan and mandelic acid merge at the catechol level.

Reprinted from *J. Bacteriol.*, **54**, 339–348 (1947)

SIMULTANEOUS ADAPTATION: A NEW TECHNIQUE FOR THE STUDY OF METABOLIC PATHWAYS

R. Y. STANIER[1]

Department of Bacteriology, Indiana University, Bloomington, Indiana

Received for publication May 21, 1947

During work on the oxidation of aromatic substances by *Pseudomonas fluorescens*, a useful technique for the elucidation of metabolic pathways by the analysis of adaptive behavior was discovered. Since it could undoubtedly be applied to many other microbial dissimilations, a brief account of its principles and applications seems merited.

METHODS

Adaptation was determined manometrically, by following the oxygen uptake after addition of the substrate to a cell suspension in the Warburg apparatus. All experiments were conducted at 30 C in an atmosphere of air, using 2.0 ml of cell suspension and 0.2 ml of 0.01 M substrate.

One strain of *Pseudomonas fluorescens* (str. A. 3.12) was used throughout. The cells were grown on agar plates at 30 C and harvested after 20 to 45 hours by suspension in M/60 phosphate buffer (pH 7.0). After centrifugation they were resuspended in the same buffer mixture. The mineral media employed for cultivation of specifically adapted cells had the following composition: specific carbon source, 0.1 to 0.25 per cent; NH_4NO_3, 0.1 per cent; K_2HPO_4, 0.1 per cent; $MgSO_4$, 0.05 per cent; and agar, 1.5 per cent; pH 7.0 to 7.2.

The precision and sensitivity of the manometric technique make it ideal for studying adaptation to nonvolatile compounds, but complications arise when such substances as benzaldehyde are tested. Even in 0.01 M solution, the vapor pressure of benzaldehyde is sufficiently high at 30 C to cause a marked distillation from the side arm into the main compartment of the Warburg vessel, and adaptation consequently begins before the contents of the side arm are added to the cell suspension. Even when the period of thermal equilibration is held to a minimum, the effect is noticeable, showing up as an apparently more rapid adaptation to benzaldehyde than to nonvolatile substrates. Hence the results with this substance cannot be strictly compared to those obtained with the remaining aromatic compounds investigated.

THEORY

If we accept the well-tested Kluyverian axiom (Kluyver, 1931) that every dissimilation is the result of a series of simple, chemically intelligible step-reactions, it follows that the complete oxidation of even a relatively small organic molecule will involve the formation of a large number of intermediate compounds. In the case of microorganisms, the further probability exists that at least some

---

[1] Present address: Department of Bacteriology, University of California, Berkeley, California.

of these intermediates will be attacked by adaptive enzymes. On the general theory of enzymatic adaptivity (cf. Karström, 1937), cells adapted to attack the primary substrate should be adapted simultaneously to attack all the intermediates formed during the oxidation of that substrate, but not to attack other substances the dissimilation of which is brought about by adaptive enzymes that fail to participate in the over-all dissimilatory process in question. Thus by growing cells on the primary substrate or on assumed intermediates and then testing for adaptation to a variety of related substances, one should be able to to obtain convincing evidence of whether or not assumed intermediates do actually occur, together (in positive instances) with information about their position in the reaction chain. The argument can be summarized in the following three postulates:

(1) If the dissimilation of a given substance A proceeds through a series of intermediates B, C, D, E, F, G ...., and if the individual steps in this chain of reactions are under adaptive enzymatic control, then growth on a medium that contains A will produce cells that are simultaneously adapted to A, B, C, D, E, F, G, ...

(2) If growth on A fails to adapt the cells to a postulated intermediate X, then X cannot be a member of the reaction chain.

(3) Growth on E will adapt the cells for F, G, ... but not necessarily for A, B, C, and D. The probability that growth on E will adapt the cells to precursors decreases with the number of intervening steps; i.e., adaptation to D is more probable than adaptation to A.

Postulate (3) perhaps requires a few additional words of explanation. In a complex dissimilation, it is conceivable that an enzyme will act at more than one stage in the dissimilatory process. Hence when two intermediates, say D and E, are separated by one enzymatic step, the possibility exists that the enzyme catalyzing that particular step (D→E) may also function later on in the oxidation of E, and that growth on E will also adapt the cells completely for the attack on D. However, if two intermediates, say B and E, are separated by several intervening steps (B→C→D→E), the probability that all three enzymes involved also take part in subsequent reactions is small, and thus growth on E is not likely to produce cells completely adapted for the oxidation of B.

ANALYSIS OF A SPECIFIC BIOCHEMICAL PROBLEM BY MEANS OF SIMULTANEOUS
ADAPTION

The application of the postulates may be illustrated with a relatively simple system, consisting of the following five compounds:

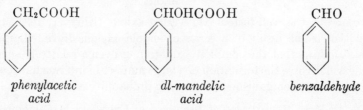

CH₂COOH   CHOHCOOH   CHO

phenylacetic   *dl-mandelic*   *benzaldehyde*
acid   *acid*

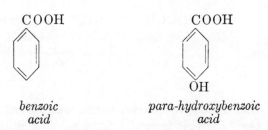

*benzoic
acid*

*para-hydroxybenzoic
acid*

Each of them is readily utilized (in the case of the acids, as the sodium or potassium salt) by a strain of *Pseudomonas fluorescens* as the sole source of energy for aerobic growth in an otherwise mineral medium.[2] Washed cell suspensions prepared from yeast extract agar are unadapted for the oxidation of these aromatic compounds: the oxygen uptake remains at the autorespiratory rate for the first 40 to 70 minutes following the addition of the substrate, and then increases exponentially to a steady maximum rate which is maintained to the point of substrate exhaustion. Cells grown in the presence of any one of

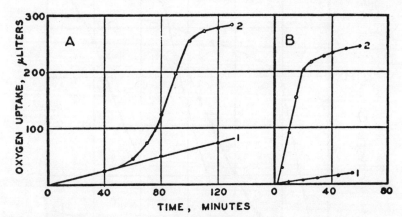

FIG. 1. OXYGEN UPTAKE WITH 2 MICROMOLES OF BENZOATE BY PSEUDOMONAS
FLUORESCENS GROWN ON YEAST EXTRACT AGAR (A) AND ON MINERAL
BENZOATE AGAR (B)
1 = autorespiration, 2 = benzoate.

the five substances show complete adaptation to that particular substance when tested in the same manner. These points are illustrated for benzoate in figure 1.

It can be seen that the system is excellently suited for analysis along the lines of the postulates enunciated above, since it consists of five closely related compounds the oxidation of which by the biological agent employed is in all cases under primary adaptive control. Inspection of the structural formulae would suggest as a provisional hypothesis that these compounds comprise five successive members of an oxidative reaction chain:

[2] Both isomers of mandelic acid are attacked at the same rate, and a racemic mixture has been used throughout the experiments herein reported.

CH₂COOH   CHOHCOOH   CHO   COOH   COOH

$\rightarrow$ $\rightarrow$ $\rightarrow$ $\rightarrow$

                                                                      OH

Analysis by simultaneous adaptation has provided conclusive evidence that this is not the case, and that in reality three separate primary oxidations are involved. The evidence for this is presented in figures 2, 3, 4, and 5. Cells

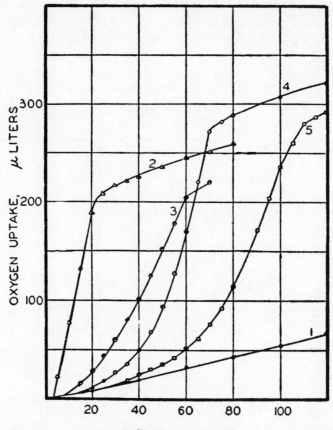

TIME, MINUTES

FIG. 2. OXYGEN UPTAKE WITH 2 MICROMOLES OF VARIOUS AROMATIC COMPOUNDS BY PSEUDOMONAS FLUORESCENS GROWN ON MINERAL BENZOATE AGAR
1 = autorespiration, 2 = benzoate, 3 = p-hydroxybenzoate, 4 = mandelate, 5 = phenyl-acetate.

were grown on four mineral agar preparations containing, respectively, benzoate, *para*-hydroxybenzoate, mandelate, and phenylacetate and then tested manometrically for adaptation to the four acids and to benzaldehyde. Only the data for the four acids are shown on the graphs.

Figure 2 demonstrates that *para*-hydroxybenzoate is not an intermediate in the oxidation of benzoate, since benzoate-grown cells are unadapted for its oxidation. The immediate attack at maximum rate on *para*-hydroxybenzoate by cells grown in its presence (figure 3) shows that the initial lag in its oxidation by benzoate-grown cells cannot be ascribed to permeability effects.

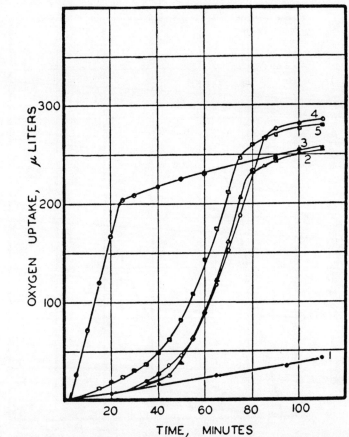

FIG. 3. OXYGEN UPTAKE WITH 2 MICROMOLES OF VARIOUS AROMATIC COMPOUNDS BY PSEUDOMONAS FLUORESCENS GROWN ON MINERAL *p*-HYDROXYBENZOATE AGAR

1 = autorespiration, 2 = benzoate, 3 = *p*-hydroxybenzoate, 4 = mandelate, 5 = phenylacetate.

Figure 4 shows that benzoate is oxidized at the same rate as mandelate by cells grown on the latter substrate, suggesting that benzoate is an intermediate in mandelate oxidation. As might be expected if this were the case, mandelate-grown cells are unadapted to *para*-hydroxybenzoate.

The results presented in figure 5 for cells grown on phenylacetate are perhaps the most interesting of all. In the first place, the typically adaptive curve for the oxidation of benzoate proves that phenylacetate cannot be oxidized along this pathway. The curve for mandelate shows a new feature: it has a double break, the initial rapid rise in oxygen uptake being followed (after a brief return to the autorespiratory rate) by an exponential rise that parallels with reasonable closeness, but at the higher absolute level initially established, the strictly adaptive curve for benzoate. The first break comes at a point that corresponds approximately to an oxygen uptake of one mole per mole of substrate. The only likely interpretation of such a curve is that growth on phenyl-

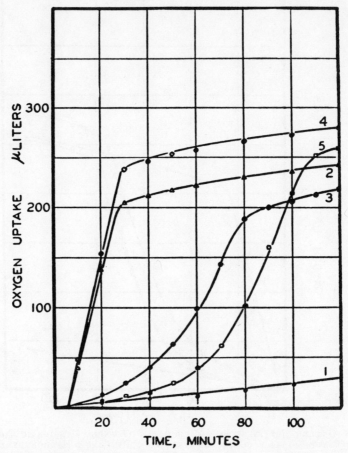

FIG. 4. OXYGEN UPTAKE WITH 2 MICROMOLES OF VARIOUS AROMATIC COMPOUNDS BY PSEUDOMONAS FLUORESCENS GROWN ON MINERAL MANDELATE AGAR
1 = autorespiration, 2 = benzoate, 3 = *p*-hydroxybenzoate, 4 = mandelate, 5 = phenylacetate.

acetate has activated the dehydrogenases involved in the initial oxidation of mandelate to benzoate—

$$CHOHCOOH + H_2O \rightarrow COOH + CO_2 + 4H$$

—but not (as shown also by the curve for benzoate) the enzyme systems operating at later stages.

The peculiar action of phenylacetate-grown cells on mandelate made possible a further experiment in substantiation of the hypothesis that benzoate really is an intermediate in the oxidation of mandelate. Adaptation to either benzoate or phenylacetate singly fails to bring about complete adaptation to mandelate (figures 2 and 5), but if the deductions drawn from the experiments above are correct, cells adapted to *both* of these substances should also be adapted, by a

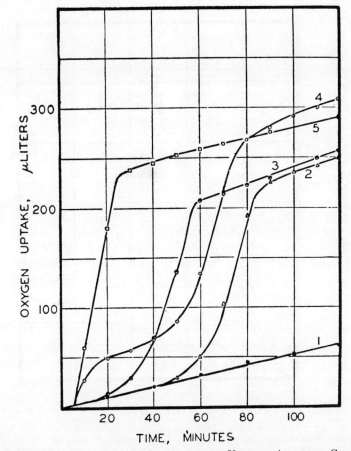

FIG. 5. OXYGEN UPTAKE WITH 2 MICROMOLES OF VARIOUS AROMATIC COMPOUNDS BY PSEUDOMONAS FLUORESCENS GROWN ON MINERAL PHENYLACETATE AGAR
1 = autorespiration, 2 = benzoate, 3 = *p*-hydroxybenzoate, 4 = mandelate, 5 = phenylacetate.

process of complementary activation, to mandelate. As shown in figure 6, this expectation is realized.

The data with benzaldehyde indicate that this substance is probably an intermediate in the oxidation of mandelate to benzoate, although for the reasons mentioned earlier the results are not so clear-cut as those with the aromatic acids. Mandelate-grown cells are completely adapted to benzaldehyde, and phenylacetate-grown cells show "semiadaptation" of the same sort as that discussed above for mandelate, with the difference that the first break in the curve for benzaldehyde oxidation comes at a level of about 0.5 moles of oxygen per mole of substrate, in accordance with the equation:

$$\text{CHO} \quad + \quad H_2O \quad \rightarrow \quad \text{COOH} \quad + \quad 2H$$

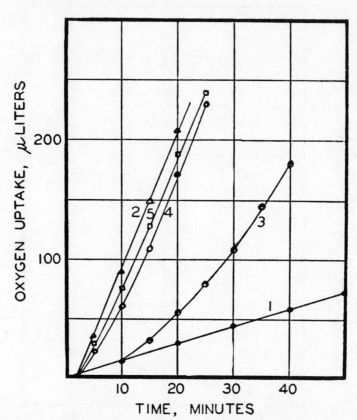

FIG. 6. OXYGEN UPTAKE WITH 2 MICROMOLES OF VARIOUS AROMATIC COMPOUNDS BY PSEUDOMONAS FLUORESCENS GROWN ON MINERAL BENZOATE AGAR AND "PREADAPTED" TO PHENYLACETATE BY INCUBATION IN THE PRESENCE OF THIS SUBSTANCE FOR 60 MINUTES PRIOR TO THE EXPERIMENT

1 = autorespiration, 2 = benzoate, 3 = p-hydroxybenzoate, 4 = mandelate, 5 = phenyl-acetate.

Interestingly enough, benzoate-grown cells show complete adaptation for benzaldehyde, suggesting that the benzaldehyde dehydrogenase also functions in the later stages of benzoate oxidation. The adaptation of benzoate-grown cells to benzaldehyde but not to mandelate is a good illustration of the third postulate.

The net result of these experiments has been to show the existence in *P. fluorescens* of three separate oxidative mechanisms involving aromatic substances:

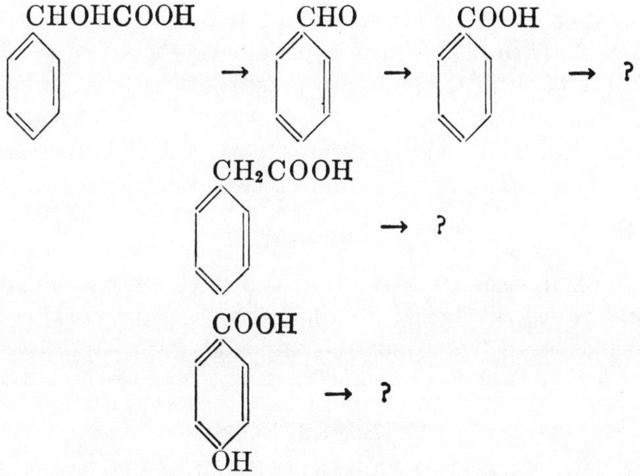

CHOHCOOH   CHO   COOH

→   →   → ?

CH₂COOH

→ ?

COOH

→ ?

OH

This information could not have been obtained from data on utilization, or even from data on absolute rates of oxidation, which are quite similar for all five compounds.

The fact that growth on phenylacetate activates the dehydrogenases involved in the oxidation of mandelate and benzaldehyde to benzoate probably indicates that these two enzymes are nonspecific, and also function at some stage in the oxidation of phenylacetate. Lack of enzymatic specificity is, of course, a limitation to the validity of the technique, and necessitates judicious evaluation of positive findings. It seems most improbable, however, that exactly the same set of enzymes would be involved in two different complex oxidative processes, so that even if growth on one substance activates nonspecifically the first step or steps in the oxidation of another substance, lack of adaptation at some later point in the chain of events will temporarily halt the attack, resulting in a "semiadapted" curve for oxygen uptake. Indeed, the occurrence of such behavior should in itself provide valuable information as to the course of the reaction. It is difficult to see how clear lack of adaptation to a postulated intermediate can be regarded as anything but conclusive negative evidence, provided that permeability effects have been ruled out by a demonstration that cells adapted to the substance in question can oxidize it immediately at the maximum rate.

One further point, at present highly speculative, deserves brief mention. It does not seem excluded that *relative rates* of adaptation may also provide indications of biochemical interrelationships. A case in point is the relatively rapid adaptation of cells grown either on benzoate or on phenylacetate to *para*-hydroxybenzoate (figures 2 and 5). A possible interpretation of this behavior is that all three substances have a common intermediate, from which *para*-hydroxybenzoate is separated by fewer steps than either of the other two, with the consequence that cells grown on benzoate or phenylacetate need to produce fewer adaptive enzymes for the attack on *para*-hydroxybenzoate than for the attack on one another.

The systematic use of simultaneous adaptation, coupled with the other kinds of data obtainable from manometric experiments, should be particularly valuable in the study of those dissimilatory processes that have so far proved least amenable to analysis—namely, rapid and complete oxidations of relatively complex substances. The only prerequisite is that the enzymatic repertoire of the biological agent employed should be largely adaptive.

SUMMARY

The theory of simultaneous adaptation as a method for the analysis of metabolic pathways is described, and its application is illustrated by a specific example: the oxidation of five aromatic compounds by a strain of *Pseudomonas fluorescens*.

REFERENCES

KARSTRÖM, H. 1937 Enzymatische Adaptation bei Mikroorganismen. Ergeb. Enzymforsch., 7, 350–376.

KLUYVER, A. J. 1931 The chemical activities of microorganisms. Univ. London Press London.

35

Reprinted from *Science*, **114**, 326–330 (1951)

The Bacterial Oxidation of Tryptophan: A Study in Comparative Biochemistry[1]

R. Y. Stanier and O. Hayaishi[2]

*Department of Bacteriology,
University of California, Berkeley*

As discovered independently by several workers (*1–3*), the analysis of adaptive patterns is of much value in the study of microbial metabolism. This technique (sometimes referred to as "simultaneous adaptation" or as "successive adaptation") is essentially an extension and refinement of the technique of kinetic analysis, and may be used to study the course of any microbial metabolic process that is under adaptive enzymatic control (*4*).

One of the specific problems that has been investigated primarily by the analysis of adaptive patterns is the pathway for the complete oxidation of tryptophan by bacteria belonging to the *Pseudomonas* group. Suda, Hayaishi, and Oda (*2*) found that an unidentified *Pseudomonas* sp.[3] adapted to oxidize tryptophan was also fully adapted to oxidize kynurenine, anthranilic acid, and catechol, but not to

[1] This work was supported by grants-in-aid from the Rockefeller Foundation, and from the American Cancer Society upon recommendation of the Committee on Growth of the National Research Council. We are indebted to R. E. Kallio, W. C. Evans, D. Bonner, T. Sakan, and the Research Division of Merck & Co., Inc., for gifts of chemicals, and to S. H. Hutner for the provision of biological material. In addition, we wish to express our thanks to Martha Tsuchida for help with many experiments.

[2] Present address: National Institutes of Health, Bethesda, Md.

[3] This organism has been subsequently identified by us as a typical member of the *P. fluorescens* species group.

TABLE 1

ADAPTIVE PATTERNS SHOWN BY 29 STRAINS BELONGING TO THE *Pseudomonas*
GROUP AFTER GROWTH IN THE PRESENCE OF DL-TRYPTOPHAN

Strains	Cells adapted (+) or unadapted (−) to oxidize				
	L-tryptophan	D-tryptophan	L-kynurenine	Anthranilic acid	Kynurenic acid
P. fluorescens (strain of Suda, Hayaishi, and Oda)	+	−	+	+	−
Pseudomonas sp. (strain of Stanier and Tsuchida)	+	+	+	−	+
Pseudomonas spp., 20 additional strains (10 belonging to the *P. fluorescens* group)	+	±[1] or −	+	+ or ±[2]	
Pseudomonas spp., 5 additional strains (none belonging to the *P. fluorescens* group)	+	+	+	−	+
Pseudomonas sp., strain Tr-14	+	−	+	−	−
P. fluorescens, strain Tr-13	+	−	−	−	−

(1) A few strains of this group can oxidize D-tryptophan at a low rate (20% or less of the rate at which they oxidize L-tryptophan).

(2) Two strains of this group show greatly impaired ability to oxidize anthranilic acid, which accumulates when they are supplied with tryptophan or kynurenine.

oxidize other, theoretically possible intermediates. The organism attacked only the L-isomer of tryptophan. Accordingly, the following pathway was proposed for the initial steps in the oxidation:

L-tryptophan → L-kynurenine →
    anthranilic acid → catechol → ?

Independently, Stanier and Tsuchida (5) conducted a similar investigation upon another unidentified *Pseudomonas* sp. This organism attacked both isomers of tryptophan, and tryptophan-adapted cells were also adapted to oxidize kynurenine and kynurenic acid, but none of a wide variety of other compounds tested, including anthranilic acid. The observed adaptive patterns implied the existence of distinct mechanisms for attack on the two stereoisomers of tryptophan and kynurenine, and hence the following initial steps were postulated:

L-tryptophan → L-kynurenine
    ↘
        kynurenic acid → ?
    ↗
D-tryptophan → D-kynurenine

In the ensuing discussion, the oxidation of tryptophan through anthranilic acid and catechol will be referred to as *the aromatic pathway,* and that through kynurenic acid as *the quinoline pathway.*

The marked differences in dissimilatory patterns of closely related bacteria revealed by these reports made a more extensive investigation desirable, and this we have recently undertaken. A large collection of tryptophan-oxidizing pseudomonads has been subjected to systematic comparative study. Adaptive patterns were determined by growing each strain on a medium containing DL-tryptophan as the energy source, harvesting the cells in phosphate buffer, and testing manometrically their ability to oxidize the following 5 compounds: D-tryptophan, L-tryptophan, L-kynurenine, anthranilic acid, and kynurenic acid. Limiting

amounts of the substrates $(2 \ \mu M)$ were used in the manometric tests to permit detection of any anomalies in total oxygen consumption. More extensive confirmatory tests, employing a wider range of compounds, were subsequently conducted with a few representative strains and gave results in accord with expectations. Table 1 summarizes the general findings, which provide confirmation of the existence of the two pathways diverging from kynurenine that had been proposed earlier by Suda, Hayaishi, and Oda and by Stanier and Tsuchida. Of 27 new strains tested, 20 followed the aromatic pathway and 5 the quinoline pathway. The difference between the two biochemical groups with respect to the oxidation of D-tryptophan has also been confirmed: every strain using the quinoline pathway oxidizes the D-isomer at a high rate, whereas strains using the aromatic pathway either do not attack it at all, or oxidize it at a rate that is low in comparison to the rate of oxidation of the L-isomer.

Two strains that decompose tryptophan through the aromatic pathway are characterized by an interesting metabolic abnormality, which proivdes additional evidence for the existence of this pathway. Their ability to oxidize anthranilic acid is severely impaired, and consequently a substantial accumulation of this compound occurs when they are fed either tryptophan or kynurenine. The severity of the metabolic block between anthranilic acid and catechol in these two strains varies somewhat, depending on the conditions of prior cultivation and the age of the cells, but in some experiments accumulations of anthranilic acid approaching 90% of the theoretical yield on a molar basis have been obtained following the addition of tryptophan or kynurenine to cell suspensions.

Two of the 29 strains tested displayed adaptive patterns after growth on tryptophan that were incompatible with an oxidation through either the aromatic or the quinoline pathway, and in both cases the total oxygen uptake per mole of tryptophan decomposed was exceptionally low, indicating an early and absolute metabolic block. The first of these strains, Tr-14, could oxidize only L-tryptophan and L-kynurenine of the substrates tested (Table 1). Spectrophotometric analysis of the supernatant liquid from a reaction vessel in which tryptophan had undergone oxidation suggested the accumulation of a mixture of anthranilic and kynurenic acids, an inference subsequently confirmed by isolation and characterization of the two compounds in an experiment conducted on a larger scale. The oxidation of either tryptophan or kynurenine by Tr-14 always results in the formation of these acids, the sum of the amounts of the two products being equal on a molar basis to the amount of substrate decomposed. Tr-14 is the only strain so far investigated in which a "mixed" dissimilation, involving the production of both benzene and quinoline derivatives, has been shown to occur; and its metabolism of tryptophan is so defective that the result could be described better as a "branched cul-de-sac" than as a "mixed pathway."

The second strain showing anomalous adaptive patterns (strain Tr-13) could metabolize only L-tryptophan of the compounds tested (Table 1); spectrophotometric analysis, followed by isolation and characterization of the product, showed that it converted tryptophan quantitatively to indole. We have not further investigated the mechanism of oxidation in this exceptional strain, which belongs to the *Pseudomonas fluorescens* species group. Ten other fluorescent pseudomonads tested all dissimilated tryptophan by the aromatic pathway.

Guided by these findings with intact cells, we then turned our attention to the enzymatic aspects of the problem. One previous report on an enzyme operative in tryptophan oxidation by the aromatic pathway had been made by Hayaishi and Hashimoto (6), who worked with the strain of *P. fluorescens* studied by Suda *et al.* (2). By extraction of acetone-dried cells grown at the expense of anthranilic acid, Hayaishi and Hashimoto obtained a catechol-oxidizing enzyme which they named pyrocatechase. After extensive purification, pyrocatechase was found to catalyze an oxidation of catechol with an uptake of 2 atoms of oxygen and with the formation of an acid which appeared to be identical with *cis-cis*-muconic acid, on the basis of melting point and elementary analysis. A crude enzyme system of very similar properties was isolated independently by Stanier *et al.* (7) from dried cells of another strain of *P. fluorescens,* grown on phenol, benzoic acid, or mandelic acid. It was shown to catalyze a conversion of catechol, again with an oxygen uptake of 2 atoms, to β-ketoadipic acid. Since it appeared improbable that two distinct enzymes catalyzing an opening of the catechol ring would be formed by *P. fluorescens,* we decided to reinvestigate catechol oxidation, using extracts from tryptophan-grown cells. A crude cell-free system was readily obtained from vacuum-dried cells, and was found to catalyze the reaction described by Stanier *et al.*—namely, an oxidation of catechol to β-keto-

adipic acid. This indicated that the enzymatic degradation of catechol might involve an initial oxidative and a subsequent nonoxidative step:

$$catechol + O_2 \longrightarrow cis\text{-}cis\text{-muconic acid} \quad (1)$$
$$(pyrocatechase)$$
$$cis\text{-}cis\text{-muconic acid} + H_2O \longrightarrow \beta\text{-ketoadipic acid} \quad (2)$$
$$(unknown\ enzyme)$$
$$catechol + O_2 + H_2O \longrightarrow \beta\text{-ketoadipic acid} \quad (1) + (2)$$
$$(crude\ extracts)$$

It was easy to test this hypothesis, since a small amount of the alleged *cis-cis*-muconic acid, isolated by Hayaishi and Hashimoto after the action of pyrocatechase on catechol, was still available. An attempt to demonstrate the conversion of this material to β-ketoadipic acid by our crude catechol-oxidizing extract gave *completely negative results.* The work of others has recently clarified this very puzzling situation. Elvidge *et al.* (8) have discovered the third geometrical isomer of muconic acid, which possesses the *cis-trans* configuration, and have further shown that the *cis-cis* isomer is unstable in aqueous solution, undergoing ready isomerization to the *cis-trans* form, from which it cannot be readily distinguished, since the physical and chemical properties of the two substances (including their melting points) are very similar. It is thus probable that most earlier chemical data reported for the *cis-cis* isomer were obtained with the *cis-trans* isomer, or with a mixture of the two. Following these chemical studies, Evans and Smith (9) examined the biological behavior of the 3 isomers of muconic acid, and found that the *cis-cis* isomer is an intermediate in the bacterial degradation of benzoic acid and phenol to β-ketoadipic acid, whereas the *cis-trans* and *trans-trans* isomers are inactive. Tests made by us on samples of the *cis-cis* and *cis-trans*-muconic acids have shown that our crude catechol-oxidizing enzyme system from tryptophan-grown cells smoothly converts the former isomer in a nonoxidative reaction to β-ketoadipic acid, but does not attack the latter isomer, thus fully confirming the conclusions of Evans and Smith. In the light of these discoveries, it is now evident that Hayaishi and Hashimoto had purified pyrocatechase to the point at which the second, nonoxidative step was eliminated; but that the *cis-cis* muconic acid produced enzymatically underwent isomerization during the the isolation procedure, which explains its inactivity when subsequently tested with the crude enzyme by us.

Although extracts from tryptophan-adapted, vacuum-dried cells of strains that follow the aromatic pathway show strong activity against catechol, they are inactive against tryptophan itself. In a search for better methods of making cell-free preparations, we found that the technique of grinding wet cells with alumina, discovered by McIlwain (10), yielded extracts containing many additional enzymes. Fresh concentrated extracts prepared in this manner from tryptophan-grown cells catalyze an oxidation of tryptophan which results in the consumption of 8 atoms of oxygen per mole of substrate and yields β-keto-

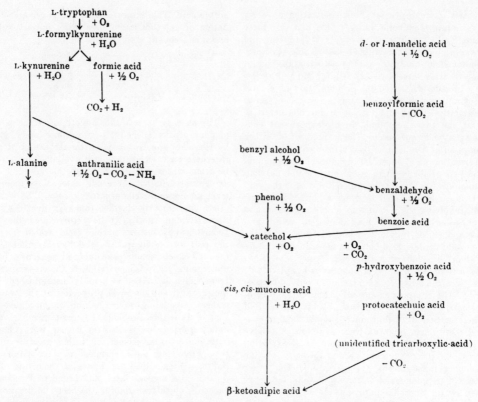

FIG. 1. A comprehensive diagram of the known bacterial metabolic pathways that converge with the formation of β-keto-adipic acid as an intermediary metabolite. Other divergent pathways from tryptophan are not shown.

adipic acid as one of the end products, demonstrating that a complete destruction of the indole nucleus must have taken place. Aging or simple dilution of such extracts results in the elimination of several oxidative steps, the total oxygen uptake per mole of tryptophan falling to 5, 3, or even 2 atoms. The oxidation of tryptophan catalyzed by such aged or diluted preparations involves the steps discovered recently by Knox and Mehler (11) for the dissimilation of tryptophan to kynurenine via formyl-kynurenine in mammalian liver extracts. With the bacterial preparations, however, kynurenine does not accumulate, since a powerful kynureninase is also present, which causes a nonoxidative cleavage of L-kynurenine to anthranilic acid and L-alanine. This enzyme, which is the only one that we have so far studied in detail, coincides in all essential properties with the mammalian kynureninase recently described by Wiss (12) and by Braunshstein, Goryachenkova, and Paskhina (13).

The work reported here permits the construction of a broad conceptual scheme that describes the oxidation of tryptophan by many bacteria, and that links up one of the possible alternate pathways for the metabolism of tryptophan with a series of other primary oxidative sequences previously known to occur in bacteria. It is now evident that the initial attack

on tryptophan most commonly involves elimination of the α carbon atom of the indole nucleus, resulting in the formation of kynurenine as an intermediary metabolite. Below kynurenine, alternate metabolic pathways are open; some bacteria degrade this compound to kynurenic acid (presumably by a specific deamination or transamination, followed by secondary ring closure), whereas others split it to alanine and anthranilic acid through the action of kynureninase. At present we do not know the nature of the later intermediates formed on the pathway through kynurenic acid; enzymatic studies have not yet been attempted, and although many benzene derivatives have been tested by analysis of the adaptive patterns of tryptophan-grown cells, the results have been uniformly negative. The outcome of these analyses suggests that the benzene moiety of the quinoline nucleus in kynurenic acid may be first destroyed, with resultant eventual oxidation via pyridine derivatives. Several of the later steps on the aromatic pathway are now firmly established. This pathway merges, near the point of final ring rupture, with oxidations of non-nitrogenous primary aromatic substrates, such as mandelic acid, phenol, and p-hydroxybenzoic acid (4); as shown in Fig. 1, the common central intermediary metabolite for all these oxidations is β-ketoadipic acid. Since the present work has also shown that the initial enzymatic steps in the breakdown of tryptophan are common to bacteria and mammals, it would not be surprising if β-ketoadipic acid proves to be an intermediate in the mammalian oxidation of tryptophan and other aromatic compounds. Full experimental details will be published shortly.

References

1. STANIER, R. Y. J. Bact., **54**, 339 (1947).
2. SUDA, M., HAYAISHI, O., and ODA, Y. Symposium on Enzyme Chemistry (Tokyo), **1**, 79 (1949) ; Med. J. Osaka University, **2**, 21 (1950).
3. KARLSSON, J. L., and BARKER, H. A. J. Biol. Chem., **175**, 913 (1948).
4. STANIER, R. Y. Bact. Revs., **14**, 179 (1950).
5. STANIER, R. Y., and TSUCHIDA, M. J. Bact., **58**, 45 (1949).
6. HAYAISHI, O., and HASHIMOTO, K. Med. J. Osaka University, **2**, 33 (1950).
7. STANIER, R. Y., et al. J. Bact., **59**, 137 (1950).
8. ELVIDGE, J. A., et al. J. Chem. Soc., 2235 (1950).
9. EVANS, W. C., and SMITH, B. S. W. Biochem. J., **49**, Proc. Biochem. Soc., x (1951).
10. MCILWAIN, H. J. Gen. Microbiol., **2**, 288 (1948).
11. KNOX, W. E., and MEHLER, A. H. J. Biol. Chem., **187**, 419 (1950) ; MEHLER, A. H., and KNOX, W. E. Ibid., 431.
12. WISS, O. Helv. Chim. Acta, **32**, 1694 (1949).
13. BRAUNSHSTEIN, A. E. GORYACHENKOVA, E. V., and PASKHINA, T. S. Biokhimiya, **14**, 163 (1949).

283

Editor's Comments on Papers 36, 37, and 38

36 **Hayaishi, Katagiri, and Rothberg:** Mechanism of the Pyrocatechase Reaction
   J. Amer. Chem. Soc., **77**, 5450–5451 (1955)

37 **Mason, Fowlks, and Peterson:** Oxygen Transfer and Electron Transport by the Phenolase Complex
   J. Amer. Chem. Soc., **77**, 2914 (1955)

38 **Mason:** Mechanisms of Oxygen Metabolism
   Science, **125**, 1185–1188 (1957)

With the new technique developed by Stanier, tremendous activity started in the field of solving the pathways of hydrocarbon utilization (Zobell, 1946, 1950). The outstanding work was, however, the discovery of the oxygenase by Hayaishi (Paper 36) and by Mason (Papers 37 and 38). Both discovered the incorporation of oxygen into the benzene molecule, causing the split of the ring structure and thus the complete breakdown of aromatic carbon compounds. They also evaluated the fact that either the whole molecule or only the atom oxygen from water is introduced; thus, oxygenases and mixed function hydroxylases became known to cause the attack on the ring structure. The present situation is well summarized by both researchers in their respective books (King et al., 1965; Block and Hayaishi, 1966) and the review article by Hayaishi (1966).

Reprinted from *J. Amer. Chem. Soc.*, **77**, 5450–5451 (1955)

MECHANISM OF THE PYROCATECHASE REACTION

O. Hayaishi, M. Katagiri, and S. Rothberg

Pyrocatechase[1,2] of *Pseudomonas* sp. catalyzes the oxidative cleavage of the aromatic ring of catechol (I) to *cis–cis*-muconic acid (II). Subsequent work has shown that pyrocatechase requires ferrous ion[3] and sulfhydryl containing compounds[4] for maximum activity, although the mechanism of electron transport as well as the nature of intermediate steps has remained unknown.

We wish to report some experimental results using O_2^{18} and H_2O^{18} which may aid in elucidating the mechanism of this unique enzymatic reaction. When the reaction was conducted in the presence of H_2O^{18}, O^{18} was not detected in the product, *cis–*

cis-muconic acid. In the presence of O_2^{18}, however, essentially all the oxygen enzymatically introduced into *cis–cis*-muconic acid was shown to be derived from molecular oxygen (Table I). The results clearly demonstrate that pyrocatechase is an

(1) O. Hayaishi and K. Hashimoto, *J. Biochem. (Japan)*, **37**, 371 (1950).

(2) O. Hayaishi and R. Y. Stanier, *J. Bact.*, **62**, 691 (1951).

(3) M. Suda, K. Hashimoto, H. Matsuoka and T. Kamahora, *J. Biochem. (Japan)*, **38**, 289 (1951).

(4) R. Y. Stanier and J. L. Ingraham, *J. Biol. Chem.*, **210**, 799 (1954).

TABLE I

ENZYMATIC INCORPORATION OF O_2^{18} INTO cis–cis-MUCONIC
ACID

Experiment I.   Catechol (0.6 mmole), 4.8 mg. of purified pyrocatechase (specific activity 112 units/mg. protein),[a] 0.6 millimole of glutathione and 4.5 millimoles of potassium phosphate buffer (pH 7.5) were incubated in a 500-ml. Erlenmeyer flask in a total volume of 60 ml. H_2O^{18}, 0.701 atom % excess. Experiment II.   A 500-ml. Büchner suction flask was modified with a high vacuum stopcock at the top; the hose connection was sealed with a rubber vaccine cap.   The same reaction components as in Expt. I were employed except that H_2O was used instead of H_2O^{18} and to the degassed container was added a O_2^{18}–N_2 mixture with an approximate ratio of O_2^{18}/N_2 of 18.2%.[b]   In Expt. II the O^{18} content of the flask was determined before the addition of the enzyme and after the completion of the reaction. The atom % excess was 1.354 and 1.331 respectively. The reactions were run at 25° with gentle mechanical shaking and the reaction rate was followed by the increased absorption at 260 mμ.   Aliquots were removed by syringe through the rubber vaccine cap in Expt. II.   After two hours of incubation 2 ml. of 2 N H_2SO_4 was added to the reaction mixture.   cis–cis-Muconic acid was isolated and was recrystallized from absolute ethanol.   The recrystallized material was pyrolyzed by the method of W. E. Doering and E. Dorfman (THIS JOURNAL, 75, 5595 (1953)[c].   The O^{18} content was determined by a Consolidated Nier Model 21-201 Mass Spectrometer, measuring $CO^{16}O^{18}/CO_2$ (46/44) ratio.

			Atom % O^{18} in cis–cis-Muconic acid[d]	Atom % excess Experiment	Theory[e]
Expt.	Medium	Catechol			
I	O_2^{16} + H_2O^{18}	0.207	0.207	0.000	0.701
			0.207	0.000	
II	O_2^{18} + H_2O^{16}	0.207	1.421	1.217	1.343
			1.433	1.229	

[a] M. Katagiri and O. Hayashi, unpublished procedure. [b] O_2^{18} was prepared by electrolysis of H_2O^{18} obtained from the Stuart Oxygen Co.   [c] We are indebted to Mr. S. Ishihara of the National Bureau of Standards for use of the pyrolysis equipment.   [d] Calculated for the oxygen atoms incorporated.   [e] Theoretical atom % excess when two oxygen atoms are derived from O^{18}.

oxygen transferase rather than a dehydrogenase and no hydration reaction is involved in the over-all process.   cis–cis-Muconic acid semialdehyde is therefore excluded as an intermediate since any known mechanism of enzymatic aldehyde oxidation involves hydration.   A compound such as (III) appears to be a more likely intermediate in the pyrocatechase reaction.   Orthobenzoquinone appears unlikely as an intermediate since H_2O_2 was previously shown not to participate in the reaction.[1,4]   This compound, however, cannot be completely ruled out as an intermediate because of the possibility of a tightly bound enzyme–H_2O_2 complex acting as a peroxidase.

The similarity of pyrocatechase to other enzymes which catalyze oxidative rupture of aromatic rings of certain phenolic compounds was recently reviewed by Crandall.[5]   In addition to pyrocatechase, homogentisicase,[6] 3-hydroxyanthranilic acid oxidase[7,8] and protocatechuic acid oxidase[4] appear to belong to this new class of metallo-protein enzymes which introduce two oxygen atoms directly across the aromatic bond adjacent to the phenolic group with simultaneous rupture of the aromatic structure.

NATIONAL INSTITUTE OF ARTHRITIS AND   OSAMU HAYAISHI
METABOLIC DISEASES AND NATIONAL HEART
INSTITUTE   MASAYUKI KATAGIRI
NATIONAL INSTITUTES OF HEALTH,   SIMON ROTHBERG
BETHESDA 14, MD.

RECEIVED AUGUST 31, 1955

(5) D. L. Crandall, "A Symposium on Amino Acid Metabolism," ed. by D. McElroy and B. Glass, Johns Hopkins Press, Baltimore, Md., 1955, p. 867.

(6) M. Suda and Y. Takeda, J. Biochem. (Japan), 37, 381 (1950).

(7) L. M. Henderson, Abstract of paper, Amer. Chem. Soc. 121st Meeting, Milwaukee, 1952, p. 23C.

(8) A. Miyake, A. H. Bockman and B. S. Schweigert, Abstract of Paper, Amer. Chem. Soc. 124th Meeting Chicago, 1953, p. 11C.

Reprinted from *J. Amer. Chem. Soc.*, **77**, 2914 (1955)

OXYGEN TRANSFER AND ELECTRON TRANSPORT BY THE PHENOLASE COMPLEX[1]

H. S. Mason, W. L. Fowlks, and E. Peterson

The metabolic role of the phenolase complex[2] is controversial, particularly in respect to an hypothesis suggesting that this enzyme system catalyses terminal transfer of electrons to oxygen.[3] In order to throw some light on the problem and to understand the molecular events occurring at the catalytic configuration of the enzyme complex, we have studied its hydroxylative phase using O^{18}_2 and H_2O^{18} as tracers.

We find that all oxygen enzymically introduced as hydroxyl into the benzene ring of the substrate comes from molecular oxygen (Table I). None comes from solvent water. Hydroxylation mechanisms inconsistent with this observation[4] must accordingly be incorrect. The phenolase complex is an *oxygen transferase*.

TABLE I

COMPARISON OF O^{18} IN 4,5-DIMETHYLCATECHOL FORMED ENZYMICALLY FROM 3,4-DIMETHYLPHENOL[a] IN O^{18}_2[b] AND H_2O AND IN O_2 AND H_2O^{18}[c]

Experiment	Found	Atom % excess O^{18}[d] theoretical for uptake of one atom	No uptake
$O^{18}_2 + H_2O$	0.52	0.59	0.00
	.51		
	.56		
$O_2 + H_2O^{18}$	.00	0.59	0.00
	.00		

[a] Twenty-five ml. reaction volumes contained 0.3 mmole ascorbic acid, 1.3 mmole KH_2PO_4, 2.15 mmole K_2HPO_4, 0.45 mmole 3,4-dimethylphenol and 4.0 mg. purified[5] mushroom phenolase having 20–80 cresolase[6] and *ca.* 1000 catecholase[7] units/mg. dry wt. 4,5-Dimethylcatechol (30–50% yield) was isolated through its lead salt, from an ether extract of the reaction mixture, m.p. 84–86°. No hydroxylation occurred in the system when heat-denatured enzyme was substituted for active protein. [b] Prepared electrolytically. [c] Obtained from the Stuart Oxygen Company, containing 1.4 atom % O^{18}. [d] Mass spectrometry was performed by the Consolidated Engineering Corporation on carbon dioxide

(1) This study has been supported by a grant from the United States Public Health Service (C-2291).

(2) We mean by "phenolase complex" that pair of enzymic activities occurring together, associated with copper-protein, and responsible for phenol *o*-hydroxylation and for dehydrogenation of *o*-diphenols to *o*-quinones.

(3) W. O. James, "Plant Respiration," Oxford Press, New York, N.Y., 1953.

(4) D. Kertesz, *Biochim. et Biophys. Acta*, **9**, 170 (1952).

(5) M. F. Mallette and C. R. Dawson, *Arch. Biochem.*, **23**, 29 (1949).

(6) M. F. Mallette and C. R. Dawson, THIS JOURNAL, **64**, 2344 (1942).

(7) W. H. Miller, M. F. Mallette, L. J. Roth and C. R. Dawson, *ibid.*, **66**, 514 (1944).

samples obtained by Unterzaucher pyrolysis[8] of 4,5-dimethylcatechol samples. Oxygen recovery was quantitative.

Since the phenolase complex is a cuprous protein[9,10,11,12] which is in the cupric form after each hydroxylation[13] and which combines with inhibitor CO in the ratio $2\,Cu^+/CO$,[9] hydroxylation by this enzyme system is describable as

$$(1)\quad \text{Protein}\begin{smallmatrix}Cu^+\\[4pt]Cu^+\end{smallmatrix} + O_2 \longrightarrow \text{Protein}\begin{smallmatrix}Cu^{\cdots}\\ \quad O\!-\!O\\ Cu^{\cdots}\end{smallmatrix}$$

$$(2)\quad \text{Protein}\begin{smallmatrix}Cu^{\cdots}\\ \quad O\!-\!O\\ Cu^{\cdots}\end{smallmatrix} + \text{Monophenol} \longrightarrow$$

$$\text{Protein}\begin{smallmatrix}Cu^{++}\\[4pt]Cu^{++}\end{smallmatrix} + \text{Diphenol} + H_2O$$

$$(3)\quad \text{Protein}\begin{smallmatrix}Cu^{++}\\[4pt]Cu^{++}\end{smallmatrix} + 2e^- \longrightarrow \text{Protein}\begin{smallmatrix}Cu^+\\[4pt]Cu^+\end{smallmatrix}$$

The hydroxylative function of phenolase (eq. 1 and 2) is thus coupled to an electron source (eq. 3), *i.e.*, oxidation of *o*-diphenol to *o*-quinone, which may be linked in turn to the common pathways of metabolism through $TPNH^+$[14] or $DPNH^+$[15], possibly by quinone reductase.[16] The function of the phenolase complex as a terminal oxidase will be in demand during the biosynthesis of *o*-diphenols from monophenols. We propose that these *o*-diphenols are subsequently utilized to form flavonoids, lignins, tannins, cuticulation diphenols of arthropods, melanoproteins of chordates, and possibly adrenaline and noradrenaline.[12] Some instances of light-irreversible inhibition of terminal respiration by carbon monoxide[17,18] may be accounted for in these terms.

(8) W. E. Doering and E. Dorfman, *ibid.*, **75**, 5595 (1953).

(9) F. Kubowitz, *Biochem. Z.*, **292**, 221 (1937); **299**, 32 (1938) *cf.* D. Keilin, *Proc. Roy. Soc., (London)*, **104B**, 206 (1929); D Keilin and T. Mann, *ibid.*, **125B**, 187 (1938).

(10) J. Doskocil, *Collection Czechoslov. Chem. Commun.*, **15**, 614 (1950).

(11) A. B. Lerner, "Advances in Enzymology," Vol. XIV, F. F. Nord, ed., 1953, p. 73.

(12) H. S. Mason, "Advances in Enzymology," Vol. XVI, F. F. Nord, ed., 1955, p. 105.

(13) Hydroxylation does not proceed in the absence of reducing agents: *cf.* R. C. Behm and J. M. Nelson, THIS JOURNAL, **66**, 711 (1944); M. Suda, N. Kimoto and S. Naono, *J. Biochem. Soc. (Japan)*, **26**, 603 (1954); A. B. Lerner, T. B. Fitzpatrick, E. Calkins and W. H. Summerson, *J. Biol. Chem.*, **191**, 799 (1951); L. P. Kendal, *Biochem. J.*, **44**, 442 (1949).

(14) F. Kubowitz, *Biochem. Z.*, **293**, 308 (1937).

(15) E. A. H. Roberts and D. J. Wood, *Biochem. J.*, **53**, 332 (1953).

(16) W. D. Wosilait and A. Nason, *J. Biol. Chem.*, **206**, 255 (1954); **208**, 785 (1954).

(17) G. K. K. Link and R. M. Klein, *Bot. Gaz.*, **133**, 190 (1951).

(18) G. C. Webster, Plant Physiol., **29**, 399 (1954).

DEPARTMENT OF BIOCHEMISTRY   H. S. MASON
UNIVERSITY OF OREGON MEDICAL SCHOOL   W. L. FOWLKS
PORTLAND, OREGON   E. PETERSON

RECEIVED APRIL 11, 1955

$$\mathscr{38}$$

Mechanisms
of Oxygen Metabolism

H. S. Mason

Application of tracer techniques to biochemistry has often been followed by fresh insight, sometimes at a level of generalization. In the study of oxygen metabolism, which has been badly prejudiced by the influence of the expression "½ O_2," the use of oxygen-18 as a tracer has become broadly feasible only recently. Formerly, it was difficult to recover oxygen quantitatively from organic compounds in a form suitable for mass spectrometric analysis, but this problem was largely solved in 1953 by Doering and Dorfman (*1*).

Since then, the mechanisms of action of a number of enzymes that catalyze reactions of molecular oxygen ("oxidases") have been examined by means of tracer oxygen. The purpose of this article (*2*) is to summarize the results which have been obtained and to show that molecular oxygen is metabolized by three broad classes of enzymes, which I have named "oxygen transferases," "mixed-function oxidases," and "electron-transfer oxidases" (*3*, p. 55C; *4*).

Oxygen Transferases

By *oxygen transferase* (*5–8*) is meant an enzyme that catalyzes the consumption of one molecule of oxygen per molecule of substrate (*9*), both atoms of consumed oxygen appearing in the product (Eq. 1; the related system described by Eq. 1a is also possible, but it has not been observed).

$$S + O_2 \rightleftharpoons O_2S \qquad (1)$$

$$2S + O_2 \rightleftharpoons 2OS \qquad (1a)$$

To identify an enzyme as an oxygen transferase, it is therefore necessary to

The author is associate professor of biochemistry at the University of Oregon Medical School, Portland. This article is based on a lecture presented at a symposium, "Enzymatic activation of oxygen," which was held 20 Sept. 1956 during the 130th meeting of the American Chemical Society at Atlantic City, N.J.

determine the amount of oxygen consumed per molecule of substrate transformed, the amount of oxygen incorporated into the product, and, by tracer experiments, the source of the incorporated oxygen. All these tests have been carried out, and the required criteria have been met by pyrocatechase (6), 3-hydroxyanthranilic oxidase (8), and tryptophan oxidase (8). Some properties of these three enzymes are listed in Table 1 along with those of enzymes which have not been completely characterized but which are probably oxygen transferases.

With the exception of lipoxidase, in which the presence of a prosthetic group is still uncertain, all these oxygen transferases are metalloproteins which are activated by reducing agents and inhibited by metal-binding reagents. When it is known that ferrous iron is essential to the oxygen-transferring activity, it is reasonable to conclude that the enzymes act as iron-oxygen complexes, since the capacity of related, reduced metalloproteins (for example, hemoglobin, myoglobin, chlorocruorin, hemerythrin, and hemocyanin) to bind oxygen is well known, and since the autoxidation of heavy metals such as ferrous iron appears to take place through the formation of intermediate complexes of iron and oxygen. In any case, molecular oxygen is transferred to substrate without exchange with solvent oxygen, so that the formation of ternary enzyme-oxygen-substrate complexes, followed by rearrangement to enzyme and product, appears probable (Eqs. 2 to 4).

$$E + O_2 \rightleftharpoons EO_2 \qquad (2)$$
$$EO_2 + S \rightleftharpoons EO_2S \qquad (3)$$
$$EO_2S \rightleftharpoons E + O_2S \qquad (4)$$

Mixed-Function Oxidases

I mean by *mixed-function oxidase* an enzyme that catalyzes the consumption of one molecule of oxygen per molecule of substrate; one atom of this oxygen molecule appears in the product, and the other undergoes a two-equivalent reduction (Eq. 5).

$$SH + O_2 + 2e \rightleftharpoons SOH + O^{--} (H_2O) \qquad (5)$$

To identify an enzyme as a mixed-function oxidase, it is necessary (i) to determine the amount of oxygen consumed per molecule of substrate transformed, (ii) to determine the amount of oxygen incorporated into the product, (iii) to determine the source of the incorporated oxygen, and (iv) to show that two reducing equivalents are also consumed during the reaction. Since enzymes of this class catalyze, in effect, two reactions of oxygen (transfer and reduction), it is particularly important, if difficult, to

Table 1. Characteristics of oxygen transferases. References, where given in column 1, identify studies made with tracer oxygen.

Name	Activators	Inhibitors	Essential groups
Homogentisate oxidase	Ascorbate, glutathione, ene-diols	Dipyridyl, CN⁻, iodoacetate, diethyldithio-carbamate (pH 5—loss of Fe^{++})	Fe^{++}, SH
Pyrocatechase (6)	Glutathione	Ag⁺, Cu⁺⁺, dialysis	Fe^{++}
3-Hydroxyanthranilic oxidase (8)	Ascorbate	Dipyridyl, CN⁻, p-chloromercuribenzoate, H_2O_2	Fe^{++}, SH
Protocatechuic acid oxidase		p-Chloromercuribenzoate	Fe^{++}, SH
Tryptophan oxidase (8)	H_2O_2 (?)	Catalase, CO (light reversible), N₃⁻, CN⁻, Cu⁺	Heme (?)
Indolylacetic oxidase	Mn⁺⁺, monophenols, aniline (peroxidase substrates)	Catalase, CO (light reversible), CN⁻	Heme
Indole oxidase	Glutathione, B₁₂, folic acid, adenylic acid	Cyanide, Azide, dipyridyl, Ag	Heavy metal
Lipoxidase			

establish the homogeneity of the active centers.

No enzyme has been shown rigorously to be a mixed-function oxidase, for this requirement has not been adequately satisfied, but a number of enzymes are probably members of this class because they possess several, if not all, of the required characteristics. These characteristics are listed in Table 2. Of this group, imidazoleacetic oxidase (8), nonspecific liver hydroxylase (10), steroid 11β-hydroxylase (11), squalene oxidocyclase I (12), and the phenolase complex (4) have been studied with heavy oxygen, as has the model hydroxylating system that consists of ferrous iron and ascorbic acid in the presence of molecular oxygen (13).

The order in which one atom of the oxygen molecule is transferred to the substrate and the other atom is reduced is an interesting problem which has not been solved for any oxidase of this class. If the electron donors function by means of two one-equivalent reduction steps, then the free radicals O_2^- or HO_2 (but not OH) may be oxygen-transferring intermediates. If the donors function by means of one two-equivalent reduction, the enzyme complexes of O_2, O_2^{--}, or O may be oxygen-transferring intermediates. These alternatives are illustrated by the following reaction types. In type i mechanisms (Eq. 6)

$$EO_2 \cdot AH \cdot DH \rightleftharpoons$$
$$AOH + E + D^+ + OH^- \qquad (6)$$

a quaternary complex, $AH \cdot E \cdot O_2 \cdot DH$, forms and dissociates into the products AOH, D, E, and OH^- (where AH represents oxygen acceptor and DH the electron donor). If the oxygen acceptor, AH, or the product of oxygen acceptance, AOH, serves as the electron donor, as

appears to be the case with the phenolase complex and p-hydroxyphenylpyruvate oxidase, only ternary complex formation is required.

According to the type ii mechanism, the oxygen-transferring intermediate is enzyme-oxygen complex, EO_2, which is transformed into EO as a result of transfer of one atom of oxygen to substrate (Eq. 7)

$$EO_2 + AH \rightleftharpoons AOH + EO \qquad (7)$$

In a second (and possibly third) step, the electron donor reduces EO to $E +$ O^{--} (Eq. 8)

$$EO + DH \rightleftharpoons E + D^+ + OH^- \qquad (8)$$

In the type iii mechanism, one oxygen atom of enzyme-oxygen complex is reduced to O^{--}, forming the oxygen-transferring intermediate, EO, Eqs. 9, 10).

$$EO_2 + DH \rightleftharpoons EO + D^+ + OH^- \qquad (9)$$
$$EO + AH \rightleftharpoons E + AOH \qquad (10)$$

In the type iv mechanism, the oxygen-transferring intermediate is the enzyme-peroxide complex, $E \cdot H_2O_2$ or its equivalent, formed by two-equivalent reduction of enzyme-oxygen complex (Eqs. 11, 12).

$$EO_2 + DH \rightleftharpoons E \cdot HO_2^- + D^+ \qquad (11)$$
$$E \cdot HO_2^- + AH \rightleftharpoons E + AOH + OH^- \qquad (12)$$

Mixed-function oxidation in which the oxygen-transferring intermediate is formed by a one-equivalent reduction step is illustrated by type v (Eq. 13).

$$EO_2 + DH \rightleftharpoons EO_2H + D \qquad (13)$$

The enzyme-oxygen complex undergoes a one-equivalent reduction to $E \cdot O_2^-$ or $E \cdot O_2H$, the oxygen-transferring intermediate. The complex EO^- or EOH

that is formed as a result of oxygen transfer (Eq. 14)

$$EO_2H + AH \rightleftharpoons EOH + AOH \quad (14)$$

undergoes a second one-equivalent reduction to free enzyme and hydroxyl anion (Eq. 15).

$$EOH + D \rightleftharpoons E + D^+ + OH^- \quad (15)$$

Evidence has developed from study of the reaction complexes of hemoproteins with peroxide (14) and from examination of the mechanisms of aromatic hydroxylation taking place in the presence of ferrous iron, oxygen, and ascorbic acid (13) or peroxidase, oxygen, and dihydroxyfumarate (15) which strongly suggests that it is possible to form positively charged oxygen-transferring species of the general structure Fe^{++}O or its equivalent, but it is not possible to generalize from this evidence to the mixed-function oxidases as a class. Much work remains to be done in this field.

Electron-Transfer Oxidases

The third major class of enzymes which catalyze reactions of molecular oxygen are the *electron-transfer oxidases*. In the presence of these enzymes and appropriate electron donors, oxygen is reduced to hydrogen peroxide (two-electron transfer, Eq. 16)

$$O_2 + 2e \rightleftharpoons O_2^{--} (= H_2O_2) \quad (16)$$

or to water (four-electron transfer, Eq. 17)

$$O_2 + 4e \rightleftharpoons 2O^{--} (= 2H_2O) \quad (17)$$

These oxidases may reduce molecular oxygen only (for example, uricase and cytochrome oxidase); in this case they are oxygen-obligative. If other electron acceptors also serve as substrates (as with glucose oxidase, xanthine oxidase, and others) they are oxygen-facultative. In order to identify an enzyme as an electron-transfer oxidase, it is necessary to show that one molecule of oxygen is consumed per two electrons transferred and that the product is hydrogen peroxide (Eq. 16) or that one molecule of oxygen is consumed per four electrons transferred and that the product is water (Eq. 17). If, as a result of electron loss, the donor molecule is ultimately oxygenated (as with uric acid and xanthine oxidations) it must be shown that the incorporated oxygen atoms arise from the solvent or from oxyanions dissolved in the solvent (Eq. 18; Eq. 19 describes one possible mechanism for this kind of reaction)

$$O_2 + DH + OH^{--} \rightleftharpoons HO_2^- + DOH \quad (18)$$

$$DH \rightleftharpoons D^+ + H^+ + 2e \quad (19)$$
$$D^+ + OH^- \rightleftharpoons DOH$$

whereas hydrogen peroxide and water

formed by these electron transfers must be derived from the atoms of molecular oxygen which have been consumed. A list of the various classes of electron-transfer oxidases follows.

Two-electron transfer, oxygen obligative. Uricase (16).

Two-electron transfer, oxygen-facultative. Xanthine oxidase (17), aldehyde oxidase, glucose oxidase (18), arabinose oxidase, pyruvic oxidase, glycolic oxidase, α-hydroxyacid oxidase, acyl CoA dehydrogenase, monamine oxidase, diamine oxidase, sarcosine oxidase, N-methylamino oxidase, diphosphopyridine nucleotide oxidase, methemoglobin reductase, triphosphopyridine nucleotide oxidase, triphosphopyridine nucleotide-cytochrome reductase, pyrimidine oxidase, and others.

Four-electron transfer oxidases. Laccase, catecholase function of phenolase complex, ascorbic acid oxidase, and cytochrome oxidase.

There are experimental obstacles which make it difficult, if not impossible, to determine whether these enzymes transfer hydrogen as well as electrons to oxygen. In the case of pyridine nucleotide acceptors for two-electron transfer oxidases, transferred hydrogen is fixed and can be detected by tracer techniques, but when molecular oxygen is the electron acceptor, hydrogen which might have been transferred during the formation of hydrogen peroxide or water is readily exchangeable with solvent protons and cannot be identified. For this reason, the expression *electron-transfer oxidase* is preferred.

During formal stepwise addition of two electrons to molecular oxygen, a very reactive free radical intermediate, O_2^- or HO_2 (perhydroxyl) may be formed, and during the formal stepwise

addition of four electrons to molecular oxygen, both perhydroxyl and free hydroxyl may form (Eqs. 20 to 23)

$$O_2 + e \rightleftharpoons O_2^- \text{ or } HO_2 \quad (20)$$

$$HO_2 + e \rightleftharpoons HO_2^- \text{ or } H_2O_2 \quad (21)$$

$$H_2O_2 + e \rightleftharpoons H_2O_2^- \text{ or } H_2O + \cdot OH \quad (22)$$

$$\cdot OH + e \rightleftharpoons OH^- \text{ or } H_2O \quad (23)$$

From a biological point of view, enzymic reduction mechanisms that form these free radicals from molecular oxygen must be disadvantageous to the organism, not only because an energetic random attack on functioning components and structures of the cell must ensue, but also because biochemically efficient utilization of the free energy of these radicals appears to be impossible. It is more likely that the whole process of oxygen reduction takes place in such a manner that intermediate unpairing of electrons, if it occurs at all, occurs under such chemical or spatial constraint that the free radicals which form are essentially independent of the random collision or mass action principle.

Since the mechanisms of enzymic two-electron and four-electron transfers to oxygen have been extensively discussed in recent articles (compare 19, 20) only brief comment on this subject is given here. Two-electron transfers to oxygen may be catalyzed by metalloproteins (for example, uricase, xanthine oxidase, aldehyde oxidase) or by coenzyme-enzyme complexes (for example, glucose oxidase, arabinose oxidase, glycolic oxidase, amino acid oxidases, and others). In the case of the copper-containing, oxygen-obligative enzyme, uricase, evidence has been reported (19) which supports the view that the metal atom provides a locus for the aggregation of both urate

Table 2. Characteristics of mixed-function oxidases.

Name	Cosubstrate	Inhibitors	Essential groups
Phenylalanine hydroxylase	Diphosphopyridine nucleotide	Dipyridyl, N$_3^-$, CN$^-$	Fe^{++}
Imidazoleacetic oxidase (8)	Diphosphopyridine nucleotide		
Nonspecific liver hydroxylase (10)	Triphosphopyridine nucleotide (not DPNH, H$_2$O$_2$, or ascorbate)	Dipyridyl, p-chloromercuribenzoate	Fe^{++}, —SH
Steroid 11-β-hydroxylase (11)	Triphosphopyridine nucleotide	Versene, CN$^-$	Unknown
Kynurenine 3-hydroxylase	Triphosphopyridine nucleotide		Unknown
p-Hydroxyphenyl-pyruvate oxidase	Substrate intermediate	p-Chloromercuribenzoate, diethyldithiocarbamate, N-ethylmaleimide	Cu, SH
Phenolase complex (4)	o-Diphenolic intermediate	CO, CN$^-$, diethyledithiocarbamate	Cu$^+$
Squalene oxidocyclase I (12)	Di- or triphosphopyridine nucleotide		Unknown
Peroxidase hydroxylating system	Dihydroxyfumarate	Mn^{++}, catalase	Heme

and oxygen in a ternary catalytic complex, permitting the transfer of electrons, either singly or in pairs, from urate to oxygen.

Beinert has recently reported that in the oxidation of substrate by the flavoprotein, fatty acyl CoA dehydrogenase, two molecules of enzyme-bound flavin appear to act together (21). They are reduced together to a semiquinonoid state by one molecule of substrate which is thereby converted directly to product without passing through a detached free radical state. It is reasonable to suppose that in the reoxidation of the semiquinonoid enzyme intermediate by oxygen, two electrons are similarly transferred to the oxygen molecule without forming a detached perhydroxyl free radical. It is of interest that the oxygen-facultative, two-electron transfer oxidase, glucose oxidase, also contains two molecules of flavin per molecule of enzyme. If these coenzymes act in concert during the reduction of molecular oxygen to hydrogen peroxide without forming detached perhydroxyl, the absence of indiscriminate radical attack during the action of the enzyme may be explained.

The enzymes which catalyze terminal four-electron transfer to molecular oxygen are all metalloproteins (laccase, ascorbic oxidase, catecholase function of the phenolase complex, and cytochrome oxidase). In these cases, it is usually considered that either four consecutive transfers of single electrons to the bound oxygen molecule occur, or that the electron-transfer oxidase is so organized with respect to substrate that groups of electrons can be transferred simultaneously. This may be accomplished by means of clusters of oxidases bound to the oxygen molecule, each undergoing one-equivalent oxidation-reductions, or by means of two-equivalent (or higher) oxidation-reductions (14).

In the case of oxidases bearing copper or iron at their active centers, this might involve valence states higher than two or three (for example, respectively Cu^{+3}, Cu^{+4}, Fe^{+4}, Fe^{+5}, or Fe^{+6}). In such a case, two-equivalent reduction of molecular oxygen becomes possible without formation of detached free radical intermediates. The evidence mentioned concerning the reactions of hemoproteins with peroxides (14), and electrophilic hydroxylations catalyzed by ferrous iron-oxygen systems (13, 15) suggests that molecular oxygen bound to cytochrome oxidase may undergo two two-electron reduction steps, each step forming a water molecule or hydroxyl anion (Eqs. 24, 25).

$$Fe_c^{++}O_2 + 2e \rightleftharpoons Fe_c^{++}O + O^{--} \quad (24)$$

$$Fe_c^{++}O + 2e \rightleftharpoons Fe_c^{++} + O^{--} \quad (25)$$

The relationship between such a mechanism for the terminal reduction of molecular oxygen to two molecules of water and mechanisms proposed for mixed-function oxidation (types ii and iii) is apparent and is being investigated. It is also apparent that such electron transfer and mixed function systems, acting in reverse with consumption rather than production of energy, afford interesting hypotheses for photosynthetic formation of molecular oxygen.

Summary

The enzymes which catalyze reactions of molecular oxygen occur in three principle classes: (i) oxygen transferases, (ii) mixed function oxidases, and (iii) electron transferases. The first class catalyzes the transfer of a molecule of molecular oxygen to substrate. The second class catalyzes the transfer of one atom of the oxygen to substrate; the other atom undergoes two-equivalent reduction. The third class catalyzes the reduction of molecular oxygen to hydrogen peroxide or to water.

References and Notes

1. W. von E. Doering and E. Dorfman, J. Am. Chem. Soc. 75, 5595 (1953).
2. An extended development and discussion of the ideas proposed here is in press (Advances in Enzymol.). I wish to thank the U.S. Public Health Service, the American Cancer Society, and the National Science Foundation for support, at the University of Oregon Medical School, of research concerned with phases of oxygen metabolism.
3. H. S. Mason, Abstr. 130th Meeting, American Chemical Society, Atlantic City, N.J., September 1956, p. 55C.
4. ———, W. L. Fowlks, E. W. Peterson, J. Am. Chem. Soc. 79, 2914 (1955).
5. The expression oxygen transferase was first used (4, 6) in the present connection in order to maintain a historical continuity in the oxidase field. The general debate on mechanisms of biological oxidation which took place between the schools of Warburg and Wieland, among many others, was concerned in part with the problem of enzymic oxygen transfer. Since tracer study has now demonstrated that oxygen transfer does occur enzymically, the expression oxygen transferase is being used categorically within the limits of a specific definition given in the text. The term oxygenase has recently been suggested for these enzymes (7, 8) because it is succinct, because it is consistent with hydrogenase and because enzymic transfer is being employed in connection with groups or radicals rather than molecules. It is hoped that a consensus of interested investigators on this matter of nomenclature will soon be reached.
6. O. Hayaishi, M. Katagiri, S. Rothberg, J. Am. Chem. Soc. 77, 5450 (1955).
7. O. Hayaishi, personal communications.
8. O. Hayaishi, S. Rothberg, A. H. Mehler, Abstr. 130th Meeting, American Chemical Society, Atlantic City, N.J., September 1956, p. 53C.
9. By substrate is meant the reagent other than molecular oxygen, which is itself a substrate.
10. S. Udenfriend, C. Mitoma, H. S. Posner, Abstr. 130th Meeting, American Chemical Society, Atlantic City, N.J., September 1956, p. 54C.
11. M. Hayano et al., Arch. Biochem. and Biophys. 59, 529 (1955); M. L. Sweat et al., Federation Proc. 15, 237 (1956).
12. T. T. Tchen and K. Bloch, J. Am. Chem. Soc. 78, 1516 (1956), Abstr. 130th Meeting, American Chemical Society, Atlantic City, N.J., September 1956, p. 56C.
13. H. S. Mason and I. Onoprienko, Federation Proc. 15, 310 (1956).
14. P. George, Currents in Biochemical Research, D. Green, Ed. (Interscience, New York, 1956), p. 338.
15. H. S. Mason, I. Onoprienko, D. Buhler, Biochim. et Biophys. Acta 24, 225 (1957).
16. R. Bentley and A. Neuberger, Biochem. J. (London) 52, 694 (1952).
17. I. Onoprienko and H. S. Mason, unpublished results.
18. R. Bentley and A. Neuberger, Biochem. J. (London) 45, 584 (1949).
19. H. R. Mahler, H. M. Baum, G. Hubscher, Science 124, 705 (1956).
20. H. R. Mahler, Advances in Enzymol. 17, 233 (1956); B. Chance and G. P. Williams, Advances in Enzymol. 17, 65 (1956); W. W. Wainio and S. J. Cooperstein, Advances in Enzymol. 17, 329 (1956).
21. H. Beinert, Biochim. et Biophys. Acta 20, 588 (1956).

Editor's Comments on Paper 39

39   **Gibson and Pittard:** Pathways of Biosynthesis of Aromatic Amino Acids and Vitamins
and Their Control in Microorganisms
Bacteriol. Rev., **32**, 465–492 (1968)

The common-pathway concept, however, can be found not only in the oxidation and degradation of aromatic amino acids and hydrocarbons, but also in the biosynthesis of cellular material. The selected paper (Paper 39) is a magnificent summary of the pathways of biosynthesis leading to aromatic amino acids and vitamins. It demonstrates both the common-pathway concept and its individual and common regulation.

$$39$$

Reprinted from *Bacteriol. Rev.*, **32**, 465–492 (1968)

Pathways of Biosynthesis of Aromatic Amino Acids and Vitamins and Their Control in Microorganisms

FRANK GIBSON AND JAMES PITTARD

John Curtin School of Medical Research, Australian National University, Canberra, Australia, and School of Microbiology, University of Melbourne, Australia

INTRODUCTION

The aims of this review are to present an outline of the metabolic pathways leading to the aromatic amino acids and vitamins and to discuss how the flow of intermediates along these pathways is controlled. The general outlines of the pathways to the aromatic amino acids, phenylalanine, tyrosine, and tryptophan have been known for some time, and they were excellently reviewed by Umbarger and Davis (162). Since then, the situation regarding the "branch points" in aromatic biosynthesis has been clarified, and much information on the biochemical genetics

and control of the biosynthesis of aromatic amino acids has accumulated. In addition, the general outlines of the pathways leading to the metabolically important compounds found in small amounts, namely, 4-aminobenzoic acid, ubiquinone, vitamin K, and 2,3-dihydroxybenzoic acid, are partially understood. The latter compounds will be referred to as vitamins.

It is these more recent studies which we intend to emphasize with one important exception, the tryptophan operon. The biochemical genetics of this operon as a whole, and the enzyme tryptophan synthetase in particular, have been studied intensively during recent years. The amount of information now available on these topics warrants a separate review; therefore, it is not our intention to deal with this work in detail. Various aspects of the work have been reviewed (171, 172); other recent general reviews on aromatic biosynthesis generally, or on specific topics, are also available (12, 48). There has been, of necessity, some selection in the papers cited, but further references may readily be found through these.

A general outline of the pathways to be discussed consists of a "common pathway" leading through shikimate to chorismate, after which there is branching to the individual pathways (Fig. 1).

INTERMEDIATES IN AROMATIC BIOSYNTHESIS

Common Pathway

The common pathway involves the condensation of two products of carbohydrate metabolism, phosphoenolpyruvate and erythrose 4-phosphate, to give a straight chain seven-carbon compound which is then cyclized and undergoes a number of reactions through shikimate to chorismate (Fig. 2).

In recent work, the main advance has been the clarification of the region of the branch point (Fig. 1) where, from chorismate, a series of individual pathways diverge. After the establishment of 3-enolpyruvylshikimate 5-phosphate as an intermediate on the common pathway (101,

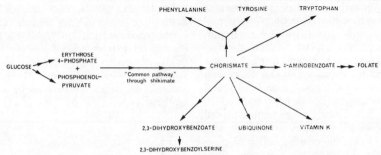

FIG. 1. *General outline of pathways for the formation of aromatic amino acids and vitamins in E. coli.*

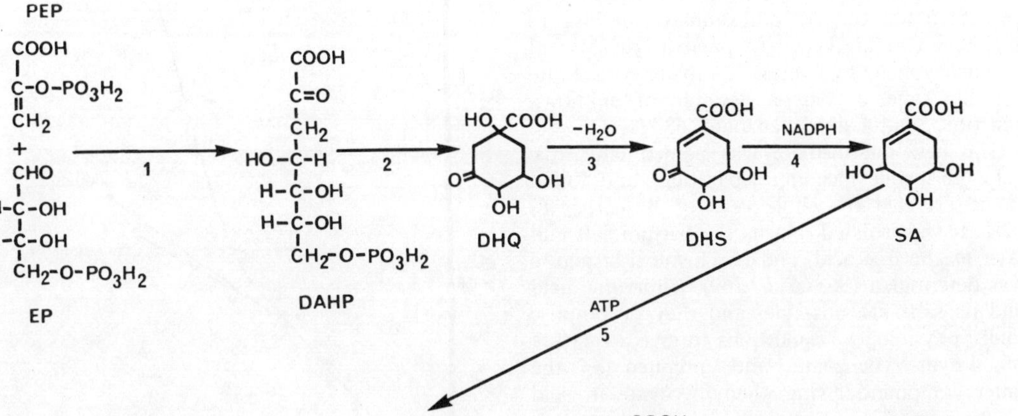

FIG. 2. *Intermediates in the common pathway of aromatic biosynthesis. Abbreviations: PEP, phosphoenolpyruvate; EP, erythrose 4-phosphate; DAHP, 3-deoxy-D-arabino-heptulosonic acid 7-phosphate; DHQ, 5-dehydroquinic acid; DHS, 5-dehydroshikimic acid; SA, shikimic acid; SAP, shikimic acid 5-phosphate; EPSAP, 3-enolpyruvylshikimic acid 5-phosphate; CA, chorismic acid. Trivial names of enzymes and some references to purification and cofactors:- (1), 3-deoxy-D-arabino-heptulosonate 7-phosphate synthetase (DAHP synthetase; 48, 154, 164); (2), 5-dehydroquinate synthetase (153); (3), dehydroshikimate reductase; (4), shikimate kinase; (5), 3-enolpyruvylshikimate 5-phosphate synthetase (102); (6), chorismate synthetase (119).*

102), two groups studying the conversion of shikimate to anthranilate showed that 3-enol-pyruvylshikimate 5-phosphate was a precursor of anthranilate, as well as of phenylpyruvate and 4-hydroxyphenylpyruvate (73, 138). It was suggested that a specific branch point compound was involved, and this compound was sought by examining a mutant in which the pathways to tryptophan, tyrosine, and phenylalanine were blocked (71, 72).

Using ultraviolet irradiation followed by penicillin selection, a strain requiring both tryptophan and tyrosine was isolated from a tryptophan auxotroph which accumulated anthranilate. The double mutant was then treated to obtain the triple mutant (*Aerobacter aerogenes* 62-1), in which tryptophan and tyrosine were essential for growth, whereas phenylalanine stimulated growth. Cell-free extracts were prepared from this strain grown with excess tryptophan to repress the enzyme system forming anthranilate. These cell extracts formed a new compound from a mixture of shikimate, ribose-5-phosphate, adenosine triphosphate (ATP), and Mg^{2+}. This compound could be converted to anthranilate in the presence of glutamine by cell extracts of a multiple aromatic auxotroph with a metabolic block immediately after 3-enol-pyruvylshikimate 5-phosphate. The new compound was readily isolated on paper chromato-grams and could be shown to be enzymically converted not only to anthranilate but also to prephenate (and thence to phenylpyruvate and 4-hydroxyphenylpyruvate), 4-hydroxybenzoate (at that time, a bacterial vitamin of unknown function), and 4-aminobenzoate (68, 71, 72).

The new intermediate was named chorismic acid (chorismic meaning separating) and found to be excreted by whole cells of *A. aerogenes* 62-1. It was isolated first as the barium salt and later as the free acid, and its chemical structure was determined (56, 66, 67, 69). Chorismic acid and its salts are unstable, and they decompose under physiological conditions to give a mixture of 4-hydroxybenzoate and prephenate, the latter compound giving phenylpyruvate in acid solution (66, 72).

Chorismate, presumably because of a permea-bility barrier, does not act as a growth factor that will replace the amino acid or vitamin require-ments of multiple aromatic auxotrophs. The instability of chorismate at 37 C (66) necessitates the detection of any growth response during a short period after its addition. Figure 3 shows the results of an experiment in which the ability of chorismate to substitute for the 4-amino-benzoate requirement of a multiple aromatic auxotroph (a mutant unable to carry out a

reaction of the common pathway) of *Escherichia coli* was tested. The concentration of 4-amino-benzoate required for half-maximal growth of such an auxotroph is about 10^{-8} M, but the addi-tion of a large excess of chorismate (5×10^{-4} M) did not support growth. The addition of dimethyl-sulfoxide (5%), which has been shown to increase cellular permeability (61), did not affect the results.

The instability of chorismate and its inability to promote growth probably were factors in the branch point compound not being discovered earlier. Metzenberg and Mitchell (115) examined a mutant of *Neurospora crassa*, which probably accumulated chorismate, in an attempt to find a branch point compound, but they found pre-phenate among other compounds.

Chorismate has also been isolated from culture fluids of *E. coli* (107), *N. crassa* (41), and *Sac-charomyces cerevisiae* (107), and it is also metabo-lized by cell extracts from *Lactobacillus arabinosus* (103), *N. crassa* (41), *Claviceps paspalis* (106), yeast (50, 104), and plants (27), indicating the general role of the compound in aromatic bio-synthesis.

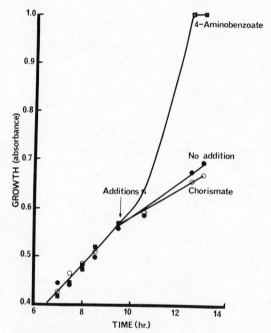

FIG. 3. *Inability of chorismate to replace the 4-aminobenzoate requirement of a multiple aromatic auxotroph (E. coli AB2839). Growth tests were carried out as described previously (174). Medium contained multiple aromatic supplement with 4-aminobenzoate limiting growth at an absorbance of about 0.6. 4-Amino-benzoate (10^{-6} M) or chorismate (5×10^{-4} M) was added at time indicated.*

Early experiments on the incorporation of ¹⁴C-glucose into aromatic amino acids in *A. aerogenes* were not consistent with the scheme as outlined, and they suggested that the shikimate ring was not used, as such, as a precursor of the aromatic amino acids (*for references, see* 149). However, similar experiments have now been carried out with *E. coli* (149), giving results which are consistent with the pathway of aromatic biosynthesis as it is now understood.

Tryptophan Pathway

No new intermediates in the tryptophan pathway have been found recently, and the pathway is as set out in Fig. 4.

The postulated intermediate, *N*-(5'-phosphoribosyl)-anthranilate, has not been isolated and chemically characterized. Its existence has been recognized by the enzymic formation of a compound with a lower intensity of fluorescence than that of anthranilate by cell extracts of *E. coli*, *A. aerogenes*, *Salmonella typhimurium*, *Saccharomyces cerevisiae*, and *Pseudomonas aeruginosa* (45, 50, 51, 57). The compound is very labile (*see* 44), particularly under acid conditions, breaking down to regenerate anthranilate. Further evidence that the labile compound is an intermediate in tryptophan biosynthesis is provided by the observation that it is formed by cell extracts from some tryptophan auxotrophs, whereas extracts from other tryptophan auxotrophs will convert it to more stable compounds further along the tryptophan pathway (51).

Because of the complexity of the reaction catalyzed by anthranilate synthetase, intermediates between chorismate and anthranilate have been proposed (102, 108, 136, 151). The enzymic evidence suggests that a protein complex metabolizes chorismate through anthranilate to *N*-(5'-phosphoribosyl)-anthranilate. Evidence that it is possible to trap an intermediate has been obtained by Somerville and Elford (147), who found that partially purified anthranilate synthetase from *E. coli* would catalyze the formation of a hydroxamate when incubated with chorismate, glutamine, and hydroxylamine. Although the structure of the hydroxamate is not yet known, the evidence obtained suggests that the overall conversion of chorismate to anthranilate may be separable into two steps, the first utilizing glutamine and the second being dependent on Mg²⁺. Several possible intermediates have been tested, but they do not serve as precursors of anthranilate (108, 151). Any mechanistic scheme for the amination of chorismate must take into account the finding of Srinivasan (151) that the amide nitrogen of glutamine is transferred to the carbon 2 of chorismate (Fig. 4). (The numbering of the carbons in compounds of the common pathway is conventionally taken from the numbering of shikimic acid, which is itself incorrect because the order of numbering should be through the double bond and not away from it.) This information was gained by growing a tryptophan auxotroph in a medium containing (3,4-¹⁴C)-glucose and determining the distribution of the ¹⁴C-labeled atoms in the excreted anthranilate. A comparison of the distribution of the ¹⁴C-label in shikimate isolated from cultures of the appropriate mutant during earlier experiments with the distribution of label in the ¹⁴C-anthranilate showed the position of insertion of the nitrogen atom.

The source of the nitrogen atom for anthranilate formation has been the subject of a number of studies. In the earlier experiments (150, 152),

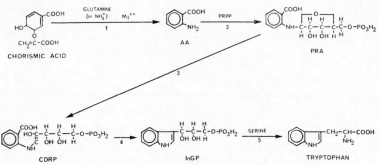

FIG. 4. *Intermediates in the tryptophan pathway. Abbreviations:- AA, anthranilic acid; PRA, N-(5'-phosphoribosyl)-anthranilic acid; CDRP, 1-(o-carboxyphenylamino)-1-deoxyribulose 5-phosphate; InGP, indoleglycerol phosphate. Trivial names of enzymes and some recent references to purification and cofactors:- (1), anthranilate synthetase (123); (2), anthranilate-5'-phosphoribosyl-1-pyrophosphate phosphoribosyl transferase (PR transferase); (3), N-(5'-phosphoribosyl)-anthranilate isomerase (35); (4), indoleglycerol phosphate synthetase (35); (5), tryptophan synthetase (34, 81, 169).*

it seemed that L-glutamine was the likely source of the nitrogen atom and that the amide nitrogen of glutamine was utilized (55, 152). A reexamination of this problem (55) showed that, if buffered at high *p*H, ammonium ions in relatively high concentrations would serve as an effective nitrogen source for anthranilate formation by crude cell extracts of *A. aerogenes*. Furthermore, it has been possible to obtain evidence that ammonium ions may be used for anthranilate formation directly in vivo rather than via glutamine as an obligate intermediate (70). Thus, cell suspensions of a double auxotroph that required tryptophan and were unable to form glutamine excreted anthranilate when incubated in a glucose-NH_4^+ salts-buffer mixture.

Pathways to Phenylalanine and Tyrosine

The intermediates between chorismate, phenylalanine, and tyrosine, namely, prephenate, phenylpyruvate and 4-hydroxyphenylpyruvate (Fig. 5), have been known for a number of years (162). These intermediates are concerned in the phenylalanine and tyrosine pathways in *E. coli*, *A. aerogenes*, *Saccharomyces cerevisiae*, and *N. crassa* (8, 105, 162).

Although no new intermediates have been discovered, it has been found that the details of the pathway in different organisms vary in the way in which the known intermediates are metabolized.

Pathway to 4-Aminobenzoic Acid

The molecule of folic acid (Fig. 6) contains a benzene moiety which is inserted as 4-aminobenzoic acid (16); the biosynthesis of the latter compound is being studied at present. Some multiple aromatic auxotrophs were shown to require 4-aminobenzoate for growth (38), and it seems that whether a requirement is shown by

such an auxotroph depends on the completeness of the metabolic block in the common pathway. "Leaky" mutants will allow sufficient flow of intermediates along the common pathway to satisfy the requirement for aromatic vitamins. Weiss and Srinivasan (166) showed that 4-aminobenzoate could be formed from shikimate 5-phosphate plus glutamine by cell-free extracts of bakers' yeast. It was then shown (155) that the amide nitrogen of glutamine was the precursor of the amino group in the aromatic amine by using ^{15}N-labeled glutamine and studying the effect of glutamine analogues on the conversion.

The fact that mutants blocked between 3-enolpyruvylshikimate 5-phosphate and chorismate required 4-aminobenzoate for growth in addition to the amino acids (40) indicated that chorismate might well be a precursor of the bacterial vitamin. Cell-free extracts of the strain which accumulated chorismate (*A. aerogenes* 62-1) were found to convert chorismate to 4-aminobenzoate in the presence of L-glutamine (68). Two different approaches to the problem of 4-aminobenzoate synthesis are currently being used. Mutants of both *N. crassa* (52) and *E. coli* (83) requiring 4-aminobenzoate for growth have been divided into two classes by genetic mapping. Hendler and Srinivasan (80) reported "cross-feeding" between the mutant strains of *N. crassa*, but no "cross-feeding" was found by Huang and Pittard (83) with the *E. coli* auxotrophs. The existence of different classes of mutants suggested that at least two reactions were involved in the specific pathway for the synthesis of the vitamin, that is, between chorismate and 4-aminobenzoate. More direct biochemical evidence now supports this concept.

Cell extracts of yeast have been fractionated by ammonium sulfate treatment yielding two

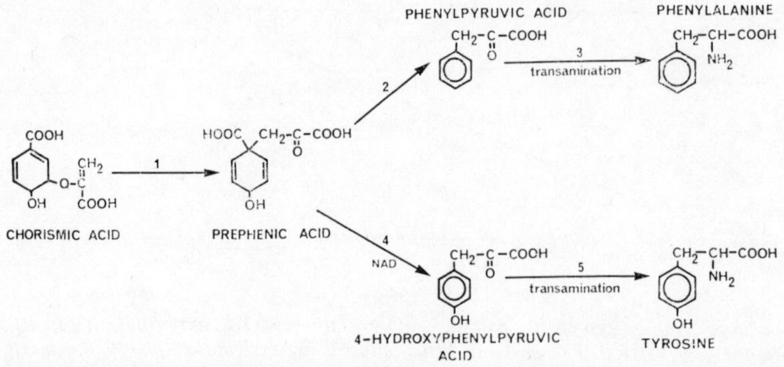

FIG. 5. *Intermediates in the biosynthesis of phenylalanine and tyrosine. Trivial names of enzymes:- (1), chorismate mutase; (2), prephenate dehydratase; (3), phenylalanine transaminase; (4), prephenate dehydrogenase; (5), tyrosine transaminase.*

fractions, neither of which alone forms 4-amino-benzoate from chorismate plus glutamine, but the two fractions do so when mixed (80). Evidence for an intermediate in *E. coli* has been obtained by the use of cell extracts from suitable mutants (M. Huang, *unpublished data*). The two mutations affecting 4-aminobenzoate synthesis have been transferred into a strain of *E. coli* K-12 unable to convert chorismate along the pathways to the amino acids. Cell extracts from the resulting strains have been tested for their ability to convert chorismate into 4-aminobenzoate. Neither extract alone will carry out the conversion, which is, however, carried out by a mixture of the two extracts. The little that is known about 4-amino-benzoate synthesis in *E. coli* is shown in Fig. 7.

Intermediates in Ubiquinone Biosynthesis

Ubiquinone occurs in a wide variety of microorganisms and other cells (32). The structure of ubiquinone is shown in Fig. 8. The number of isoprenoid units in the side chain varies with the species (32), although ubiquinones with varying numbers of isoprenoid units may be isolated

FOLIC ACID

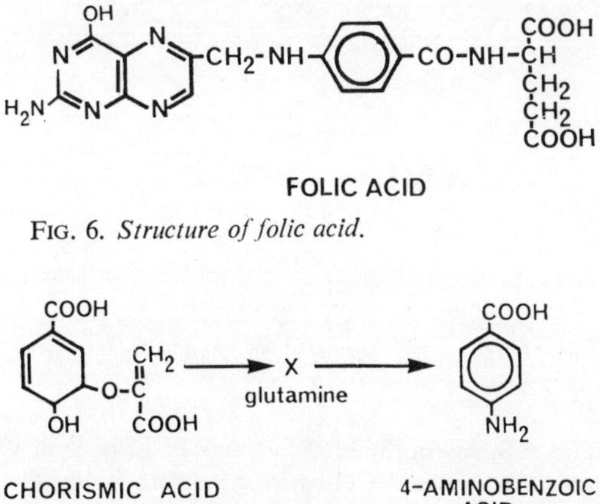

FIG. 6. *Structure of folic acid.*

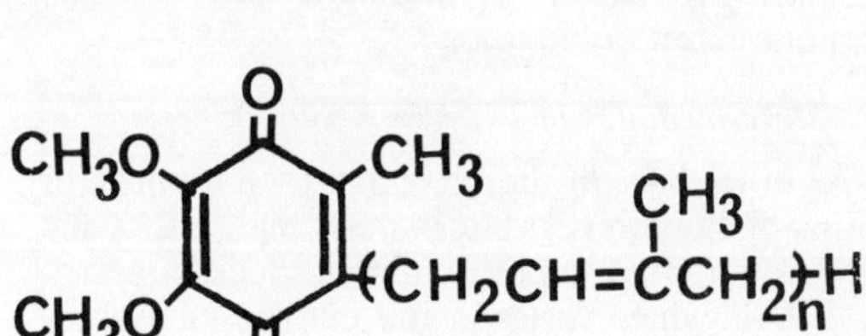

CHORISMIC ACID   **4-AMINOBENZOIC ACID**

FIG. 7. *Biosynthesis of 4-aminobenzoic acid.*

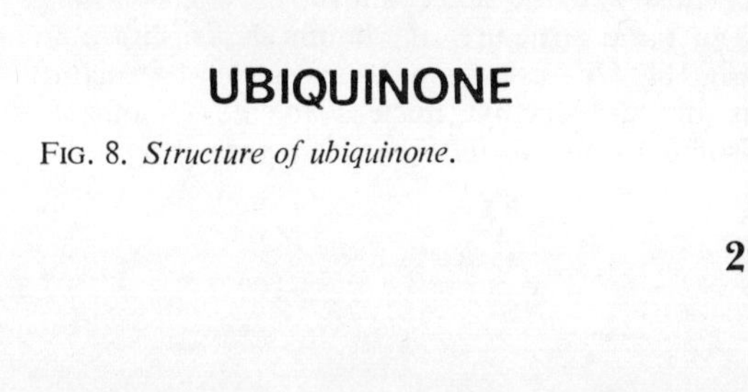

UBIQUINONE

FIG. 8. *Structure of ubiquinone.*

from the one organism (64, 92). In *E. coli* and *A. aerogenes*, the ubiquinone with a forty-carbon atom side chain is the predominant form. We are concerned here with the quinone nucleus of ubiquinone, which is derived from an aromatic precursor.

The observation of Rudney and Parson (139) that ^{14}C-4-hydroxybenzaldehyde was incorporated into the benzoquinone ring of ubiquinone in *Rhodospirillum rubrum* provided the first definite evidence for an intermediate in ubiquinone biosynthesis. ^{14}C-4-Hydroxybenzoic acid, as well as the aldehyde, was then shown to be incorporated into ubiquinone in *Azotobacter vinelandii*, bakers' yeast and rat kidney (129) and *R. rubrum* (130). The relationship of ubiquinone to the shikimic acid pathway was shown by the demonstration that ^{14}C-shikimic acid was incorporated into ubiquinone in *E. coli* (28). In the latter experiments, it was shown that an excess of unlabeled 4-hydroxybenzoate in the medium together with the ^{14}C-shikimate "swamped" the labeling of ubiquinone, providing further evidence that 4-hydroxybenzoate lay on the pathway.

4-Hydroxybenzoate had been shown to have vitamin-like activity for multiple aromatic auxotrophs of *E. coli* many years before (37), although the requirement was not an absolute one. Multiple aromatic auxotrophs of *E. coli* growing on a glucose-mineral-salts medium supplemented with the aromatic amino acids and 4-aminobenzoate formed ubiquinone only when 4-hydroxybenzoic acid was added (29). However, in similar experiments with multiple aromatic auxotrophs of *A. aerogenes*, ubiquinone was formed, suggesting that an alternative pathway to ubiquinone may exist in these cells. Experiments with cell-free extracts of *A. aerogenes* (29; F. Gibson and R. Bayly, *unpublished data*) indicate 4-hydroxybenzoate is formed from tyrosine (Fig. 9), although the conversion of 4-hydroxyphenylpyruvate to 4-hydroxybenzaldehyde occurs spontaneously at physiological *p*H; it is not known whether there is an enzyme carrying out this step (130). Under conditions where extracts of *A. aerogenes* readily convert 4-hydroxybenzaldehyde to 4-hydroxybenzoate, extracts of *E. coli* K-12 are unable to do so, probably accounting for the inability of the multiple aromatic auxotrophs of the latter strain to form ubiquinone, although there is tyrosine in the medium.

The pathway from 4-hydroxybenzoate to ubiquinone is not well established, but the complete sequence shown in Fig. 10 has been proposed (63). A number of isoprenoid compounds have been isolated from cells of *R. rubrum* and *P. ovalis* (63, 65, 128, 129), and the plausible scheme of Fig. 10 has been advanced. However, it should

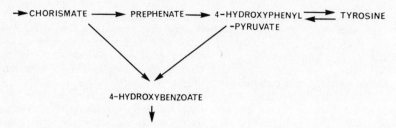

FIG. 9. *Alternative pathways of 4-hydroxybenzoate formation.*

be emphasized that not all of the compounds set out in Fig. 10 have been isolated; furthermore, other related compounds not in the scheme have been isolated (65). The only reaction which has been studied with cell-free extracts is the conversion of chorismate into 4-hydroxybenzoate (71). Recently, this reaction was studied in greater detail and the enzyme was partially purified (I. G. Young, *unpublished data*). The results of investigation of other reactions of the proposed pathway, with cell-free enzymes, are awaited with interest.

Another approach to the problem of the biosynthesis of ubiquinone is to isolate mutants unable to carry out specific reactions in the pathway and to look for accumulated precursors. This approach has been used with *E. coli* K-12, but ubiquinone does not give a growth response and is not required for growth in a glucose-mineralsalts medium. Hence, the usual methods of mutant selection cannot be used. However, an indirect method of selection has been developed (31) which is based on the assumption that ubiquinone is essential for electron transport and that, therefore, a ubiquinoneless strain of *E. coli* would grow fermentatively on a glucose medium but be unable to grow on a reduced substrate such as malate or succinate as sole source of carbon. By testing strains of the desired phenotype for their ability to form ubiquinone, a number of ubiquinoneless strains were isolated (31; G. B. Cox, *unpublished data*). One of the strains contains two mutations affecting ubiquinone biosynthesis (31). These mutations have been separated, by conjugation, into different strains. Examination of these strains for accumulated intermediates has shown that one of them (*ubiA⁻*) accumulates 4-hydroxybenzoate and the other (*ubiB⁻*) accumulates octaprenylphenol (G. B. Cox, *unpublished data*). The continuation of this approach should yield further information about the biosynthesis of ubiquinone.

The methyl group of methionine has been shown to serve as the source of the methoxymethyl groups and the ring-methyl group of ubiquinone in *Mycobacterium phlei* and *E. coli* (90, 91).

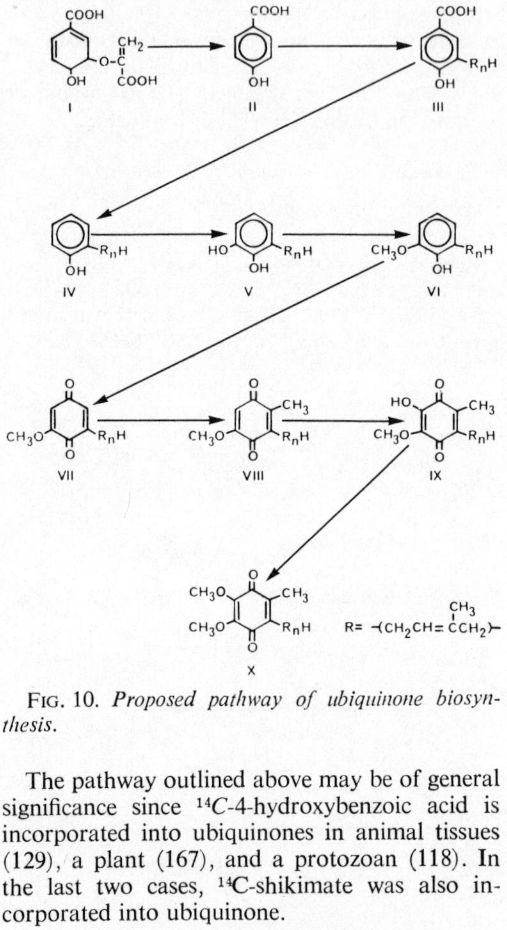

FIG. 10. *Proposed pathway of ubiquinone biosynthesis.*

The pathway outlined above may be of general significance since ^{14}C-4-hydroxybenzoic acid is incorporated into ubiquinones in animal tissues (129), a plant (167), and a protozoan (118). In the last two cases, ^{14}C-shikimate was also incorporated into ubiquinone.

Intermediates in Vitamin K Biosynthesis

As in the case of the ubiquinones, a number of forms of vitamin K occur in microbial cells. They have a common naphthoquinone nucleus and a side chain which varies in the number of isoprenoid units and the degree of saturation and stereochemistry of the side chain (6, 32, 53, 86, 143). The basic structure of vitamin K is shown in Fig. 11. One exception to this general structure is the 2-desmethyl nucleus in the vitamin K isolated from *Haemophilus influenzae* (100).

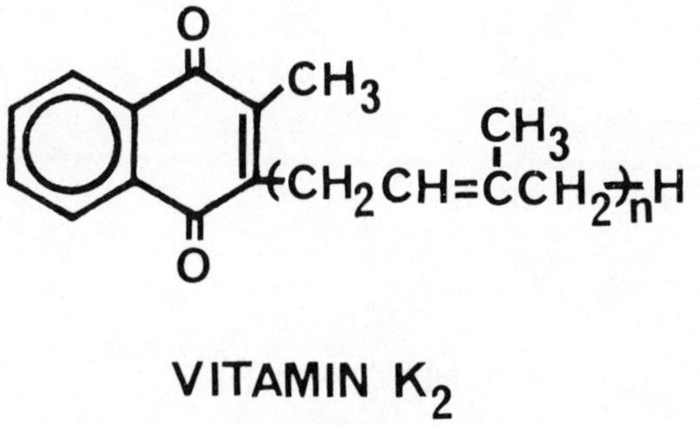

VITAMIN K$_2$

FIG. 11. *Structure of vitamin K$_2$.*

Virtually nothing was known about the biosynthesis of the naphthoquinone nucleus of vitamin K until 1964, when it was observed that *E. coli* growing in the presence of ^{14}C-shikimate incorporated the label into the naphthoquinone nucleus (28). It was later shown that the shikimate was incorporated into the benzene ring of the naphthoquinone (29). More recently, evidence has been obtained that the carboxyl group of shikimate is incorporated into vitamin K (19) and also into a plant naphthoquinone (177).

It is likely that the branch point from the common pathway for vitamin K biosynthesis is at chorismate, although the fact that chorismate does not act as a growth factor means that incorporation of ^{14}C-chorismate by the use of whole cells cannot be tested. However, a multiple aromatic auxotroph of *A. aerogenes* blocked between 3-enolpyruvylshikimate 5-phosphate and chorismate did not form vitamin K (29), and an excess of unlabeled phenylpyruvate or 4-hydroxyphenylpyruvate did not "swamp" the labeling of vitamin K formed from ^{14}C-shikimate. The possibility still remains that the branch point is at prephenate.

The pathway from the branch point to vitamin K is at present unknown. Two compounds, 3,4-dihydroxybenzaldehyde and α-naphthol, have been suggested as possible intermediates. In early experiments, it was found that a compound with some growth factor activity for multiple aromatic auxotrophs, 3,4-dihydroxybenzaldehyde (39), would "swamp" the incorporation of ^{14}C-shikimate into vitamin K, although the effect was not as marked as the effect of 4-hydroxybenzoate on the incorporation of label into ubiquinone (28). Recently, it has been shown that ^3H-3,4-dihydroxybenzaldehyde is not incorporated into vitamin K in *E. coli*, *Bacillus subtilis*, or *M. phlei* (19, 98), although the results of the swamping experiment in *E. coli* were confirmed (98). α-Naphthol has been suggested as a precursor of vitamin K (98), following the observation that

^{14}C-α-naphthol is incorporated into vitamin K. Further evidence is needed, preferably with cell-free systems, to establish that α-naphthol is directly on the pathway of vitamin K biosynthesis and to clarify the effects observed with 3,4-dihydroxybenzaldehyde. No satisfactory system for the formation of the naphthoquinone nucleus of vitamin K by cell-free extracts has been devised, despite one promising report (4, 5).

It has been established for a number of organisms that the 2-methyl group of the quinone nucleus of vitamin K, like that of ubiquinone, is derived from methionine (4, 90, 91, 97).

As in studies of ubiquinone biosynthesis, the isolation of suitable mutants would assist in the search for possible intermediates. One mutant of *E. coli* K-12 unable to form vitamin K was isolated during a search for ubiquinoneless mutants (31) and is being examined for possible accumulation products, but a rational procedure for the isolation of mutants blocked in the specific pathway of biosynthesis of vitamin K has yet to be devised.

Pathways Involving 2,3-Dihydroxybenzoate

The importance of 2,3-dihydroxybenzoate in bacterial metabolism was emphasized recently with the observation that it is an essential growth factor for some multiple aromatic auxotrophs of *E. coli* (30, 174). However, it has been known for some time that 2,3-dihydroxybenzoate and certain compounds containing the phenolic acid are formed by microbial cells. Ito and Neilands (88) isolated 2,3-dihydroxybenzoylglycine from the culture media of *B. subtilis* growing in an iron-deficient medium. Since then, 2,3-dihydroxybenzoate and related compounds have been identified as metabolic products formed by other organisms including *A. aerogenes* (132), *C. paspali* (3), *Aspergillus niger* (160), *Streptomyces griseus* (54), *S. rimosus* (21) and *E. coli* (15, 174). In *C. paspali* (161) and *Aspergillus niger* (156), it appears that 2,3-dihydroxybenzoate may be formed from tryptophan, but in *A. aerogenes* and *E. coli*, it is formed more directly from chorismate. Crude cell extracts of *A. aerogenes* 62-1 (174) or of a similar mutant of *E. coli* K-12 (R. K. J. Luke, *unpublished data*) form 2,3-dihydroxybenzoate when incubated with chorismate, Mg^{2+} and nicotinamide mononucleotide (NAD). The pathway in *A. aerogenes* has been examined in detail (Fig. 12). Evidence for at least two steps in the conversion of chorismate to 2,3-dihydroxybenzoate was provided by the observation that crude extracts of *A. aerogenes* continued to form 2,3-dihydroxybenzoate after all the chorismate had been removed. When NAD was not added

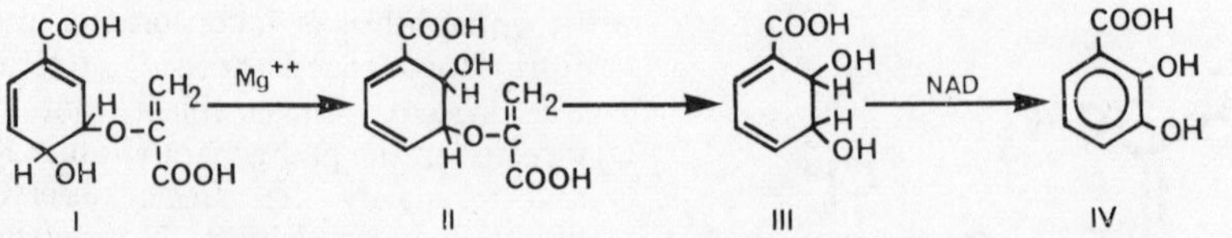

FIG. 12. *Conversion of chorismate (I) to 2,3-dihydroxybenzoate (IV) through isochorismate (II) and 2,3-dihydro-2,3-dihydroxybenzoate (III).*

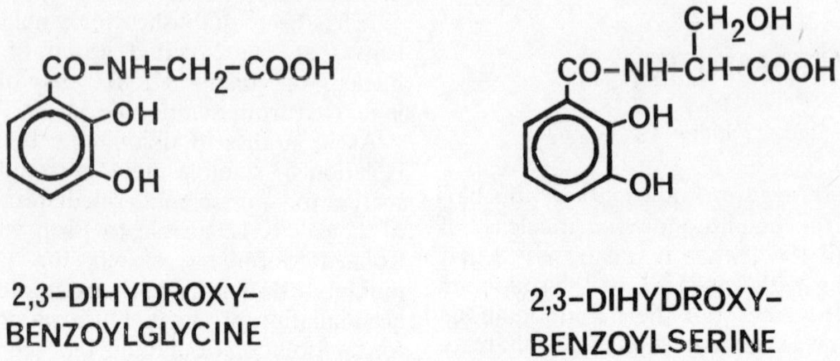

2,3-DIHYDROXY-
BENZOYLGLYCINE

2,3-DIHYDROXY-
BENZOYLSERINE

FIG. 13. *Structures of 2,3-dihydroxybenzoylglycine and 2,3-dihydroxybenzoylserine.*

to the reaction mixture, chorismate was removed at about the same rate as when NAD was added. The compound formed by metabolism of chorismate in the absence of NAD was isolated, examined by nuclear magnetic resonance and mass spectrometry (175; I. G. Young, *unpublished data*), and identified as 2,3-dihydro-2,3-dihydroxybenzoic acid (Fig. 12).

Fractionation of crude extracts of *A. aerogenes* 62-1 by chromatography on diethylaminoethyl (DEAE) cellulose gave a fraction which formed an intermediate capable of being converted to 2,3-dihydro-2,3-dihydroxybenzoate and to 2,3-dihydroxybenzoate (I. G. Young, *unpublished data*). The new intermediate, for which the trivial name isochorismic acid is suggested, is very unstable but has been isolated and identified (I. G. Young, T. J. Batterham, and F. Gibson, *unpublished data*) as the compound II of Fig. 12.

The functional form of 2,3-dihydroxybenzoate is not known. As mentioned above, 2,3-dihydroxybenzoylglycine (Fig. 13) is formed by *B. subtilis*. A similar compound formed by *E. coli* was tentatively identified as 2,3-dihydroxybenzoylserine (15). The structure of the serine conjugate (Fig. 13) excreted by *E. coli* and *A. aerogenes* has recently been established by synthesis and by comparison with the natural product (I. G. O'Brien, *unpublished data*).

It has been observed that these compounds are formed in large quantities when cells are grown in iron-deficient media (14, 88; B. R. Byers and C. E. Lankford, Bacteriol. Proc., p. 43, 1967). The enzymes forming 2,3-dihydroxybenzoate in *A.*

aerogenes (174) and the enzyme system converting 2,3-dihydroxybenzoate to 2,3-dihydroxybenzoylserine in *E. coli* (14) are strongly repressed by iron or cobalt ions. Iron (or in one case, manganese ions) will replace the 2,3-dihydroxybenzoate requirement of multiple aromatic auxotrophs (174). These observations support the suggestion of Ito and Neilands that the glycine conjugate might play an important role in iron transport (88). However, the effects of other metals may mean that these phenolic compounds are also important in the metabolism of metals other than iron.

Mutants of *E. coli* K-12 requiring 2,3-dihydroxybenzoylserine have been isolated to aid in the study of the biosynthetic pathway and for studies on function (R. K. J. Luke, *unpublished data*).

Other Phenolic Growth Factors

Other phenols have been found to act as growth factors. Tyrosine or lower concentrations of phenols such as protocatechuic acid or catechol acted as growth factors for a species of *Sarcina* (77) or *Micrococcus lysodeikticus* (140). The pathways to these compounds are not known in the above organisms; however, in *N. crassa*, protocatechuic acid is formed from the common pathway intermediate, 5-dehydroshikimic acid (78). This compound has also been shown as the source of both protocatechuic acid and catechol in *A. aerogenes* by experiments with whole cells (133) and cell extracts (A. F. Egan, *unpublished data*).

A species of *Pseudomonas* can convert anthranilate into catechol (157).

ISOENZYMES AND PROTEIN AGGREGATES CONCERNED IN AROMATIC BIOSYNTHESIS

Although not all of the reactions concerned in aromatic biosynthesis have been studied in detail, a number of interesting features have been revealed. These include the occurrence of isoenzymes, protein aggregates carrying out more than one reaction, and the catalysis of two reactions by one polypeptide. A brief survey of the occurrence of these features in the various pathways follows, and some aspects will be dealt with in more detail when discussing metabolic regulation of the various pathways of biosynthesis.

Common Pathway

Isoenzymes have been found for three of the reactions of the common pathway. 3-Deoxy-D-*arabino*-heptulosonate 7-phosphate synthetase (DAHP synthetase), the first enzyme, has an important function in the regulation of aromatic biosynthesis and will be discussed in detail. Inhibitor studies, ammonium sulfate fractionation, and column chromatography have provided evidence for the presence of isoenzymes of DAHP synthetase (often three) in a wide variety of microorganisms (17, 48, 49, 62, 93, 94, 145, 163, 164), of which the best studied are *E. coli* and *N. crassa*. In *B. subtilis*, however, only a single DAHP synthetase is present (96), as judged by the results of enzyme purification, inhibitors, and the isolation of auxotrophic mutants lacking DAHP synthetase activity, which are the result of single-step revertible mutations.

Although multiple aromatic auxotrophs of *N. crassa* that lack shikimate kinase activity may be isolated (74), no similar mutants have been reported from the widely studied species of *E. coli*, *A. aerogenes*, *S. typhimurium*, and *B. subtilis*. The presence of two distinct shikimate kinases in *S. typhimurium* (120), and possibly in *B. subtilis* (125), probably accounts for the lack of shikimate kinase mutants in this species, and a similar explanation may apply to the other species. In *N. crassa*, however, no auxotrophs lacking dehydroquinase were isolated, and again it was possible to demonstrate the presence of two enzymes (75); one of the enzymes was constitutive and the other was inducible.

In two organisms, *B. subtilis* and *N. crassa*, protein aggregates carrying out more than one reaction on the common pathway have been described. A single revertible mutation in one strain of *B. subtilis*, resulting in loss of chorismate mutase activity, gave a strain which simultaneously lost DAHP synthetase activity. Gel filtration of cell extracts suggested that one of the shikimate kinases might also be complexed with the two enzymes mentioned (125). All the enzymes of the common pathway, with the exception of the first (DAHP synthetase) and the last (chorismate synthetase), are associated as a multienzyme complex in *N. crassa* (74).

Tryptophan Pathway

One of the best examples studied of a protein aggregate is the terminal enzyme in tryptophan biosynthesis in *E. coli*, tryptophan synthetase, which can be separated into two proteins, A and B (34, 171). Tryptophan synthetase from *S. typhimurium* is also dissociable, but that from *N. crassa* is not dissociable, although it shows many similarities to the *E. coli* enzyme (13). Although there are five recognizable reactions in the specific pathway of tryptophan biosynthesis, it seems that in *E. coli* there are only three enzymic steps, since anthranilate synthetase and 5'-phosphoribosyl-1-pyrophosphate phosphoribosyl (PR) transferase activities are associated

TABLE 1. *Combination of PR transferase from A. aerogenes with anthranilate synthetase from E. coli*

Strain[a]	Anthranilate synthetase		PR transferase	
	Approx molecular weight	Inhibition by tryptophan	Approx molecular weight	Inhibition by tryptophan
A. aerogenes (wild type)	170,000	+	170,000	+
A. aerogenes NC3	Activity not detectable		90,000	−
E. coli K-12 (wild type)	170,000	+	170,000	+
A. aerogenes NC3, and *E. coli* D 9778[b]	170,000	+	170,000	+

[a] Anthranilate synthetase activity was not detectable in *A. aerogenes* NC3. No activity was detectable in *E. coli* D 9778.
[b] *E. coli* D 9778 was obtained from C. Yanofsky.

in a protein complex (89), *N*-(5'-phosphoribosyl)-anthranilate isomerase and indoleglycerol phosphate synthetase activities are carried by the same polypeptide (35), and tryptophan synthetase carries out the final step.

Anthranilate synthetase is evidently associated with PR transferase in *E. coli* (89) and *S. typhimurium* (10, 11), since the two activities travel together during ultracentrifugation in sucrose gradients. Also, it was observed (89) that a nonsense mutation affecting the *D* gene coding for PR transferase activity in *E. coli* affected anthranilate synthetase activity, although the latter could be detected on mixing extracts of such cells with extract from cells in which the anthranilate synthetase was affected by a mutation affecting the *E* gene. Purification of the protein complex from *E. coli* results in loss of PR transferase activity because of instability (C. Yanofsky, *personal communication*). However, purification of anthranilate synthetase from *A. aerogenes* simultaneously purifies the second activity (57; A. F. Egan, *unpublished data*). Furthermore, it is possible to obtain evidence that anthranilate synthetase from *E. coli* K-12, which is inactive alone, will combine with the PR transferase from *A. aerogenes* to form an active complex (89; A. F. Egan, *unpublished data*). This evidence is summarized in Table 1. Thus, anthranilate synthetase and PR transferase in wild-type cells of these strains form a protein aggregate with a molecular weight of about 170,000, and both reactions are inhibited by tryptophan. The mutant of *A. aerogenes* (NC3) lacking anthranilate synthetase activity contains PR transferase activity which has a lower molecular weight, as judged by sucrose gradient centrifugation, than that in extracts from wild type, and it has lost its sensitivity to tryptophan. The mutant strain of *E. coli* used (D9778) has lost PR transferase activity and anthranilate synthetase activity owing to a mutation in the gene coding for PR transferase activity (89). When crude cell extracts from the mutants are incubated together and examined by centrifugation in a sucrose gradient, there is found a peak of anthranilate synthetase—PR

transferase activity with the molecular weight and sensitivity to tryptophan of the aggregate from wild type *A. aerogenes* or *E. coli*.

It has recently been found that PR transferase activity is not necessary for anthranilate synthetase activity in *P. putida* and that anthranilate synthetase itself in this organism is separable into two components (S. W. Queener and I. C. Gunsalus, Bacteriol. Proc., p. 136, 1968).

It can be seen that in *E. coli* (89) and *S. typhimurium* (10) anthranilate synthetase activity is the result of aggregation of two polypeptides. Similar combinations of polypeptides have been demonstrated for enzymes of the tryptophan pathway in a variety of organisms, but the relationships between the genes and the enzymes vary with the species. This point is well illustrated by reference to an extensive study by Hütter and DeMoss (84) of the biochemistry and genetics of a variety of microorganisms, particularly fungi.

Phenylalanine and Tyrosine Pathways

Examination of chorismate mutase activity in *A. aerogenes* by chromatography of cell extracts showed that there were two enzymes (24). One of these activities (chorismate mutase P) was associated with the next enzymic activity on the phenylalanine pathway, namely, prephenate dehydratase (*see* Fig. 5), and both activities were absent in a phenylalanine auxotroph. The protein carrying out these activities was named the P protein. The second chorismate mutase (T) is associated with prephenate dehydrogenase. This protein aggregate from *A. aerogenes* has been highly purified (R. G. H. Cotton, *unpublished data*) and is dissociable into two subunits, neither of which alone has either chorismate mutase or prephenate dehydrogenase activity (25, 26). Both activities of the T protein may be lost as the result of a single revertible mutation (24). The pathways in *A. aerogenes* 62-1 may be represented as in Fig. 14. The pathways in *E. coli* appear to be the same as in Fig. 14, but a mutant has been found in *E. coli* that has lost prephenate de

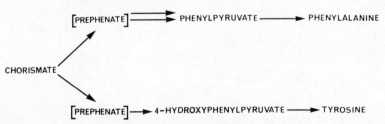

FIG. 14. *The pathways to phenylalanine and tyrosine in E. coli K-12 and A. aerogenes 62-1. There is a second prephenate dehydratase in A. aerogenes 62-1.*

hydratase activity but still has two chorismate mutases (134).

In *A. aerogenes* 62-1, the strain which accumulates chorismate, there is a second prephenate dehydratase (A) which is still present in phenylalanine auxotrophs (28; Fig. 14). No specific function can be ascribed to this enzyme and it is not present in the only other strain of *A. aerogenes* examined (R. G. H. Cotton, *unpublished data*). *A. aerogenes* 62-1 has lost both T and P protein activities, but a reversion to tyrosine independence also removes the phenylalanine requirement. The simplest explanation is that the prephenate formed by the T protein is then converted by the remaining prephenate dehydratase A into phenylpyruvic acid, thus bypassing the metabolic block.

Other organisms that have been examined differ from *E. coli* and *A. aerogenes*. In *N. crassa* (8) and the bean (*Pisum sativum*) (27), there appears to be one chorismate mutase activity with branching of the pathways at prephenate (as in Fig. 5). In extracts of one strain of *B. subtilis*, three distinct species (CM₁, CM₂, and CM₃) of chorismate mutase could be separated by chromatography on DEAE-cellulose, whereas extracts of another strain contained only the CM₃ species (109). Unlike the *E. coli* and *A. aerogenes* system, there was no association of chorismate mutase with either of the subsequent activities.

REGULATION OF THE COMMON PATHWAY

Enzymes of the common pathway provide an intermediate, chorismic acid, which is a common precursor molecule of tyrosine, phenylalanine, tryptophan, folic acid, ubiquinone, vitamin K, and 2,3-dihydroxybenzoylserine (or 2,3-dihydroxybenzoylglycine). Of these end-products only the three amino acids appear to play an important role in controlling the rate of synthesis of chorismic acid. In different microorganisms, this control is affected either by feedback inhibition alone or by a combination of feedback inhibition and repression.

In feedback inhibition, it would be possible for the various end products to effectively control the common pathway by one of at least four different mechanisms. (i) In "cumulative inhibition", as reported by Woolfolk and Stadtman for glutamine synthetase (170), each inhibitor adds its effect to the total inhibition of the enzyme, in which, however, the combined effect of any two inhibitors is less than the sum of their single inhibitions. (ii) In "concerted or multivalent inhibition" (36), two end products are required together before any significant inhibition occurs. (iii) "Sequential feedback inhibition" is carried out by a single molecule whose accumulation

TABLE 2. *Percentage of inhibition of DAHP synthetase isoenzymes of Escherichia coli K-12 by the aromatic amino acids*[a]

DAHP synthetase	Tyrosine		Phenylalanine		Tryptophan	
	10^{-3} M	10^{-5} M	10^{-3} M	10^{-5} M	10^{-3} M	10^{-5} M
(Tyr)	95	50	5	0	0	0
(Phe)	40	0	95	60	0	0
(Trp)[b]	0	0	0	0	60	20

[a] Data taken from unpublished results of B. J. Wallace and J. Pittard. Single isoenzymes were assayed in crude cell-free extracts obtained from mutant strains possessing only one functional DAHP synthetase isoenzyme. The reaction mixture contained erythrose-4-phosphate (0.5 μmole), phosphoenolpyruvate (0.5 μmole), sodium phosphate buffer (pH 6.4; 25 μmoles), a rate-limiting amount of enzyme and inhibitors at the final concentrations shown above.

[b] Co^{2+} 10^{-3} M was added to the reaction mixture.

is in turn controlled by several end products (124). (iv) In "feedback inhibition of isoenzymes," the reaction is carried out by more than a single enzyme, and a balanced control is possible because an inhibitable isoenzyme exists for each major end product. In this case, it is expected that the inhibition caused by two end products will equal the sum of the inhibitions caused by each one separately. If extensive cross-inhibitions occur, this result will not be obtained and the final distinction between (i) and (iv) may depend on the physical separation of different isoenzymes.

Theoretically, similar possibilities exist for the repression of the formation of the enzymes of the common pathway. If there is no duplication of enzymes, a system of multivalent repression could ensure that only in the presence of all the end products of the terminal pathways would the enzymes of the common pathway be repressed. Alternatively, if multiple enzymes are formed for any particular reaction, repression of the formation of individual enzymes by individual end products offers a reasonably efficient system of control.

Studies on the regulation of the common pathway of aromatic biosynthesis in a number of different microorganisms suggest that the control of the first reaction of the pathway, the conversion of erythrose-4-phosphate and phosphoenolpyruvate to DAHP, by inhibition or repression, or both, is an important factor in the control of the common pathway. Therefore, this reaction will be considered separately from the other reactions of the common pathway. The control of this first reaction has also recently been reviewed by Doy (48).

Feedback Inhibition of DAHP Synthetase

Smith et al. (145) demonstrated the existence of two DAHP synthetase isoenzymes in *E. coli*, DAHP synthetase (tyr) and DAHP synthetase (phe); DAHP synthetase (tyr) was inhibited by tyrosine and DAHP synthetase (phe) was inhibited by phenylalanine. Brown and Doy (17), also working with *E. coli* W, demonstrated the existence of a third isoenzyme, DAHP synthetase (trp), the activity of which was apparently not inhibited by either phenylalanine, tyrosine, or tryptophan, but the formation of which was repressed by tryptophan. The presence of three isoenzymes in *E. coli* K-12 has been confirmed by the isolation of mutants which have lost one or more of their isoenzymes, and by the identification of these three activities using chromatography on DEAE-cellulose (163, 164; K. D. Brown and W. K. Maas, Federation Proc., p. 338, 1966).

With *E. coli* W, DAHP synthetase (phe) and DAHP synthetase (tyr) activities have been separated by ammonium sulfate fractionations of crude cell-free extracts (49). With *E. coli* K-12, recombinant strains have been isolated which contain only one of the three isoenzymes (164). In these strains, the activity of a single isoenzyme can be assayed in crude cell-free extracts. In both systems, the sensitivities of DAHP synthetase (tyr) and DAHP synthetase (phe) to inhibition by phenylalanine, tyrosine, and tryptophan have been determined (49). Similar results have been obtained with both organisms, and the results of studies of inhibition with *E. coli* K-12 are summarized in Table 2.

There have been many reports to the effect that DAHP synthetase (trp) from either *E. coli* W or *E. coli* K-12 is not inhibited by tryptophan (49, 94, 107, 164). However, Doy has recently reported a 32% inhibition of this enzyme from *E. coli* W (46). Because of the early difficulties in establishing in vitro inhibition of DAHP synthetase (trp), experiments have recently been carried out to demonstrate inhibition of this enzyme in whole cells (*unpublished data*). When the *trypR⁻* gene is present in a strain of *E. coli* K-12 which possesses only DAHP synthetase (trp), this enzyme and the enzymes of the tryptophan operon are synthesized constitutively; i.e., their rate of synthesis is no longer affected by the presence or absence of tryptophan. These strains rely entirely on DAHP synthetase (trp) to carry out the first reaction of the pathway, and they have a mean generation time in minimal medium of 3 hr, compared with 80 min for the wild-type cells. When tryptophan is added to the medium, even though it has no effect on the formation of DAHP synthetase (trp), the mean generation time of these strains is increased to 12 hr. When a further mutation which prevents the conversion of DAHP to dehydroquinate is introduced into these strains, added tryptophan (5×10^{-4} M) reduces the rate of accumulation of DAHP by 80%. The cells in both instances, however, contain the same levels of the enzyme DAHP synthetase (trp). Further studies with extracts have shown that in the presence of Co^{2+} (10^{-3} M) DAHP synthetase (trp) is inhibited 60% by 10^{-3} M L-tryptophan (*unpublished data*).

Using strains that each possess only one of the isoenzymes, it has been possible to isolate feedback-resistant mutants. The DAHP synthetase (trp) of one mutant isolated shows an inhibition of 20% at 10^{-3} M L-tryptophan, compared with 60% inhibition of the wild-type enzyme. The DAHP synthetase (phe) of another feedback resistant mutant shows an inhibition of 30% at 10^{-4} M L-phenylalanine, compared with 92% for the wild-type enzyme (J. Pittard, *unpublished data*). Ezekiel has also reported the isolation of mutant strains from *E. coli* K-12, in which DAHP synthetase (phe) is no longer inhibited by phenylalanine (59). Although there have been no reports yet of mutant strains in which DAHP synthetase (tyr) is feedback-resistant, there is no reason to believe that these should be difficult to isolate.

In *S. typhimurium*, the situation would appear to be very similar to that existing in the case of *E. coli* (76). In crude cell-free extracts, inhibitions by phenylalanine and tyrosine are found to be additive when both amino acids are added together, suggesting the presence of two separate isoenzymes. Furthermore, DAHP synthetase (tyr) and DAHP synthetase (phe), inhibitable by tyrosine and phenylalanine, respectively, can be separated by ammonium sulfate fractionation.

Evidence for the existence of a third isoenzyme, DAHP synthetase (trp), comes from the isolation of mutant strains unable to grow in minimal medium supplemented with phenylalanine and tyrosine but able to grow in minimal medium. Mutant strains lacking DAHP synthetase (tyr) or DAHP synthetase (phe) have also been isolated in this organism (76). No fraction of the DAHP synthetase activity of *S. typhimurium* has yet been found to be inhibited by tryptophan (76, 93). In view of the difficulty experienced in *E. coli*, however, this failure to demonstrate inhibition in vitro may not reflect the true in vivo situation.

A survey of the inhibition of DAHP synthetase

from a variety of gram-negative and gram-positive organisms by phenylalanine, tyrosine, and tryptophan has recently been carried out (94). In some cases (e.g., *Hydrogenomonas* sp.) phenylalanine and tyrosine exerted a cumulative feedback inhibition on DAHP synthetase. In other organisms, the effects of the individual amino acids were additive. Therefore, it was concluded that each amino acid was inhibiting a different isoenzyme. Many cases in which tryptophan could inhibit part of the DAHP synthetase activity were described, and there were some strains which appeared to possess only a single enzyme inhibited by a single amino acid. As the authors point out, the dilemma posed by these last mentioned strains, which are able to grow in the presence of the amino acid which totally inhibits DAHP synthetase in vitro, may well be resolved when they are studied in more detail.

In *Saccharomyces cerevisiae*, results suggest (47, 105) that there are only two DAHP synthetase isoenzymes, one inhibited by tyrosine [DAHP synthetase (tyr)] and one inhibited by phenylalanine [DAHP synthetase (phe)]. Mutants lacking either enzyme have also been isolated (117). The growth of these strains is inhibited by phenylalanine or tyrosine, respectively, confirming the existence of only two isoenzymes. Furthermore, a recombinant strain which has neither isoenzyme is unable to grow on minimal medium and possesses no detectable DAHP synthetase activity (116).

In *N. crassa*, there are three isoenzymes, one inhibited by tyrosine, one by phenylalanine, and one by tryptophan (46, 48, 93). One fraction, which can be isolated by chromatography on Sephadex G-100, has been shown to be inhibited 100% by tryptophan (93). Studies of the regulation of aromatic amino acid biosynthesis in *C. vaspali* reveal the presence of three isoenzymes (106). One of these is inhibited by phenylalanine, one by tyrosine, and one by tryptophan. In this case the tryptophan-inhibitable isoenzyme constitutes approximately 60% of the total activity.

B. subtilis and a number of other strains of *Bacillus* have a different means of inhibiting the first reaction of the pathway (95). In these strains, there appears to be only a single DAHP synthetase enzyme which is inhibited by either chorismic acid or prephenic acid. The accumulation of chorismate and prephenate is, in turn, controlled by the amino acids phenylalanine, tyrosine, and tryptophan, acting on the reactions of the terminal pathways which utilize chorismate (124). These reactions will be dealt with in a later section. In addition to the various strains of *Bacillus*, strains of *Staphylococcus*, *Gaffkya*, *Flavobacterium*,

Achromobacter, and *Alcaligenes* show sequential feedback inhibition of DAHP synthetase by either prephenate or chorismate. The DAHP synthetase from *Xanthomonas*, on the other hand, is inhibited approximately 86% by chorismate, but it shows 10% or less inhibition by prephenate (94).

Repression of DAHP Synthetase

The early work from two laboratories (17, 145) established that in *E. coli* W there were three DAHP synthetase isoenzymes and that the formation of each was repressed by a single amino acid, e.g., DAHP synthetase (tyr) by tyrosine, DAHP synthetase (phe) by phenylalanine, and DAHP synthetase (trp) by tryptophan. In addition, cross repression of DAHP synthetase (tyr) by phenylalanine and tryptophan and DAHP synthetase (phe) by tryptophan was also reported (18). Recently, the derepression of the DAHP synthetase isoenzymes has been studied by growing an aromatic auxotroph of *E. coli* K 12 in a chemostat under conditions in which single aromatic amino acids, in turn, limit the growth rate (K. D. Brown, 1968. Genetics, *in press*). When either tryptophan or phenylalanine limits growth, DAHP synthetase (phe) is derepressed, and it is inferred from these results that phenylalanine and tryptophan together are required for the repression of DAHP synthetase (phe). DAHP synthetase (tyr) is only derepressed when tyrosine is the limiting amino acid and when phenylalanine and tryptophan are present at 10^{-4} M. If these last two amino acids are present in higher concentrations (10^{-3} M), derepression of DAHP synthetase (tyr) is greatly reduced. DAHP synthetase (trp), measured as DAHP synthetase activity not inhibited by either phenylalanine or tyrosine, is derepressed when the growth rate is limited by tryptophan (K. D. Brown. 1968. Genetics, *in press*). Studies carried out on the repression of DAHP synthetase (tyr) in strains containing only this isoenzyme confirm the finding that DAHP synthetase (tyr) is repressed in the presence of high concentrations of phenylalanine and tryptophan (B. J. Wallace, *unpublished data*).

It has been known for some time that a mutation in a gene, *trpR*, can cause derepression of the enzymes of the tryptophan operon (23). Studies of *trpR⁻* strains of *E. coli* K-12 which either possess all three DAHP synthetase isoenzymes or possess only the single isoenzyme, DAHP synthetase (trp), have demonstrated that DAHP synthetase (trp) is also produced constitutively in *trpR⁻* strains (K. D. Brown. 1968. Genetics, *in press*).

A second class of mutants has been isolated (*unpublished data*) in which the control of DAHP synthetase (trp) has been altered. These mutants also make this enzyme constitutively but still possess a normally repressible tryptophan operon. Since the mutations conferring this change are closely linked to the structural gene for DAHP synthetase (trp), these mutants may turn out to be operator constitutive mutants. In these mutants, DAHP synthetase (trp) is not only produced constitutively, but is much less sensitive to inhibition by tryptophan. This pattern resembles that of certain 5-methyl tryptophan-resistant mutants of *E. coli* possessing mutations in the anthranilate synthetase gene, as reported by Somerville and Yanofsky (148). Mutations in a third gene, the *trpS* gene, have an indirect effect on the levels of DAHP synthetase (trp) and the enzymes of the tryptophan operon; this will be discussed later.

The tyrosine analogues 4-aminophenylalanine and 3-thianaphthenealanine have been found to repress the formation of DAHP synthetase (tyr), although they are not activated by tyrosyl-tRNA synthetase. Since these compounds can per se repress the formation of DAHP synthetase (tyr), it has been proposed that tyrosine uncomplexed to any transfer RNA molecule should also function as corepressor (137).

4-Aminophenylalanine at relatively low concentrations (10^{-4} M) completely inhibits the growth of a recombinant strain of *E. coli* K-12 possessing only DAHP synthetase (tyr). Since 4-aminophenylalanine does not inhibit the activity of this enzyme (146), the inhibition of growth is presumably caused by the repression of its formation. Using this system, it is a simple matter to isolate mutant strains in which DAHP synthetase (tyr) is no longer repressed by tyrosine. Several of these strains have been isolated, and one group in particular has been studied in detail (B. J. Wallace and J. Pittard, J. Bacteriol., *in press*). In this case, a mutation in a gene designated as *tyr*R, which is situated in the general region of the tryptophan operon (*see* Fig. 15), causes derepression of DAHP synthetase (tyr), chorismate mutase T and its associated prephenate dehydrogenase, and transaminase A. It also has an effect on the repression of the shikimate kinase enzyme. In other words, those enzymes normally repressible by tyrosine are made constitutively by these mutants. The sensitivity of DAHP synthetase (tyr) to feedback inhibition by tyrosine is, however, unchanged, as would be expected from the fact that the *tyr*R gene and the *aroF* gene, the structural gene for DAHP synthetase (tyr), are widely separated on the chromosome.

TABLE 3. *Repressed and derepressed levels of the DAHP synthetase isoenzymes in mutant strains of E. coli K-12 possessing only a single DAHP synthetase isoenzyme[a]*

DAHP synthetase	Specific activities in extracts prepared from[b]	
	Fully repressed cells	Fully derepressed cells
(Tyr)	0	50
(Phe)	11	18
(Trp)	0.4	5–10

[a] Conditions under which the cells were grown are described in the text. Values obtained in the case of strains possessing *trpR⁻* or *tyrR⁻* mutations are: DAHP synthetase (tyr) in a strain possessing *tyrR⁻*, 150; DAHP synthetase (trp) in a strain possessing *trpR⁻*, 4.

[b] Specific activity = 0.1 μmole of DAHP formed per mg of protein per 20 min at 37 C.

In strains possessing the *tyrR⁻* mutation, high concentrations of phenylalanine and tryptophan no longer repress DAHP synthetase (tyr), indicating that the gene product of the *tyrR* gene is involved in this apparent cross-repression (B. J. Wallace, *unpublished data*). No strains have yet been reported that are derepressed for the DAHP synthetase (phe) isoenzyme.

One interesting feature of the production of each of the isoenzymes in *E. coli* K-12 and in *E. coli* W (K. D. Brown, Genetics, *in press;* 18) is to be found in the differences between fully repressed and fully derepressed values for each one. In studies carried out in our laboratories, repressed values have been determined by growing mutants containing single isoenzymes in the presence of the three aromatic amino acids plus shikimic acid (10^{-6} M), to satisfy the requirement for aromatic vitamins, and harvesting cells in late exponential phase. Derepressed values have been obtained using strains containing only a single isoenzyme, which were also unable to convert DAHP to 5-dehydroquinic acid (DHQ) because of a mutation in the *aroB* gene. These were grown, either in limiting shikimic acid or in a mixture of the three amino acids in which the relevant amino acid was present in growth limiting concentrations. In the latter case, shikimic acid (10^{-6} M) was also added.

The results of this study are indicated in Table 3. Two interesting points emerge from this table. The first is that under derepressed conditions DAHP synthetase (tyr) activity is much higher than that of either DAHP synthetase (phe) or DAHP synthetase (trp). The second point of interest is that the variation in levels of DAHP synthetase (phe) from repressed to derepressed state is very small by comparison with DAHP synthetase (tyr). Furthermore, although DAHP synthetase (tyr) and DAHP synthetase (trp) are repressed to very low values, DAHP synthetase (phe) exhibits much higher values for maximally repressed conditions.

Inhibition appears to play a much more important role in the regulation of DAHP synthetase (phe) activity than does repression. Recombinant strains possessing only DAHP synthetase (phe) are unable to grow in minimal medium supplemented with phenylalanine or with phenylalanine plus tryptophan. Mutant strains, however, in which the DAHP synthetase (phe) is feedback-resistant suffer no reduction in growth rate when these amino acids are added to the medium, even though the enzyme is as repressible in these strains as in the parent (J. Pittard, *unpublished data*). Therefore, repression by itself exerts little control on the in vivo activity of DAHP synthetase (phe). By contrast, however, 4-aminophenylalanine, which acts only as a corepressor, can completely inhibit growth of a strain possessing only DAHP synthetase [(tyr) B. J. Wallace and J. Pittard, J. Bacteriol., *in press*], and a strain possessing only a feedback-resistant DAHP synthetase (trp) isoenzyme has its growth rate halved by the addition of tryptophan (J. Pittard and J. Camakaris, *in preparation*).

In *S. typhimurium*, at least a 10-fold derepression of the total DAHP synthetase activity occurs when cells are transferred from medium containing excess phenylalanine and tyrosine to one in which these amino acids are present in very low (1 μg/ml) concentration (76). However, whereas DAHP synthetase (tyr) is derepressed about 10-fold in a "leaky" multiple aromatic auxotroph derived from *S. typhimurium* strain LT2, DAHP synthetase (phe) is not derepressed (189). In contrast, in a mutant strain of LT2 resistant to β-2-thienylalanine a 12-fold derepression of DAHP synthetase (phe) was observed (176). Other studies involving different strains of *S. typhimurium* indicate that when cells are grown in minimal medium, DAHP synthetase (tyr) is the predominant isoenzyme, but both DAHP synthetase (tyr) and DAHP synthetase (phe) can be derepressed about 10-fold by making suitable changes in the growth conditions (93).

In *Saccharomyces cerevisiae*, it has been reported that the formation of neither of the two DAHP synthetases is repressed by phenylalanine, tyrosine, or tryptophan (47, 105).

In *N. crassa*, there appear to be three distinct DAHP synthetase isoenzymes. Although their formation is not repressed by either tyrosine,

phenylalanine, or tryptophan to levels lower than those found in wild-type strains growing in minimal medium, derepression can be demonstrated by the use of auxotrophic strains, thus demonstrating that some form of specific control does exist (48).

In *B. subtilis*, the formation of the single DAHP synthetase enzyme is repressed by the aromatic amino acids (125), but no detailed studies of this repression have yet been reported.

Inhibition of Other Enzymes of the Common Pathway

Studies of the control of a number of biosynthetic pathways have shown that when feedback inhibition occurs, it almost always affects the enzyme carrying out the first reaction in a particular biosynthetic sequence. Since the net result of feedback inhibition is to stop the wasteful flow of intermediates along a pathway, it is not surprising that the enzyme of the first reaction normally functions as the major control point.

There is currently only one reported case of feedback inhibition of an enzyme of the common pathway other than DAHP synthetase, and it is interesting to note that in this case the affected enzyme is found in close association with DAHP synthetase. In *B. subtilis*, three enzymes, DAHP synthetase, chorismate mutase, and shikimate kinase, form a protein aggregate (125). The activity of both DAHP synthetase and shikimate kinase is feedback-inhibited by both chorismate and prephenate.

Repression of Other Enzymes of the Common Pathway

Relatively little work has been carried out on the repressibility of the enzymes of the common pathway other than DAHP synthetase. Studies involving the growth of an aromatic auxotroph of *E. coli* K-12 in a chemostat under various conditions failed to show any significant repression or derepression of either dehydroquinate synthetase or dehydroquinase (K. D. Brown. 1968. Genetics, *in press*). Fewster (60) failed to find any variation in the level of shikimate kinase activity in many strains of *E. coli* when grown in the presence or absence of the aromatic amino acids. Similarly, in *S. typhimurium* it has recently been reported that the addition of excess aromatic amino acids to wild-type cells growing in minimal medium failed to repress any of the enzymes involved in converting DAHP to chorismate (76).

In contrast to these results, it has recently been shown (J. Pittard et al., *in preparation*) that under certain conditions the shikimate kinase activity of *E. coli* K-12 can be considerably derepressed. When a wild-type strain is grown in the presence of the aromatic amino acids, only a twofold repression of this activity occurs, in comparison with extracts from cells grown in minimal medium. When, however, strains possessing only DAHP synthetase (trp), which are either *trpR*⁺ or *trpR*⁻, are grown in minimal medium, the shikimate kinase activity is derepressed seven- to eightfold by comparison with fully repressed wild-type values. A similar result is obtained when a strain which possesses the *tyrR*⁻ mutation and has only DAHP synthetase (tyr) is grown in minimal medium. The addition of the aromatic amino acids to the minimal medium represses the formation of kinase activity in every case, although in strains containing either the *trpR*⁻ or the *tyrR*⁻ mutations, the fully repressed values are approximately double those obtained in the corresponding *trpR*⁺ and *tyrR*⁺ strains. These results are summarized in Table 4. It can also be seen from Table 4 that when either shikimic acid, tyrosine, or tryptophan limits the growth of an aromatic auxotroph, in contrast to when these aromatic amino acids are present in excess, a three- to fourfold derepression of the kinase activity occurs. When, however, phenylalanine limits growth, there is no derepression of kinase activity. Although these results do not indicate any simple system of control, they do clearly demonstrate that the levels of this particular enzymic activity can be subject to considerable variations. Before these studies can be interpreted in terms of any specific model, it is necessary to establish whether the activity that is measured in crude cell-free extracts represents one or more than one shikimate kinase enzyme. It has recently been demonstrated that in *S. typhimurium* there are two shikimate kinase enzymes which can be separated from each other by chromatography on DEAE-cellulose (120).

REGULATION OF THE TRYPTOPHAN PATHWAY

Feedback Inhibition

In *E. coli* (89), anthranilate synthetase and PR transferase have been shown to form an enzyme aggregate such that, although the PR transferase activity can function by itself, only the aggregate has appreciable anthranilate synthetase activity.

Both anthranilate synthetase and PR transferase activity are inhibited by tryptophan. Feedback-resistant mutants have been obtained by the use of tryptophan analogues such as 5-methyl tryptophan. In a number of cases, these strains are found to be both feedback-resistant and to produce the enzymes of the tryptophan pathway constitutively (121, 148; C. Cordaro and E. Balbinder, Bacteriol. Proc., p. 51, 1967).

TABLE 4. *A comparison of the specific activities of shikimate kinase in different strains of E. coli K-12 grown under different conditions*[a]

Phenotype	Specific activities in extracts prepared from cells grown in	
	Minimal medium	Minimal medium plus phenylalanine, tyrosine, and tryptophan (each, 10^{-3} M)
Wild type	3.4	1.6
Multiple aromatic auxotroph	—[b]	1.2[c]
Prototroph possessing only DAHP synthetase (trp)	12.0	2.5
As above, but possessing the *trpR*⁻ mutation	12.1	3.9
Prototroph possessing only DAHP synthetase (tyr)	4.9	1.7[c]
As above, but possessing the *tyrR*⁻ mutation	10.7	3.0

[a] Specific activity = 0.1 μmole of substrate utilized per 20 min per mg of protein at 37 C.

[b] When the aromatic auxotroph was grown in limiting shikimate, limiting tryptophan, limiting tyrosine, and limiting phenylalanine, respectively, specific activities were 3.5, 4.1, 5.4, and 0.5.

[c] 4-Aminobenzoic acid and 4-hydroxybenzoic acid (10^{-6} M) were also added to the medium.

These examples occur in *E. coli* K-12, *E. coli* W, and *S. typhimurium*. Only in the *E. coli* K-12 mutants, however, has it been established that both changes were the result of a single mutation (148).

In *Chromobacterium violaceum* (J. Wegman and I. P. Crawford, Bacteriol. Proc., p. 115, 1967), *P. putida* (33), *B. subtilis* (124), *Saccharomyces cerevisiae* (50, 105), and *N. crassa* (42), tryptophan acts as a feedback inhibitor of anthranilate synthetase, although in *C. paspali* (106), tryptophan does not inhibit the activity of anthranilate synthetase.

Repression

In *E. coli*, the structural genes for the enzymes of the tryptophan pathway are organized into the now well-characterized tryptophan operon. Studies of various operator-constitutive mutants have shown that the expression of all these genes is controlled by a single operator locus (112, 113, 148). Furthermore, it has been shown (87) that all the enzymes of the tryptophan pathway are repressed or derepressed in a coordinate fashion. The regulation of these enzymes is controlled by the *trpR* gene, which was originally described by Cohen and Jacob (23).

In the biosynthesis of at least two other amino acids, histidine and valine (58, 122, 142), it has been demonstrated that histidyl-transfer ribonucleic acid (tRNA)$_{(his)}$ and valyl-tRNA$_{(val)}$ are the active corepressors and not the amino acids themselves. Consequently, mutations affecting tRNA molecules or amino acid activating enzymes can also cause derepression of enzymes in a biosynthetic pathway. Furthermore, in diploids these mutations would be expected to be recessive in the same way in which a mutation which caused the formation of a nonfunctional aporepressor is expected to be recessive. Hirst and DeMoss (Bacteriol. Proc., p. 114, 1967) have studied the relationship between the size of the free tryptophan pool and the repression of tryptophan synthetase in *E. coli*. They find that changes in this pool do not affect repression of tryptophan synthetase, and they conclude that either there is more than a single intracellular pool of tryptophan or that tryptophan itself is not the corepressor.

A class of mutant strains which require tryptophan for growth has recently been described (43, 82, 111) in which the mutations causing tryptophan dependence map in the *trpS* gene, which is located between the *aroB* and the *pabA* genes and far away from the tryptophan operon. In spite of the inability of these strains to grow without added tryptophan, all of the enzymes of the tryptophan operon can be detected in their cell-free extracts. The levels of these enzymes in extracts prepared from derepressed *trpS⁻* cells are, however, only one-third or less of the levels obtained in extracts from derepressed *trpS⁺* cells (82). The level of DAHP synthetase (trp) is similarly lowered in *trpS⁻* strains (J Pittard and J. Camakaris, *in preparation*). Because of these observations, it seemed possible that the *trpS⁻* strains may be producing a super-repressor analogous to the *iˢ* mutants of the *lac* operon (82, 111). Doolittle and Yanofsky (43), however, have recently demonstrated that the *trpS* gene codes for the tryptophanyl-tRNA synthetase enzyme, and that *trpS⁻* mutants have a greatly reduced ability to charge tryptophan-specific tRNA. By contrast with the histidyl-tRNA synthetase mutants, in which the poor charging of histidyl-tRNA causes derepression of the histidine enzymes, the enzymes of the tryptophan pathway are not derepressed in the tryptophanyl-tRNA synthetase mutants. Therefore, it has been suggested that tryptophan, and not tryptophanyl-tRNA, is the active corepressor for the tryptophan operon (43). The low values which have been observed for enzymes of the

tryptophan operon and for DAHP synthetase (trp) in *trpS⁻* strains is probably, therefore, a direct consequence of an internal accumulation of tryptophan by these strains.

In *S. typhimurium*, a single tryptophan operon exists, although it has been suggested that in this organism the tryptophan operon contains two separate promoter genes instead of one as in *E. coli* (10). Mutant strains resistant to 5-methyl tryptophan and derepressed for enzymes of the tryptophan pathway have been isolated, but the mutations have not yet been mapped (176). Preliminary studies in both *Saccharomyces cerevisiae* and *N. crassa* (50) indicate that repression plays an important role in these organisms. No repression of the tryptophan enzymes has been found in *C. paspali* (106), and it has been reported that tryptophan synthetase formation is specifically induced in *P. putida* by indoleglycerolphosphate (33).

REGULATION OF THE TYROSINE PATHWAY

Feedback Inhibition

In *A. aerogenes* and *E. coli*, the first two reactions of the tyrosine pathway are carried out by a single enzyme (24). Tyrosine is a feedback inhibitor of the second of these activities, prephenate dehydrogenase (90% inhibition at 10^{-3} M), but it does not affect the first, chorismate mutase T (24; B. J. Wallace, *unpublished data*). In strains of *B. subtilis*, there are one or more chorismate mutase enzymes and a separate prephenate dehydrogenase enzyme. Chorismate mutase is not inhibited by tyrosine, but this amino acid does inhibit the prephenate dehydrogenase enzyme [90% at 10^{-3} M (124)].

In *S. cerevisiae*, prephenate dehydrogenase activity is activated by phenylalanine (105). In *C. paspali*, prephenate dehydrogenase is inhibited by tyrosine (106).

Repression

In *A. aerogenes* and *E. coli*, the formation of chorismate mutase T and its associated prephenate dehydrogenase activity are strongly repressed by tyrosine (24). In *E. coli*, tyrosine has also been shown to repress the formation of transaminase A, an enzyme which converts 4-hydroxyphenylpyruvate to tyrosine (144). Mutations in a gene (*tyrR*) which is located at some distance on the chromosome from *tyrA* (the structural gene for chorismate mutase T) and its associated prephenate dehydrogenase cause constitutive synthesis of chorismate mutase T and prephenate dehydrogenase, transaminase A, and DAHP synthetase [(tyr) B. J. Wallace and J. Pittard, *in preparation*].

AroF, the structural gene for DAHP synthetase (tyr), and *tyrA* are closely linked in the *E. coli* chromosome and may be part of an operon. The isolation of a mutant strain which has lost DAHP synthetase (tyr) activity and which produces greatly reduced levels of chorismate mutase T and prephenate dehydrogenase (B. J. Wallace, *unpublished data*) lends support to this possibility. No operator constitutive mutants have yet been found. In *S. cerevisiae* (105), tyrosine does not repress prephenate dehydrogenase or chorismate mutase. In this strain, however, prephenate dehydrogenase is induced by phenylalanine. The genetic units involved in this process of induction have not yet been studied.

REGULATION OF THE PHENYLALANINE PATHWAY

Feedback Inhibition

In *A. aerogenes* and *E. coli*, phenylalanine feedback inhibits prephenate dehydratase activity (90 to 100% inhibition at 10^{-3} M). Although phenylalanine has no effect on the associated chorismate mutase P in *E. coli* (J. Pittard, *unpublished data*), it causes 65% inhibition of the chorismate mutase P of *A. aerogenes* (24). In *B. subtilis*, phenylalanine inhibits prephenate dehydratase (124). Mutant strains of *B. subtilis* have been isolated that are resistant to β-2-thienylalanine. In some of these mutants, phenylalanine activates prephenate dehydratase instead of inhibiting it (22). In *N. crassa* and *C. paspali*, there appears to be a single chorismate mutase enzyme. The activity of this enzyme is inhibited by phenylalanine and by tyrosine, but the inhibition is reversed and the enzyme is activated by L-tryptophan (7, 106). In *C. paspali*, phenylalanine also inhibits prephenate dehydratase activity (106).

Repression

In *A. aerogenes* and *E. coli*, phenylalanine represses the formation of chorismate mutase P and its associated prephenate dehydratase. The variation in activity between maximally repressed and derepressed levels is much less in the case of chorismate mutase P than in that of chorismate mutase T (24; B. J. Wallace and J. Pittard, *unpublished data*), and a transaminase enzyme which is involved in the formation of phenylalanine is found not to be repressed by phenylalanine (144). DAHP synthetase (phe) shows similar small variations in activity between maximally repressed and derepressed conditions. No regulator genes associated with the control of this pathway have yet been identified.

REGULATION OF THE PATHWAYS OF VITAMIN BIOSYNTHESIS

Although there is no doubt that the relative amounts of any aromatic vitamin formed by bacterial cells can vary as a result of mutations or changes in growth conditions, little information is available concerning the mechanisms that normally control their synthesis. In part, this lack of information is due to the fact that the details of the pathways leading to the biosynthesis of the aromatic vitamins are still being worked out.

Mutant strains of *Staphylococcus aureus* which overproduce and excrete 4-aminobenzoic acid have been reported (168). The formation of 2,3-dihydroxybenzoate and related compounds has been shown to be markedly influenced by the medium in which the cells are grown. Thus the amount of 2,3-dihydroxybenzoate and 2,3-dihydroxybenzoylglycine produced in cultures of *B. subtilis* is inversely proportional to the iron content of the growth medium (88). The formation of enzymes concerned in the biosynthesis of 2,3-dihydroxybenzoate by *A. aerogenes* (174) and 2,3-dihydroxybenzoylserine by *E. coli* (14) is repressed by the presence of iron or cobalt in the growth medium.

The presence of the aromatic amino acids also inhibits the production of 2,3-dihydroxybenzoate and 3,4-dihydroxybenzoate by washed cell suspensions of *A. aerogenes* (133). These effects in *A. aerogenes* can be explained by feedback inhibition of the DAHP synthetase system (A. F. Egan, *unpublished data*).

Vitamin K and ubiquinone levels are affected by conditions of aeration (135), and in mutants which are unable to form one of the quinones, there is a several-fold increase in the level of the remaining quinone (31).

There is no indication that the aromatic vitamins play any effective role in the control of the common pathway. On the other hand, since a strain of *E. coli* K-12 which has mutations in the structural genes for DAHP synthetase (tyr), DAHP synthetase (phe), and DAHP synthetase (trp) possesses no detectable DAHP synthetase activity, there does not appear to be a fourth DAHP synthetase isoenzyme which is concerned with vitamin biosynthesis. The results of these in vitro tests are confirmed by the observation that this same strain grows slowly with a mean generation time of 280 min in a medium containing phenylalanine, tyrosine, and tryptophan. When, however, either shikimic acid (10^{-6} M) or 4-aminobenzoic acid, 4-hydroxybenzoic acid, and 2,3-dihydroxybenzoic acid (each at 10^{-6} M) are also added to the medium, the growth rate is returned to normal with a mean generation time of 80 min (B. J. Wallace and J. Pittard, *in preparation*).

There are indications that not all of the DAHP synthetase isoenzymes play an equal role in vitamin biosynthesis. When a mutant strain of

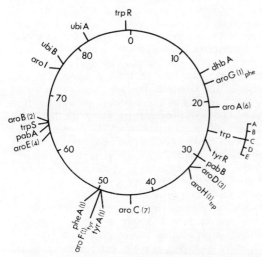

FIG. 15. *A map of the E. coli chromosome showing the relative positions of genes concerned with aromatic biosynthesis. The chromosomal locations of the genes ubiA, ubiB, aroI, and tyrR are based solely on the data of interrupted mating experiments. The exact order of the genes pheA, aroF, tyrA and aroH, aroD has not been determined. Genes coding for enzymes of the common pathway have the prefix aro. Genes coding for enzymes of the tryptophan, phenylalanine, or tyrosine pathways have the prefixes trp, phe, and tyr, respectively. Genes concerned with the biosynthesis of ubiquinone have the prefix ubi. Genes concerned with the biosynthesis of p-aminobenzoic acid have the prefix pab, and those concerned with the biosynthesis of 2,3-dihydroxybenzoic acid, dhb. Two genes concerned with regulation which affect both the common pathway and one of the terminal pathways have been given the prefix relevant to the terminal pathway, e.g., trpR, tyrR. The uppercase letters given to the genes have no significance with regard to the relative positions of the enzymes in the biosynthetic sequences. For example, aroA does not code for the first enzyme of the common pathway. The numbers in parenthesis describe the particular reaction with which the gene is concerned. For example, tyrA (1) codes for the first reaction in the terminal pathway of tyrosine biosynthesis and aroF (1)$_{tyr}$ codes for one of the three isoenzymes involved in the first reaction of the common pathway. The subscript tyr denotes that it codes for DAHP synthetase (tyr); aroG (1)$_{phe}$ codes for DAHP synthetase (phe) and aroH (1)$_{trp}$ codes for DAHP synthetase (trp). The function of aroI is yet to be determined. The gene trpS is the structural gene for tryptophanyl-tRNA synthetase. The formal representation of the chromosome is in accordance with the recommendations of Taylor and Trotter (159).*

E. coli containing only DAHP synthetase (tyr) is inoculated into minimal medium supplemented with phenylalanine, tyrosine, and tryptophan, in the presence and absence of 10^{-6} M shikimate, its growth rate in the absence of shikimate is very slow (mean generation time of 9 hr). In the presence of 10^{-6} M shikimate, however, it grows with a mean generation time of 120 min. In a strain containing only DAHP synthetase (trp), the addition of shikimate to medium containing phenylalanine, tyrosine, and tryptophan causes only a slight stimulation of growth rate, whereas in the strain containing DAHP synthetase (phe), this addition makes no difference to the growth rate. In medium not containing shikimate but containing phenylalanine, tyrosine, and tryptophan, the mean generation times of strains containing only DAHP synthetase (trp) and DAHP synthetase (phe) are 114 and 130 min, respectively (B. J. Wallace and J. Pittard, *in preparation*). It would appear, therefore, that either DAHP synthetase (phe) or DAHP synthetase (trp) can provide enough DAHP synthetase activity for vitamin synthesis even in the presence of phenylalanine, tyrosine, and tryptophan.

A mutant strain of *N. crassa* lacking DAHP synthetase (tyr), however, exhibits a growth requirement for 4-aminobenzoic acid in the presence of phenylalanine, tyrosine, and tryptophan. Since wild-type *N. crassa* does not exhibit this requirement in the presence of these amino acids, it would appear that in this organism it is probably DAHP synthetase (tyr) which provides enough DAHP synthetase activity for vitamin synthesis under repressed conditions (48). Since the enzymes of the common pathway other than the DAHP synthetases do not appear to be repressed to such levels as would interfere with vitamin biosynthesis, no special controls are required to ensure the supply of chorismate for vitamin syntheses. However, systems of control of each of the terminal pathways to the vitamins must exist to ensure the production of less of the vitamins than of the aromatic amino acids.

CHROMOSOMAL DISTRIBUTION OF GENES CONCERNED WITH AROMATIC BIOSYNTHESIS

In *E. coli* K-12, genetic analyses of mutant strains that have been carried out over the last few years permit many of the genes concerned with aromatic biosynthesis to be given specific map locations (23, 31, 43, 82, 83, 111, 134, 158, 163, 173; R. Luke, *unpublished data*). The position of these genes on the *E. coli* chromosome is shown in Fig. 15.

Although the function of the *aroI* gene has not yet been determined, a mutant strain has been isolated which requires phenylalanine, tyrosine, and tryptophan for growth at 42 C. A genetic analysis of this strain shows that the mutation maps in the position designated by the *aroI* gene (J. Pittard and E. M. Walker, *unpublished data*). The gene product of the *aroI* gene has not yet been identified.

The normal functions of the regulator genes, *trpR* and *tyrR*, have not yet been determined, and structural genes for shikimate kinase(s) and one or more transaminases have yet to be identified.

For the genes coding for the tryptophan pathway, organization into a single operon is well established (87, 112, 113). As can be seen from Fig. 15, the only other genes which, as a result of position and function, show a possibility of such an arrangement are the *aroF* and *tyrA* genes and possibly the *aroH* and *aroD* genes. In neither pair, however, has contiguity been established, and in the latter pair it can already be calculated that under conditions in which *aroH* is repressed *aroD* is not affected.

On the other hand, it is possible that *aroF* and *tyrA* may constitute an operon. In general, however, the gene distribution is such that any system of control affecting several genes will probably resemble that already described for arginine biosynthesis (110) for which the term regulon has been proposed.

Genetic studies of *S. typhimurium* have so far concentrated on genes coding for enzymes of the common pathway and of the terminal pathways of phenylalanine, tyrosine, and tryptophan biosynthesis. The general distribution of these genes resembles that found for *E. coli* (76, 126, 141; E. Gollub et al., Federation Proc., p. 337, 1966), although minor discrepancies between the two maps still exist (134). Although mutants that are derepressed for enzymes of the tryptophan pathway have been isolated in *Salmonella*, the mutations causing this change have not yet been studied (176).

In *B. subtilis*, all the genes concerned with the tryptophan pathway are closely linked to each other on the chromosome (2, 20, 123, 125). Moreover, genes for dehydroquinate synthetase, prephenate dehydrogenase, 3-enolpyruvyl-shikimate 5-phosphate synthetase, and one form of the chorismate mutase enzyme are located on the same transforming molecule of deoxyribonucleic acid (DNA) as the tryptophan cluster. There is, however, no evidence at the moment to suggest that these genes form an operon like structure. A gene for DAHP synthetase, *aroA*, and one for a second chorismate mutase, *aroG*, are closely

linked on another molecule of transforming DNA (123). In the latter case, there is also a close association of the two gene products, DAHP synthetase and chorismate mutase, in an enzyme aggregate. Genes for dehydroshikimate reductase, dehydroquinase, chorismate synthetase, and prephenate dehydratase have also been mapped but are not linked to each other or to the tryptophan cluster.

In *N. crassa*, the structural genes for enzymes of the tryptophan pathway are unlinked to each other (1), although the gene products of two of these genes combine to form a molecular aggregate (42). Genes coding for enzymes for each of the reactions of the common pathway, with the exception of the third step for which there are two dehydroquinase enzymes (74), have all been mapped. Genes coding for dehydroshikimate reductase, shikimate kinase, dehydroquinate synthetase, and 3-enolpyruvyl-shikimate 5-phosphate synthetase have been shown to be closely linked on linkage group II (74, 79). A study of a class of polarity mutants suggests that these four genes and a gene for dehydroquinase activity form a single unit of transcription (74). It was originally postulated that this gene cluster may in fact constitute an operon, but neither operator nor regulator mutants have been found to substantiate this proposal (74). Mutant strains lacking each of the three DAHP synthetase isoenzymes have also been isolated and the mutations have been mapped. The gene for DAHP synthetase (tyr) is located on linkage group VI, the gene for DAHP synthetase (phe) on linkage group I, and the gene for DAHP synthetase (trp) either on linkage group I or II (48).

Conclusion

In recent years, knowledge of the pathways of biosynthesis of the aromatic amino acids has been extended, and it is probable that most, if not all, of the intermediates concerned are now known. The emphasis has now changed from the determination of the pathways themselves to the study of the biochemical genetics related to the pathways and to a detailed examination of certain key reactions. The branched pathways leading to the aromatic amino acids have provided a valuable system for experiments on enzyme repression and feedback inhibition. The isolation of mutant strains possessing only a single DAHP synthetase, DAHP synthetase (tyr), DAHP synthetase (phe), or DAHP synthetase (trp) has greatly simplified the study of the role of these enzymes in the regulation of metabolism. Only some of the genes concerned with the regulation of aromatic biosynthesis have so far been identified, and the normal function of these genes has yet to be determined. Even after all the genes and their products have been identified, the understanding of the interplay between these various systems in wild-type cells in vivo will require a great deal more work involving new and sensitive experimental approaches.

In all of the organisms in which the regulation of aromatic biosynthesis has been studied, the rate of synthesis of chorismic acid (the end product of the common pathway) appears to be affected primarily by control of the first reaction of the common pathway. At least three different systems have evolved to allow a balanced control of the common pathway by the major end products, tyrosine, phenylalanine, and tryptophan. (i) In the gram-negative enteric microorganisms, and in *N. crassa*, *S. cerevisiae*, and *C. paspali*, the first reaction of the common pathway is carried out by isoenzymes (usually three). Each of these DAHP synthetases appears to be end product inhibited and repressed, primarily by one of the aromatic amino acids, although the effects of the amino acids are not completely specific. (ii) In many strains of *Bacillus*, *Staphylococcus*, *Flavobacterium*, *Achromobacter*, and *Alcaligenes*, a single enzyme carries out the first reaction of the common pathway. This DAHP synthetase activity is sensitive to inhibition by chorismate or prephenate. Control of the common pathway in these organisms is apparently exerted by "sequential feedback inhibition," in which the amino acids inhibit reactions on their particular pathways causing the accumulation of chorismate or prephenate, or both; these, in turn, inhibit DAHP synthetase activity. (iii) *Hydrogenomonas* sp. appear to possess a single DAHP synthetase enzyme which is subject to "cumulative end product inhibition" by phenylalanine and tyrosine.

The control of the terminal pathways differs in detail from organism to organism, but it may involve feedback inhibition or repression, or both. Feedback inhibition is exerted on anthranilate synthetase (by tryptophan), prephenate dehydrogenase (by tyrosine), and prephenate dehydratase (by phenylalanine). Chorismate mutase is inhibited by phenylalanine or tyrosine, or by both, in some organisms, and in *N. crassa* and *C. paspali* it is stimulated by tryptophan which also reverses inhibition by the end products.

At present, there is no evidence, apart from the repression (by iron) of the enzymes concerned in 2,3-dihydroxybenzoate synthesis to suggest that the biosynthesis of the aromatic vitamins is controlled by repression or end product inhibition. More work will have to be done on the regulation of formation of the aromatic vitamins before any generalization can be made.

The pathways of biosynthesis of the aromatic vitamins are being clarified, and the isolation of mutants unable to form ubiquinone, vitamin K, or the 2,3-dihydroxybenzoate group of compounds will assist in studying the biosynthetic pathways leading to, and the function of, these compounds.

The comparative biochemistry of the pathways and control mechanisms will no doubt continue to be studied actively. Experiments with bacteria have thus far played a major role in the elucidation of the pathways, but work with other microorganisms and higher plants has indicated that, although the intermediates are likely to be the same, there may be differences in details of organization and control of the pathways within different cells.

ACKNOWLEDGMENTS

We are grateful to our colleagues for permission to use their unpublished data and, in particular, to G. B. Cox, B. J. Wallace, and I. G. Young for helpful discussions.

This investigation was supported by a research grant from the Australian National Health and Medical Research Council and by Public Health Service grant AM 4632 from the National Institute of Arthritis and Metabolic Diseases.

LITERATURE CITED

1. Ahmad, M., and D. G. Catcheside. 1960. Physiological diversity amongst tryptophan mutants in *Neurospora crassa*. Heredity **15**:55–64.

2. Anagnostopoulos, C., and I. P. Crawford. 1961. Transformation studies on the linkage of markers in the tryptophan pathway in *Bacillus subtilis*. Proc. Natl. Acad. Sci. U.S. **47**:378–390.

3. Arcamone, F., E. B. Chain, A. Ferretti, and P. Pennella. 1961. Formation of 2,3-dihydroxybenzoic acid in fermentation liquors during the submerged culture production of lysergic acid α-hydroxyethylamide by *Claviceps paspali* Stevens and Hall. Nature **192**:552–553.

4. Azerad, R., R. Bleiler-Hill, F. Catala, O. Samuel, and E. Lederer. 1967. Biosynthesis of dihydromenaquinone-9 by *Mycobacterium phlei*. Biochem. Biophys. Res. Commun. **27**:253–257.

5. Azerad, R., R. Bleiler-Hill, and E. Lederer. 1965. Biosynthesis of a vitamin K_2 by cell-free extracts of *Mycobacterium phlei*. Biochem. Biophys. Res. Commun. **19**:194–197.

6. Azerad, R., M. O. Cyrot, and E. Lederer. 1967. Structure of the dihydromenaquinone-9 of *Mycobacterium phlei*. Biochem. Biophys. Res. Commun. **27**:249–252.

7. Baker, T. I. 1966. Tryptophan: A feedback

activator for chorismate mutase from *Neurospora*. Biochemistry **5**:2654–2657.

8. Baker, T. I. 1968. Phenylalanine-tyrosine biosynthesis in *Neurospora crassa*. Genetics **58**:351–359.

9. Baker, T. I., and I. P. Crawford. 1966. Anthranilate synthetase. Partial purification and some kinetic studies on the enzyme from *Escherichia coli*. J. Biol. Chem. **241**:5577–5584.

10. Bauerle, R. H., and P. Margolin. 1966. A multifunctional enzyme complex in the tryptophan pathway of *Salmonella typhimurium*. Comparison of polarity and pseudopolarity mutations. Cold Spring Harbor Symp. Quant. Biol. **31**:203–214.

11. Bauerle, R. H., and P. Margolin. 1966. The functional organization of the tryptophan gene cluster in *Salmonella typhimurium*. Proc. Natl. Acad. Sci. U.S. **56**:111–118.

12. Bohm, B. A. 1965. Shikimic acid (3,4,5-trihydroxy-1-cyclohexene-1-carboxylic acid). Chem. Rev. **65**:435–466.

13. Bonner, D. M., J. A. DeMoss, and S. E. Mills. 1965. The evolution of an enzyme, p. 305–318. *In* V. Bryston and H. J. Vogel (ed.), Evolving genes and proteins. Academic Press, Inc., New York.

14. Brot, N., and J. Goodwin. 1968. Regulation of 2,3-dihydroxybenzoylserine synthetase by iron. J. Biol. Chem. **243**:510–513.

15. Brot, N., J. Goodwin, and H. Fales. 1966. *In vivo* and *in vitro* formation of 2,3-dihydroxybenzoylserine by *Escherichia coli* K-12. Biochem. Biophys. Res. Commun. **25**:454–461.

16. Brown, G. M. 1967. Folic acid, p. 341–343. *In* R. J. Williams and E. M. Lansford (ed.), Encyclopedia of biochemistry. Reinhold Publishing Corp., New York.

17. Brown, K. D., and C. H. Doy. 1963. Endproduct regulation of the general aromatic pathway in *Escherichia coli* W. Biochim. Biophys. Acta **77**:170–172.

18. Brown, K. D., and C. H. Doy. 1966. Control of three isoenzymic 7-phospho-2-oxo-3 deoxy-D-*arabino*-heptonate-D-erythrose-4-phosphate lyases of *Escherichia coli* and derived mutants by repression and "inductive" effects of the aromatic amino acids. Biochim. Biophys. Acta **118**:157–172.

19. Campbell, I. M., C. J. Coscia, M. Kelsey, and R. Bentley. 1967. Origin of the aromatic nucleus in bacterial menaquinones. Biochem. Biophys. Res. Commun. **28**:25–29.

20. Carlton, B. C. 1966. Fine-structure mapping by transformation in the tryptophan region of *Bacillus subtilis*. J. Bacteriol. **91**:1795–1803.

21. Catlin, E. R., C. H. Hassall, and B. C. Pratt. 1968. Biosynthesis of phenols. XIV. Isolation of some shikimic acid-derived metabolites from mutant strains of *Streptomyces rimosus* unable to produce oxytetracycline. Biochim. Biophys. Acta **156**:109–118.

22. Coats, J. H., and E. W. Nester. 1967. Regulation reversal mutation: Characterization of end product-activated mutants of *Bacillus subtilis*. J. Biol. Chem. **242**:4948–4955.

23. Cohen, G., and F. Jacob. 1959. Sur la répression de la synthése des enzymes intervenant dans le formation du tryptophane chez *Escherichia coli*. Compt. Rend. **248**:3490–3492.

24. Cotton, R. G. H., and F. Gibson. 1965. The biosynthesis of phenylalanine and tyrosine; enzymes converting chorismic acid into prephenic acid and their relationships to prephenate dehydratase and prephenate dehydrogenase. Biochim. Biophys. Acta **100**:76–88.

25. Cotton, R. G. H., and F. Gibson. 1967. The biosynthesis of tyrosine in *Aerobacter aerogenes*: Partial purification of the T proteih. Biochim. Biophys. Acta **147**:222–237.

26. Cotton, R. G. H., and F. Gibson. 1968. The biosynthesis of tyrosine in *Aerobacter aerogenes*: Evidence for a subunit structure of the protein converting chorismate into 4-hydroxyphenylpyruvate. Biochim. Biophys. Acta **160**:188–195.

27. Cotton, R. G. H., and F. Gibson. 1968. The biosynthesis of phenylalanine and tyrosine in the pea (*Pisum sativum*): Chorismate mutase. Biochim. Biophys. Acta **156**:187–189.

28. Cox, G. B., and F. Gibson. 1964. Biosynthesis of vitamin K and ubiquinone. Relation to the shikimic acid pathway in *Escherichia coli*. Biochim. Biophys. Acta **93**:204–206.

29. Cox, G. B., and F. Gibson. 1966. The role of shikimic acid in the biosynthesis of vitamin K_2. Biochem. J. **100**:1–6.

30. Cox, G. B., and F. Gibson. 1967. 2,3-Dihydroxybenzoic acid, a new growth factor for multiple aromatic auxotrophs. J. Bacteriol. **93**:502–503.

31. Cox, G. B., F. Gibson, and J. Pittard. 1968. Mutant strains of *Escherichia coli* K-12 unable to form ubiquinone. J. Bacteriol. **95**:1591–1598.

32. Crane, F. L. 1965.. Distribution of ubiquinones, p. 183–206. *In* R. A. Morton (ed.), Biochemistry of quinones. Academic Press, Inc., New York.

33. Crawford, I. P., and I. C. Gunsalus. 1966. Inducibility of tryptophan synthetase in *Pseudomonas putida*. Proc. Natl. Acad. Sci. U.S. **56**:717–724.

34. Crawford, I. P., and C. Yanofsky. 1958. On the separation of the tryptophan synthetase of *Escherichia coli* into two protein components. Proc. Natl. Acad. Sci. U.S. **44**:1161–1170.

35. Creighton, T. E., and C. Yanofsky. 1966. Indole-3-glycerol phosphate synthetase of *Escherichia coli*, an enzyme of the tryptophan operon. J. Biol. Chem. **241**:4625–4637.

36. Datta, P., and H. Gest. 1964. Alternative patterns of end-product control in biosynthesis of amino acids of the aspartic family. Nature **203**:1259–1261.

37. Davis, B. D. 1950. p-Hydroxybenzoic acid: A new bacterial vitamin. Nature **166**:1120–1121.

38. Davis, B. D. 1952. Aromatic biosynthesis. IV. Preferential conversion, in incompletely

blocked mutants, of a common precursor of several metabolites. J. Bacteriol. **64**:729–748.

39. Davis, B. D. 1952. Intermediates in the biosynthesis of proline, ornithine, histidine, lysine and the aromatic amino acids. Congr. Intern. Biochim. 2nd, Paris, 1952, p. 32–40.

40. Davis, B. D., and E. S. Mingioli. 1953. Aromatic biosynthesis. VII. Accumulation of two derivatives of shikimic acid by bacterial mutants. J. Bacteriol. **66**:129–136.

41. DeMoss, J. A. 1965. The conversion of shikimic acid to anthranilic acid by extracts of *Neurospora crassa*. J. Biol. Chem. **240**:1231–1235.

42. DeMoss, J. A., and J. Wegman. 1965. An enzyme aggregate in the tryptophan pathway of *Neurospora crassa*. Proc. Natl. Acad. Sci. U.S. **54**:241–247.

43. Doolittle, W. F., and C. Yanofsky. 1968. Mutants of *Escherichia coli* with an altered tryptophanyl-transfer ribonucleic acid synthetase. J. Bacteriol. **95**: 1283–1294.

44. Doy, C. H. 1961. Lability of N-*o*-carboxylphenylribosylamine as a factor in the study of tryptophan biosynthesis. Nature **189**:461–463.

45. Doy, C. H. 1964. The biochemical difference between certain phenotypically similar, but genotypically different, tryptophan auxotrophs of *Pseudomonas aeruginosa*. Biochim. Biophys. Acta **90**:180–183.

46. Doy, C. H. 1967. Tryptophan as an inhibitor of 3-deoxy-*arabino*-heptulosonate 7-phosphate synthetase. Biochem. Biophys. Res. Commun. **26**:187–192.

47. Doy, C. H. 1968. Aromatic biosynthesis in yeast. II. Feedback inhibition and repression of 3-deoxy-D-*arabino*-heptulosonic acid 7-phosphate synthase. Biochim. Biophys. Acta **151**:293–295.

48. Doy, C. H. 1968. Control of aromatic biosynthesis particularly with regard to the common pathway and the allosteric enzyme, 3-deoxy-D-*arabino*-heptulosonate 7-phosphate synthetase. Rev. Pure Appl. Chem. **18**:41–78.

49. Doy, C. H., and K. D. Brown. 1965. Control of aromatic biosynthesis: The multiplicity of 7-phospho-2-oxo-3-deoxy-D-*arabino*-heptonate D-erythrose-4-phosphate-lyase (pyruvate phosphorylating) in *Escherichia coli* W. Biochim. Biophys. Acta **104**:377–389.

50. Doy, C. H., and J. M. Cooper. 1966. Aromatic biosynthesis in yeast. I. The synthesis of tryptophan and the regulation of this pathway. Biochim. Biophys. Acta **127**:302–316.

51. Doy, C. H., A. Rivera, and P. R. Srinivasan. 1961. Evidence for the enzymatic synthesis of N-(5′-phosphoribosyl) anthranilic acid, a new intermediate in tryptophan biosynthesis. Biochem. Biophys. Res. Commun. **4**:83–88.

52. Drake, B. 1956. Evidence for two loci governing paraaminobenzoic acid synthesis in *Neurospora crassa*. Genetics **41**:640.

53. Dunphy, P. J., D. L. Gutnick, P. G. Phillips, and A. F. Brodie. 1968. A new natural naphthoquinone in *Mycobacterium phlei*.

cis-Dihydromenaquinone-9, structure and function. J. Biol. Chem. **243**:398–407.

54. Dyer, J. R., H. Heding, and C. P. Schaffner. 1964. Phenolic metabolite of "low-iron fermentation" of *Streptomyces griseus*. Characterization of 2,3-dihydroxybenzoic acid. J. Org. Chem. **29**:2802–2803.

55. Edwards, J. M., F. Gibson, L. M. Jackman, and J. S. Shannon. 1964. The source of the nitrogen atom for the biosynthesis of anthranilic acid. Biochim. Biophys. Acta **93**:78–84.

56. Edwards, J. M., and L. M. Jackman. 1965. Chorismic acid. A branch point intermediate in aromatic biosynthesis. Australian J. Chem. **18**:1227–1239.

57. Egan, A. F., and F. Gibson. 1966. Anthranilate synthetase and PR-transferase from *Aerobacter aerogenes* as a protein aggregate. Biochim. Biophys. Acta **130**:276–277.

58. Eidlic, L., and F. C. Neidhardt. 1965. Role of valyl-sRNA synthetase in enzyme repression. Proc. Natl. Acad. Sci. U.S. **53**:539–543.

59. Ezekiel, D. H. 1965. False feedback inhibition of aromatic amino acid biosynthesis by β-2-thienylalanine. Biochim. Biophys. Acta **95**:54–62.

60. Fewster, J. A. 1962. Phosphorylation of shikimic acid by ultrasonic extracts of micro-organisms. Biochem. J. **85**:388–393.

61. Fowler, A. V., and I. Zabin. 1966. Effects of dimethylsulfoxide on the lactose operon in *Escherichia coli*. J. Bacteriol. **92**:353–357.

62. Fradejas, R. G., J. M. Ravel, and W. Shive. 1961. The control of shikimic acid synthesis by tyrosine and phenylalanine. Biochem. Biophys. Res. Commun. **5**:320–323.

63. Friis, P., G. Doyle-Daves, and K. Folkers. 1966. Complete sequence of biosynthesis from *p*-hydroxybenzoic acid to ubiquinone. J. Amer. Chem. Soc. **88**:4754–4756.

64. Friis, P., G. Doyle-Daves, and K. Folkers. 1966. Isolation of ubiquinone-5, new member of ubiquinone group. Biochem. Biophys. Res. Commun. **24**:252–256.

65. Friis, P., J. Lars, G. Nilsson, G. Doyle-Daves, and K. Folkers. 1967. New multiprenylquinones in the biosynthesis of ubiquinone. Biochem. Biophys. Res. Commun. **28**:324–327.

66. Gibson, F. 1964. Chorismic acid: Purification and some chemical and physical studies. Biochem. J. **90**:256–261.

67. Gibson, F. 1968. Chorismic acid. Biochemical Prep. **12**:94–97.

68. Gibson, F., M. Gibson, and G. B. Cox. 1964. The biosynthesis of *p*-aminobenzoic acid from chorismic acid. Biochim. Biophys. Acta **82**:637–638.

69. Gibson, F., and L. M. Jackman. 1963. Structure of chorismic acid, a new intermediate in aromatic biosynthesis. Nature **198**:388–389.

70. Gibson, F., J. Pittard, and E. Reich. 1967. Ammonium ions as the source of nitrogen for tryptophan biosynthesis in whole cells of

Escherichia coli. Biochim. Biophys. Acta **136**:573–576.

71. Gibson, M. I., and F. Gibson. 1962. A new intermediate in aromatic biosynthesis. Biochim. Biophys. Acta **65**:160–163.

72. Gibson, M. I., and F. Gibson. 1964. Preliminary studies on the isolation and metabolism of an intermediate in aromatic biosynthesis: chorismic acid. Biochem. J. **90**:248–256.

73. Gibson, M. I., F. Gibson, C. H. Doy, and P. Morgan. 1962. The branch point in the biosynthesis of the aromatic amino acids. Nature **195**:1173–1175.

74. Giles, N. H., M. E. Case, C. W. H. Partridge, and S. I. Ahmed. 1967. A gene cluster in *Neurospora crassa* coding for an aggregate of five aromatic synthetic enzymes. Proc. Natl. Acad. Sci. U.S. **58**:1453–1460.

75. Giles, N. H., C. W. H. Partridge, S. I. Ahmed, and M. E. Case. 1967. The occurrence of two dehydrogenases in *Neurospora crassa*, one constitutive and one inducible. Proc. Natl. Acad. Sci. U.S. **58**:1930–1937.

76. Gollub, E., H. Zalkin, and D. B. Sprinson. 1967. Correlation of genes and enzymes, and studies on regulation of the aromatic pathway in *Salmonella*. J. Biol. Chem. **242**:5323–5328.

77. Gorini, L., and R. Lord. 1956. Nécessité des orthodiphénols pour la croissance de Coccus P (*Sarcina* sp.). Biochim. Biophys. Acta **19**:84–90.

78. Gross, S. R. 1958. The enzymatic conversion of 5-dehydroshikimic acid to protocatechuic acid. J. Biol. Chem. **233**:1146–1151.

79. Gross, S. R., and A. Fein. 1960. Linkage and function in *Neurospora*. Genetics **45**:885–904.

80. Hendler, S., and P. R. Srinivasan. 1967. An intermediate in the conversion of chorismate to p-aminobenzoate. Biochim. Biophys. Acta **141**:656–658.

81. Henning, U., D. R. Helinski, F. C. Chao, and C. Yanofsky. 1962. The A protein of the tryptophan synthetase of *Escherichia coli*. Purification, crystallization and composition studies. J. Biol. Chem. **237**:1523–1530.

82. Hiraga, S., K. Ito, K. Hamada, and T. Yura. 1967. A new regulatory gene for the tryptophan operon of *Escherichia coli*. Biochem. Biophys. Res. Commun. **26**:522–527.

83. Huang, M., and J. Pittard. 1967. Genetic analysis of mutant strains of *Escherichia coli* requiring p-aminobenzoic acid for growth. J. Bacteriol. **93**:1938–1942.

84. Hütter, R., and J. A. DeMoss. 1967. Organization of the tryptophan pathway; a phylogenetic study of the fungi. J. Bacteriol. **94**:1896–1907.

85. Imamoto, S., and S. Senoh. 1967. Two new metabolites, 2-nonaprenylphenol and 2-nonaprenyl-3-methyl-6-methoxy-1,4-benzoquinone from *Pseudomonas ovalis*. Tetrahedron Letters **13**:1237–1240.

86. Isler, O., R. Rüegg, L. H. Chopard-Dit-Jean, A. Winterstein, and O. Wiss. 1958. Synthese und Isolienung won Vitamin K₂ und Isopreno-logen verbindungen. Helv. Chim. Acta **41**:786–807.

87. Ito, J., and I. P. Crawford. 1965. Regulation of the enzymes of the tryptophan pathway in *Escherichia coli*. Genetics **52**:1303–1316.

88. Ito, T., and J. B. Neilands. 1958. Products of "low-iron fermentation" with *Bacillus subtilis*: Isolation, characterization and synthesis of 2,3-dihydroxybenzoylglycine. J. Am. Chem. Soc. **80**: 4645–4647.

89. Ito, J., and C. Yanofsky. 1966. The nature of the anthranilic acid synthetase complex of *Escherichia coli*. J. Biol. Chem. **241**:4112–4114.

90. Jackman, L. M., I. G. O'Brien, G. B. Cox, and F. Gibson. 1967. Methionine as the source of methyl groups for ubiquinone and vitamin K: A study using nuclear magnetic resonance and mass spectrometry. Biochim. Biophys. Acta **141**:1–7.

91. Jaureguiberry, G., M. Lenfant, B. C. Das, and E. Lederer. 1966. Sur le mécanisme des C-méthylations biologiques par le methionine. Tetrahedron Suppl. **8**:27–32.

92. Jeffries, L., M. A. Cawthorne, M. Harris, A. T. Diplock, J. Green, and S. A. Price. 1967. Distribution of menaquinones in aerobic *Micrococcaceae*. Nature **215**:257–259.

93. Jensen, R. A., and D. S. Nasser. 1968. Comparative regulation of isoenzymic 3-deoxy-D-*arabino*-heptulosonate 7-phosphate synthetases in microorganisms. J. Bacteriol. **95**:188–196.

94. Jensen, R. A., D. S. Nasser, and E. W. Nester. 1967. Comparative control of a branch point enzyme in microorganisms. J. Bacteriol. **94**:1582–1593.

95. Jensen, R. A., and E. W. Nester. 1965. The regulatory significance of intermediary metabolites: Control of aromatic acid biosynthesis by feedback inhibition in *Bacillus subtilis*. J. Mol. Biol. **12**:468–481.

96. Jensen, R. A., and E. W. Nester. 1966. Regulatory enzymes of aromatic biosynthesis in *Bacillus subtilis*. I. Purification and properties of 3-deoxy-D-*arabino*-heptulosonate 7-phosphate synthetases. J. Biol. Chem. **241**:3365–3372.

97. Lederer, E. 1964. The origin and function of some methyl groups in branched chain fatty acids, plant sterols and quinones. Biochem. J. **93**:449–468.

98. Leistner, E., J. H. Schmitt, and M. H. Zenk. 1967. α-Naphthol a precursor of vitamin K₂. Biochem. Biophys. Res. Commun. **28**:845–850.

99. Lester, G. 1961. Repression and inhibition of indole-synthesizing activity in *Neurospora crassa*. J. Bacteriol. **82**:215–223.

100. Lester, R. L., D. C. White, and S. L. Smith. 1964. The 2-desmethyl vitamin K₂'s. A new group of naphthoquinones isolated from *Haemophilus parainfluenzae*. Biochemistry **3**:949–954.

101. Levin, J. G., and D. B. Sprinson. 1960. The formation of 3-enolpyruvyl shikimate 5-phos-

phate in extracts of *Escherichia coli*. Biochem. Biophys. Res. Commun. **3**:157–163.

102. Levin, J. G., and D. B. Sprinson. 1964. The enzymatic formation and isolation of 3-enolpyruvylshikimate 5-phosphate. J. Biol. Chem. **239**:1142–1150.

103. Lingens, F., W. Goebel, and H. Grimminger. 1967. Über die Biosynthese Aromatischer Aminosäuren in *Lactobacillus arabinosus*. Naturwissenschaften **54**:91–92.

104. Lingens, F., W. Goebel, and H. Uesseler. 1966. Regulation der Biosynthese der Aromatischen Aminosäuren in *Saccharomyces cerevisiae*. I. Hemmung der Enzymaktivitäten (Feedback-wirkung). Biochem. Z. **346**:357–367.

105. Lingens, F., W. Goebel, and H. Uesseler. 1967. Regulation der Biosynthese der Aromatischen Aminosäuren in *Saccharomyces cerevisiae*. 2. Repression, Induktion und Activierung. European J. Biochem. **1**:363–374.

106. Lingens, F., W. Goebel, and H. Uesseler. 1967. Regulation der Biosynthese der Aromatischen Aminosäuren in *Claviceps paspali*. European J. Biochem. **2**:442–447.

107. Lingens, F., and G. Müller. 1967. Über die Akkumulation von Chorisminsäure bei Mutanten und Wildstämmen von *Escherichia coli* und *Saccharomyces cerevisiae*. Z. Naturforsch. **22**:991.

108. Lingens, F., B. Sprössler, and W. Goebel. 1966. Zur Biosynthese der Anthranilsäure in *Saccharomyces cerevisiae*. Biochim. Biophys. Acta **121**:164–166.

109. Lorence, J. H., and E. W. Nester. 1967. Multiple molecular forms of chorismate mutase in *Bacillus subtilis*. Biochemistry **6**:1541–1553.

110. Maas, W. K., and A. J. Clark. 1964. Studies on the mechanism of repression of arginine biosynthesis in *Escherichia coli*. II. Dominance of repressibility in diploids. J. Mol. Biol. **8**:365–370.

111. Matsushiro, A., and Y. Kano. 1967. Isolation and characterization of the novel regulatory mutants of the tryptophan system in *E. coli*. Intern. Congr. Biochem. 7th Tokyo, p. 669.

112. Matsushiro, A., S. Kida, J. Ito, K. Sato, and F. Imamoto. 1962. The regulatory mechanism of enzyme synthesis in the tryptophan biosynthetic pathway of *Escherichia coli* K-12. Biochem. Biophys. Res. Commun. **9**:204–207.

113. Matsushiro, A., K. Sato, J. Ito, S. Kido, and F. Imamoto. 1965. On the transcription of the tryptophan operon in *Escherichia coli*. I. The tryptophan operator. J. Mol. Biol. **11**:54–63.

114. Meister, A. 1965. Biochemistry of the amino acids, p. 359–362. Academic Press Inc., New York.

115. Metzenberg, R. L., and H. K. Mitchell. 1958. The biosynthesis of aromatic compounds by *Neurospora crassa*. Biochem. J. **68**:168–172.

116. Meuris, P. 1967. Mise en évidence et séparation génétique de deux PODH aldolases soumises

à la rétroinhibition chez *S. cerevisiae*. Compt. Rend. **264**:1197–1199.

117. Meuris, P., F. Lacroute, and P. P. Slonimski. 1967. Etude systematique de mutants inhibes par leurs propres metabolites chez la levure *Saccharomyces cerevisiae*. 1. Obtention et caracterisation des differentes classes de mutants. Genetics **56**:149–161.

118. Miller, J. E. 1965. Biosynthesis of the benzoquinone ring of ubiquinone in *Tetrahymena pyriformis*. Biochem. Biophys. Res. Commun. **19**:335–339.

119. Morell, H., M. J. Clark, P. F. Knowles, and D. B. Sprinson. 1967. The enzymic synthesis of chorismic and prephenic acids from 3-enolpyruvylshikimic acid 5-phosphate. J. Biol. Chem. **242**:82–90.

120. Morell, H., and D. B. Sprinson. 1968. Shikimate kinase isoenzymes in *Salmonella typhimurium*. J. Biol. Chem. **243**:676–677.

121. Moyed, H. S. 1960. False feedback inhibition. Inhibition of tryptophan biosynthesis by 5-methyltryptophan. J. Biol. Chem. **235**:1098–1102.

122. Nass, G. 1967. Regulation of histidine biosynthetic enzymes in a mutant of *Escherichia coli* with an altered histidyl-tRNA synthetase. Mol. Gen. Genetics **100**:216–224.

123. Nasser, D., and E. W. Nester. 1967. Aromatic amino acid biosynthesis: gene-enzyme relationships in *Bacillus subtilis*. J. Bacteriol. **94**:1706–1714.

124. Nester, E. W., and R. A. Jensen. 1966. Control of aromatic biosynthesis in *Bacillus subtilis*: sequential feedback inhibition. J. Bacteriol. **91**:1594–1598.

125. Nester, E. W., J. H. Lorence, and D. S. Nasser. 1967. An enzyme aggregate involved in the biosynthesis of aromatic amino acids in *Bacillus subtilis*. Its possible function in feedback regulation. Biochemistry **6**:1553–1563.

126. Nishioka, Y., M. Demerec, and A. Eisenstark. 1967. Genetic analysis of aromatic mutants of *Salmonella typhimurium*. Genetics **56**:341–351.

127. Olsen, R. K., G. Doyle-Daves, H. W. Moore, K. Folkers, W. W. Parson, and H. Rudney. 1966. 2-Multiprenylphenols and 2-decaprenyl-6-methoxyphenol, biosynthetic precursors of ubiquinones. J. Am. Chem. Soc. **88**:5919–5923.

128. Olsen, R. K., J. L. Smith, G. Doyle-Daves, H. W. Moore, K. Folkers, W. W. Parson, and H. Rudney. 1965. 2-Decaprenylphenol, biosynthetic precursor of ubiquinone-10. J. Am. Chem. Soc. **87**:2298–2300.

129. Parson, W. W., and H. Rudney. 1964. The biosynthesis of the benzoquinone ring of ubiquinone from p-hydroxybenzaldehyde and p-hydroxybenzoic acid in rat kidney, *Azotobacter vinelandii*, and baker's yeast. Proc. Natl. Acad. Sci. U.S. **51**:444–450.

130. Parson, W. W., and H. Rudney. 1965. The biosynthesis of ubiquinone and rhodoquinone

from p-hydroxybenzoate and p-hydroxy-benzaldehyde in *Rhodospirillum rubrum*. J. Biol. Chem. **240**:1855–1863.

131. Peters, W. J., and R. A. J. Warren. 1968. Itoic acid synthesis in *Bacillus subtilis*. J. Bacteriol. **95**:360–366.

132. Pittard, A. J., F. Gibson, and C. H. Doy. 1961. Phenolic compounds accumulated by washed cell suspensions of a tryptophan auxotroph of *Aerobacter aerogenes*. Biochim. Biophys. Acta **49**:485–494.

133. Pittard, A. J., F. Gibson, and C. H. Doy. 1962. A possible relationship between the formation of *o*-dihydric phenols and tryptophan biosynthesis by *Aerobacter aerogenes*. Biochim. Biophys. Acta **57**:290–298.

134. Pittard, J., and B. J. Wallace. 1966. Distribution and function of genes concerned with aromatic biosynthesis in *Escherichia coli*. J. Bacteriol. **91**:1494–1508.

135. Polglase, W. J., W. T. Pun, and J. Withaar. 1966. Lipoquinones of *Escherichia coli*. Biochim. Biophys. Acta **118**:425–426.

136. Ratledge, C. 1964. Relationship between the products of aromatic biosynthesis in *Mycobacterium smegmatis* and *Aerobacter aerogenes*. Nature **203**:428–429.

137. Ravel, J. M., M. N. White, and W. Shive. 1965. Activation of tyrosine analogues in relation to enzyme repression. Biochem. Biophys. Res. Commun. **20**:352–359.

138. Rivera, A., and P. R. Srinivasan. 1962. 3-Enol-pyruvylshikimate 5-phosphate, an intermediate in the biosynthesis of anthranilate. Proc. Natl. Acad. Sci. U.S. **48**:864–867.

139. Rudney, H., and W. W. Parson. 1963. The conversion of p-hydroxybenzaldehyde to the benzoquinone ring of ubiquinone in *Rhodospirillum rubrum*. J. Biol. Chem. **238**:3137–3138.

140. Salton, M. R. J. 1964. Requirement of dihydroxyphenols for the growth of *Micrococcus lysodeikticus* in synthetic media. Biochim. Biophys. Acta **86**:421–422.

141. Sanderson, K. E., and M. Demerec. 1965. The linkage map of *Salmonella typhimurium*. Genetics **51**:897–913.

142. Schlesinger, S., and B. Magasanik. 1964. Effect of α-methyl histidine on the control of histidine synthesis. J. Mol. Biol. **9**:670–682.

143. Scholes, P. B., and H. K. King. 1965. Isolation of a naphthoquinone with a partly hydrogenated side chain from *Corynebacterium diphtheriae*. Biochem. J. **97**:766–768.

144. Silbert, D. F., S. E. Jorgensen, and E. C. C. Lin. 1963. Repression of transaminase A by tyrosine in *Escherichia coli*. Biochim. Biophys. Acta **73**:232–240.

145. Smith, L. C., J. M. Ravel, S. R. Lax, and W. Shive. 1962. The control of 3-deoxy-D-*arabino*-heptulosonic acid 7-phosphate synthesis by phenylalanine and tyrosine. J. Biol. Chem. **237**:3566–3570.

146. Smith, L. C., J. M. Ravel, S. R. Lax, and W. Shive. 1964. The effects of phenylalanine and tyrosine analogues on the synthesis and activity of 3-deoxy-D-*arabino*-heptulosonic acid 7-phosphate synthetases. Arch. Biochem. Biophys. **105**:424–430.

147. Somerville, R. L., and R. Elford. 1967. Hydroxamate formation by anthranilate synthetase of *Escherichia coli* K-12. Biochem. Biophys. Res. Commun. **28**:437–444.

148. Somerville, R. L., and C. Yanofsky. 1965. Studies on the regulation of tryptophan biosynthesis in *Escherichia coli*. J. Mol. Biol. **11**:747–759.

149. Sprecher, M., P. R. Srinivasan, D. B. Sprinson, and B. D. Davis. 1965. The biosynthesis of tyrosine from labeled glucose in *Escherichia coli*. Biochemistry **4**:2855–2860.

150. Srinivasan, P. R. 1959. The enzymatic synthesis of anthranilic acid from shikimic acid-5-phosphate and L-glutamine. J. Am. Chem. Soc. **81**:1772–1773.

151. Srinivasan, P. R. 1965. The biosynthesis of anthranilate from (3,4-¹⁴C)glucose in *Escherichia coli*. Biochemistry **4**:2860–2865.

152. Srinivasan, P. R., and A. Rivera. 1963. The enzymatic synthesis of anthranilate from shikimate 5-phosphate and L-glutamine. Biochemistry **2**:1059–1062.

153. Srinivasan, P. R., J. Rothschild, and D. B. Sprinson. 1963. The enzymic conversion of 3-deoxy-D-*arabino*-heptulosonic acid 7-phosphate to 5-dehydroquinate. J. Biol. Chem. **238**:3176–3182.

154. Srinivasan, P. R., and D. B. Sprinson. 1959. 2-Keto-3-deoxy-D-*arabino*-heptonic acid 7-phosphate synthetase. J. Biol. Chem. **234**:716–722.

155. Srinivasan, P. R., and B. Weiss. 1961. The biosynthesis of *p*-aminobenzoic acid: studies on the origin of the amino group. Biochim. Biophys. Acta **51**:597–599.

156. Subba Rao, P. V., K. Moore, and G. H. N. Towers. 1967. The conversion of tryptophan to 2,3-dihydroxybenzoic acid and catechol by *Aspergillus niger*. Biochem. Biophys. Res. Commun. **28**:1008–1012.

157. Taniuchi, H., M. Hatanaka, S. Kuno, O. Hayaishi, M. Nakajima, and N. Kurihara. 1964. Enzymatic formation of catechol from anthranilic acid. J. Biol. Chem. **239**:2204–2211.

158. Taylor, A. L., and M. S. Thoman. 1964. The genetic map of *Escherichia coli* K-12. Genetics **50**:659–677.

159. Taylor, A. L., and C. D. Trotter. 1967. Revised linkage map of *Escherichia coli*. Bacteriol. Rev. **31**:332–353.

160. Terui, G., T. Enatzu, and S. Tabota. 1961. Dissimilative metabolism of anthranilate by *Aspergillus niger*. Hakko Kogaku Zasshi **39**:724–731.

161. Tyler, V. E., K. Mothes, and D. Gröger. 1964. Conversion of tryptophan to 2,3-dihydroxy-

benzoic acid by *Claviceps paspali*. Tetrahedron Letters **11**:593–598.

162. Umbarger, E., and B. D. Davis. 1962. Pathways of amino acid biosynthesis, p. 168–251. *In* I. C. Gunsalus and R. Y. Stanier (ed.), The bacteria, vol. 3. Academic Press Inc., New York.

163. Wallace, B. J., and J. Pittard. 1967. Genetic and biochemical analysis of the isoenzymes concerned in the first reaction of aromatic biosynthesis in *Escherichia coli*. J. Bacteriol. **93**:237–244.

164. Wallace, B. J., and J. Pittard. 1967. Chromatography of 3-deoxy-D-arabinoheptulosonic acid 7-phosphate synthetase (trp) on diethylaminoethyl cellulose: a correction. J. Bacteriol. **94**:1279–1280.

165. Weber, H. L., and A. Böck. 1968. Comparative studies on the regulation of DAHP synthetase in blue-green and green algae. Archiv. Mikrobiol. **61**:159–168.

166. Weiss, B., and P. R. Srinivasan. 1959. The biosynthesis of *p*-aminobenzoic acid. Proc. Natl. Acad. Sci. U.S. **45**:1491–1494.

167. Whistance, G. R., D. R. Threlfall, and T. W. Goodwin. 1966. Incorporation of (G-¹⁴C) shikimate and (U-¹⁴C) parahydroxybenzoate into phytoquinones and chromanols. Biochem. Biophys. Res. Commun. **23**:849–853.

168. White, P. J., and D. D. Woods. 1965. The synthesis of *p*-aminobenzoic acid and folic acid by Staphylococci sensitive and resistant to sulphonamides. J. Gen. Microbiol. **40**:243–253.

169. Wilson, D. A., and I. P. Crawford. 1965. Purification and properties of the B component of *Escherichia coli* tryptophan synthetases. J. Biol. Chem. **240**:4801–4808.

170. Woolfolk, C. A., and E. R. Stadtman. 1964. Cumulative feedback inhibition in the multiple end product regulation of glutamine synthetase activity in *Escherichia coli*. Biochem. Biophys. Res. Commun. **17**:313–319.

171. Yanofsky, C. 1960. The tryptophan synthetase system. Bacteriol. Rev. **24**:221–245.

172. Yanofsky, C. 1967. Gene structure and protein structure. Harvey Lectures Ser. 61, p. 145.

173. Yanofsky, C., and E. S. Lennox. 1959. Transduction and recombination study of linkage relationships among the genes controlling tryptophan synthesis in *Escherichia coli*. Virology **8**:425–447.

174. Young, I. G., G. B. Cox, and F. Gibson. 1967. 2,3-Dihydroxybenzoate as a bacterial growth factor and its route of biosynthesis. Biochim. Biophys. Acta **141**:319–331.

175. Young, I. G., L. M. Jackman, and F. Gibson. 1967. 2,3-Dihydro-2,3-dihydroxybenzoic acid: An intermediate in the biosynthesis of 2,3-dihydroxybenzoic acid. Biochim. Biophys. Acta **148**:313–315.

176. Zalkin, H. 1967. Control of aromatic amino acid biosynthesis in *Salmonella typhimurium*. Biochim. Biophys. Acta **148**:609–621.

177. Zenk. M. H., and E. Leistner. 1967. On the mode of incorporation of shikimic acid into 2-hydroxy-1,4-naphthoquinone (lawsone). Z. Naturforsch. **22**:460.

Erratum: The legend for Fig. 2 should read: ... (1) 3-deoxy-D-arabinoheptulosonate 7-phosphate synthetase (DAHP synthetase; 48, 154, 164); (2) 5-dehydroquinate synthetase (153); (3) dehydroquinase; (4) dehydroshikimate reductase; (5) shikimate kinase; (6) 3-enolpyruvylshikimate 5-phosphate synthetase (102); (7) chorismate synthetase (119).

V
Anaerobic Fermentation

Editor's Comments on Papers 40, 41, and 42

40 Stickland: The Chemical Reactions by Which *Cl. sporogenes* Obtains Its Energy
Biochem. J., **28**, 1746–1759 (1934)

41 Swick and Wood: The Role of Transcarboxylation in Propionic Acid Fermentation
Proc. Natl. Acad. Sci. U.S., **46**, 28–41 (1960)

42 Stephenson and Stickland: The Bacterial Formation of Methane by the Reduction of One-Carbon Compounds by Molecular Hydrogen
Biochem. J., **27**, 1517–1527 (1933)

Clostridia, in particular the proteolytic clostridia, are strict anaerobes that obtain their energy by utilizing amino acids as their sole carbon source. It was Stickland who found that energy can be derived from chemical reactions involving either pairs of amino acids or one amino acid and one keto acid. The necessary energy for growth is obtained by reducing one carbon source and oxidizing the other (Paper 40). This "Stickland reaction" was certainly an important discovery helping to clarify the metabolism of anaerobic proteolytic clostridia (Stickland, 1935; Nisman et al., 1948; Nisman, 1954).

A second discovery was in the field of propionic acid fermentation. Although propionic acid formation from carbohydrates was known for a long time (Wood and Werkman, 1936), the conversion from succinate to propionic acid was unknown. Using labeled ^{13}C (Paper 17; Carson and Ruben, 1940; Wood et al., 1940), the existence of part of the tricarboxylic acid cycle was confirmed, but no decarboxylase was detectable until Swick and Wood (Paper 41) found the transcarboxylation system in these bacteria. Its great potential is the possibility for transferring carboxyl groups as ester phosphates, a very important aspect from the point of view of economy and control of cellular reactions.

The last paper of this group (Paper 42) marks the start of investigations into those bacteria that are able to produce methane under anaerobic conditions. These microorganisms are of great importance in applied microbiology (e.g., sewage disposal). Until now, little had been known about their taxonomy and metabolic events.

Reprinted from *Biochem. J.*, **28**, 1746–1759 (1934)

CCXXXII. STUDIES IN THE METABOLISM OF THE STRICT ANAEROBES (GENUS *CLOSTRIDIUM*).

I. THE CHEMICAL REACTIONS BY WHICH *CL. SPOROGENES* OBTAINS ITS ENERGY.

By LEONARD HUBERT STICKLAND[1].

From the Biochemical Laboratory, Cambridge.

(*Received August 19th, 1934.*)

OUR knowledge of the metabolism of the bacteria of the genus *Clostridium* (the strict anaerobes) is at present very scanty. It has been recently reviewed [Topley and Wilson, 1929; McLeod, 1930; Stephenson, 1930], so only a brief summary will be given here, including facts discovered since the above reviews were published. Special reference will be made to *Cl. sporogenes*, which has been used by many workers as a type species, and of which our knowledge is the fullest. The present position is as follows.

(1) These bacteria cannot grow in media containing an appreciable concentration of free oxygen. The degree of tolerance to low concentrations of oxygen varies from species to species. With regard to the reason for this lack of tolerance of oxygen no final decision has been reached. McLeod and Gordon [see McLeod, 1930] claim that it is due to production of hydrogen peroxide, while Quastel and Stephenson [1926] believe that oxygen acts by preventing the culture from reaching a sufficiently low oxidation-reduction potential.

(2) They are unable to grow except in media containing protein or amino-acids. Carbohydrates, if present in addition, are fermented, but are neither sufficient nor essential for growth.

(3) A compound containing the —SH group, or one from which the bacteria can produce an —SH group, is essential for growth (Quastel and Stephenson [1926] for *Cl. sporogenes*, and Burrows [1933] for *Cl. botulinum*).

(4) Tryptophan is an "essential" amino-acid for *Cl. sporogenes* [Fildes and Knight, 1933]. With other species opinions differ; for instance, with *Cl. botulinum* Fildes and Knight say that tryptophan is "essential," Burrows [1933] that it is not. The word "essential" is here used in the special sense that the bacteria require it because they are unable to synthesise it.

(5) In the case of *Cl. sporogenes* growth depends also on the presence in the medium of a trace of a vitamin-like substance [Knight and Fildes, 1933].

(6) Burrows [1933] showed that *Cl. botulinum* can grow on a synthetic medium containing no amino-acids except glycine, alanine, leucine, proline, lysine and cysteine.

(7) Wolf and Harris [1917; 1918–19] analysed the products of the action of *Cl. sporogenes* on various natural media, but could deduce little as to the reactions by which the products had been formed.

[1] Beit Memorial Research Fellow.

It is evident that the quantitatively most important part of the chemical action of bacteria on the medium during growth must be the chemical reactions by which they obtain their energy. As the above summary shows, we know nothing so far of this aspect of the metabolism of the strict anaerobes, and it forms the subject of the present communication.

THE CHEMICAL REACTIONS BY WHICH *CL. SPOROGENES* OBTAINS ITS ENERGY.

The simplest medium on which *Cl. sporogenes* will grow consists of an acid hydrolysate of gelatin with the addition of traces of cysteine (or thiolacetic acid), tryptophan and vitamin [Knight and Fildes, 1933]. This medium contains practically nothing but amino-acids, so the source of energy must lie in anaerobic reactions involving only amino-acids. It is difficult to picture any reaction by which a single amino-acid molecule could break down anaerobically to yield energy, so the most likely type of reaction is one between two molecules of amino-acids, probably involving oxidation of one molecule and reduction of the other, as in the hypothetical equation

$$R^1.CHNH_2.COOH + R^2.CHNH_2.COOH + H_2O \rightarrow R^1.CO.COOH + R^2.CH_2.COOH + 2NH_3.$$

R^1 and R^2 may theoretically be the same group or two different groups.

A reaction of this type would be similar to certain anaerobic energy-yielding reactions of *Bact. coli, e.g.* sodium lactate and sodium fumarate reacting to give sodium pyruvate and sodium succinate [Quastel *et al.*, 1925]. If such a reaction between amino-acids were catalysed by *Cl. sporogenes*, it would be expected that some amino-acids would react as hydrogen donators (*i.e.* would reduce methylene blue in the presence of the bacteria) while others would act as hydrogen acceptors (*i.e.* would oxidise leucomethylene blue). These theoretical considerations have been tested by experiment, and found to provide a satisfactory explanation of the method by which *Cl. sporogenes* obtains its energy.

EXPERIMENTAL.
Preparation of bacterial suspensions.

All the experiments described in this paper were done with washed suspensions of *Cl. sporogenes*. The culture was obtained from the National Collection of Type Cultures (No. 533, *B. sporogenes* Bellette), and was maintained on a meat medium. To prepare the washed suspensions, 800 ml. of tryptic digest of caseinogen in a one litre flask were inoculated directly with a loopful of the meat culture, and incubated for 40–45 hours in a McIntosh and Fildes anaerobic jar. The culture was then centrifuged, and the bacteria were washed twice by centrifuging with Ringer's solution and finally suspended in 10–20 ml. of Ringer's solution. The enzymic activity of such suspensions was very unstable, and experiments had to be carried out within a few hours of the washing of the bacteria; within 24 hours the activity had completely disappeared, even if the suspension were kept anaerobically in the ice-chest. Microscopic examination of many of the suspensions prepared in this way showed that they almost always contained nothing but vegetative cells, though rarely a few spores were visible.

Detection of hydrogen donators.

The usual method was employed. 1 ml. of phosphate buffer at p_H 7·5, 1 ml. of methylene blue or brilliant cresyl blue $M/2000$, 1 ml. of water and 1 ml. of the substances under investigation in neutralised $M/10$ solutions were added to a series of Thunberg tubes. After the addition to each in turn of 1 ml. of a

L. H. STICKLAND.

suitably diluted bacterial suspension, the tubes were evacuated and incubated in a water-bath at 40°, and the rate of reduction of the dye was observed. The averages of the results of a large number of such experiments are given in Table I. It will be noted first that those substances which are the most active

Table I. *Relative velocities of oxidation by dyes of various substrates.*
Velocity with alanine is taken as standard (= 100).

Substrate	Rate of oxidation	Substrate	Rate of oxidation
Sodium formate	0	*l*-Leucine	100
Sodium acetate	0	*l*-Phenylalanine	10
Sodium propionate	0	*l*-Aspartic acid	5
Sodium lactate	0	*d*-Glutamic acid	2
Sodium succinate	0	*d*-Arginine	0
Sodium pyruvate	40	*d*-Lysine	0
Glucose	0	*l*-Histidine	<2
		l-Proline	0
Glycine	0	*l*-Hydroxyproline	0
d-Alanine	100	*dl*-Serine	0
l-Alanine	0	*l*-Tyrosine	<2
d-Valine	60	*l*-Tryptophan	<2

hydrogen donators in the case of facultative anaerobes and aerobes (*e.g.* glucose, formate, lactate and succinate) were not oxidised at all by *Cl. sporogenes*. On the other hand, among the amino-acids were several very active hydrogen donators, especially the simple aliphatic monoamino-acids, *d*-alanine, *d*-valine and *l*-leucine. The only compound among those tried, apart from the amino-acids, which could be oxidised at all was sodium pyruvate.

The oxidation of alanine.

Before proceeding further, a few experiments on the reaction between alanine and methylene blue or cresyl blue must be described.

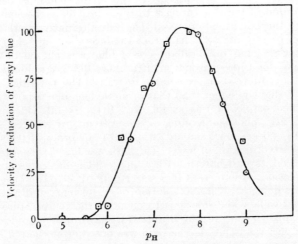

Fig. 1. Relation between activity of alanine dehydrogenase and p_H.

(a) *The relation between rate of oxidation and* p_H. A series of Thunberg tubes containing 1 ml. $M/10$ *d*-alanine, 1 ml. $M/2000$ cresyl blue, 1 ml. water, 1 ml. suspension of bacteria and 1 ml. of buffer (phthalate, phosphate or borate according to the p_H) at different p_H values was incubated at 40° and the reduction time of the dye noted. The optimum p_H was found to lie at about 7·6 (see Fig. 1). A similar result was obtained with *l*-leucine.

(b) *The relation between rate of oxidation and concentration of alanine.* A similar series of tubes, all at p_H 7·5, with different concentrations of *d*-alanine was incubated at 40° and the reduction time of the dye observed. It was found that the affinity of alanine dehydrogenase for *d*-alanine was rather low (K = $10^{-2·5}$ M), so that maximum velocity is not obtained unless the concentration of alanine is about $M/30$.

(c) *Stereochemical specificity.* *l*-Alanine hydrochloride was prepared from the commercial *dl*-product by the method of Fischer [1899]. The sample of *l*-alanine prepared was too small to permit of a measurement of its rotation, which is very low, but the rotation of the benzoyl-*l*-alanine was measured before hydrolysis, and found to be of the right order (found $[\alpha]_{5461}^{16·5°} = -36°$; Fischer [1899] gives $[\alpha]_{D}^{20°} = -37·4°$). As the result was a complete negative, exact proof of the optical purity of the specimen was unnecessary. A neutralised $M/10$ solution was added to a Thunberg tube in the usual way and was found not to reduce methylene blue. To eliminate the unlikely possibility of some toxic material being present in the preparation, a control experiment was carried out as below:

	Reduction time (min.)
1 ml. *d*-alanine $M/10$	$7\frac{1}{2}$
1 ml. *l*-alanine hydrochloride $M/10$	<120
1 ml. *d*-alanine + 1 ml. *l*-alanine hydrochloride	$9\frac{1}{2}$

Specimens of the enantiomorphs of other natural amino-acids have not yet been obtained, but it seems likely that only the natural isomerides are oxidised.

(d) *The course and extent of oxidation of alanine.* The usual method of measuring the extent of oxidation of a substrate, *viz.* manometric measurement of oxygen uptake, was not available in this case. Even in the presence of a dye as hydrogen carrier no oxygen was used. This might be due to peroxide formation, but addition of purified catalase to the solutions in the manometer vessel did not enable the oxidation to proceed. The only alternative method of following the oxidation was to allow the bacteria to reduce a strong solution of an indicator, and for this purpose brilliant cresyl blue was chosen in preference to methylene blue for three reasons: (a) it is more quickly reduced, (b) it is less toxic, (c) its leuco-form is more soluble in water. The potential of cresyl blue (+0·043 v.) is slightly higher than that of methylene blue (+0·011 v.).

The method employed was as follows. In a 100 ml. Büchner flask were placed 5 ml. $M/5$ phosphate buffer p_H 7·5, 10 ml. of a thick suspension of *Cl. sporogenes* and a known amount (usually of the order of 0·005 millimol) of *d*-alanine dissolved in 5 ml. of water. The flask was fitted with a rubber stopper carrying a 10 ml. tapped burette with a fine jet. The flask was now thoroughly evacuated, sealed and immersed in a water-bath at 40°. The burette was filled with a freshly de-aerated $M/200$ solution of cresyl blue, and after an interval of 5 minutes to allow the solutions to come to the temperature of the bath, this solution was run in drop by drop, a further drop being added as soon as the previous one was reduced. The time was noted after the reduction of each 0·2 ml. With every such experiment a control was carried out, differing only in the omission of the alanine.

In Fig. 2 are shown graphically the results of one experiment. It will be noted that the reduction in the control is very large, so that the end-point of the oxidation of the alanine is rather vague. Fig. 3 gives the results of a series of experiments, all corrected for the blank. These curves show that for each molecule of alanine two molecules of the dye are reduced rapidly. In some

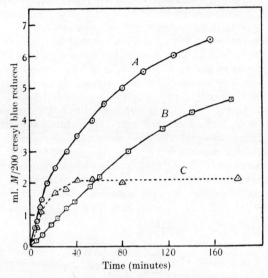

Fig. 2. Course of oxidation of d-alanine by cresyl blue. Curve A, 1 ml. $M/200$ alanine; curve B, no alanine; curve $\check{C}$, difference between A and B.

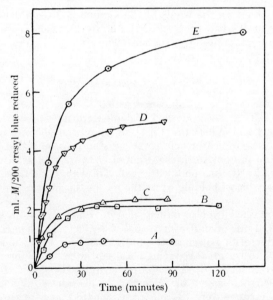

Fig. 3. Course of oxidation of d-alanine by cresyl blue. A, 0·4 ml., B and C, 1·0 ml., D, 2·0 ml. and E 4·0 ml. of $M/200$ d-alanine, all corrected for blank.

cases there appears to be a further very slow oxidation, but on account of the large correction that has to be made for the blank it is very doubtful whether this has any significance.

It was found impossible to reduce this "blank" reduction by further washing of the bacteria, or to remove it by chemical treatment of the suspensions. For instance, toluene treatment, which is so useful with *Bact. coli*, completely destroys the enzymes of *Cl. sporogenes*. In these particular experiments the blank is, of course, greatly exaggerated, as the substrate concentration is so small ($M/4000$). At higher substrate concentrations the blank would be proportionately much smaller both in amount and in rate, but higher concentrations of alanine could not be used on account of the toxic properties of large amounts of cresyl blue.

(*e*) *The deamination of alanine during oxidation.* From experiments such as those described in the preceding paragraph it is possible to learn at what stage in the oxidation of alanine its amino-group is eliminated as ammonia. For this purpose an experiment and its control were taken down when the (corrected) amount of dye reduced was rather more than the molecular equivalent of the alanine present. The dye was removed with kieselguhr, and the ammonia estimated in aliquot portions of the filtrates. Other experiments were carried out with excess of alanine in the flask (5 ml. $M/10$). When a certain amount of the dye had been reduced, the solutions were treated as above, and the ammonia was estimated. One result from each type of experiment is given in Table II. It is

Table II.

Alanine present	Cresyl blue reduced (corrected for blank) ml. $M/100$	Ammonia found (corrected for blank) ml. $M/100$
5 ml. $M/100$	7·0	5·3
10 ml. $M/20$	3·75	3·40

clear that in the first case the whole of the alanine had been deaminated while only 40 % excess of dye had been reduced, and in the second case the ammonia corresponded to the amount of dye reduced. The alanine is therefore deaminated during the first step of the oxidation.

Detection of hydrogen acceptors.

A hydrogen acceptor is a substance which, in the presence of cells, will oxidise leuco-dyes. The easiest method of demonstrating such substances is that devised by Quastel and Whetham [1924], in which the bacteria themselves are allowed to reduce the indicator before the substance to be tested is added from a side-tube. In the present work the original U-tube of Quastel and Whetham was replaced by the Keilin modification of the Thunberg tube, which has a hollow stopper capable of holding up to 0·5 ml. of the solution of the substance under investigation.

Each tube contained 1 ml. of buffer, $M/5$ p_H 7·5, 1 ml. of a thick suspension of *Cl. sporogenes*, 1 ml. of indicator (usually $M/2000$, but sometimes less, according to the tinctorial power of the indicator), and 1 ml. of leucine $M/100$ (sometimes, owing to the great reducing blank of the thick bacterial suspensions, the leucine could be omitted). The stopper contained 0·2 ml. of a neutralised $M/2$ solution of the substance to be tested, or else the equivalent amount of the dry solid. The tubes were thoroughly evacuated, special care being taken that no dissolved air remained in the solution in the stopper, and incubated at 40° until the dye was completely reduced. At this point the solution in the stopper was tipped into the tube and the whole left for a further 2 hours to observe any reoxidation of the indicator. In the first series of experiments the traditional methylene blue was used, and no substance was found capable of oxidising leucomethylene blue in the presence of *Cl. sporogenes*. This meant that, if hydrogen acceptors with respect to *Cl. sporogenes* exist, they must lie at a considerably more negative point on the potential scale than methylene blue, and consequently experiments were carried out with more negative dyes. It was obviously useless to employ dyes so negative that the dehydrogenases of *Cl. sporogenes* were incapable of reducing them, so a rough colorimetric determination was made of the reducing level of the alanine dehydrogenase system. It was found that all dyes down to benzyl viologen were easily reduced (r_H 3 at p_H 7·5), and a partial reduction even of methyl viologen at p_H 8·0 (r_H 1) was observed.

Another series of experiments was therefore carried out with benzyl viologen. It was now found that proline and hydroxyproline caused a rapid and complete reoxidation of this dye, while glycine caused a rapid partial reoxidation. No other substance tried had any effect, and it is noteworthy that, as in the case of hydrogen donators, substances which are active with facultative anaerobes (*i.e.* nitrate and fumarate) are inactive with *Cl. sporogenes* (see Table III).

Table III. Hydrogen acceptors.

Substance	Indicator	r_H of indicator	Reoxidation
Sodium nitrate	Benzyl viologen	3 (at p_H 7·5)	–
Sodium fumarate	,,	,, ,,	–
dl-Serine	Benzyl viologen	3 (at p_H 7·5)	–
l-Aspartic acid	,,	,, ,,	–
d-Glutamic acid	,,	,, ,,	–
d-Arginine	,,	,, ,,	–
d-Lysine	Neutral red	,,	–
l-Histidine	Benzyl viologen	,, (at p_H 7·5)	–
l-Tyrosine	,,	,, ,,	–
l-Proline	Benzyl viologen	3 (at p_H 7·5)	+ +
,,	Neutral red	,,	+ +
,,	Rosinduline	4·5	+ +
,,	Phenosafranine	5·5	+ +
,,	Ethyl Capri blue	11·5	–
l-Hydroxyproline	Benzyl viologen	3 (at p_H 7·5)	+ +
,,	Neutral red	,,	+ +
Glycine	Methyl viologen	1 (at p_H 8·0)	+ +
,,	Benzyl viologen	3 (at p_H 7·5)	+
,,	Phenosafranine	5·5	–

+ + indicates complete reoxidation.   + indicates partial reoxidation.

A few further experiments were done to determine the oxidising level of glycine and proline (Table III). Glycine oxidised methyl viologen completely, benzyl viologen partially, and phenosafranine not at all, so it lies somewhere near the range of benzyl viologen (r_H 3 at p_H 7·5). Proline reoxidised all the leuco-dyes up to phenosafranine (−0·25 v.), but failed to oxidise leuco-Capri blue (−0·08 v.), so it lies somewhere between these two values. No suitable indicator between these exists, since *Cl. sporogenes* is unable to reduce Nile blue (−0·125 v.) or cresyl violet (−0·15 v.).

The reduction of glycine and proline.

The study of the reduction of hydrogen acceptors by a method analogous to that used in following the oxidation of alanine, *i.e.* by letting the bacteria oxidise a strong standard solution of a leuco-dye, presents great technical difficulties and has not been attempted. There are accounts in the literature however of the reduction of these substances by mixed cultures of bacteria, which suggest the probable course of the reductions in the present experiments. Brasch [1909] showed that glycine was converted by putrefying bacteria into acetic acid and ammonia; this is indeed the only way in which glycine can be reduced, unless the biologically abnormal reduction of the carboxyl group is considered. Neuberg [1911] allowed mixed putrefying bacteria to act on proline and isolated from the products δ-aminovaleric acid and *n*-valeric acid. The first stage of the reduction in this case apparently breaks the ring, without deamination. Ackermann [1911] also obtained the same products from proline. Keil and Günther [1933], from similar experiments with hydroxyproline, isolated only δ-aminovaleric acid.

Direct reactions between hydrogen donators and hydrogen acceptors.

It has so far been demonstrated that *Cl. sporogenes* is able to activate certain amino-acids, some as hydrogen donators (*e.g.* alanine, valine and leucine) and some as hydrogen acceptors (proline, hydroxyproline and glycine). For the provision of energy for the bacteria it is obviously not sufficient that these substances should react with dyes and leuco-dyes respectively; they must be able to react directly with one another, without the intervention of an artificial hydrogen carrier. For detecting such reactions between hydrogen-donating and hydrogen-accepting amino-acids, a useful test is provided in the fact, already demonstrated, that the amino-group of alanine is eliminated as ammonia during the first stage of oxidation. Hence if, for instance, alanine is oxidised by proline, ammonia will be liberated.

Experiments were carried out in the following way. In a Thunberg tube were placed 0·5 ml. of a $M/10$ solution of the hydrogen donator, 0·5 ml. of a $M/10$ solution of the hydrogen acceptor, 0·5 ml. of $M/5$ phosphate buffer, p_H 7·5, and 1 ml. of a suspension of *Cl. sporogenes*. Control tubes contained (*a*) hydrogen donator alone, (*b*) hydrogen acceptor alone and (*c*) neither amino-acid. The tubes were evacuated and incubated at 40° for a period of usually 2–6 hours. After incubation the free ammonia was estimated in each tube. 2 ml. of the solution were measured into 25 ml. of 50 % alcohol in a Kjeldahl flask, which was connected through a condenser to a receiver containing 5 ml. of $N/100$ sulphuric acid. The solution was made alkaline by the addition of 10 ml. of borate buffer ($M/5$, p_H 10), and raised to the boiling-point, while the ammonia was removed to the receiver by a current of ammonia-free air. The excess of acid was titrated with $N/100$ CO$_2$-free NaOH. A typical result with alanine and proline is shown in Table IV. This shows that only when hydrogen donator

Table IV.

	Ammonia found ml. $N/10$	Ammonia (corrected for blank) ml. $N/10$
Blank	0·07	—
0·5 ml. $M/10$ *d*-alanine	0·06	0·00
0·5 ml. $M/10$ *l*-proline	0·05	0·00
0·5 ml. alanine + 0·5 ml. proline	0·42	0·35

and hydrogen acceptor were present together was any ammonia liberated, and this is good evidence that the reaction proceeding was indeed an oxidation of alanine and reduction of proline. Further evidence on this point will be given later.

It can further be shown that any one of the hydrogen-accepting amino-acids will react in the same way with any one of the hydrogen-donating amino-acids. Experiments with d-alanine, d-valine and l-leucine on the one hand, and glycine, l-proline and l-hydroxyproline on the other, carried out in the way described above, gave the results shown in Table V. None of the amino-acids alone is deaminated, but any mixture of hydrogen donor and acceptor produces ammonia.

Table V. *Direct reactions between pairs of amino-acids.*

0·5 ml. of $M/10$ solution of each amino-acid was used.
The figures represent ammonia liberated (ml. $N/10$ per tube) corrected for the blank experiment.
The first figure is for the hydrogen acceptor alone, the second for the hydrogen donor alone, and the third for both together.

Hydrogen acceptors	Hydrogen donors		
	d-Alanine	d-Valine	l-Leucine
l-Proline	0·00	0·00	0·00
	0·00	0·00	0·02
	0·35	0·33	0·20
l-Hydroxyproline	0·00	0·00	0·00
	0·00	0·00	0·02
	0·28	0·41	0·15
Glycine	0·01	0·04	0·04
	0·00	0·00	0·01
	0·26	0·55	0·31

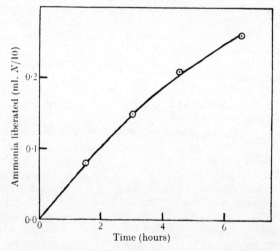

Fig. 4. Course of reaction between glycine and d-alanine.

(*a*) *The course of the reaction.* It is necessary to exclude the possibility that the bacteria were growing during these rather long experiments; this is, of course, unlikely as *Cl. sporogenes* has never been shown to grow on such simple mixtures, and has, even when growing on tryptic broth, a lag period of about 24 hours. A set of Thunberg tubes was prepared containing 0·5 ml. of buffer, 0·5 ml. $M/10$ d-alanine, 0·5 ml. $M/10$ glycine and 1 ml. of bacterial suspension, and another set with 1 ml. of water replacing the two amino-acids. These were incubated at 40°, and the ammonia liberated was estimated at various times up to 6 hours. The result is shown in Fig. 4 (ammonia liberated, corrected for control, plotted against time), and it is clear that the reaction started with no lag period and proceeded with slowly diminishing velocity.

Another similar experiment showed that the glycine and alanine were both completely deaminated.

	Ammonia found (6½ hours) (corrected for control) ml. $N/10$
0·5 ml. $M/10$ glycine + 0·5 ml. $M/10$ alanine	0·95

It can further be shown, in the same way, that just as one molecule of alanine can reduce two of cresyl blue, so it can reduce two molecules of glycine.

	Ammonia found (22 hours) (corrected for control) ml. $N/10$
1·0 ml. $M/10$ glycine + 0·5 ml. $M/10$ alanine	1·46

(b) *Energy of reaction and rates of reaction.* It is clear now that *Cl. sporogenes* is able to carry out various oxidation-reduction reactions anaerobically between pairs of amino-acids. To decide whether these reactions are of quantitative significance in the metabolism of the bacteria two further points must be considered: (a) the amount of energy liberated by the reactions and (b) the rates at which they proceed, relative to the amount of cell material present. Unfortunately the data are not available for calculating the change of free energy in any of these reactions, so for the time being this point must be passed over, but experiments on the rates of the reactions show that they proceed at a speed comparable with those of other bacterial oxidations. That some energy is liberated by the reactions is of course demonstrated by the fact that they do proceed spontaneously.

The velocity of the reaction between glycine and *d*-alanine or *l*-proline and *d*-alanine was measured by estimating the rate of ammonia production as described above, and the nitrogen content of the bacterial suspension was determined by a micro-Kjeldahl method. Using the fact that 10 % of the dry weight of *Cl. sporogenes* is nitrogen, the dry weight of the bacteria used in the experiment was calculated. The results are most conveniently expressed in terms of $Q_{O_2}^{\text{alanine}}$, this being taken to mean in the present case the number of μl. of oxygen which would be used per mg. dry weight of bacteria per hour if the oxidation had been aerobic. Allowing for the fact that in the reaction between alanine and glycine only one-half of the ammonia is derived from the alanine, it was found in nine experiments that $Q_{O_2}^{\text{alanine}}$ with glycine as oxidant varied from 5 to 12. Considering the great instability of the enzymes concerned, it appears justifiable to take the highest value recorded as a minimum, and on that assumption the values given in Table VI were obtained. These may be compared with the figures of Cook and Haldane [1931] for aerobic oxidations with *Bact. coli*, viz. $Q_{O_2}^{\text{formate}} = 40$, $Q_{O_2}^{\text{lactate}} = 12$ etc.

Table VI. *Rates of oxidation in terms of dry weight of bacteria.*

	Hydrogen donators		
	d-Alanine	*d*-Valine	*l*-Leucine
Hydrogen acceptors	Q_{O_2}	Q_{O_2}	Q_{O_2}
Glycine	12	12	8
l-Proline	50	—	30
l-Hydroxyproline	40	—	—

112—2

(c) *Reactions between other amino-acids.* The fact that glycine when reduced, and alanine when oxidised, liberate ammonia, can be used to confirm the identity of hydrogen donators and hydrogen acceptors. The indicator experiments already described, though useful as a starting-point, are not physiological, and cases are known in which substances which do not react with indicators do react with natural substrates, *e.g. Bact. coli* oxidises acetate rapidly by means of oxygen but not at all by means of methylene blue. A large number of amino-acids were therefore tested as hydrogen donators by estimation of the ammonia produced when they were incubated anaerobically with glycine and a suspension of *Cl. sporogenes*, and as hydrogen acceptors by estimation of the ammonia production when they were incubated with *d*-alanine. The experiments were carried out as before, *i.e.* 0·5 ml. of $M/10$ solution of each amino-acid, 0·5 ml. of buffer at p_H 7·5 and 1 ml. of suspension of bacteria were incubated anaerobically in Thunberg tubes at 40°. After 2–5 hours' incubation, the ammonia was estimated in 2 ml. of the solution. The usual controls with neither amino-acid and with each separately were performed.

The results of incubation of various amino-acids with glycine are shown in Table VII. It will be seen that there is a fairly close agreement between the

Table VII. *Hydrogen donators.*

	By reduction of indicator	By ammonia from glycine		By reduction of indicator	By ammonia from glycine
Glycine	0	0	d-Arginine	0	0
d-Alanine	100	100	d-Lysine	0	0
d-Valine	60	100	l-Histidine	<2	55
l-Leucine	100	70	l-Proline	0	0
l-Phenylalanine	10	30	l-Hydroxyproline	0	0
l-Aspartic acid	5	25	l-Tryptophan	<2	10
d-Glutamic acid	2	15			

indicator method and the glycine method, but that some amino-acids, notably glutamic acid and histidine, react relatively more quickly with glycine than with the indicator.

The tests for hydrogen acceptors by incubation with alanine gave the results shown in Table VIII. The agreement is complete, and only glycine, proline and hydroxyproline can oxidise either alanine or leuco-dyes in the presence of *Cl. sporogenes*.

Table VIII. *Hydrogen acceptors.*

	By oxidation of leuco-indicators	By ammonia from alanine		By oxidation of leuco-indicators	By ammonia from alanine
Glycine	+	+	d-Arginine	-	-
d-Alanine	-	-	d-Lysine	-	-
d-Valine	-	0	l-Histidine	-	-
l-Leucine	-	-	l-Proline	+	+
l-Aspartic acid	-	-	l-Hydroxyproline	+	-
d-Glutamic acid	-	-	l-Tryptophan	0	-

0 = not tested.

Serine and tyrosine.

It was found in the course of the above experiments that serine and tyrosine behaved exceptionally in liberating ammonia when incubated alone with *Cl. sporogenes*. Neither amino-acid reacted with dyes either as a hydrogen donator or as a hydrogen acceptor, except for a very slight hydrogen-donating activity of tyrosine. The production of ammonia from serine was demonstrated by experiments similar to those already described, but, since only *dl*-serine was available, 0·5 ml. of an $M/5$ solution of this compound was used. The following is a typical experimental result:

	Ammonia production in 7 hours ml. $N/10$ per tube
0·5 ml. $M/10$ glycine	0·04
0·5 ml. $M/10$ *d*-alanine	0·00
0·5 ml. $M/5$ *dl*-serine	0·35
0·5 ml. glycine + 0·5 ml. serine	0·53
0·5 ml. alanine + 0·5 ml. serine	0·35

Thus serine, apart from yielding ammonia by itself, donates hydrogen to glycine to give extra ammonia, but does not accept hydrogen from alanine. The rate of production of ammonia from serine is about the same as that from a mixture of glycine and alanine. Tyrosine gives ammonia at about one-fifth of this rate, and does not yield extra ammonia with either glycine or alanine. The slow rate may be caused by the small solubility of tyrosine in water (this amino-acid was added as a $M/10$ suspension).

The chemistry of the reactions.

Preliminary results show that the complete reaction between *d*-alanine and glycine is

$$CH_3.CHNH_2.COOH + 2CH_2NH_2.COOH + 2H_2O \rightarrow 3CH_3COOH + 3NH_3 + CO_2.$$

The evidence for this will be presented in a later paper. Work is proceeding on the chemistry of the oxidation of *l*-leucine and the reduction of *l*-proline, and also on the application of these results to growth experiments with *Cl. sporogenes*.

DISCUSSION.

The experiments described in this paper show that washed cells of *Cl. sporogenes* are able to catalyse a hitherto unknown type of chemical reaction, *viz.* the oxidation and reduction of certain pairs of amino-acids. Whether these reactions play an important quantitative part in the provision of energy for the growth of the bacteria on protein media has not yet been determined experimentally, but there can be little doubt that they do. The results of Burrows [1933] are in support of this view. He found that *Cl. botulinum* grew well on a mixture of amino-acids containing only glycine, *d*-alanine, *l*-leucine, *l*-proline, *d*-lysine, *l*-cysteine and *l*-tryptophan. It is significant that, excluding the two "essential" amino-acids cysteine and tryptophan, two of the remaining five are hydrogen donators (alanine and leucine) and two hydrogen acceptors (glycine and proline). Burrows [1932; 1933] interpreted his results as showing that all these amino-acids were "essential," *i.e.* the bacteria needed their presence in the medium because they were unable to synthesise them, but this seems improbable, especially in the case of such simple molecules as glycine and alanine. It is far more likely that they are needed to provide energy by their chemical interaction.

It was stated in the introduction to this paper that "it is difficult to picture any reaction by which a single amino-acid molecule could break down anaerobically to yield energy." It now seems possible that the case of serine is an example of this type of reaction, though it is equally possible that this is an example of a reaction between two molecules of the same amino-acid. It is useless to speculate on the chemistry of the breakdown of serine, and the author hopes to study the matter experimentally.

Bessey and King [1934] have recently described experiments in which washed suspensions of *Cl. sporogenes* were allowed to act aerobically on various amino-acids. They found that the amino-acids were deaminated, some completely. These results are not comparable with those described in the present paper, since, apart from the aerobic conditions, the reactions were very slow (alanine deaminated in 5 days, arginine in 3 days, glutamic acid in 7 days, *etc.*), and there was in every case a considerable lag period before the reaction started. The significance of such deaminations is not yet clear.

Two interesting points should be mentioned in connection with the oxidation of alanine by *Cl. sporogenes*. Krebs [1933] in studying the aerobic oxidation of amino-acids by mammalian tissue slices found that though the natural optical isomerides were oxidised their enantiomorphs were oxidised with much greater velocity by kidney slices. This is the opposite of the case with *Cl. sporogenes*, where the non-natural isomeride is not oxidised at all. Yeast [Ehrlich, 1906] and moulds [Schultze and Bosshard, 1906] also attack only the natural isomerides. Wurmser and Mayer-Reich [1933] calculated the free energy change of the reaction

$$CH_3.CO.COO^- + NH_4^+ + 2H \rightarrow CH_3.CHNH_2.COOH + H_2O$$

and showed that an alanine dehydrogenase system should reduce indicators down to about -0.06 v. (r_H 12) but no further. The alanine dehydrogenase of *Cl. sporogenes* reduces dyes down to -0.35 v. (r_H 2), so the only conclusion is that pyruvic acid is not in this case the oxidation product of alanine. Experimental evidence on this point will be given in a later paper.

SUMMARY.

Washed suspensions of *Cl. sporogenes* activate certain amino-acids as hydrogen donators (especially alanine, valine and leucine) and others as hydrogen acceptors (glycine, proline and hydroxyproline).

One molecule of alanine reduces two molecules of cresyl blue; the amino-acid is deaminated during the first step of the oxidation.

Direct reactions occur between the hydrogen-donating and hydrogen-accepting amino-acids, any one of one group reacting with any one of the other.

The rates of these reactions are of the same order as those of aerobic oxidations with other bacteria, *e.g.* $Q_{O_2}^{alanine + proline} = 50$.

The probable significance of these reactions in the metabolism of the bacteria is discussed.

The author wishes to thank Sir F. G. Hopkins and Miss M. Stephenson for their interest and help in this work.

REFERENCES.

Ackermann (1911). *Z. Biol.* **57**, 104.
Bessey and King (1934). *J. Inf. Dis.* **54**, 123.
Brasch (1909). *Biochem. Z.* **22**, 403.
Burrows (1932). *J. Inf. Dis.* **51**, 298.
—— (1933). *J. Inf. Dis.* **52**, 126.
Cook and Haldane (1931). *Biochem. J.* **25**, 880.
Ehrlich (1906). *Biochem. Z.* **1**, 8.
Fildes and Knight (1933). *Brit. J. Exp. Path.* **14**, 343.

Fischer (1899). *Ber. deutsch. chem. Ges.* **32**, 2451.

Keil and Günther (1933). *Z. physiol. Chem.* **221**, 10.

Knight and Fildes (1933). *Brit. J. Exp. Path.* **14**, 112.

Krebs (1933). *Z. physiol. Chem.* **217**, 191.

McLeod (1930). A system of bacteriology, **1**, 269–274. (H.M. Stationery Office, London.)

Neuberg (1911). *Biochem. Z.* **37**, 490.

Quastel and Stephenson (1926). *Biochem. J.* **20**, 1125.

—— —— and Whetham (1925). *Biochem. J.* **19**, 304.

—— and Whetham (1924). *Biochem. J.* **18**, 519.

Schultze and Bosshard (1906). *Z. physiol. Chem.* **10**, 134.

Stephenson (1930). Bacterial metabolism, pp. 77–82. (Longmans, Green and Co., London.)

Topley and Wilson (1929). Principles of bacteriology and immunity, **1**, 67–70. (Arnold, London.)

Wolf and Harris (1917). *J. Path. Bact.* **21**, 386.

—— —— (1918–19). *J. Path. Bact.* **22**, 270.

Wurmser and Mayer-Reich (1933). *Compt. Rend. Soc. Biol.* **112**, 1648.

41

Reprinted from *Proc. Natl. Acad. Sci., U.S.*, **46**, 28–41 (1960)

THE ROLE OF TRANSCARBOXYLATION IN PROPIONIC ACID FERMENTATION*

By ROBERT W. SWICK† AND HARLAND G. WOOD

DEPARTMENT OF BIOCHEMISTRY, WESTERN RESERVE UNIVERSITY, SCHOOL OF MEDICINE, AND DIVISION OF BIOLOGICAL AND MEDICAL RESEARCH, ARGONNE NATIONAL LABORATORY

Communicated November 25, 1959

The evidence that propionibacteria form propionate by the direct decarboxylation of succinyl CoA[1] has been reviewed by Wood *et al.*[2] It has generally been considered that carbohydrates, e.g., glucose, glycerol, etc. are catabolized to pyruvate which is then converted to oxalacetate by the fixation of carbon dioxide. Oxalacetate is reduced to succinate, which in turn is esterified with CoA and decarboxylated to propionyl CoA and CO_2. Therefore the reduction of one mole of pyruvate to propionate would be expected to involve the fixation and release of one mole of CO_2.

Because succinate is symmetrical, half of the CO_2 released would be derived from the original fixation, and the other half from pyruvate. However, in isotope experiments designed to measure these reactions, the observed turnover of CO_2 was insufficient to account for the propionate formed and it was concluded that a one-carbon unit other than free CO_2 was a product of the cleavage.[2, 3] Delwiche et al.[4] and Phares et al.[5] also obtained evidence suggesting that a one-carbon unit was formed during the decarboxylation of succinate; isotopic propionyl CoA was incorporated into succinyl CoA by extracts of Propionibacterium pentosaceum more rapidly than labeled CO_2. Further evidence for the formation of a C_1 compound other than CO_2 was obtained in studies of the randomization of the C^{14} of propionate-3-C^{14} to propionate-2,3-C^{14} by resting cell suspensions of P. arabinosum.[2] This conversion presumably occurred via a carboxylation yielding a catalytic amount of a symmetrical C_4 dicarboxylic acid followed by decarboxylation. On the other hand there was little fixation of CO_2 during this reaction, nor was there loss of C^{14} from the carboxyl group of $C^{14}H_3$—CH_2—$C^{14}OOH$ during the randomization of the C^{14} in carbons 2 and 3. However, Pomerantz,[6] by the mass analysis of the products formed from C^{13} triply-labeled propionate, was able to show that there is cleavage between carbons 1 and 2 yielding a C_1, presumably by formation of a C_4 dicarboxylic acid, randomization, and subsequent cleavage.

Succinate has also been shown to be involved in the catabolism of propionate in animal tissues. Lardy and Peanasky[7] and Lardy and Adler[8] showed with extracts of liver mitochondria that CO_2 is fixed in an ATP-dependent reaction with propionyl CoA yielding succinate. Flavin and Ochoa[9] demonstrated that the primary product of the carboxylation of propionyl CoA was not succinyl CoA but methylmalonyl CoA, and that succinyl CoA was only formed in a subsequent reaction from methylmalonyl CoA.

The elucidation of this pathway in animal tissues raised the question whether succinate was directly decarboxylated or whether methylmalonate was an intermediate in the formation of propionate by propionic acid bacteria. Therefore the present studies were designed to investigate the pathway of propionate formation in cell-free extracts of P. shermanii and to ascertain the fate of the one-carbon unit. P. shermanii was chosen because Wood, Kulka, and Edson[10] have shown that extracts from this culture fix CO_2, bring about the randomization of C^{14} in propionate formed from glucose-1-C^{14}, and remain active for several hours at 30°.

The results indicate that succinyl CoA is not decarboxylated but is first converted to methylmalonyl CoA and that it is the latter compound which is cleaved to propionyl CoA. This cleavage occurs with transfer of the carboxyl carbon to pyruvate, forming oxalacetate, and the C_1 unit does not equilibrate with free CO_2. Thus it is not CO_2 as such but a C_1 unit which combines with pyruvate to form oxalacetate, while the fixation of CO_2 per se, may occur with phosphenol pyruvate.[11, 12]

The results may be summarized by the following set of equations:

$$\text{Succinyl CoA} \rightleftarrows \text{Methylmalonyl CoA} \tag{1}$$

$$\text{E*} + \text{Methylmalonyl CoA} \rightleftarrows \text{Propionyl CoA} + \text{E—C}_1 \tag{2a}$$

$$\text{E—C}_1 + \text{Pyruvate} \rightleftarrows \text{Oxalacetate} + \text{E} \tag{2b}$$

$$\text{Oxalacetate} + 4\text{H} \rightleftarrows \text{Succinate} \qquad (3)$$

$$\text{Succinate} + \text{Propionyl CoA} \rightleftarrows \text{Succinyl CoA} + \text{Propionate} \qquad (4)$$

$$\text{Net: Pyruvate} + 4\text{H} \rightleftarrows \text{Propionate} \qquad (5)$$

* E = Enzyme. ————————

Reactions 2a and b involve a transcarboxylation, which is a novel biochemical reaction.

Methods.—*Propionibacterium shermanii* (52W) was maintained in lactate-glucose stab cultures and grown for 3 days at 30° in 900 ml of glucose-yeast extract medium[13] in 1-liter flasks fitted with cotton plugs. The cells were harvested by centrifugation and washed with 10 volumes of distilled water. The yield was 4–5 gm (wet wt.) of cells/liter of medium and the cells were lyophilized and stored at −10°.

A cell-free extract was prepared with the aid of the Nossal shaker.[14] Each gram of dry cells was suspended in 16 ml of a solution of KCl (0.12 M) and L-cysteine (0.001 M) at pH 7, mixed with an equal volume of glass beads (Ballotini No. 13). The mixture was then shaken for 15 sec and recooled for 5 min; the process was repeated 4–6 times. The glass beads were removed by centrifugation at 13,000 × g for 15 min and the remainder of the cell debris by centrifugation at 35,000 × g for 30 min. The supernatant solution was passed through a column of Dowex 1-Cl⁻ (0.5 gm/ml of extract) to remove nucleotides.[15] The eluate was next brought to 90 per cent saturation with neutralized ammonium sulfate, centrifuged, and the precipitate was washed once with 20 volumes of 90 per cent ammonium sulfate solution. The precipitate was dissolved in 5 volumes of 0.1 M potassium phosphate buffer at pH 7 containing 0.001 M cysteine. This solution was dialyzed overnight against 20 volumes of the same buffer; after the first 3 hours the dialyzing fluid was replaced by fresh buffer All operations were carried out at 0–4° and the extract contained about 15–20 mg of protein per ml as measured by the biuret reaction.[16] The extracts were stored at −12° and remained active for a month or longer.

Sodium propionate-3-C[14] and succinic acid-1,4-C[14] were obtained from Volk Radiochemical Co. Propionic acid anhydride-C[14] was prepared by the method of Orshansky and Bograchov.[17] Dry sodium propionate (1.1 gm) was thoroughly stirred with sulfur (0.055 g) dissolved in bromine (0.6 gm). The anhydride was distilled under reduced pressure and was 90 per cent pure. The yield was 70–80 per cent. Succinic acid anhydride-C[14] was prepared by refluxing succinic acid-C[14] with acetic anhydride. The acetic anhydride was removed by distillation and the last traces were removed by briefly washing with cold ether. Methylmalonic acid was synthesized from methyl iodide and sodium diethylmalonate[18] and isolated by partition chromatography on Celite.[19] The coenzyme A derivatives were prepared from the appropriate acid anhydrides by a modification[20] of the method of Simon and Shemin.[21] When only the acid was available, the mixed anhydride method described by Beck *et al.*[22] was employed.

Oxalacetate-4-C[14] was prepared from oxalacetate by an exchange with $C^{14}O_2$ in the presence of Mn^{++}, ITP, and phosphoenol pyruvate carboxykinase.[23] Carrier oxalacetic acid was added and the product was isolated by elution from Celite with $CHCl_3$ containing 15 per cent of *n*-butanol.[19]

In order to measure the incorporation of propionyl-C^{14} CoA into the mixed dicarboxylic acids (succinate and methylmalonate), the appropriate compounds were incubated in potassium phosphate buffer at pH 7 at 30°. The reaction was stopped by the addition of 2 drops of 2 N NaOH, and the CoA derivatives were hydrolyzed for 5–10 min in a boiling water bath. The reaction mixture was made acid with 2 drops 6 N HCl, mixed with 2–3 gm of Celite and packed into a column 15 mm in diameter. The organic acids were eluted with 25 ml of ether and transferred into 1 ml of dilute alkali containing bromthymol blue by evaporating the ether. The alkaline solution was evaporated to dryness on planchets under an infrared lamp and the radioactivity was measured in a gas flow counter. The mixture was next made acid with dilute HCl and re-evaporated, whereupon propionic acid distilled off quantitatively leaving only the non-volatile, dicarboxylic acids to be counted.

When it was desired to isolate propionic, methylmalonic, and succinic acids individually, 5–10 μmoles of each acid was added as carrier to the alkaline reaction mixture and evaporated to dryness. The residue was dissolved in 0.5 ml of 0.5 N H_2SO_4, mixed with 1 gm of Celite, and packed into a 5-gm column of Celite prepared according to the procedure of Swim and Krampitz.[19] Propionic acid was eluted with 50 ml of $CHCl_3$, methylmalonic acid with 50 ml of $CHCl_3$ containing 7.5 per cent of n-butanol, and succinic acid with 50 ml of $CHCl_3$ containing 10 per cent of n-butanol. The compounds were located by titration, and the alkaline layer was removed and evaporated to dryness on planchets for measurement of the radioactivity.

Results.—Exchange of propionate-C^{14} with succinate: It has been observed with resting cells,[2, 3] and with extracts of propionibacteria[4, 5] that propionate is "equilibrated" with succinate. It is seen in Table 1 that the present extracts bring about a similar exchange; however, the conversion is believed to occur by reactions 1 and

TABLE 1

THE CARBOXYLATION OF PROPIONYL-C^{14} CoA BY SUCCINATE OR CO_2

Exp. No.	Substrate*	C^{14}-Dicarboxylic Acid Formed† μMoles
1	Propionyl-C^{14} CoA + succinyl CoA	0.084
2	Propionate-C^{14} + succinate + CoA + ATP	0.090
3	Propionate-C^{14} + succinate + ATP	0.002
4	Propionate-C^{14} + succinate + CoA	0.033
5	Propionate-C^{14} + KHCO$_3$ + ATP + CoA	0.030

* When indicated the system contained (in μmoles): propionate-C^{14} or propionyl-C^{14} CoA, 0.3; succinate or succinyl CoA, 1; KHCO$_3$, 50; ATP, 3; CoA, 1 and in addition potassium phosphate, pH 7, 50; enzyme with 4 mg of protein. Final volume, 0.5 ml.; incubated 30 min at 30°.
† Presumably a mixture of succinic and methylmalonic acids. The μmoles are calculated from the total non-volatile radioactivity and the specific activity of the propionate.

2a. In Exp. 1, Table 1, the incorporation of C^{14} is consistent with conversion of the succinyl CoA to methylmalonyl CoA (reaction 1) and exchange of propionyl-3-C^{14} CoA with the methylmalonyl CoA (reaction 2a). In Exp. 2 when CoA derivatives were not added, the derivatives were synthesized in the presence of CoA and ATP. Omission of CoA (Exp 3) or ATP (Exp 4) greatly decreased the reaction. Exp. 5 with CO_2, ATP, CoA, and propionate-3-C^{14} involves a net synthesis of dicarboxylic acids, presumably with conversion of the CO_2 to the active C_1. When extracts were prepared from lyophilized cells which had been stored for several months, there was no activity with CO_2 but there was transfer of the C_1 from methylmalonyl CoA to pyruvate (reaction 2). This observation lends support to the postulate that the transcarboxylation reaction involves a C_1 unit which is not CO_2.

Formation of dicarboxylic acids from propionyl CoA and oxalacetate: Reaction 2a involves the formation of the C_1 unit from methylmalonyl CoA. It was of interest to learn whether other compounds which were known to yield Co_2 during their catabolism would also form a C_1 unit which would be transferred to propionyl CoA. It is seen in Table 2 that in the presence of succinate, ATP, and CoA there was con-

TABLE 2

THE CARBOXYLATION OF PROPIONYL-C^{14} CoA BY VARIOUS
COMPOUNDS

Additions*	C^{14} in Dicarboxylic Acids Formed† μMoles
Succinate	0.036
Oxalacetate	0.117
Oxalacetate + malonate	0.120
Malate	0.016
Fumarate	0.006
Isocitrate	0.002
α-Ketoglutarate	0.003
$KHCO_3$‡	0.014

* The system contained (in μmoles): potassium phosphate, pH 7, 50; propionate-C^{14}, 0.3; CoA, 1; ATP, 1; enzyme with mg of protein; and where indicated, succinate, oxalacetate, isocitrate, α-ketoglutarate, malate, fumarate, 1; malonate, 3; $KHCO_3$, 50. Final volume, 0.5 ml; incubated 30 min at 30°.
† Calculated as described in footnote to Table 1.
‡ 3 μmoles of ATP were present in this case.

version of propionate-C^{14} to dicarboxylic acids, thus confirming Exp. 2, Table 1. However, oxalacetate was much more effective than succinate. Forty per cent of the propionate was converted to nonvolatile acids in the presence of oxalacetate and higher yields have been observed in subsequent trials. These results are in accord with reaction 2b in which a C_1 unit would be formed from oxalacetate and transferred to propionyl CoA to form methylmalonyl CoA, reaction 2a. Other experiments in Table 2 indicate that oxalacetate probably was not converted to succinate prior to transcarboxylation with propionyl CoA. The presence of 3 μmoles of malonate was not inhibitory. Also, several of the possible intermediates in the reduction of oxalacetate to succinate were tested and none was as active as oxalacetate itself. It is not likely that oxalacetate was first decarboxylated and the free CO_2 fixed with propionyl CoA since the yield of dicarboxylic acids was only about one-tenth as great with bicarbonate as with oxalacetate. Furthermore, other extracts, which were prepared from aged cells and which would not fix CO_2, readily utilized oxalacetate for the formation of the dicarboxylic acids from propionyl CoA. Formaldehyde, formate, pyruvate. and 6-phosphogluconate were also inactive in the transcarboxylation. It is not known, however, whether these compounds are metabolized by the extracts; therefore, the results may be negative because the required enzymes were not present to form the C_1 compound which is transferred to propionyl CoA.

The final products of the transcarboxylation reaction between propionyl CoA and oxalacetate are succinyl CoA and pyruvate (reactions 2b, 2a, and 1, right to left). Succinyl CoA was demonstrated by the preparation and chromatographic separation of radioactive succinhydroxamic acid.[24]   The pyruvate was determined by the oxidation of DPNH with lactic dehydrogenase (Table 3).   Although there

TABLE 3

THE FORMATION OF PYRUVATE FROM OXALACETATE AND PROPIONYL CoA

Substrate*	Pyruvate Formed† μMoles
Oxalacetate + propionyl CoA	0.56
Oxalacetate	0.17

*The system contained (in μmoles): oxalacetate, 2; propionyl CoA, 1; sodium phosphate, pH 7, 50; and enzyme with 4 mg of protein.   Final volume, 1 ml; incubated 10 min at 30°.

† Reaction was stopped by the addition of TCA to give a concentration of 2 per cent and the preparation was centrifuged and neutralized.   Pyruvate was assayed in an aliquot by observing the change in O.D. at 340 mμ after the addition of 0.4 μmole of DPNH and lactic dehydrogenase.

was considerable decarboxylation of oxalacetate to pyruvate in the absence of propionyl CoA, the addition of propionyl CoA markedly increased the formation of pyruvate.   No phosphoenol pyruvate was detected by enzymic assay with pyruvic kinase, ADP, DPNH, and lactic dehydrogenase.

The formation of oxalacetate from pyruvate and a C_1 unit (reaction 2b) was investigated using succinyl-1,4-C^{14} CoA as the C_1 donor, i.e., via methylmalonyl CoA.   The oxalacetate formed was separated from the residual pyruvate by partition chromatography and degraded as follows.[25]   The β-carboxyl group was released by treatment with 0.1 volume of 0.1 M Al$_2$(SO$_4$)$_3$ for 60 min.   The resulting pyruvate was isolated by elution from Dowex 1-Cl$^-$ with 0.02 N HCl and was decarboxylated with Ce(SO$_4$)$_2$.   The CO$_2$ formed in each degradation was collected in alkali and plated as BaCO$_3$.   All of the radioactivity in the oxalacetate carboxyl groups was present in the β-carboxyl moiety.   Had oxalacetate arisen from succinate by oxidation, radioactivity would have been present in both carboxyl groups.

In addition to oxalacetate, propionyl CoA should be formed in the over-all reaction of succinyl CoA with pyruvate.   There was some formation of propionyl-C^{14} CoA from succinyl-1,4-C^{14} CoA in the absence of pyruvate, but the addition of pyruvate increased the yield of propionyl C^{14} CoA almost two-fold.   In addition to propionyl CoA and oxalacetate some $C^{14}O_2$ was produced and the amount was increased in the presence of pyruvate.   The $C^{14}O_2$ presumably was formed by decarboxylation of oxalacetate.   In the absence of added pyruvate the $C^{14}O_2$ may have arisen by conversion of the C_1 unit of reaction 2a to CO$_2$ or by transcarboxylation to trace amounts of pyruvate, reaction 2b, and subsequent enzymatic decarboxylation of oxalacetate.   Phosphenol pyruvate was much less active than pyruvate in promoting the decarboxylation of succinyl CoA.

Demonstration of methylmalonyl CoA as a reactant: Flavin and Ochoa[9] showed in mammalian tissue preparations that methylmalonyl CoA is the primary product of the carboxylation of propionyl CoA by CO$_2$.   This compound has now been shown to be the primary product of the transcarboxylation reaction in propionic acid bacteria (reactions 2a and 2b).   Propionyl CoA and oxalacetate-4-C^{14} were incubated with the bacterial extract for various periods, the reaction was halted, and carrier methylmalonate and succinate were added to the reaction mixture and re-isolated chromatographically.

TABLE 4

RELATIVE YIELDS WITH TIME OF METHYLMALONATE AND SUCCINATE FORMED
FROM PROPIONYL CoA AND OXALACETATE-4-C[14]

Duration of Incubation min	Methylmalonate Formed μMoles*	Succinate Formed μMoles*	Total Acids Formed μMoles
1	0.139	0.032	0.171
5	0.170	0.071	0.241
20	0.125	0.125	0.250
40	0.058	0.247	0.305

* Calculated on the basis of the total radioactivity recovered and from the specific activity of the oxalacetate.

The complete system contained (in μmoles): potassium phosphate, pH 7, 50; propionyl CoA, 0.4; oxalacetate-4-C[14], 1; and enzyme with 4 mg. of protein. Final volume, 0.5 ml; incubated as indicated at 30°.

As shown in Table 4, both labeled methylmalonate and succinate were present, indicating that the CoA esters had been formed from oxalacetate-C[14] and propionyl CoA. Maximum methylmalonate formation occurred within 5 min and thereafter decreased, while succinate formation, which initially lagged behind that of methylmalonate increased continuously. After 1 min methylmalonate constituted 82 per cent of the total dicarboxylic acid while at 45 min it was only 19 per cent of the total.

Further evidence that methylmalonyl CoA and not succinyl CoA is the reactant in the transcarboxylation was obtained by incubating extract and pyruvate and either methylmalonyl CoA or succinyl CoA for 1 min and measuring oxalacetate formation with malic dehydrogenase. Table 5 shows that more than 10 times as much

TABLE 5

FORMATION OF OXALACETATE FROM PYRUVATE AND METHYLMALONYL CoA
OR SUCCINYL CoA

Substrate*	Oxalacetate Formed† μMoles
Pyruvate + methylmalonyl CoA (0.65 μmole)‡	0.325
Pyruvate + methylmalonyl CoA (0.4 μmole)‡	0.203
Pyruvate + succinyl CoA (0.58 μmole)	0.022
Pyruvate + succinyl CoA (0.58 μmole)	0.020

* System contained potassium phosphate, pH 7, 50 μmoles; pyruvate, 10 μmoles; methylmalonyl CoA or succinyl CoA as indicated and enzyme with 2 mg of protein. Final volume, 0.5 ml; incubated 1 min at 30°.

† Reaction was stopped by the addition of TCA to give a concentration of 2 per cent and the preparation was centrifuged and neutralized. Oxalacetate was assayed in an aliquot by observing the change in O.D. at 340 mμ after the addition of 0.4 μmole of DPNH and malic dehydrogenase.

‡ As active isomer.[26]

oxalacetate was formed from methylmalonyl CoA as from succinyl CoA during the brief reaction period. Therefore, it seems reasonable to conclude that the compound which is the immediate C_1 donor is methylmalonyl CoA rather than succinyl CoA. It also seems clear that the rate-limiting reaction is the conversion of succinyl CoA to methylmalonyl CoA, since upon longer incubation the yield of oxalacetate from succinyl CoA was similar to that obtained with methylmalonyl CoA.

The role of biotin: Delwiche[27] has shown that resting cells of *P. pentosaceum* grown on a medium low in biotin decarboxylate succinate slowly and that the addition of biotin stimulates this decarboxylation. Therefore experiments were performed to ascertain the effect of avidin, an inhibitor of biotin activity, on the exchange between succinate and propionyl CoA and on the transcarboxylation

TABLE 6

EFFECT OF AVIDIN AND BIOTIN ON THE CARBOXYLATION OF PROPIONYL-
C^{14}CoA BY OXALACETATE OR SUCCINATE

	C^{14}-Dicarboxylic Acids Formed in the Presence of	
Additions*	Oxalacetate μMoles†	Succinate μMoles†
None	0.129	0.054
Avidin	0.002	0.002
Avidin + biotin	0.140	. . .
Biotin	0.122	. . .

* The system contained (in μmoles): potassium phosphate, pH 7, 50; propionyl-C^{14}CoA 0.3; oxalacetate or succinate, 1; enzyme containing 4 mg of protein; and, where indicated, biotin, 0.08, avidin, 200 μg. Final volume, 0.5 ml; incubated 30 min at 30°.
† Calculated as described in footnote to Table 1.

between oxalacetate and propionyl CoA in extracts of *P. shermanii*. It is seen in Table 6 that the addition of 200 μg of avidin (0.5 units of activity) almost completely inhibited the transfer of a carboxyl moiety from oxalacetate or from succinate (via methylmalonyl CoA). This inhibition was prevented by the addition of 0.08 μmole of biotin simultaneously with the avidin. The addition of biotin to the extract in the absence of avidin did not enhance the transcarboxylation reaction. A similar relationship between avidin and biotin has been reported by Wakil *et al.*[28] in their studies of the formation of malonyl CoA from acetyl CoA and CO_2. Recently, Lynen *et al.*[29] have presented evidence of the formation of a CO_2-biotin-enzyme complex as an intermediate in the fixation of CO_2 with β-methylcrotonyl CoA. The inhibition by avidin indicates that biotin also functions as a cofactor in the transcarboxylation reaction and it may be mediated by a complex similar to that formulated by Lynen *et al.*

The isomerization of methylmalonyl CoA and succinyl CoA (reaction 1): It has been suggested that the mechanism of conversion of methylmalonyl CoA to succinyl CoA is a transcarboxylation reaction, i.e., that the unesterified carboxyl group of methylmalonyl CoA is transferred to the β-carbon of propionyl CoA to form succinyl CoA.[26] If this were also the mechanism in the bacterial system, it seemed possible that both the formation of methylmalonyl CoA and its subsequent conversion to succinyl CoA might be inhibited by avidin. However, that was not the case. Table 7 summarizes the results of two experiments in which methyl-

TABLE 7

THE EFFECT OF AVIDIN ON THE FORMATION OF METHYLMALONATE AND SUCCINATE FROM
PROPIONYL CoA AND OXALACETATE-C^{14}

Exp. No.	Conditions‡	Methylmalonate Formed* μMoles	Succinate Formed* μMoles
1	Complete system + avidin, 5 min	0.002	0.001
2a	Complete system, 5 min	0.155	0.104
2b	Complete system, 5 min,† fresh enzyme, 30 min	0.020	0.377
2c	Complete system, 5 min,† fresh enzyme + avidin, 30 min	0.014	0.246
3a	Complete system, 5 min	0.195	0.027
3b	Complete system, 5 min,† fresh enzyme, 30 min	0.019	0.320
3c	Complete system, 5 min,† fresh enzyme + avidin, 30 min	0.013	0.208

* Calculated as described in footnote to Table 4.
‡ The complete system contained (in μmoles): potassium phosphate, pH 7, 50; propionyl CoA, 0.5; oxalacetate-4-C^{14}, 1; enzyme with 4 mg of protein in Exp. 1 and 2, with 2 mg of protein in Exp. 3 and 200 μg of avidin where indicated.
† The incubation was stopped after 5 min by the addition of acid, the preparation was neutralized, and fresh enzyme was added with or without 200 μg of avidin. Incubation was then continued for 30 min at 30°.

malonyl CoA was synthesized from oxalacetate-4-C^{14} and propionyl CoA by a 5-min incubation with the extract. The reaction was stopped by the addition of acid. An aliquot of the preparation was fractionated to determine the amount of methylmalonyl CoA and succinyl CoA formed during the initial incubation. Two aliquots of the mixture were then neutralized and incubated with fresh extract, one portion of which had been pre-incubated with avidin for 5 min. The two reactions were then allowed to proceed for 30 min and the methylmalonate and succinate were isolated. It is seen that during the 30-min incubation, the methylmalonyl CoA was utilized in both the presence and absence of avidin. In the presence of avidin the increase in succinate was equivalent to the decrease of the methylmalonate. In the absence of avidin the amounts of succinate and of total dicarboxylic acids were greater than in the avidin-treated mixture because additional transcarboxylation from oxalacetate was occurring during the 30 min.

Flavin *et al.*[30] obtained complete inhibition of the conversion of methylmalonyl CoA to succinyl CoA by the addition of malonate. However, when extracts of propionibacteria were incubated with propionyl CoA and oxalacetate-C^{14}, the amount of succinate formed was the same with or without malonate. The possibility exists that the failure of malonate to inhibit the isomerization was due to the demonstrated inability of these extracts to convert malonate to malonyl CoA, a compound which would be more likely to inhibit the reaction.

Recently Smith and Monty[31] have reported that the methylmalonyl isomerase activity is considerably lower in vitamin B_{12}-depleted rats than in control rats. Barker *et al.*[32] have found that the conversion of glutamate to β-methylaspartate requires a heat stable coenzyme containing pseudovitamin B_{12}. The coenzyme could be removed from their enzyme preparation by treatment with charcoal. In view of the results of Smith and Monty it seemed possible that the isomerase might involve a B_{12} coenzyme; however, treatment of extracts of propionibacteria with charcoal failed to inhibit isomerization of methylmalonyl CoA.

Formation of CoA derivatives of succinate, propionate, and methylmalonate: Assay of the enzymes involved in the esterification of these acids showed that there was negligible formation of the CoA derivatives of succinate and methylmalonate while propionate was readily esterified (Table 8). These results are in contrast to those

TABLE 8

ESTERIFICATION OF PROPIONATE, METHYLMALONATE, AND SUCCINATE BY CoA AND ATP AS MEASURED BY HYDROXAMATE FORMATION

Acid	Hydroxamate Formed μMoles
Succinate	~0.1, 0.2
Methylmalonate	~0
Propionate	7.1, 9.5

The system contained (in μmoles): Tris buffer, pH 7.4, 250; CoA, 0.5; ATP, 10; $MgCl_2$, 8; glutathione, 20; hydroxylamine, 1,000; propionate, succinate, or methylmalonate, 100; and enzyme with 4 mg of protein. Final volume, 2.0 ml; incubated 30 min at 30°. Hydroxamic acid was determined by the method of Lipmann and Tuttle.[33]

previously reported by Delwiche *et al.*[34] in which activation of succinate was observed in cell-free extracts of *P. pentosaceum;* however, the preparation of their extracts differed somewhat from that used in the present experiments.

The transfer of CoA between the dicarboxylic acids and propionate was studied by measuring the incorporation of propionyl-C^{14} CoA into dicarboxylic acids via reversible reactions 4, 1, and 2a (Table 9). It is seen that there was considerable

TABLE 9

CoA Transfer as Measured by the Carboxylation of Propionyl-C^{14}CoA

Substrate	C^{14}-Dicarboxylic Acids Formed* μMoles
Propionyl-C^{14}CoA + methylmalonate	0.001
Propionyl-C^{14}CoA + methylmalonate + ATP + CoA	0.003
Propionyl-C^{14}CoA + methylmalonyl CoA	0.084
Propionyl-C^{14}CoA + succinate	0.060
Propionate-C^{14} + succinyl CoA	0.072

* Calculated as described in footnote of Table 1.
  The system contained (in μmoles): potassium phosphate, pH 7, 50; propionyl-C^{14} CoA or propionate-C^{14},[26] 0.3; methylmalonate, succinate, succinyl CoA, 1; methylmalonyl CoA (active isomer),[26] 0.5; CoA, 1; ATP, 3; enzyme containing 4 mg of protein. Final volume, 0.5 ml; incubated 30 min at 30°.

incorporation of C^{14} from propionyl-C^{14} CoA into the dicarboxylic acids with either methylmalonyl CoA or succinyl CoA. With propionyl-C^{14} CoA and methylmalonate the incorporation of C^{14} was negligible but with succinate it was comparable to that with succinyl CoA. The succinate apparently may be activated by a transfer of CoA from propionyl CoA (reaction 4), as previously reported,[34] but there appears to be little transfer of CoA between propionyl CoA and methylmalonate. Methylmalonate likewise was not activated by ATP plus CoA. The transfer of CoA between propionyl CoA and succinate apparently is reversible, since there was incorporation of C^{14} into the dicarboxylic acids from succinyl CoA and free propionate-C^{14}. These results also demonstrate that methylmalonate must be esterified with CoA before it can be converted to succinate.

There is no *a priori* reason for the transcarboxylation reaction to be confined to the compounds discussed so far. A few preliminary experiments were performed with the extracts of propionibacteria using other acceptors and donors. Since acetyl CoA[35, 36] and butyryl CoA[37] have now been shown to be carboxylated with CO_2 in animal tissues, the ability of these two compounds to act as acceptors in the transcarboxylation reaction was tested. Oxalacetate and acetyl CoA gave rise to malonyl CoA, while oxalacetate and butyryl CoA gave rise to ethylmalonyl CoA. In addition malonyl CoA and ethylmalonyl CoA will transcarboxylate with propionyl CoA, presumably yielding methylmalonyl CoA. Whether or not these transcarboxylations are all catalyzed by the same enzyme is not known at present.

Discussion.—Although the pathway of propionate formation in propionibacteria involves the same compounds as propionate catabolism in animal tissues, there appear to be some differences in the enzyme mechanisms. Tietz and Ochoa[38] reported that the carboxylation of propionyl CoA by pig heart is a one-step reaction involving CO_2 and ATP and that it is catalyzed by an enzyme apparently containing no biotin. However, more recent work has shown that the reaction can be inhibited by avidin.[39] In propionibacteria the carboxylation of propionyl CoA involves a transcarboxylation reaction which also can be inhibited by avidin but which requires no ATP. The fixation of CO_2 into methylmalonyl CoA by propropionibacteria, however, does involve ATP. Whether the carboxylation of propionyl CoA with CO_2 is accomplished by formation of E-C_1 from CO_2 or indirectly by carboxylation of catalytic amounts of phosphoenol pyruvate and subsequent transcarboxylation from oxalacetate is uncertain. Nevertheless, the transfer of a carboxyl group occurs without involvement of ATP and provides a mechanism for the transfer of a carboxyl group from one compound to another without the expenditure of energy. It is possible that a similar transfer may occur during fatty acid synthesis as illustrated in reactions 6 and 7. Since this sequence avoids the formation of free CO_2 and does not require its activation, it may provide more favorable kinetics for the fatty acid synthesis.

$$
\begin{matrix}
COOH & & COOH \\
| & & | \\
CH_3COSCoA + CH_2COSCoA & \rightarrow & CH_3COCHCOSCoA + HSCoA
\end{matrix} \quad (6)
$$

$$
\begin{matrix}
COOH & & \\
| & & \\
CH_3COCHCOSCoA + CH_3COSCoA & \rightarrow & CH_3COCH_2COSCoA +
\end{matrix}
$$

$$
\begin{matrix}
& COOH \\
& | \\
& CH_2COSCoA
\end{matrix} \quad (7)
$$

Lynen *et al.*[29] have suggested that in *Mycobacterium* the initial step in CO_2 fixation is a kinase-like reaction whereby ATP reacts with a biotin-enzyme complex to form an ADP $\sim$ biotin-enzyme complex and orthophosphate. The ADP is then displaced "irreversibly" by CO_2. If this mechanism operates in propionic acid bacteria, the loss of activity for CO_2 fixation in our extracts may reflect the loss of the kinase, apparently due to aging of the lyophilized cells. It is possible that the CO_2 fixation occurs by a complex enzyme and that part of the single enzyme becomes inactive. It appears from our results that a C_1-biotin-enzyme may be formed without participation of ATP when the C_1 is transferred from the proper donor. The structural requirements for a donor compound, apparently, are that it have a carbonyl group β to the carboxyl group being donated and adjacent either to another carboxyl group, as in oxalacetate, or to coenzyme A, as in methylmalonyl CoA.

Biotin appears to be firmly bound to the enzyme in some intricate fashion as shown by our failure to inactivate the extracts after several different kinds of treatment. When *P. shermanii* was grown on a medium low in biotin[27] we observed that the extract had low transcarboxylation activity which was not stimulated by the addition of biotin *in vitro*,[40] suggesting that the formation of the biotin complex may not be a simple process.

It was of interest to determine whether transcarboxylation is a widespread reaction, and a cursory examination was made of several preparations of animal tissues. Ammonium sulfate fractions of ox liver, dog heart muscle, dog skeletal muscle, and a preparation of rat liver mitochondria disrupted by sonic treatment were tested for activity. Although all were able to fix CO_2 with propionyl CoA and ATP, only the dog skeletal muscle preparation catalyzed the formation of dicarboxylic acid from propionyl CoA and oxalacetate.[41] The magnitude of the reaction was about one-thirtieth that of the bacterial extract per mg of protein; nevertheless, the results suggest that transcarboxylation is not confined to propionibacteria.

The mechanism of the conversion of methylmalonyl CoA to succinyl CoA is somewhat uncertain. Beck and Ochoa[26] presented evidence from isotope experiments that in animal tissues methylmalonyl CoA transfers a carboxyl group to the β-carbon of propionyl CoA forming succinyl CoA and regenerating a molecule of propionyl CoA. However the mechanism is perplexing for the following reason. Presumably methylmalonyl CoA is the initial carboxylation product because only the α-carbon of propionyl CoA is sufficiently reactive to combine with the C_1 unit. Yet in the isomerase reaction as formulated by Beck and Ochoa the β-carbon of propionyl CoA is now active as an acceptor of a carboxyl group from methylmalonyl CoA. Our studies show that the transfer of a carboxyl group of methylmalonyl CoA to the α-position of propionyl CoA to form a new molecule of methylmalonyl CoA (i.e., exchange) is susceptible to inhibition by avidin (Table 6) while "transfer" to the β-position of propionyl CoA to form succinyl CoA (i.e., rearrangement) is unaffected by avidin (Table 7). Therefore it seems possible that the isomerization may occur by a mechanism differing from the transcarboxylation.

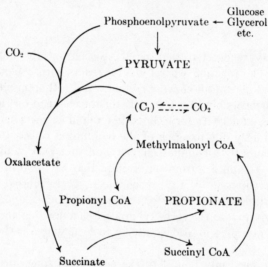

FIG. 1.—Formation of propionate by interlocked reactions involving a C_1 transcarboxylation cycle and a CoA transfer cycle.

The earlier failure to obtain the expected turnover of CO_2 during propionate synthesis *in vivo* in *P. shermanii*[3] now has a demonstrable explanation. The unesterified carboxyl group of methylmalonyl CoA need not be released as free CO_2 but may be transferred to pyruvate with the formation of oxalacetate which can be reduced to succinate, etc. Thus, only catalytic amounts of oxalacetate need be produced by fixation of CO_2. Likewise, coenzyme A may be recycled and only catalytic amounts of the acyl derivatives need be formed by *de novo* synthesis requiring the expenditure of ATP. The transfer of CoA between propionate and succinate has been demonstrated directly by Delwiche *et al.*[34] and indirectly by the present experiments. Indeed, in *P. shermanii* the principal pathway of succinate activation may be by transfer from propionyl CoA.

The scheme shown in Figure 1 is consistent with the results of this study and is proposed as the pathway of propionate formation from pyruvate in propionibacteria.

Summary.—The pathway of propionic acid synthesis in *P. shermanii* has been studied in cell-free extracts and appears to involve the following reactions. Pyruvate is converted to oxalacetate by the transcarboxylation of a one-carbon unit which is derived from methylmalonyl CoA and which is not in equilibrium with free CO_2. Transcarboxylation is inhibited by avidin and occurs in the absence of fixation of CO_2. Oxalacetate is reduced to succinate which is esterified by the transfer of coenzyme A from propionyl CoA. Succinyl CoA is converted to methylmalonyl CoA by an isomerization which is not inhibited by avidin, malonate, or by treatment with charcoal. The transcarboxylation of methylmalonyl CoA yields propionyl CoA. These interlocked reactions therefore involve a "one-carbon cycle" and a CoA cycle. Thus pyruvate is reduced to propionate with a minimum expenditure of energy and without fixation of CO_2.

The authors are indebted to Dr. M. F. Utter for his criticism and many helpful suggestions and to Dr. Rune Stjernholm and Dr. Joseph R. Stern for their interest and assistance.

* Supported in part by a grant from the U.S. Public Health Service and performed in part under the auspices of the U.S. Atomic Energy Commission. A preliminary report was presented at the 136th Meeting of the American Chemical Society, Atlantic City, September 13–18, 1959.

† Post-doctoral Research Fellow in the National Institute of Arthritis and Metabolic Diseases, U.S. Public Health Service. Present address: Argonne National Laboratory, Lemont, Illinois.

[1] Abbreviations used are CoA (coenzyme A), ATP (adenosine triphosphate), ADP (adenosine diphosphate), ITP (inosine triphosphate), DPNH (diphosphopyridine nucleotide, reduced), TCA (trichloroacetic acid), Tris (tris(hydroxymethyl)methylamine).

[2] Wood, H. G., R. Stjernholm, and F. W. Leaver, *J. Bact.*, **72**, 142 (1956).

[3] Wood, H. G., and F. W. Leaver, *Biochim. et Biophys. Acta*, **12**, 207 (1953).

[4] Delwiche, E. A., E. F. Phares, and S. F. Carson, *Federation Proc.*, **12**, 194 (1952).

[5] Phares, E. F., E. A. Delwiche, and S. F. Carson, *J. Bact.*, **71**, 604 (1956).

[6] Pomerantz, S. H., *J. Biol. Chem.*, **231**, 505 (1958).

[7] Lardy, H. A., and R. Peanasky, *Physiol. Rev.*, **33**, 560 (1953).

[8] Lardy, H. A., and J. Adler, *J. Biol. Chem.*, **219**, 933 (1956).

[9] Flavin, M., and S. Ochoa, *J. Biol. Chem.*, **229**, 965 (1957).

[10] Wood, H. G., R. G. Kulka, and N. L. Edson, *Biochem. J.*, **63**, 177 (1956).

[11] Bandurski, R. S., and C. M. Greiner, *J. Biol. Chem.*, **204**, 781 (1953).

[12] Utter, M. F., and K. Kurahashi, *J. Biol. Chem.*, **207**, 821 (1954).

[13] Stjernholm, R., *Acta Chem. Scand.*, **12**, 646 (1958).

[14] Nossal, P. M., *Austral. J. Exptl. Biol. Med. Sci.*, **31**, 583 (1953).

[15] Stadtman, E. R., G. D. Novelli, and F. Lipmann, *J. Biol. Chem.*, **191**, 365 (1951).

[16] Gornall, A. G., C. J. Bardawill, and M. M. David, *J. Biol. Chem.*, **177**, 751 (1949).

[17] Orshansky, J., and E. Bograchov, *Chem. and Indust.*, **1944**, 382 (1944).

[18] Gilman, H., and A. H. Blatt, *Org. Syntheses*, **1**, 250 (1941).

[19] Swim, H. E., and L. O. Krampitz, *J. Bact.*, **67**, 426 (1954).

[20] Stadtman, E. R., in *Methods in Enzymology*, eds. S. P. Colowick and N. O. Kaplan (New York: Academic Press, 1957), vol. 3, pp. 931–941.

[21] Simon, E. J., and D. Shemin, *J. Am. Chem. Soc.*, **75**, 2520 (1953).

[22] Beck, W. S., M. Flavin, and S. Ochoa, *J. Biol. Chem.*, **229**, 997 (1957).

[23] Utter, M. F., K. Kurahashi, and I. A. Rose, *J. Biol. Chem.*, **207**, 803 (1954).

[24] Stadtman, E. R., and H. A. Barker, *J. Biol. Chem.*, **184**, 769 (1950).

[25] Utter, M. F., *J. Biol. Chem.*, **188**, 847 (1951).

[26] Beck, W. S., and S. Ochoa, *J. Biol. Chem.*, **232**, 931 (1958).

[27] Delwiche, E. A., *J. Bact.*, **59**, 439 (1950).

[28] Wakil, S. J., E. B. Titchener, and D. M. Gibson, *Biochim. et Biophys. Acta*, 29, 225 (1958).

[29] Lynen, F., J. Knappe, E. Lorch, G. Jutting, and E. Ringelmann, *Angew. Chem.*, 71, 481 (1959).

[30] Flavin, M., P. J. Ortiz, and S. Ochoa, *Nature*, 176, 823 (1955).

[31] Smith, R. M., and K. J. Monty, *Biochem. Biophys. Research Communications*, 1, 105 (1959).

[32] Barker, H. A., H. Weissbach, and R. D. Smyth, these PROCEEDINGS, 44, 1093 (1958).

[33] Lipmann, F., and L. C. Tuttle, *J. Biol. Chem.*, 159, 21 (1945).

[34] Delwiche, E. A., E. F. Phares, and S. F. Carson, *J. Bact.*, 71, 598 (1956).

[35] Wakil, S. J., *J. Am. Chem. Soc.*, 80, 6465 (1958).

[36] Formica, J. V., and R. O. Brady, *J. Am. Chem Soc.*, 81, 752 (1959).

[37] Stern, J. R., D. L. Friedman, and G. K. K. Menon, *Biochim. et Biophys. Acta*, 36, 299 (1959).

[38] Tietz, A., and S. Ochoa, *J. Biol. Chem.*, 234, 1394 (1959).

[39] Ochoa, S., Personal communication.

[40] Swick, R. W., and H. G. Wood (unpublished data).

[41] Swick, R. W., and J. R. Stern (unpublished data)).

Reprinted from *Biochem. J.*, **27**, 1517–1527 (1933)

CCVII. HYDROGENASE.

III. THE BACTERIAL FORMATION OF METHANE BY THE REDUCTION OF ONE-CARBON COMPOUNDS BY MOLECULAR HYDROGEN.

By MARJORY STEPHENSON
AND LEONARD HUBERT STICKLAND[1].

From the Biochemical Laboratory, Cambridge.

(*Received August 18th, 1933.*)

THE production of methane from a 1-carbon compound was first observed by Sohngen in his classical work on methane formation from fatty acids [Sohngen, 1910], calcium formate being quantitatively decomposed to give methane and calcium carbonate. The same culture also effected the reduction of carbon dioxide. It is important to notice that Sohngen worked with mixed cultures which produced methane also from the higher fatty acids. More recently Fischer *et al.* [1931] have obtained from mud a culture (not claimed by them to be pure) which reduces carbon monoxide to methane, the reaction being accelerated by various colloids. These authors suggest that carbon dioxide is an intermediate product, some evidence being adduced for the occurrence of the reaction

$$CO + H_2O \rightarrow CO_2 + H_2.$$

They also showed [1932] that if the ratio of carbon monoxide to hydrogen exceeded one-third, carbon dioxide and methane both resulted, while in higher proportions of hydrogen methane alone was produced.

In the work about to be described we have obtained an organism which we believe to be in pure culture. This differs from the mixed cultures of previous workers in attacking, so far as we have been able to observe, only 1-carbon compounds.

The culture.

The culture used by us was originally obtained from the River Ouse, which had been recently subjected to an influx of fermentable carbohydrate material from a beet-sugar factory and had given a visible fermentation with evolution of gas in the river itself. By subculturing on a medium containing the usual salts [Stephenson, 1930] with 0·5 % formic acid in the form of the sodium salt as the sole source of carbon, and incubating anaerobically, a culture was obtained which decomposed formic acid according to equation (1)

$$4H.COOH \rightarrow CH_4 + 3CO_2 + 2H_2O + 39 \text{ kg. cals.} \qquad \ldots\ldots(1).$$

The culture was continued on this medium for upwards of three years, involving some hundreds of subcultivations, and there seems to be no doubt that growth depends on the decomposition of the formic acid as above and is not due to any extraneous source of carbon. After a large number of subcultures on this medium

---

[1] Beit Memorial Research Fellow.

the culture appeared morphologically homogeneous, but very numerous attempts to get growth on agar plates failed, and the earlier experiments here described were carried out with no certainty as to whether we were dealing with a pure culture or with an association of organisms of similar physiological properties. Subsequently we resorted to the single cell technique[1] and by this means obtained a culture descended from one cell. The experiments were then repeated with the pedigree culture, the results obtained being identical with those from the crude culture.

As the physiology of the organism is peculiar and not yet fully worked out, we propose to incorporate its full description in a subsequent paper and to confine ourselves here to the chemical aspect of the subject.

Cultivation of the organism.

In our early experiments we found that very large inoculations (1 cc. in 10) were necessary to get certain growth; later we showed that if the old medium were sterilised by passing through a Seitz filter and added to the new medium at the time of sowing a small inoculation served. Finally we found that the Seitz filtrate could be replaced by sulphide (which it always contained owing to the reduction of sulphate). Our final procedure was as follows. The medium to be inoculated was sterilised by autoclaving; immediately before sowing a solution of sodium sulphide in similar medium readjusted to p_H 7 and sterilised by filtration was added, the concentration of the sulphide being arranged to give a final concentration of 0·035 % $Na_2S, 9H_2O$. Immediately after this addition the culture was inoculated and the anaerobic conditions established; delay results in the rapid oxidation of the sulphide. The culture is able to grow indefinitely without the addition of sulphide, provided the sowings are large enough. This is explained by the fact that the bacteria can reduce the sulphate of the medium to sulphide, as is shown in Exp. 7 on p. 1523. Cysteine and reduced glutathione cannot take the place of sulphide in promoting the growth of the culture.

In order to grow the bacteria in bulk six boiling-tubes each containing 30 cc. of medium were first inoculated; when growth was obtained (8 to 14 days) the whole of the contents of the tubes were sown into one litre of medium. A small quantity of sterile mud results in quicker growth at all stages, but is open to the objection that constituents of the mud may be entering into the subsequent reactions. We have tested this point experimentally, and found that the objection is not valid (see Exp. 8, p. 1524); further evidence is given by the fact that identical results are obtained whether the growth of the bacteria has been aided by mud or not. When the culture was well grown, as shown by vigorous effervescence, it was centrifuged and washed with 0·9 % sodium chloride solution or Ringer's solution with full sterile precautions. The growth from one litre of medium was used for each experiment, but it must be realised that the growth is very scanty as compared with that of most organisms grown on broth.

Apparatus.

This consisted of a bolt-headed flask of about 250 cc. capacity attached to a manometer (see Fig. 1). The method used for sterilisation is fully described in a previous communication [Stephenson and Stickland, 1931, 2].

Exp. 1. The decomposition of formic acid into methane and carbon dioxide. This is the reaction occurring during the growth of the organism on the formate

---

[1] One of us (M. S.) owes Prof. Morton Kahn of Cornell University and his assistant Mrs Schwarz-kopf the warmest thanks for instruction and help in the use of this method.

BACTERIAL FORMATION OF METHANE 1519

medium; the quantitative nature of the process was established by the use of washed suspensions as follows.

Into the flask were put 10 cc. of phosphate buffer, p_H 6·4, 10 cc. of 0·25 N sodium formate, 10 cc. bacterial suspension (from one litre of medium) and 10 cc. of water. The flask was then attached to the mano-
meter as previously described; nitrogen passed over heated copper was then introduced and the process repeated. After filling with nitrogen for the second time the manometer was connected to the flask by turning the tap T_1 and the apparatus placed at 37°. When the manometer reading was constant (after 1½–2 hours) the initial reading was taken, together with the temperature and pressure. When the reaction was complete (4–5 days), i.e. when no further change of pressure took place, the final readings of manometer, temperature and barometer were taken, and a sample of gas was removed through tap T_3 for analysis.

The carbon dioxide remaining bound in the solution as bicarbonate was estimated by acidi-

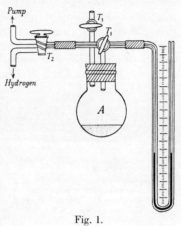

Fig. 1.

fying an aliquot part and blowing the carbon dioxide into standard baryta by means of a current of air. The complete figures for one experiment are given in Table I and the results of three similar experiments in Table II.

Table I.

Formic acid decomposed (mg.)	115
Volume of gas space of flask (cc.)	168
Final temperature	35°
Final barometric pressure (mm.)	763·0
Final manometer reading (mm.)	+108·0
Final composition of gas	H_2 0·0 %; CO_2 6·35 %; CH_4 8·7 %; N_2 (by difference) 84·95 %
Final CO_2 in solution	28·2 cc. of 0·0977 N acid
Volumes of gas formed at N.T.P. (cc.)	CO_2 41·1; CH_4 14·1

Table II.

	Formic acid decomposed (millimols)	CO_2 formed (millimols)	CH_4 formed (millimols)	Formic acid / 4 (millimols)	CO_2 formed / 3 (millimols)
1	2·00	1·53	0·46	0·50	0·51
2	2·00	1·47	0·45	0·50	0·49
3*	2·50	1·83	0·63	0·625	0·61

* Indicates experiment with pure culture.

Thus a washed suspension of the culture decomposes formic acid quantitatively in accordance with equation (1) (p. 1517). (The last two columns in Table II are added to show the extent of the agreement more clearly.)

Exp. 2. The reduction of carbon dioxide by hydrogen to methane. We next investigated whether the culture responsible for the reaction described in the last section could also effect the reduction of carbon dioxide to methane by molecular hydrogen, as Sohngen's did. The same apparatus was used and in the flask were placed 10 cc. buffer p_H 7·0, 10 cc. bacterial suspension and 20 cc. water. After connection to the manometer, the flask was evacuated; pure carbon dioxide from a Kipp's apparatus was then let in to a pressure of about 60 mm.

(bringing the p_H of the solution to 6·5, the optimum), and this pressure was read off accurately on the manometer attached to the pump; the flask was then completely filled with pure hydrogen, and the tap turned to connect it with its own manometer. Finally, the manometer readings, the barometric pressure and the room temperature were taken; from these data the absolute volumes of carbon dioxide and hydrogen in the flask could be calculated. The whole apparatus was then placed at 37°, and when the uptake of gas had finished (in about 6 days) the temperature and manometer and barometer readings were again taken and a sample of gas withdrawn for analysis. The complete results of a typical experiment are given in Table III, and the condensed results of four experiments in Table IV.

Table III.

Original pressure of CO_2 (mm.)	65·5		
Volume of gas space in flask (cc.)	176		
Final composition of gas	CO_2 0·0 %; H_2 86·7 %; CH_4 13·5 %		

	Initial	Final	Difference
Temperature	20°	36°	
Barometric pressure (mm.)	757·5	761·5	
Manometer reading (mm.)	+19·5	−198·5	
Volume of CO_2 at N.T.P. (cc.)	14·2	0·0	−14·2
Volume of H_2 at N.T.P. (cc.)	150·0	92·0	−58·0
Volume of CH_4 at N.T.P. (cc.)	0·0	14·3	+14·3

Table IV.

	Hydrogen used (millimols)	Carbon dioxide used (millimols)	Methane formed (millimols)	$\dfrac{\text{Hydrogen used}}{4}$ (millimols)
1	2·59	0·64	0·64	0·65
2	2·56	0·63	0·61	0·65
3	2·85	0·70	0·69	0·71
4*	4·48	1·00	0·97	1·12

* Indicates experiment with pure culture.

The theoretical equation is

$$CO_2 + 4H_2 \rightarrow CH_4 + 2H_2O \qquad \ldots\ldots(2),$$

and the results obtained agree with this, so we must conclude that the same culture which decomposes formic acid to methane and carbon dioxide is also capable of reducing carbon dioxide to methane by means of molecular hydrogen.

It will be remembered that Sohngen carried out the fermentation of a number of fatty acids in the presence of hydrogen and obtained greater yields of methane with uptake of hydrogen. We therefore allowed our culture to decompose formate in an atmosphere of hydrogen, and estimated the methane formed and the hydrogen used.

Exp. 3. The reduction of formic acid with hydrogen. The same method was used as in Exp. 1, but only 5 cc. of 0·25 N formate were taken, and the apparatus was filled with hydrogen. After about six days there was no further movement of the manometer, and the usual readings were taken, a sample of gas was withdrawn and the residual formic acid estimated. The results of three experiments are given in Table VI, with complete details of one of them in Table V.

The equation is

$$H.COOH + 3H_2 \rightarrow CH_4 + 2H_2O \qquad \ldots\ldots(3).$$

From these experiments it is clear that if the change of formic acid into methane is carried out in an atmosphere of hydrogen no carbon dioxide is produced, but the carbon of the formic acid is completely reduced to methane.

Table V.

	Formic acid decomposed (mg.)	56·2		
	Volume of gas space in flask (cc.)	170		
	Final composition of gas	H_2 72·6 %; CH_4 27·4 %		

	Initial	Final	Difference
Temperature	36°	36°	
Barometric pressure (mm.)	767·0	743·5	
Manometer reading (mm.)	+ 36·0	− 227·5	
Volume of H_2 at N.T.P. (cc.)	150·0	69·0	− 81·0
Volume of CH_4 at N.T.P. (cc.)	0·0	26·0	+ 26·0

Table VI.

	Formic acid decomposed (millimols)	Hydrogen used (millimols)	Methane formed (millimols)	$\dfrac{\text{Hydrogen used}}{3}$ (millimols)
1	1·22	3·62	1·16	1·21
2	1·25	3·91	1·22	1·30
3*	1·11	3·36	1·16	1·12

* Indicates experiment with pure culture.

Exp. 4. The reduction of carbon monoxide by hydrogen to methane. The usual phosphate buffer and cell suspension were placed in the flask in a total volume of 40 cc., and the flask was evacuated and filled with a gas mixture containing about 95 % hydrogen and 5 % carbon monoxide, accurately analysed in the Haldane apparatus. The gas was freed from oxygen first by heating a coil of platinum wire in it and then by bubbling it through alkaline pyrogallol on its way to the flask; the former of these two treatments reduced the oxygen content below that detectable in the Haldane apparatus, *viz.* 0·02 %. When the apparatus was incubated at 37°, the gas volume diminished rather slowly, and after several weeks the hydrogen uptake stopped considerably short of the theoretical amount. At the end of the experiment the usual readings were taken, and a sample of gas was withdrawn for estimation of hydrogen, carbon monoxide and methane.

The distinction between carbon monoxide and methane in this mixture depended on the estimation of the oxygen remaining after burning the gas, and as the total amount of $(CO + CH_4)$ was only roughly 6 % of the gas, and the analyses had to be done on samples of 0·8 cc., the results were less accurate than usual. These particular gas samples were always analysed in triplicate, and the values agreed as well as could be expected. Further, a mixture of carbon monoxide and hydrogen, containing no methane, on analysis by this method, gave values for methane between + 0·1 % and − 0·5 %.

Table VII. *Analyses of mixture of H_2 and CO, to test accuracy of analyses of mixtures of H_2, CO and CH_4.*

			(1) %	(2) %				(1) %	(2) %
(a) By ordinary method		H_2	80·9	80·3	(b) By special method		H_2	81·3	80·8
		CO	19·1	19·4			CO	19·2	20·0
			100·0	99·7			CH_4	0·1	−0·5
								100·6	100·3

The results of experiments on the reduction of carbon monoxide are given in Tables VIII and IX. The equation representing the reaction is

$$CO + 3H_2 \rightarrow CH_4 + H_2O \qquad \ldots\ldots(4),$$

1522   M. STEPHENSON AND L. H. STICKLAND

and the results are sufficiently close to show that this is actually the reaction
that takes place; the experimental error is greater than in the previous experiments.

Table VIII.

Volume of gas space in flask (cc.)	170		
Initial composition of gas	H_2 91·6 %; CO 7·3 %; CH_4 0·0 %.		
Final composition of gas	H_2 90·8 %; CO 3·6 %; CH_4 4·1 %.		

	Initial	Final	Difference
Temperature	36°	37°	
Barometric pressure (mm.)	755·0	751·0	
Manometer reading (mm.)	+ 82·0	− 15·0	
Volume of H_2 at N.T.P. (cc.)	143·5	123·2	− 20·3
Volume of CO at N.T.P. (cc.)	11·4	4·9	− 6·5
Volume of CH_4 at N.T.P. (cc.)	0·0	5·6	+ 5·6

Table IX.

	Hydrogen used (millimols)	CO reduced (millimols)	CH_4 produced (millimols)	$\frac{H_2 \text{ used}}{3}$ (millimols)
1	0·91	0·29	0·25	0·30
2*	0·61	0·18	0·175	0·20

* Indicates experiment with pure culture.

Exp. 5. The reduction of formaldehyde by hydrogen. Formaldehyde is far too
toxic for use in our apparatus, as the smallest amount the reduction of which
could be measured would be sufficient to kill the bacteria and destroy their
enzymes. The only possibility was to use some very slightly dissociated compound of formaldehyde, such as hexamethylenetetramine, and this was done.

10 cc. of 0·63 % hexamethylenetetramine were placed in the flask with the
usual buffer and bacterial suspension in a total volume of 40 cc., and the
apparatus was filled with hydrogen and incubated at 37°. Hydrogen uptake
continued for two to three weeks, when the gas was analysed and the remaining
hexamethylenetetramine estimated. This was done by converting the hexamethylenetetramine into formaldehyde by treatment with dilute sulphuric acid,
allowing the aldehyde to react with sodium bisulphite (in excess) and titrating
the bound sulphite with standard iodine in the usual way. The method is
unsatisfactory, owing to the fact that the reaction of hexamethylenetetramine
with dilute acids produces, besides formaldehyde and ammonia, methylamine,
dimethylamine and other products; too low results in the initial and final
hexamethylenetetramine estimations would partly account for the low value for
"formaldehyde reduced."

The results (Tables X and XI) are sufficient to show that the reaction

$$H.CHO + 2H_2 \rightarrow CH_4 + H_2O \qquad \qquad ......(5)$$

does really occur.

Table X.

Formaldehyde disappeared (mg.)	40		
Volume of gas space in flask (cc.)	162		
Final composition of gas	H_2 70·1 %; CH_4 29·8 %		

	Initial	Final	Difference
Temperature	35°	37°	
Barometric pressure (mm.)	764·0	769·0	
Manometer reading (mm.)	+ 81·0	− 146·0	
Volume of H_2 at N.T.P. (cc.)	151·4	73·5	− 75·9
Volume of CH_4 at N.T.P. (cc.)	0·0	32·1	+ 32·1

Table XI.

	Formaldehyde reduced (millimols)	Hydrogen used (millimols)	Methane formed (millimols)	$\dfrac{H_2 \text{ used}}{2}$ (millimols)
1	1·34	3·39	1·43	1·69
2*	0·215	0·46	0·20	0·23

* Indicates experiment with pure culture.

Exp. 6. The reduction of methyl alcohol to methane by hydrogen. This was carried out in the usual way except that special precautions were taken to avoid loss of methyl alcohol vapour during the evacuation of the flask. 10 cc. of buffer at p_H 6·3, 7 cc. of water and 20 cc. of bacterial suspension were placed in the flask, which was then twice evacuated and filled with hydrogen, leaving at the end a diminished pressure of about 20 mm. of mercury. 1 cc. of the methyl alcohol solution was then added through the tap, care being taken that no air was admitted, and washed down twice with 1 cc. of water, and the flask was then completely filled with hydrogen and the whole apparatus incubated at 37°. Theoretically, if the reaction taking place is

$$CH_3OH + H_2 = CH_4 + H_2O \qquad \ldots\ldots(6),$$

no change of pressure should occur. The results are given in Tables XII and XIII; in Exps. 1 and 2 excess of methyl alcohol was present, and the amount left was not estimated, but the agreement between hydrogen used and methane formed is good, and in Exp. 3 the methyl alcohol was completely accounted for as methane.

Table XII.

Volume of gas space in flask (cc.)	180		
Final composition of gas	H_2 91·2 %; CH_4 8·6 %		
	Initial	Final	Difference
Temperature	34°	36°	
Barometric pressure (mm.)	753·0	761·0	
Manometer reading (mm.)	+ 74·0	+ 73·0	
Volume of H_2 at N.T.P. (cc.)	165·5	151·0	− 14·5
Volume of CH_4 at N.T.P. (cc.)	0·0	14·2	+ 14·2

Table XIII.

	Methyl alcohol reduced (millimols)	Hydrogen used (millimols)	Methane formed (millimols)
1	—	0·65	0·64
2	—	0·30	0·29
3*	0·62	0·54	0·59

* Indicates experiment with pure culture.

Exp. 7. The reduction of sulphate to sulphide by hydrogen. This experiment was carried out in the same way as those previously described [Stephenson and Stickland, 1931, 2]. The results show that the methane-forming culture can also carry out the reaction

$$H_2SO_4 + 4H_2 = H_2S + 4H_2O.$$

The experimental results are summarised in Table XIV.

Table XIV.

Na_2SO_4 reduced (millimols)	Hydrogen used (millimols)	$\dfrac{H_2 \text{ used}}{4}$ (millimols)	Hydrogen sulphide formed (millimols)
0·42	1·60	0·40	0·35

Exp. 8. Control. The bacteria from a litre of medium together with the mud of the medium on which they had grown were placed in the manometer apparatus as usual, but without the addition of any carbon compound. After incubation with hydrogen for fourteen days no methane was found in the gas, showing that the results of the quantitative experiments are not invalidated by the presence of mud. This result received confirmation in experiments in which various 2-carbon compounds were added and in which no methane was formed.

Experiments on reaction velocity.

Of the six reactions described in which carbon compounds are converted into methane, the three involving carbon dioxide and formic acid proceed easily and rapidly and are completed in our manometer apparatus in a few days. The reductions of carbon monoxide, formaldehyde and methyl alcohol, on the other hand, are relatively very slow and are usually incomplete in twenty-one days, even with low initial concentrations. This difference of velocity has been confirmed by experiments in Barcroft apparatus, in which a thick suspension of bacteria (pure culture) was allowed to act on carbon dioxide, formic acid, hexamethylenetetramine and methyl alcohol in an atmosphere of hydrogen. The substrate concentration was in each case $N/30$, and the p_H 6.5; for carbon dioxide the p_H was adjusted by using a mixture of 50 % hydrogen and 50 % carbon dioxide in equilibrium with $N/30$ sodium bicarbonate. The results showed that formic acid and carbon dioxide are reduced at roughly the same rate, while hexamethylenetetramine is reduced at a rate too slow for measurement in the conditions of such experiments. Values for the rate of reaction in terms of the dry weight of bacteria present cannot be given, as the suspension of bacteria is always mixed with a small amount of mud which makes estimations of dry weight or nitrogen content useless.

In these experiments the reaction curve starts immediately in a straight line, which—especially in the case of a very slow-growing organism—precludes the idea that cell multiplication is interfering appreciably with the results.

Experiments on the course of the reactions.

The mechanism involved in the production of methane from these compounds must now be considered. The decomposition of formic acid into hydrogen and carbon dioxide ($H.COOH \rightarrow H_2 + CO_2$) is a common property of many organisms and has recently been shown to be due to a particular enzyme (formic hydrogenlyase) distinct from formic dehydrogenase catalysing the reaction $H.COOH \rightarrow 2H + CO_2$ [Stephenson and Stickland, 1932]. An organism possessing this enzyme together with hydrogenase (activating molecular hydrogen) [Stephenson and Stickland, 1931, 1] and at the same time capable of reducing carbon dioxide might well bring about reaction (1) (p. 1517) in a stepwise manner, by the preliminary decomposition of formic acid into carbon dioxide and hydrogen, followed by a reduction of carbon dioxide by hydrogen as in reaction (2) (p. 1520). Our organism possesses hydrogenase, as is shown by the reduction of methylene blue by hydrogen with a suspension of washed cells:

	Reduction time (min.)
1 cc. 1/5000 methylene blue, p_H 6.3, *in vacuo*	>60
1 cc. 1/5000 methylene blue, p_H 6.3, in hydrogen	6

Moreover, we have obtained evidence for the presence of formic hydrogenlyase; a series of test-tubes containing Durham tubes and formic inorganic medium was sown in the usual way and gas withdrawn from the Durham tubes for analysis at different stages in the growth of the culture. It is seen from the figures in Table XV that in the early stages hydrogen as well as methane was present, but that if the reaction was allowed to continue methane alone was the final product.

Table XV.

Amount of gas (mm.)	Composition of gas	
	CH_4 %	H_2 %
2	64	36
6	86	14
7	92	8
8	71	29
21	98·5	1·5
31	99·5	0·5

The extent of growth of the culture was measured by the length of the column of gas in the Durham tube, given in the Table in mm.

The same conclusion was reached from experiments carried out in Barcroft manometers. A thick cell suspension was shaken in this apparatus with $M/10$ formate in buffer at p_H 6·5 in an atmosphere of nitrogen; the results showed a brief rapid evolution of gas followed by a slower prolonged evolution. When the gas in the cups was analysed at the end of the first period it was found to contain (besides nitrogen) mainly hydrogen and carbon dioxide with a little methane; after further reaction had taken place the analysis showed decreased hydrogen and carbon dioxide and increased methane.

Analysis of gas in Barcroft cups.

	Total evolution mm.^{3}	H_2 %	CO_2 %	CH_4 %
After 1 hour	448	0·9	1·1	0·1
After 26 hours	1666	0·6	0·3	3·9

This suggests that formic acid undergoes a preliminary decomposition to carbon dioxide and hydrogen, and methane is then synthesised by reaction (2) (p. 1520). This would involve, not a direct reduction of formic acid, but a reduction by excess hydrogen of the carbon dioxide produced in the first reaction. It must be admitted, however, that we are offering here a plausible hypothesis and no proof.

In respect of reactions (4), (5) and (6) (pp. 1521, 1522 and 1523 respectively) we are in the dark. Possibly a preliminary reduction of all three initial compounds to formic acid and a decomposition of this first to carbon dioxide and hydrogen and thence to methane is as plausible as any. It should be noted that recent workers [Fischer *et al.*, 1932], have suggested that in the case of carbon monoxide a decomposition of water takes place thus

$$CO + H_2O \rightarrow CO_2 + H_2.$$

Their evidence rests on the appearance of 13·4 cc. of hydrogen in a bacterial decomposition of 1100 cc. of carbon monoxide in the presence of mud, giving 323 cc. of methane and 724 cc. of carbon dioxide. Without a control experiment in nitrogen no evidence exists to decide whether carbon monoxide is transformed to methane *via* this reaction

$$CO + H_2O \rightarrow CO_2 + H_2$$

or by hydration to formic acid

$$CO + H_2O \rightarrow H.COOH.$$

As an alternative it is possible that formic acid is a stage in the reduction of carbon dioxide to methane by a stepwise process thus:

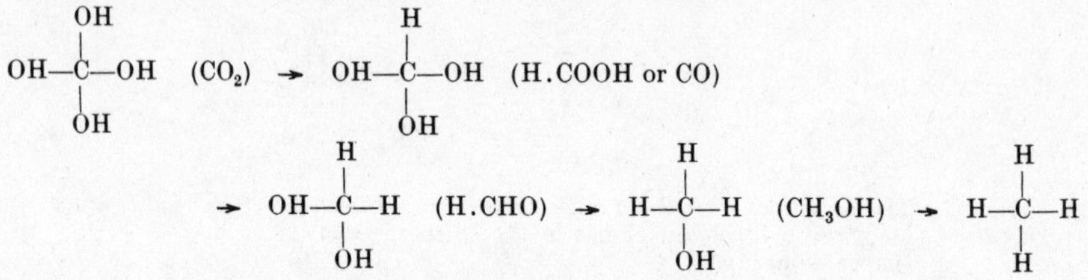

On this view formic hydrogenlyase would be competing with the enzyme concerned in the reduction of formic acid, and the hydrogen produced by its action in the initial stages would be finally used up again in the reduction.

The reduction of other carbon compounds.

We have shown that five simple 1-carbon compounds are reduced by our organism to methane. On the other hand the following compounds were not attacked: acetic, propionic, butyric and caprylic acids (which were all decomposed to methane and carbon dioxide by Sohngen's mixed culture), ethyl alcohol, acetaldehyde and glucose. These compounds were tested in conditions where they formed the sole source of carbon for the organism, and also in broth cultures; in the former case no growth occurred, and in the latter the bacteria grew on the broth but failed to produce any methane from the added compound. In addition acetic acid, acetaldehyde and ethyl alcohol were tested in the manometer apparatus, with washed suspensions, with negative results. As far as we have tested, therefore, only compounds with one carbon atom are reduced by our culture.

SUMMARY.

1. An organism has been isolated by the single cell technique which is able to live anaerobically on an inorganic medium with formate as sole source of carbon.

2. The formic acid is decomposed as follows:

$$4H.COOH = CH_4 + 3CO_2 + 2H_2O + 39 \text{ kg. cals.}$$

This reaction has been shown to occur in two stages, *viz.*

$$(1) \quad H.COOH = H_2 + CO_2,$$

and

$$(2) \quad 4H_2 + CO_2 = CH_4 + 2H_2O,$$

and is therefore the work of two enzymes, formic hydrogenlyase (1) and hydrogenase (2) with an additional mechanism for the activation of carbon dioxide as a hydrogen acceptor.

3. The organism (tested in washed suspensions) reduces the following 1-carbon compounds to methane by means of molecular hydrogen (*i.e.* hydro-

genase reactions): carbon dioxide, formic acid, carbon monoxide, formaldehyde (as hexamethylenetetramine) and methyl alcohol.

4. No compounds so far tested containing more than one carbon atom are reduced by this organism with production of methane.

We take this opportunity of thanking Sir Frederick Hopkins for his interest in this work.

REFERENCES.

Fischer, Lieske and Winzer (1931). *Biochem. Z.* **236**, 247.
—— —— —— (1932). *Biochem. Z.* **245**, 2.
Sohngen (1910). *Rec. Trav. Chim. Pays Bas.* **29**, 238.
Stephenson (1930). Bacterial metabolism (Longmans, London).
—— and Stickland (1931, 1). *Biochem. J.* **25**, 205.
—— —— (1931, 2). *Biochem. J.* **25**, 215.
—— —— (1932). *Biochem. J.* **26**, 712.

Editor's Comments on Paper 43

43 Tatum: Amino Acid Metabolism in Mutant Strains of Microorganisms
Federation Proc., **8**, 511–517 (1949)

As soon as it was established that amino acids can be degraded to their respective keto acids with the release of ammonia (Krebs, 1934), it was also realized that these deaminations could occur without the appearance of ammonia (Herbst and Engel, 1934; Braunstein and Kritzmann, 1937). The reversal of the deamination step, together with the discovery of transamination, formed the basis for amino acid and protein biosynthesis research (David, 1955; Meister, 1955). Autotrophs and heterotrophs are thus able to form the amino acids necessary for protein biosynthesis by utilizing keto acids formed during their catabolic or anabolic events. The paper selected (Paper 43) is not a historical one but was chosen to demonstrate the biochemical unity of amino acid metabolism.

43

Reprinted from *Federation Proc.*, **8**, 511–517 (1949)

AMINO ACID METABOLISM IN MUTANT STRAINS OF MICROORGANISMS

E. L. TATUM

From the Department of Biological Sciences, Stanford University

STANFORD, CALIFORNIA

THIS discussion of some aspects of amino acid metabolism in microorganism is necessarily limited in scope. It will deal primarily with metabolic relations which have been found to be of general significance in both higher and lower organisms and with certain new relations, probably also of general significance, which have been suggested by studies with microorganisms. In both instances, the discussion will center around the results obtained with the help of mutant strains.

Mutations which have as biochemical consequences defective biosyntheses of essential cellular constituents, such as vitamins and amino acids, are being produced in steadily increasing numbers of types of microorganisms. These now include representative bacteria, yeasts and fungi.

In order to give some idea of how nutritionally-deficient mutant strains of microorganisms are produced and isolated, a brief summary of various techniques now available is given in table 1. Basically, mutations in a microorganism are produced by exposing the culture to the action of a mutagen; x-rays, ultra-violet radiation, or chemicals such as mustard-gas. Pure genetic lines of the treated material are derived from single spores with fungi, or from single vegetative cells with bacteria, by growing them on a 'complete' medium which supplies a variety of growth-factors, both known and unknown. A nutritionally deficient mutant among these cultures is detected by its failure to grow in a 'minimal' synthetic medium; and its defective biosynthesis is identified by testing its growth in variously supplemented synthetic media. This method has been used with *Neurospora* (1) and with *E. coli* (2) and other microorganisms. Several less laborious methods for selecting mutants from large popula-

tions have recently been developed. These are also summarized in table 1. All of these modifications are based on the failure of a mutant to metabolize and grow normally without its specific essential supplement. When this supplement is added after a period of incubation, mutant cells of bacteria only then form colonies which at a given time are smaller than those from normal cells (3). Fries has successfully increased the proportion of mutant spores of the mold *Ophiostoma* in mixtures by removing the germinated normal mycelia by filtration (4). With *Ophiostoma* (4) and with *Neurospora* (5) mutants have been visually selected from populations of spores cultured on minimal agar media on the basis that a mutant fails to grow or grows very slowly under these conditions. Even more efficient are methods based on the more rapid death of normal cells due in one case to exhaustion of endogeneous reserves in a minimal medium lacking a growth-factor required by the normal strain (6) and due in the other instance to the growth and consequent sterilization of normal cells in minimal medium containing penicillin (7, 8).

If the B-vitamins and the amino acids are metabolically essential for microorganisms, and if random mutation in nature or in the laboratory results in defective syntheses of these substances, we would expect to find a close correlation between the growth factor requirements of strains as isolated from nature and mutant strains produced experimentally. This expectation is fairly well fulfilled.

The requirements of mutant strains which have now been found in bacteria and fungi do include most of the known water soluble vitamins and the amino acids. This widespread range is summarized most easily by listing those substances not yet so represented. It can be seen from table 2 that deficiencies in mutant strains of fungi include riboflavin, pantothenic acid,

TABLE 1. TECHNIQUES FOR ISOLATING
NUTRITIONAL MUTANTS OF
MICROORGANISMS

DESCRIPTION OF METHOD	ORGANISM USED	REFERENCE
Isolation on complete medium, testing on minimal	*Neurospora*	(1)
	E. coli	(2)
Incubated in minimal, later supplemented as desired	*E. coli*	(3)
Incubated in minimal, non-mutants removed by filtration	*Ophiostoma*	(4)
Incubated on minimal, mutants selected by observation	*Ophiostoma* *Neurospora*	(4) (5)
Incubated in minimal, with selective survival of mutants	*Ophiostoma*	(6)
Incubation in minimal with penicillin, with selective survival of mutants	*E. coli*	(7, 8)

TABLE 2. COMPARISON OF NUTRITIONAL
REQUIREMENTS OF MUTANT AND
WILD-TYPE STRAINS OF
MICROORGANISMS

FILAMENTOUS FUNGI		BACTERIA	
Strains from nature	*Mutant strains*	*Strains from nature*	*Mutant strains*
B-vitamins not required			
B_2	B_{12}	Inositol	B_2
Pantothenic acid	Folic acid	Choline	Inositol
Nicotinic acid			Choline
p-amino benzoic acid			B_{12}
Choline			Folic acid
B_{12}			
Folic acid			
Amino acids not required			
?	Alanine Hydroxy-proline	Alanine Hydroxy-proline	Alanine Hydroxy-proline

nicotinic acid, *p*-aminobenzoic acid and choline, which are not required by any filamentous fungi yet isolated from nature. So far as is known, folic acid and vitamin B_{12} are not required either

by fungi from nature or by mutant strains. For the bacteria, inositol is not yet known to be required but all the other vitamins except riboflavin, folic acid, B_{12} and choline are included in the requirements of mutant strains.

A similar comparison for amino acids suggests that in nature few spontaneously arising amino acid-requiring mutants of non-pathogenic fungi survive. However, mutant strains of fungi have been found with requirements for all the well-established amino acids except alanine and hydroxyproline. The same is true for strains of both classes of bacteria.

There is therefore available a wealth of experimental material in mutant strains of bacteria and fungi. In the strains to be considered, for example, single reactions in the biosyntheses of amino acids are blocked by gene mutations in a more specific manner than possible with enzyme inhibitors. The use of mutant strains as tools in the biochemical analysis of synthetic mechanisms is evident. However, before discussing specific examples of this, I want to mention briefly a phenomenon which has been found fairly frequently in mutant strains requiring amino acids. This phenomenon is one of a specific and often extreme susceptibility to growth inhibitions caused by certain amino acids, usually not the ones required for growth. These inhibitions are important both because they may indicate previously unsuspected interrelations between amino acids, and because they must be taken into account in the interpretation of studies of biosyntheses. To illustrate the diversity of antagonistic amino acid relations in Neurospora some examples are shown in table 3. Similar antagonisms have been invoked by Bonner to explain the double requirement of a mutant strain of Neurospora for isoleucine and valine (15). In this case an accumulated precursor of isoleucine appears to inhibit the synthesis of valine, and both are therefore required.

I now want to discuss some of the biochemical interrelations which have been found in amino acid metabolism in microorganisms. Three general considerations should be emphasized for this discussion: first, the validity of the viewpoint of comparative biochemistry, that the biochemical processes of microorganisms, higher plants, and animals are fundamentally similar; secondly, the contributions of studies with mutant strains of microorganisms to the analysis of the biochemical steps involved in reactions and relations between amino acids; thirdly, the importance of mutant strains of microorganisms in discovering hitherto unknown reactions and unsuspected amino acid interrelations.

Since amino acid metabolism has been most thoroughly studied in mutants of *Neurospora* and of *E. coli*, the examples used in this discussion for the most part will come from work with these two microorganisms.

As shown in figure 1, one of the best examples of the essential similarity of amino acid metabolism in different organisms is the synthesis of arginine, in which the same steps of the orni-

TABLE 3. SOME AMINO-ACID ANTAGONISMS IN NEUROSPORA

GROWTH-FACTOR	GROWTH INHIBITOR	REFERENCE
Isoleucine + valine	Excess of either	(9)
Lysine	Arginine	(10)
D-α-aminoadipic acid	Arginine, asparagine, glutamic acid	(11)
Glycine or serine	Asparagine	(12)
Methionine or threonine	Excess methionine	(13)
None (reversed by arginine)	Canavanine	(14)
Histidine	'Complete' medium	(5)
Adenine	Indole	(5)

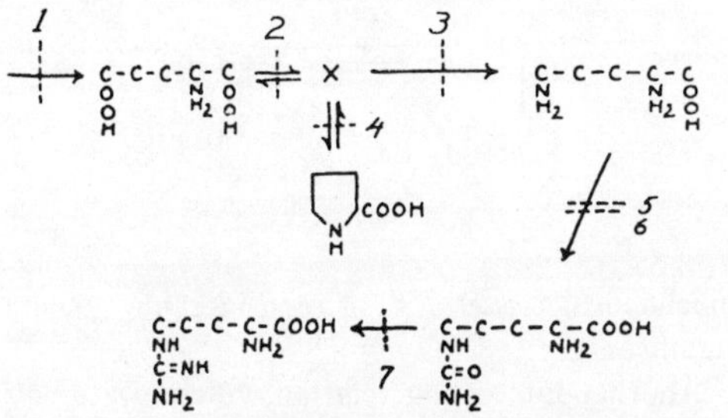

FIG. 1

thine cycle are involved in mammals, in *Neurospora* (16), in *Penicillium* (17), and in bacteria (18, 19). Further probable relations of arginine to glutamic acid and to proline are indicated by *reactions 1, 2,* and *4.* One mutant strain of *E. coli* is apparently blocked at *step 1* and another at *4,* resulting in requirements for glutamic acid or proline, and for proline, respectively (2). A block at *reaction 2* in *Penicillium* apparently explains a requirement for proline or for arginine (17).

Another excellent example of the essential similarity in different organisms is in the metab-

olism of the sulfur-containing amino acids. As shown in figure 2, the relation of cystathionine to cysteine and methionine first established for higher animals by du Vigneaud and collaborators holds also for *Neurospora* (20) and *E. coli* (21). Some minor differences exist, however. In *Neurospora* serine as such seems not to be formed from cystathionine (13). In *E. coli* the reactions leading from methionine to cysteine apparently do not operate in that direction, and this bacterium differs from Neurospora in being able to use D-allocystathionine as a source of methionine (21).

Investigations with mutant strains of *Neurospora* have also indicated unsuspected relations between homoserine and threonine (13), as pic-

FIG. 2

FIG. 3

tured diagrammatically in figure 3. Strain 51504 grows with either amino acid. A similar relation has been found in mutant strains of *B. subtilis* by Teas (22). An even more surprising relation is suggested by a mutant strain of *Neurospora* with an alternative requirement for isoleucine or threonine (22). These intriguing amino acid interconversions remain to be elucidated.

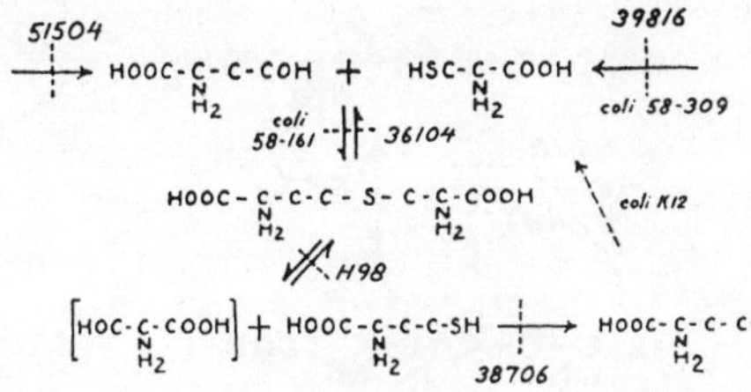

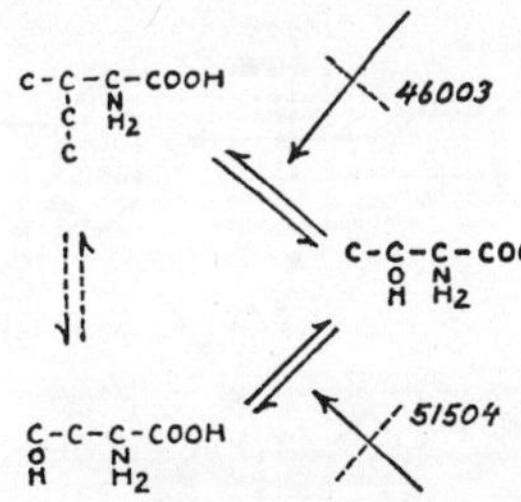

The metabolic relation between lysine and α-aminoadipic acid found in the rat by Borsook and collaborators (23) and shown in figure 4, has been found also in *Neurospora* since α-amino adipic acid has recently been shown to be a precursor of lysine for strain 33933 (11).

Although antranilic acid, indole, and tryptophane have for some time been known to be metabolically related, convincing evidence that anthranilic acid is a precursor of tryptophane was first obtained with mutant strains of *Neurospora* (24). This is shown in figure 5. The mechanism of the conversion of indole to tryptophane has likewise been analyzed with *Neurospora*, and has been shown to involve a hitherto unsuspected condensation of indole with the amino acid serine (25). There seems to be at least two steps involved in the conversion of anthranilic acid to indole, since two genetically different mutants are unable to carry out this reaction. A clue to the mechanism of this conversion has been given by

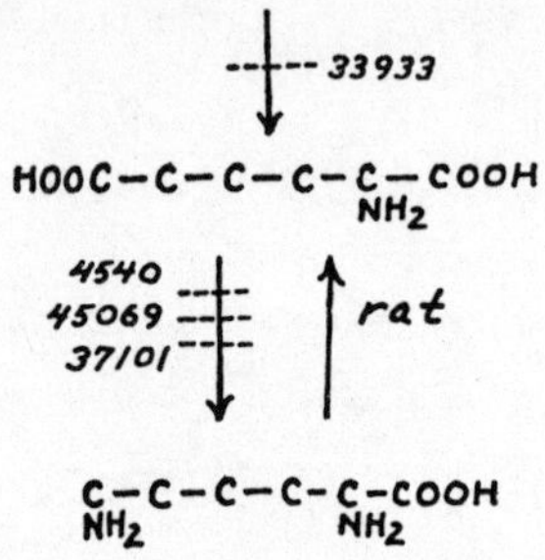

FIG. 4

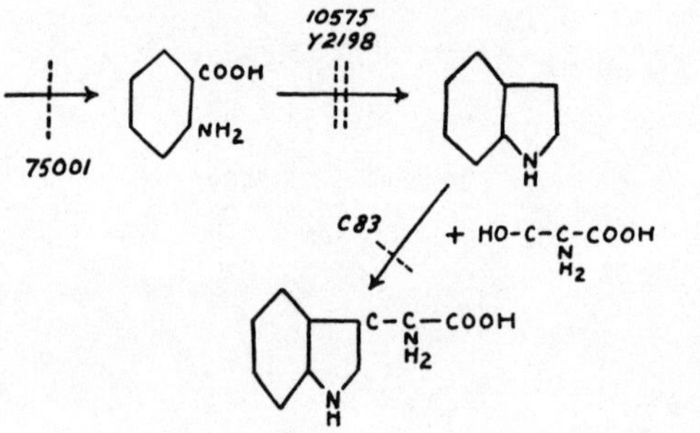

FIG. 5

Nyc *et al.* (26) who have found by isotopic techniques that the carboxyl carbon of anthranilic acid is not present in the formed tryptophane. The conversion of indole to tryptophane has been shown to be an enzymatic reaction involving pyridoxine (27). Recently a mutant strain of *Neurospora* which requires tryptophane and which apparently lacks this enzyme has been described (28). This evidence provides excellent supporting evidence that a gene-enzyme relation is involved in the genetic control of biosynthetic reactions.

An interesting relation between an amino acid and a vitamin is the conversion of tryptophane to nicotinic acid. This relation has been substan-

tiated and clarified with mutant strains of *Neurospora*. As shown in figure 6, some strains of *Neurospora* are known which require either tryptophane or nicotinic acid. This conversion is most readily explained by steps involving kynurenine, the hypothetical compound hydroxykynurenine and the established intermediate 3-hydroxyanthranilic acid. This latter compound is converted to nicotinic acid by strains 40008 and 65001 and by strain Y31881. (29–31). The production of this last intermediate by strain 4540 has been demonstrated by Bonner (31). The evidence obtained with these strains of microorganisms thus lends excellent support to the relation of tryptophane and nicotinic acid suggested first by animal studies. In addition, this conversion has been shown to involve several new

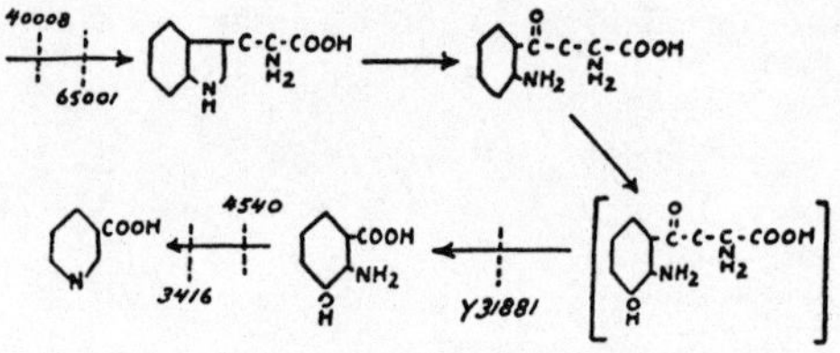

FIG. 6

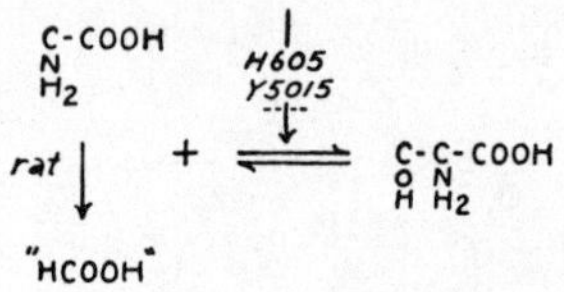

FIG. 7

biochemical reactions of considerable general significance.

Another interesting relation which exists both in animals and in microorganisms is that of the interconversion of glycine and serine. Strains of bacteria (18, 19) and of *Neurospora* (12) are known which have alternative requirements for either glycine or serine. The relation of these two amino acids has been demonstrated in higher animals by Shemin (32) and the mechanism illustrated diagramatically in figure 7 has been recently suggested by Sakami (33). Sakami's evidence, based on the use of marked glycine, suggests that glycine gives rise to formate, which then reacts with another molecule of glycine to form serine. This reaction may be involved in the interconversion of these amino acids in microorganisms. The arrow marked with the two strain numbers on the figure represents the reaction chain leading into this series. There seem to be at least two steps which have been genetically blocked in the synthesis of glycine and serine. Evidence now available suggests that the rat and *Neurospora* may metabolize glycine in somewhat different fashions. Shemin has presented evidence that in the rat glycine is not particularly active in transamination reactions. In *Neurospora*, glycine apparently very readily supplies amino nitrogen for the formation of several other amino acids, including tryosine, histidine, aspartic acid, and glutamic acid, as indicated by the use of nitrogen labelled glycine with a glycine requiring strain (34).

Some other extremely interesting relations between amino acids have been found which deal with the aromatic compounds phenylalanine, tyrosine, anthranilic acid and para-aminobenzoic acid. The precise mechanisms of these interrelations remain to be investigated. As diagramatically represented in figure 8, mutant strains with re-

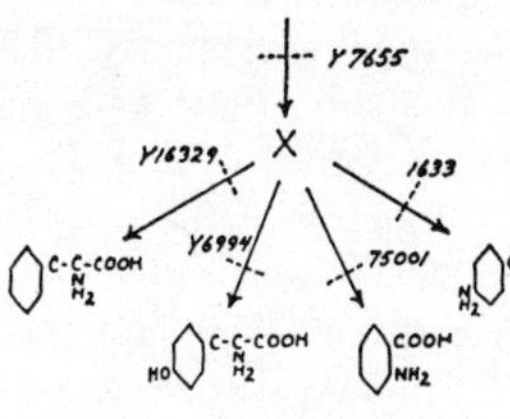

phatic amino acid may not be directly involved in its biosynthesis. Working with a mutant strain of *Neurospora* which requires isoleucine and valine (9, 15) E. A. Adelberg, in our laboratory, has recently isolated and identified a new intermediate in the biosynthesis of isoleucine. The structure of this compound and a tentative suggestion of its part in the synthesis of isoleucine are indicated in figure 9. The keto acid analogue of isoleucine is perhaps only indirectly related to the biosynthesis of isoleucine in microorganisms. The evidence for this includes the inactivity of the keto acid in releasing the valine inhibition of growth of wild-type *E. coli*. In addition, some mutant strains of bacteria have been found capable of using the dihydroxy or the keto-acid analogue instead of isoleucine, while other mutant strains can use only the dihydroxy analogue in place of isoleucine. This evidence apparently provides a new clue to the mechanism of synthesis of aliphatic α-amino acids.

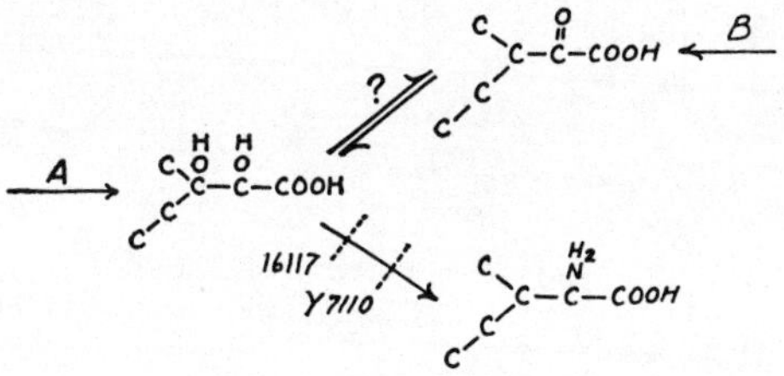

FIG. 8

FIG. 9

quirements for each one of the indicated aromatic compounds are known in *E. coli* (18, 19, 35) and in *Neurospora* (24, 36, 37). In *E. coli* recovery experiments have indicated that phenylalanine and tyrosine are synthesized independently, perhaps from a common precursor (35). The synthesis of all four compounds from a common precursor (x) is suggested by the existence of a mutant strain of Neurospora, Y7655, which requires all four substances (36) and by the existence of similar multiple-requiring mutants in *E. coli* (19). The relations existing in these mutant strains provide extremely interesting possibilities for further biochemical investigations of the biosynthesis of aromatic compounds.

Shemin (32) has suggested that the non-essential amino acids may be synthesized in the rat by amino acid interconversions rather than by amination of their keto acid analogues. Recent investigations with *Neurospora* have suggested that the keto acid of at least one essential ali-

As mentioned earlier, there is now a considerable body of evidence suggesting that many amino acids may be synthesized by interconversions rather than directly from their keto acid analogues. In addition, evidence is now available that some keto acids are biologically inactive in certain microorganisms. These two lines of evidence cast some doubt on the general significance of direct amination reactions as terminal steps in the bio-syntheses of certain amino acids in microorganisms. Some examples are summarized in table 4. In the first group of examples listed, the most probable syntheses are by way of mechanisms other than amination of the keto acids, perhaps those indicated in the last column of the table. In several instances the keto acids have been found to be inactive for mutant strains of microorganisms. It might be concluded that perhaps the only amino acids which are formed *de novo* by direct amination or transamination are those directly related to known intermediates in carbohydrate metabolism, notably alanine, aspartic acid and glutamic acid.

Some of the known amino acid relations which have been found to be common to both microorganisms and animals are summarized in table

TABLE 4. KETO-ACID AND AMINO ACID RELATIONS IN MUTANT STRAINS OF MICROORGANISMS

AMINO ACID	ACTIVITY OF KETO-ACID ANALOGUE	PROBABLE SYNTHESIS FROM:
Arginine	?	Citrulline (16)
Lysine	?	α-aminoadipic acid (11)
Serine	?	Glycine (12)
Glycine	?	Serine (12)
Cysteine	?	Cystathionine (20)
Methionine	+	Cystathionine (20)
Isoleucine	−, +	Dihydroxyacid analogue
Tyrosine	± (10%)	Phenylalanine or common precursor (35)
Aminoadipic acid	− (11)	?
Tryptophane	−	Indole + serine (25)
Histidine	?	
	− (Hydroxy- acid, 34)	?

TABLE 5. REACTIONS COMMON TO MICROORGANISMS AND ANIMALS

Ornithine ⟶ citrulline ⟶ arginine
cystathionine ⇌ homocysteine + [serine]
cystathionine ⇌ homoserine + cysteine
glycine ⇌ serine
α-aminoadipic acid ⇌ lysine
tryptophane ⟶ nicotinic acid
tryptophane ⟶ kynurenine

TABLE 6. REACTIONS AND INTERRELATIONS ESTABLISHED WITH MICROORGANISMS

indole + serine ⟶ tryptophane
threonine ⇌ homoserine
anthranilic acid ($-CO_2+$?) ⟶ indole
kynurenine ⟶ 3-hydroxyanthranilic acid
3-hydroxyanthranilic acid ⟶ nicotinic acid
$α,β$, dihydroxy, $β$-ethyl-butyric acid ⟶ isoleucine

croorganisms and animals are summarized in table 5. These reactions, which have already been discussed, include those of the ornithine cycle, the relation of cystathionine to methionine and cysteine, the interconversion of glycine and serine, the relation of alpha-aminoadipic acid to lysine,

and the conversion of tryptophane to nicotinic acid, and to kynurenine.

As the result of examinations of the mechanisms of these and other biosynthetic reactions with mutant strains of microorganisms, a number of new reactions and relations have been established. These include the reactions summarized in table 6. The involvement of serine in the synthesis of tryptophane has been discussed. The relationship of threonine to homoserine suggested by studies with microorganisms remains to be elucidated. Similarly, the exact steps in the conversion of anthranilic acid to indole are as yet unknown. The essential outline of the biochemical steps involved in the conversion of kynurenine to 3-hydroxyanthranilic acid, and of this compound to nicotinic acid has been suggested. Finally, a role of $α,β$-dihydroxy-$β$-ethyl-butyric acid in the biosynthesis of isoleucine has been fairly adequately established by studies with microorganisms.

It may be expected that future investigations with microorganisms, particularly with mutant strains, will reveal other new and unsuspected relations between amino acids, and that these strains will prove highly useful tools for the elucidation of the mechanisms of reactions involved in the biosyntheses of these amino acids. It may also be anticipated that further studies correlating enzyme activity with gene mutation will add additional information regarding the role of the gene and of gene mutations in determining enzyme specificity. The first clear-cut example of this relationship in *Neurospora* is the enzyme involved in tryptophane synthesis from indole and serine. Information is now available which should permit the extension of this analysis of gene-enzyme relations to other biosyntheses. These include the syntheses of the amino acids arginine, proline, glycine, and serine. It may be expected that other reactions will become available for such studies as the precise mechanisms of the biosyntheses of other amino acids are established.

In summary, we have discussed various aspects of amino acid metabolism in the examination of which microorganisms have been of primary value Judging from past experience we may anticipate that additional discoveries coming from studies from microorganisms will be of general metabolic significance. The principles of comparative biochemistry thus adequately justify the use of microorganisms in investigations of amino acid metabolism. In these investigations mutant strains of microorganisms should prove of significant value in future developments.

REFERENCES

1. BEADLE, G. W., AND E. L. TATUM. *Am J. Botany* 32: 678, 1945.
2. TATUM, E. L. *Cold Spring Harbor Symposia Quant. Biol.* 11: 113, 1946.
3. LEDERBERG, J. AND E. L. TATUM. *J. Biol. Chem.* 165: 381, 1946.
4. FRIES, N. *Nature* 159: 199, 1947.
5. LEIN, J., H. K. MITCHELL AND M. B. HOULAHAN. *Proc. Nat. Acad. Sc.* 34: 435, 1948.
6. FRIES, N. *Physiologia Plantarum* 1: 330, 1948.
7. DAVIS, B. D. *J. Am. Chem. Soc.* 70: 4267, 1948.
8. LEDERBERG, J. AND N. ZINDER. *J. Am. Chem. Soc.* 70: 4267, 1948.
9. BONNER, D. M., E. L. TATUM AND G. W. BEADLE. *Arch. Biochem.* 3: 71, 1943.
10. DOERMANN, A. H. *Arch Biochem.* 5: 373, 1944.
11. MITCHELL, H. K. AND M. B. HOULAHAN. *J. Biol. Chem.* 174: 883, 1948.
12. HUNGATE, F. Stanford University thesis.
13. TEAS, H. J., N. H. HOROWITZ AND M. FLING. *J. Biol. Chem.* 172: 651, 1948.
14. HOROWITZ, N. H. AND A. M. SRB. *J. Biol. Chem.* 174: 371, 1948.
15. BONNER, D. *J. Biol. Chem.* 166: 545, 1946.
16. SRB, A. M. AND N. H. HOROWITZ. *J. Biol. Chem.* 154: 129, 1944.
17. BONNER, D. *Cold Spring Harbor Symposia Quant. Biol.* 11: 14, 1946.
18. ROEPKE, R. R. *J. Bact.* 52: 504, 1946.
19. DAVIS, B. D. Unpublished results.
20. HOROWITZ, N. H. *J. Biol. Chem.* 171: 255, 1947.
21. SIMMONDS, S. *J. Biol. Chem.* 174: 717, 1948.
22. TEAS, H. J. Unpublished results.
23. BORSOOK, H., C. L. DEASY, A. J. HAAGEN-SMIT, G. KEIGHLEY AND P. H. LOWY. *J. Biol. Chem.* 176: 1383, 1948.
24. TATUM, E. L., D. BONNER AND G. W. BEADLE. *Arch. Biochem.* 3: 477, 1944.
25. TATUM, E. L. AND D. M. BONNER. *Proc. Nat. Acad. Sci.* 30: 30, 1944.
26. NYC, J. F., H. K. MITCHELL, LEIFER AND LAUGHAM. *J. Biol. Chem.* In press.
27. UMBREIT, W. W., W. A. WOOD AND I. C. GUNSALUS. *J. Biol. Chem.* 165: 731, 1946.
28. MITCHELL, H. K. AND J. LEIN. *J. Biol. Chem.* 175: 481, 1948.
29. BEADLE, G. W., H. K. MITCHELL AND F. J. NYC. *Proc. Nat. Acad. Sc.* 33: 155, 1947.
30. MITCHELL, H. K. AND J. F. NYC. *Proc. Nat. Acad. Sc.* 34: 1, 1948.
31. BONNER, D. *Proc. Nat. Acad. Sc.* 34: 5, 1948.
32. SHEMIN, D. *J. Biol. Chem.* 162: 297, 1946.
33. SAKAMI, W. *J. Biol. Chem.* 176: 999, 1948.
34. SHEMIN, D. AND E. L. TATUM. Unpublished results.
35. SIMMONDS, S., E. L. TATUM AND J. S. FRUTON. *J. Biol. Chem.* 169: 91, 1947.
36. TATUM, E. L. Unpublished results.
37. TATUM, E. L. AND G. W. BEADLE. *Proc. Nat. Acad. Sc.* 28: 234, 1943.

Editor's Comments on Paper 44

44 **Buchanan:** The Enzymatic Synthesis of the Purine Nucleotides
The Harvey Lectures, **54**, 104–130 (1958–1959)

The last large group of compounds necessary for the life of a microorganism are the purine nucleotides, which form the genetic material DNA (Moat and Friedman, 1960). Purine nucleotides branch off from three main catabolic intermediates: ribose 5-phosphate, erythrose 4-phosphate (see HMP pathway), and the amino acid glycine, which is derived from the amination of pyruvate. The selected publication (Paper 44) shows in a very clear and precise form the utilization of amino acids and catabolic intermediates for the synthesis of these essential purine nucleotides.

Reprinted from *The Harvey Lectures*, **54**, 104–130 (1958–1959)

THE ENZYMATIC SYNTHESIS OF
THE PURINE NUCLEOTIDES*†

JOHN M. BUCHANAN

*Division of Biochemistry, Department of Biology,
Massachusetts Institute of Technology, Cambridge, Massachusetts*

I N the era of biochemical research in the field of intermediary metabolism preceding the use of isotopic tracers, speculation concerning the biological synthesis of purine compounds was largely guided by models of organochemical reactions. This was in large part due to the vast literature on purine structure and synthesis which had appeared from the laboratories of the great German masters of organic chemistry during the last century. Since organic chemistry at that time was closely tied to the study of natural products it was appropriate that the first attempts to understand the synthesis of compounds of the physiological system should have derived their origin from this source. For lack

---

* Lecture delivered December 18, 1958.

† The following are the trivial and corresponding systematic names with abbreviations in parentheses of intermediates of purine biosynthesis: glycinamide ribotide (GAR), 2-amino-N-ribosylacetamide-5'-phosphate; formylglycinamide ribotide (FGAR), 2-formamido-N-ribosylacetamide-5'-phosphate; formylglycinamidine ribotide (FGAM), 2-formamido-N-ribosylacetamidine-5'-phosphate; 5-aminoimidazole ribotide (AIR), 5-amino-1-ribosylimidazole-5'-phosphate; 5-amino-4-imidazolecarboxylic acid ribotide (CAIR), 5-amino-1-ribosyl-4-imidazolecarboxylic acid 5'-phosphate; 5-amino-4-imidazole-N-succinocarboxamide ribotide (SAICAR), N-(5-amino-1-ribosyl-4-imidazolecarbonyl)-L-aspartic acid 5'-phosphate; 5-amino-4-imidazolecarboxamide ribotide (AICAR), 5-amino-1-ribosyl-4-imidazolecarboxamide-5'-phosphate; 5-formamido-4-imidazolecarboxamide ribotide (FAICAR), 5-formamido-1-ribosyl-4-imidazolecarboxamide-5'-phosphate; and adenylosuccinic acid (AMPS), 6-(succinylamino)-9-(ribofuranosyl 5'-phosphate) purine.

Other abbreviations are as follows: AMP, ADP, and ATP, the 5'-phosphate, 5'-diphosphate, and 5'-triphosphate of adenosine, respectively; GDP and GTP, the 5'-diphosphate and 5'triphosphate of guanosine, respectively; THFA, tetrahydrofolic acid; DPN and DPNH, the oxidized and reduced forms of diphosphopyridine nucleotide; TPN and TPNH, the oxidized and reduced forms of triphosphopyridine nucleotide; IMP, inosinic acid.

of a definite experimental approach, Wiener's proposal (1) that uric acid was synthesized from dialuric acid and urea in living systems remained the most acceptable hypothesis for the biosynthesis of the purines for a period of thirty-five years. Attempts to prove or disprove this theory or to establish that certain dietary materials were possible contenders as precursors in the biological system were inconclusive. However, with the appearance of N^{15}, the investigators at the Department of Biochemistry at Columbia University clearly established that purine compounds of the tissues and the excreta are rapidly synthesized from simple metabolic units. The experiments of Barnes and Schoenheimer (2) with N^{15}-labeled ammonium salts as well as those of Bloch (3) and of Tesar and Rittenberg (4) excluded such preformed substances as arginine, urea, and histidine as direct precursors of the purines.

The efforts of Krebs and his colleagues (5, 6) to synthesize purines *de novo* in pigeon liver slices represented the first major advance in the direction of the study of the synthesis at an enzymatic level. They found that hypoxanthine accumulated in their incubations rather than uric acid because of the absence of xanthine oxidase in this tissue. As was later confirmed, this finding emphasized the relative importance of the reduced purine compounds as the first purine structures to be formed in the *de novo* synthesis. Glutamine and oxalacetate stimulated hypoxanthine synthesis *de novo* possibly in the role of precursors, but without the use of isotopes it was difficult to ascertain their exact function.

Our own decision to begin experiments in purine chemistry was prompted by this background and by the appearance of Dr. John C. Sonne, then a sophomore in the University of Pennsylvania Medical class, with a request to undertake a thesis. This capable collaborator was in a large way responsible for the initial progress in developing the degradation procedures needed to trace the origin of individual carbon and nitrogen atoms of uric acid. In these initial experiments this purine compound was isolated from the excreta of pigeons fed various C^{13}- and N^{15}-labeled compounds.

To summarize briefly the results found in the summer of 1946 in collaboration with Dr. Adelaide Delluva (Fig. 1): CO_2 is the precursor of carbon atom 6; formate, of carbon atoms 2 and 8;

and the carboxyl carbon of glycine, of carbon atom 4 (7–10). This left carbon atom 5 and nitrogen atom 7 as quite likely derived from the α-carbon and nitrogen of glycine. Their origin was soon determined directly with C^{14}- and N^{15}-labeled glycine (11, 12).

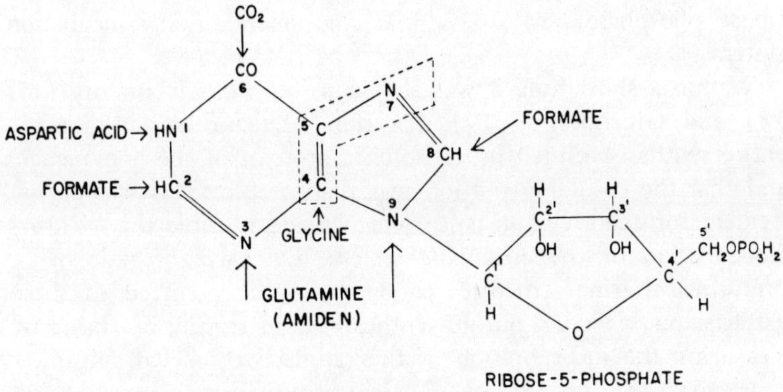

FIG. 1. Precursors of inosinic acid.

Because of the rapid interchange and loss *in vivo* of N^{15} from N^{15}-labeled compounds suspected to being the precursors of nitrogen atoms 1, 3, and 9, research was deferred on this aspect of the problem until an *in vitro* system could be obtained where the magnitude of these side reactions was negligible. Also it was necessary to develop an independent degradation procedure for uric acid (or purines) by which nitrogen atoms 1 and 3 could be separated or with which the N^{15} concentration of these nitrogen atoms could be calculated when this procedure was used in combination with other methods (13, 14).

The successful development of a cell-free system of pigeon liver capable of carrying out hypoxanthine synthesis was achieved by G. R. Greenberg (15), then at Western Reserve University. With C^{14}-labeled CO_2 or formate as a tracer he showed that pigeon liver homogenates could synthesize not only hypoxanthine, but also another intermediate in small amounts but with high specific activity (16). This new compound proved to be the phosphoribosyl derivative of hypoxanthine, inosinic acid. By a study of the variation of specific activities of inosinic acid and hypoxanthine with time, Greenberg came to the conclusion that inosinic acid was the first purine compound formed and that it was catabolized successively to inosine and hypoxanthine. This work strongly suggested that purine bases were synthesized from phosphoribosyl derivatives of nonpurine precursors and that ribose phosphate was an essential component of any incubation system.

Within a short time it was shown in both our laboratory (17, 18) and Greenberg's (19) that the enzymatic activity for the entire synthesis resided in the soluble proteins of the homogenate and that the insoluble portion was dispensable. This was an extremely fortunate circumstance which made possible the eventual fractionation of the enzymatic system. Extensive breakdown of preformed purine structures to hypoxanthine occurred in these extracts, but *de novo* purine synthesis could readily be traced by measuring the incorporation of the radioactive labeled substrates CO_2, formate, and glycine. Their utilization for hypoxanthine synthesis in the ratio of 1:2:1 was proof that *de novo* purine formation was taking place (18). With this same approach Sonne *et al.* (20, 21) demonstrated that two nitrogen atoms were derived from the amide nitrogen of glutamine and that aspartic acid (or glutamic acid) contributed one nitrogen to the synthesis of the purine ring. Subsequent extension of this work by Levenberg *et al.* (22) demonstrated conclusively that nitrogen 1 was derived from aspartic acid nitrogen and nitrogen atoms 3 and 9 from the amide nitrogen of glutamine. Nitrogen 7 of the purine ring originates, as was previously shown, from glycine.

I. Enzymatic Steps in the Synthesis of Inosinic Acid

With this information on hand the separation of the enzymatic system into its component enzymatic steps to determine the pathway of purine biosynthesis (Figs. 2 and 3) became possible. Concurrently with these studies attempts had been made to relate to purine biosynthesis an important compound which, from structural considerations, seemed to be a likely precursor of the purines.

This compound was isolated by Stetten and Fox (23) from cul-

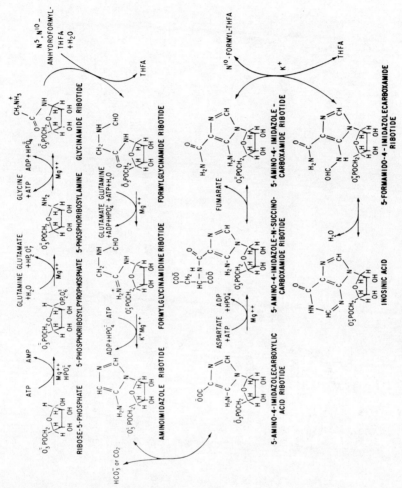

Fig. 2. Enzymatic synthesis of inosinic acid *de novo*.

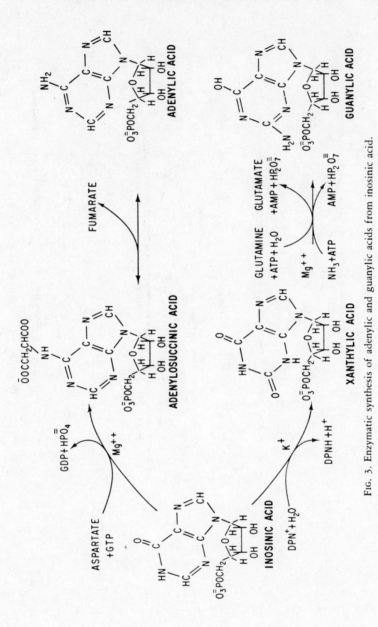

FIG. 3. Enzymatic synthesis of adenylic and guanylic acids from inosinic acid.

tures of *Escherichia coli* poisoned by sulfonamides and was identified by Shive *et al.* (24) as 5-amino-4-imidazolecarboxamide (Fig. 4). Its metabolic activity in bacterial systems at first seemed unpromising, but experiments with animal systems were more encouraging. At the University of Pennsylvania the carboxamide compound, labeled with C^{14}, was demonstrated to be a precursor

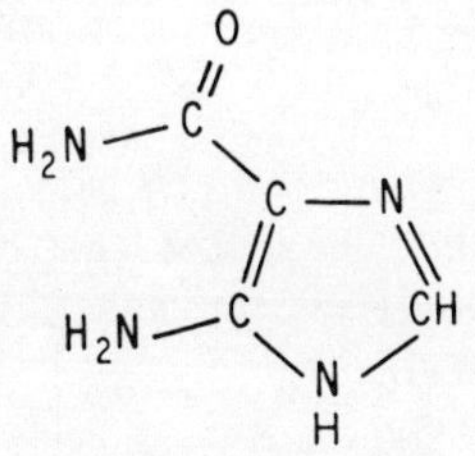

FIG. 4. Structure of 5-amino-4-imidazolecarboxamide.

of nucleic acid-adenine and -guanine in rat tissues (25) and a precursor of uric acid in the pigeon (26). At the enzymatic level, it was possible to demonstrate its conversion to inosinic acid, inosine, and hypoxanthine in pigeon liver homogenates or extracts (27). The labeling of these products again suggested that inosinic acid was the first purine compound formed and indicated that the 5'-phosphoribosyl derivative of 5-amino-4-imidazolecarboxamide was an intermediate not only in the conversion of the carboxamide to inosinic acid, but also in the *de novo* synthesis of the purine nucleotide from glycine.

Subsequent experiments fully bore out the essential role of 5-amino-4-imidazolecarboxamide ribotide in purine synthetic reactions. The riboside was finally isolated from cultures of *E. coli* by Greenberg (28–30) and converted enzymatically to the ribotide and to inosinic acid in the presence of a suitable formyl donor and ATP. The carboxamide ribotide could be formed from inosinic acid by reversal of this reaction (31) and also from 5-amino-4-imidazolecarboxamide itself by two separate enzymatic pathways (Fig. 5) (32, 33). Involved in the addition and removal of formyl groups was the compound, tetrahydrofolic acid, which is now known to be the coenzyme of transformylation reactions.

Fortunately at this juncture Greenberg's laboratory and our own took two entirely different approaches to aspects of the same problem, i.e., the initial steps in purine biosynthesis. The finding that inosinic acid was the first purine structure formed in the synthesis indicated to us that more information was required about the reactions of phosphoribose compounds in nucleotide synthesis from bases. At the time these studies were initiated no information was

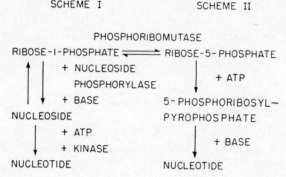

FIG. 5. Alternate pathways for the synthesis of nucleotides from heterocyclic bases.

available on these reactions in purine synthesis *de novo* and knowledge of the conversion of purine bases to nucleotides was incomplete. Kalckar (34) had reported the interconversion of the nucleosides, guanosine and inosine, with their respective bases through the action of nucleoside phosphorylase and ribose-1-phosphate. However, there was no enzyme system in pigeon liver which could effect the conversion of either of these nucleosides to nucleotides, although a kinase was known to phosphorylate adenosine in the 5' position (35). In pigeon liver extracts an active system was discovered, however, for the synthesis of inosinic acid from hypoxanthine, ribose-5-phosphate, and ATP. This enzyme system was fractionated by Drs. Williams and Korn and their colleagues (36, 37) into two components. Upon purification of these components it could be shown that neither contained nucleoside phosphorylase or phosphoribomutase and that the purified enzymatic system could not utilize ribose-1-phosphate as a ribose source. This clearly demonstrated that the pathway of nucleotide synthesis from bases under investigation did not involve the nucleoside as an intermediate nor enzymes concerned with nucleoside metabolism. By sequential incubation of the two enzymes with selected substrates it was shown that a new intermediate (38) could be formed from ATP and ribose-5-phosphate (reaction 1)

ATP + ribose-5-phosphate → 5-phosphoribosylpyrophosphate + AMP   (1)

in the presence of one enzyme and that the second enzyme condensed this intermediate with hypoxanthine to yield inosinic acid. By this time Kornberg and his collaborators (39) had taken up the study of a similar enzymatic reaction, i.e., the synthesis of orotidylic acid from orotic acid. They isolated this same compound in their system and were first to identify it as 5-phosphoribosyl-pyrophosphate (Fig. 6).

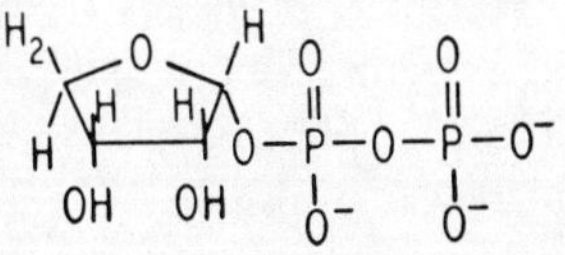

FIG. 6. Structure of 5-phosphoribosylpyrophosphate.

5-Phosphoribosylpyrophosphate has now been demonstrated to participate in a multitude of reactions, among them the *de novo* synthesis of purines. These experiments leading to the discovery of 5-phosphoribosylpyrophosphate were soon to be coordinated to the second line of investigation concerned with the first steps in purine synthesis. Goldthwait, Peabody, and Greenberg (40) found that upon incubating ribose-5-phosphate, ATP, glutamine, and glycine with pigeon liver preparations a new nucleotide accumulated which could be isolated by paper or resin chromatography followed by precipitation as the barium salt. This compound, upon digestion or hydrolysis in acid solution, yielded glycine (ammonia, ribose, and phosphate in the ratio of 1:1:1:1 (41, 42). From these data it was concluded that the new intermediate had the structure of glycinamide ribotide (Fig. 7). When the above incubation was carried out in the presence of a formyl donor a second compound was formed. By similar procedures the structure of this second intermediate was determined as α-N-formylglycinamide ribotide.

By virtue of the discovery of 5-phosphoribosylpyrophosphate and the two acyclic ribotides it was possible to unravel within a short time the mechanism of synthesis of glycinamide ribotide

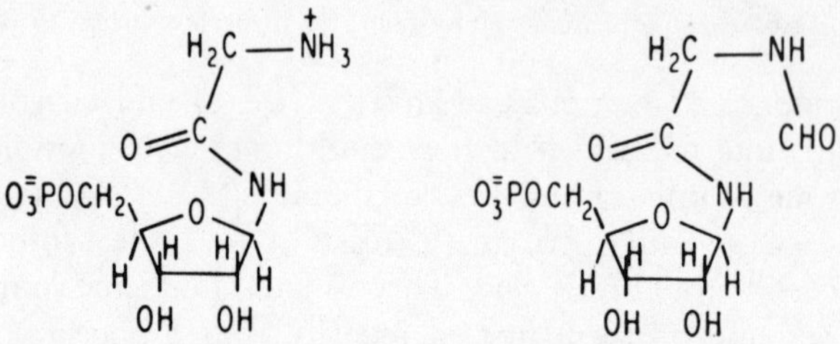

FIG. 7. Structures of glycinamide ribotide and formylglycinamide ribotide.

from its precursors. Hartman et al. (43) showed that in a partially fractionated enzyme system from which the enzyme responsible for the synthesis of 5-phosphoribosylpyrophosphate had been removed, ribose-5-phosphate could no longer support the synthesis of glycinamide ribotide. However, glycinamide ribotide could be formed enzymatically from glycine, glutamine, 5-phosphoribosylpyrophosphate and ATP. ATP thus had a dual function in the reaction, serving to pyrophosphorylate ribose-5-phosphate in one step and also to react in an unknown fashion in a later step. Hartman (44, 45) was able to fractionate the enzyme system for the synthesis of glycinamide ribotide into two components and to purify these fractions to some extent. Shortly thereafter Goldthwait et al. (46, 47) demonstrated that the first of the two reactions involved glutamine and 5-phosphoribosylpyrophosphate to yield probably 5-phosphoribosylamine and pyrophosphate (reaction 2).

$$\text{glutamine} + \text{5-phosphoribosylpyrophosphate} + H_2O \xrightarrow{Mg^{++}}$$
$$\text{glutamic acid} + \text{5-phosphoribosylamine} + \text{pyrophosphate} \quad (2)$$

The second concerned the further reaction of 5-phosphoribosylamine, glycine, and ATP to yield glycinamide ribotide, ADP, and inorganic phosphate (reaction 3).

5-phosphoribosylamine + glycine + ATP $\rightleftarrows$
$$\text{glycinamide ribotide} + \text{ADP} + \text{HPO}_4^{--} \quad (3)$$

Reaction 3 is reversible but reaction 2 is not.

Further discussion of the work on these two reactions as well as the experiments on the formylation of glycinamide ribotide will be reserved for a later section in favor of the question of the conversion of formylglycinamide ribotide to inosinic acid.

The study of the further reactions of formylglycinamide ribotide was greatly facilitated by the finding that a number of purine precursors to which it is converted are aminoimidazoles. These compounds may be diazotized with nitrous acid and then coupled with N-(1-naphthyl)-ethylenediamine according to the method of Bratton and Marshall (48). This procedure results in the formation of colored products with characteristic absorption maxima between 500 and 560 mμ. The variation of the different imidazoles in their response to this color reaction has been an invaluable factor in following the individual enzymatic steps (Table 1). Another property which has been useful in analysis of the enzymatic reactions has been the relative acid stability of the aglycones of some of the imidazole ribotides. Thus one of the stable amines may readily be determined by the Bratton and Marshall procedure in the presence of an unstable amine by heating the solution of the two for a short time at pH 1. Certain of the imidazole derivatives may also be distinguished by their absorption spectra in the ultraviolet region. The properties of the five imidazole compounds are summarized in Table 1. A sixth intermediate to be discussed is an acyclic ribotide which may be determined by enzymatic conversion to one of the imidazole amines.

The general pathway of the reactions between formylglycinamide ribotide and inosinic acid was established by Dr. Bruce Levenberg (49) in our laboratory, which was by now established at the Massachusetts Institute of Technology. To complete the series of reactions between formylglycinamide ribotide and inosinic acid it was necessary to incorporate CO_2, formate, an amide nitrogen from glutamine and the nitrogen of aspartic acid. By a simple procedure of incubating certain of these substrates with an enzyme system obtained from pigeon liver extract by ethanol fractionation,

TABLE 1

PROPERTIES OF IMIDAZOLE COMPOUNDS OF PURINE SYNTHESIS

Imidazole Intermediare of Purine Synthesis	I AIR	II CAIR	III SAICAR	IV AICAR	V FAICAR
Stability of aglycone to acid hydrolysis	−	−	+	+	a
Absorption maximum (mμ)	None	249	268	267	267
Color of product formed in Bratton-Marshall reaction	Salmon-orange	Purple-red	None (25°) Purple (0°)	Purple	None
Absorption maximum of product (mμ)	500	519	560	540	---

a Forms IV on acid hydrolysis.

he was able to detect the synthesis of one imidazole derivative and to demonstrate its conversion first to another imidazole compound and finally to inosinic acid (Fig. 8). This experiment was of considerable practical value because it permitted the division of the series of reactions into three major groups which could be studied separately. By fractionation of either pigeon or chicken liver ex-

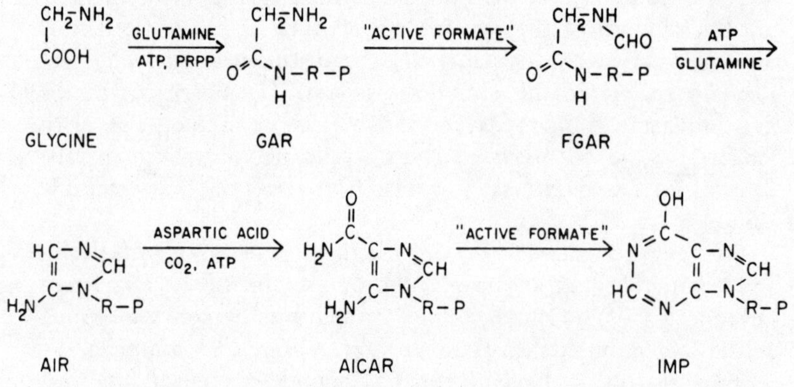

FIG. 8. Abbreviated scheme of purine biosynthesis.

tracts the demonstration of the existence of the other intermediates listed in Table 1 became possible. All of the intermediates have been isolated by resin chromatography and further purified by precipitation as the barium salt. Several of the enzymes which catalyze these reactions have been extensively purified and the mechanism of the reactions studied in some detail.

The further metabolism of formylglycinamide ribotide (50, 51) is initiated by its reaction with glutamine and ATP to yield formylglycinamidine ribotide, glutamic acid, ADP, and inorganic phosphate (reaction 4):

formylglycinamide ribotide $+$ ATP $+$ glutamine $+$ H$_2$O $\rightarrow$
formylglycinamidine ribotide $+$ ADP $+$ HPO$_4^{--}$ $+$ glutamic acid   (4)

In the presence of ATP and potassium ions in high concentration, formylglycinamidine ribotide undergoes enzymatic cyclization to yield 5-aminoimidazole ribotide, ADP, and inorganic phosphate (reaction 5):

formylglycinamidine ribotide $+$ ATP $\rightarrow$
aminoimidazole ribotide $+$ ADP $+$ HPO$_4^{--}$ (5)

5-Aminoimidazole ribotide may be readily distinguished by the fact that it yields a bright salmon orange color by reaction with the Bratton and Marshall reagents.

The next reaction, which has been studied by Dr. L. N. Lukens (52) involves the reversible carboxylation of 5-aminoimidazole ribotide to the 4-carboxylic acid derivative (reaction 6):

aminoimidazole ribotide $+$ HCO$_3^-$ $\rightleftharpoons$
aminoimidazolecarboxylic acid ribotide $+$ H$_2$O   (6)

No components other than the carboxylase enzyme are involved. Relatively high concentrations of bicarbonate are required for this reaction to proceed to a significant extent unless a mechanism for removal of the product of the reaction is provided. 5-Amino-4-imidazolecarboxylic acid ribotide is the first of the intermediates of the purine series to have a distinct absorption maximum (at 249 mμ) in the ultraviolet region. The reaction is best followed by measurement of the increase in absorbance at 265 mμ since 5-aminoimidazole ribotide has a considerable "end absorption" at the lower wavelengths.

The next step of purine synthesis (52) concerns the reversible reaction of 5-amino-4-imidazolecarboxylic acid ribotide, aspartic acid, and ATP to yield 5-amino-4-imidazole-N-succinocarbox-amide ribotide, ADP, and inorganic phosphate (reaction 7):

5-amino-4-imidazolecarboxylic acid ribotide + aspartate + ATP →
  5-amino-4-imidazole-N-succinocarboxamide ribotide + ADP + HPO_4^{--} (7)

The succinocarboxamide ribotide is unique among the aminoimida-zole compounds in that it does not give a positive response in the Bratton and Marshall color test when the procedure is carried out in the usual manner at room temperature. This is probably due to destruction of the diazotized amine by an intramolecular reaction since, if the procedure is carried out at zero degrees, diazotiza-tion and coupling with N-(1-naphthyl)-ethylenediamine hydro-chloride occurs to yield a colored product. The activity of the enzyme which catalyzes reaction 7 is best followed by measuring the splitting of the succinocarboxamide ribotide to the carboxylic acid ribotide in the presence of ADP and inorganic phosphate or arsenate. If the reaction is followed by the Bratton and Marshall reaction at *room temperature*, the product of the enzymatic re-action yields a colored derivative, whereas the reactant, the suc-cinocarboxamide ribotide, does not.

Miller and Lukens (53) have shown that the next reaction in the direction of inosinic acid synthesis involves the splitting of the succinocarboxamide ribotide to 5-amino-4-imidazolecarbox-amide ribotide and fumaric acid (reaction 8):

5-amino-4-imidazolesuccinocarboxamide ribotide $\rightleftarrows$
  5-amino-4-imidazolecarboxamide ribotide + fumarate   (8)

This is also a reversible reaction with an equilibrium constant of 2.4×10^{-3} moles per liter in the direction written. The reaction is easily followed by measuring the production of a product which yields a purple color in the Bratton and Marshall test carried out at room temperature.

The final steps of inosinic acid biosynthesis involving formyla-tion of 5-amino-4-imidazolecarboxamide ribotide and closure of the ring have been discussed in an earlier section of this paper. A formyl derivative of tetrahydrofolic acid participates as a formylat-

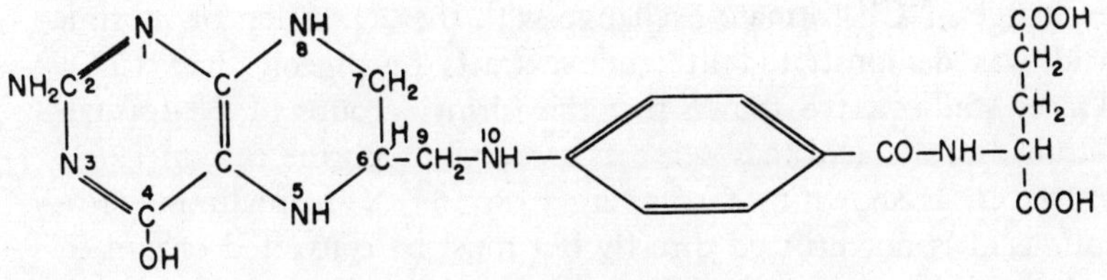

5,6,7,8 – Tetrahydrofolic acid (THFA)

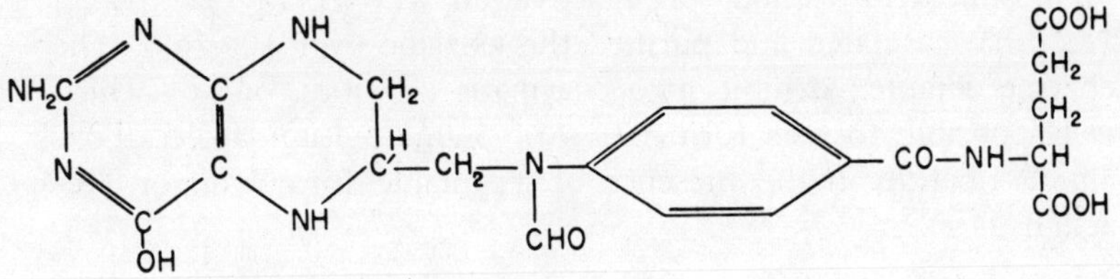

N^{10} – Formyltetrahydrofolic acid

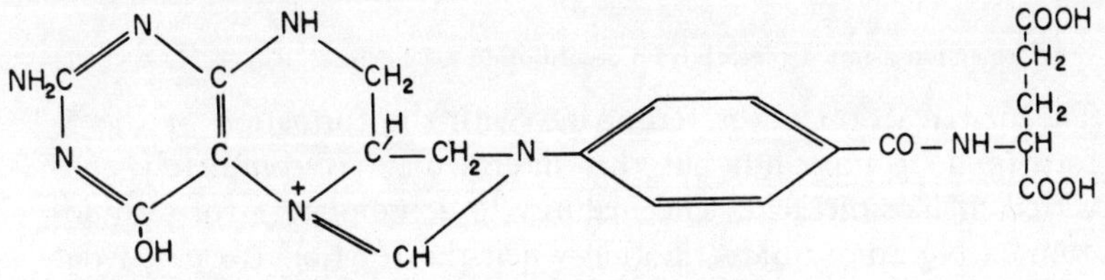

N^{5},N^{10} – Anhydroformyltetrahydrofolic acid *

FIG. 9. Formyl derivatives of tetrahydrofolic acid involved in purine nucleotide synthesis (*N^5, N^{10}-anhydroformyltetrahydrofolic acid has also been called N^5, N^{10}-methenyltetrahydrofolic acid).

ing cofactor in this reaction (27, 54) as well as in the conversion of glycinamide ribotide to formylglycinamide ribotide (Fig. 9) (40). These are the only two reactions where a coenzyme is involved in purine biosynthesis.

The function of N^5-formyltetrahydrofolic acid in catalyzing an exchange of C^{14}-formate exchange with the 2 position of inosinic acid was demonstrated in crude extracts of pigeon liver (27). Tracer studies have shown that the formyl groups of N^5-formyl-tetrahydrofolic acid may serve as a source of purine carbon (28). However, as shown by Greenberg (28, 55) N^5-formyltetrahydro-folic acid is not utilized directly but must be converted enzymatically in the presence of ATP to the actual transformylation agent. In his system, both N^{10}-formyltetrahydrofolic acid and the N^5, N^{10}-anhydroformyltetrahydrofolic acid could function in the enzymatic conversion of 5-amino-4-imidazolecarboxamide ribotide to inosinic acid without prior activation with ATP. Flaks *et al.* (56) have isolated and purified this enzyme over 100-fold. The enzyme complex exhibits two enzymatic activities, one of which is responsible for the formylation of 5-amino-4-imidazolecarbox-amide ribotide in the presence of a suitable formyl donor (reaction 9):

$$N^{10}\text{-formyl-THFA} + 5\text{-amino-4-imidazolecarboxamide ribotide} \rightleftarrows$$
$$5\text{-formamido-4-imidazolecarboxamide ribotide} + \text{THFA} \quad (9)$$

The second is concerned with the conversion of 5-formamido-4-imidazolecarboxamide ribotide to inosinic acid (reaction 10):

$$5\text{-formamido-4-imidazolecarboxamide ribotide} \rightleftarrows \text{inosinic acid} + H_2O \quad (10)$$

The first reaction never terminates with the formation of the 5-formamido compound, but this intermediate is completely converted to inosinic acid. The inability to accumulate 5-formamido-4-imidazolecarboxamide ribotide when the reaction is carried out enzymatically is due to the fact that the two enzymatic activities, i.e., the transformylase and inosinicase, have not as yet been separated. However, 5-formamido-4-imidazolecarboxamide ribotide may be obtained for study by the chemical formylation of 5-amino-4-imidazolecarboxamide ribotide. Although, as a substituted amine, it does not react in the Bratton and Marshall procedure, it may be converted to the free amine by a short period of hydrolysis in 0.1 N HCl at 100°C. This distinguishing feature of the formamido compound has provided an excellent means for its determination. There is in fact some evidence for the belief that one enzyme may catalyze both reactions 9 and 10. Mutants of *Neurospora crassa*, class J, of Giles and Partridge may lack both enzyme activities, although a few have been studied which have the cyclization activity (inosinicase) but lack the transformylase. The transformylase activity requires potassium ions but inosinicase does not.

The synthesis of inosinic acid from the carboxamide ribotide is a reversible reaction. The equilibrium constant of reaction 10 may be determined by incubating inosinic acid in high concentration with purified inosinicase. Under these conditions a small amount of 5-formamido-4-imidazolecarboxamide ribotide is formed (57). At equilibrium the ratio of inosinic acid to formamido compound is 16,000 to 1. The reversibility of the transformylation reaction may be studied by reacting the formamido compound with tetrahydrofolic acid. Detectable amounts of 5-amino-4-imidazolecarboxamide ribotide were formed in such an incubation, but the equilibrium constant of the reaction was difficult to measure because of enzymatic and nonenzymatic side reactions.

In the presence of TPNH, potassium ions, a crude enzyme system from pigeon liver, and a formyl acceptor such as glycine, the transfer of formyl units may be demonstrated as shown in reaction 11 (31).

inosinic acid + glycine + TPNH + H^+ + H_2O $\rightleftharpoons$
$\qquad$ 5-amino-4-imidazolecarboxamide ribotide + TPN + serine   (11)

Reaction 11 consists of a complex series of reactions ending in the formation of serine. Another formyl transfer reaction which is catalyzed by pigeon liver enzymes is shown in reaction 12 (57).

inosinic acid + glycinamide ribotide + H_2O $\rightarrow$
$\qquad$ 5-amino-4-imidazolecarboxamide ribotide + formylglycinamide ribotide   (12)

Here glycinamide ribotide is such an effective acceptor that the reaction goes to completion and for all practical purposes is irreversible.

These studies concerning formate transfer systems have posed another important question which has been settled only recently. This is the question of the actual donor of the two transformylation reactions. With partially purified enzymic systems it had previously not been possible to distinguish between the two active forms of the transformylation cofactor, i.e., between N^{10}-formyl-tetrahydrofolic acid and the N^5, N^{10}-anhydroformyltetrahydrofolic acid. This confusion results from the fact that less purified preparations contain an enzyme *cyclohydrolase* (58) which catalyzes the interconversion of the two formyl derivatives of tetrahydrofolic acid according to reaction 13.

$$N^5,\ N^{10}\text{-anhydroformyl-THFA} + H_2O \rightleftharpoons N^{10}\text{-tetrahydrofolic acid} + H^+ \quad (13)$$

When both transformylases (56, 59) were purified with attention to the elimination of this particular enzymatic component it could be shown by Dr. Hartman (60) that the two transformylation reactions require different and specific formyl donors. The formation of glycinamide ribotide takes place according to reactions 14.

$$N^5,\ N^{10}\text{-anhydroformyl-THFA} + \text{glycinamide ribotide} + H_2O \rightarrow$$
$$\text{formylglycinamide ribotide} + THFA \quad (14)$$

This reaction is specific for the N^5, N^{10}-anhydroformyltetrahydrofolic acid and is essentially irreversible. On the other hand the formylation of 5-amino-4-imidazolecarboxamide ribotide requires the N^{10}-formyl derivative of tetrahydrofolic acid (see reaction 9). It is at present unknown why these two closely related reactions should require different derivatives of tetrahydrofolic acid.

II. Synthesis of Adenylic and Guanylic Acids from Inosinic Acid

The synthesis of adenosine 5'-phosphate and guanosine 5'-phosphate from inosinic acid (Fig. 3) involves reactions of the same type found in the *de novo* synthesis of inosinic acid. The origin of the extra ring nitrogen atoms of adenylic and guanylic acids in animal systems has been shown by Abrams and Bentley (61) to be aspartic acid nitrogen and the amide nitrogen of glutamine, respectively. The study of the enzymatic synthesis of these two nucleotides has been pursued by a number of laboratories (61–68).

The synthesis of adenylic from inosinic acid (61–63) takes place in two steps (reactions 15 and 16).

$$\text{inosinic acid} + GTP + \text{aspartic acid} \rightleftharpoons$$
$$\text{adenylosuccinic acid} + GDP + HPO_4^{--} \quad (15)$$
$$\text{adenylosuccinic acid} \rightleftharpoons \text{adenylic acid} + \text{fumaric acid} \quad (16)$$

As may be seen both reactions 15 and 16 have counterparts in the reactions concerned with the introduction of nitrogen atom 1 into the purine ring.

Guanylic acid synthesis from inosinic acid (61, 64–68) also proceeds in two steps (reactions 17 and 18).

$$\text{inosinic acid} + DPN^+ + H_2O \rightarrow \text{xanthylic acid} + DPNH + H^+ \quad (17)$$
$$\text{xanthylic acid} + \text{glutamine} + ATP + H_2O \rightarrow$$
$$\text{guanylic acid} + \text{glutamic acid} + AMP + \text{pyrophosphate} \quad (18)$$

III. Purine Nucleotide Synthesis in Microorganisms

The question has often been raised whether the pathway of purine biosynthesis in other systems is the same as that found in avian liver. To determine whether the reactions shown in Figs.

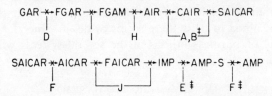

FIG. 10. Mutants of *Neurospora crassa* with genetic blocks in purine biosynthesis. Letters refer to classes of adenineless mutants obtained from N. G. Giles and collaborators; †, order not determined; ‡, determined by N. H. Giles and C. W. H. Partridge.

2 and 3 apply to microorganisms, Mr. Thayer French has assayed extracts of *Neurospora crassa*, *E. coli*, and *Salmonella typhimurium*. The most complete analysis has been carried out with wild-type *Neurospora crassa* together with a number of mutants which have been classified genetically by Dr. Norman Giles and his group (69). Not only have all the reactions of inosinic acid synthesis been demonstrated in wild-type *Neurospora crassa*, but certain mutants have been shown to lack definite enzymes of purine synthesis. These results are summarized in Fig. 10.

A similar though not so complete a study has been made with *E. coli*, *S. typhimurium*, *Saccharomyces cerevisiae*. All three systems contain the enzymes responsible for the conversion of formylglycinamide ribotide to formylglycinamidine ribotide, the succinocarboxamide ribotide to 5-amino-4-imidazolecarboxamide ribotide and adenylosuccinic acid to adenylic acid (70). Several of the other enzymes are found in one organism or another of the three (71). To date one minor difference demonstrated between the reactions of purine synthesis in microorganisms and animal systems has been the finding of Moyed and Magasanik (67) that ammonia is the source of nitrogen in the amination of xanthylic acid to guanylic acid in *Aerobacter aerogenes*. The enzyme derived from animal sources may utilize both glutamine or ammonia but prefers the former at physiological pH values. On the other hand the bacterial enzyme cannot utilize glutamine.

Revel and Magasanik (72) have also shown that carbon atom 2 of purines formed *de novo* by *Pseudomonas fluorescens* is not derived from formate whereas carbon atom 8 is. Both carbon atoms of purines may become labeled from glycine-2-C^{14} but only carbon atom 8 is labeled from histidine-2-C^{14}. With these few exceptions noted to date, there seems to be, in general, a striking uniformity of purine synthesis in the several systems which have been studied.

IV. ENZYMATIC MECHANISMS

From a mechanistic point of view several of the enzymatic reactions bear a strong resemblance to each other and to closely related reactions of intermediary metabolism.

The first category of reactions deserving special considerations is that which includes (a) the synthesis of glycinamide ribotide (45), (b) the synthesis of glutamine (73), and (c) the synthesis of glutathione (74). These three reactions have much in common from a mechanistic point of view. The properties of these reactions are as follows:

1. All three concern the formation of an amide bond from amino and carboxyl reactants. At the same time an equivalent of ATP is broken down to ADP and inorganic phosphate. The reactions are reversible, the amide bond cleavage taking place with the formation of ATP from ADP.

2. Although the three enzymes have been purified extensively (45, 74, 75), there is no indication of the separation of any one of the enzymes into more than one component.

3. In the same manner there has been no evidence of the

formation of discrete covalent intermediates of any of the reactions. In fact the evidence is all to the contrary.

4. Arsenate may replace phosphate in the cleavage of the amide bond but ADP is still required as an essential participant of the reaction. This argues against any carboxyl arsenate compound, and hence a carboxyl phosphate, as an intermediate since the properties of other such compounds would predict that its spontaneous decomposition should take place in the absence of ADP. Thus the function of ADP as an arsenate acceptor would be made unnecessary.

5. When inorganic phosphate is labeled with O^{18}, O^{18} is transferred to the carboxyl carbon of glycine formed by the phosphorolysis of glycinamide ribotide. It would be expected that the transfer of oxygen from glycine to the terminal phosphate of ATP would occur (i.e., the one which becomes inorganic phosphate) if the reaction were carried out in the direction of amide bond synthesis.

These facts have led to the postulation of a mechanism of reaction (Fig. 11) in which all three substrates react at the enzyme surface, ATP exerting an electrophilic attraction on the oxygen of the carboxyl group simultaneously with the attack of the nucleophilic agent, 5-phosphoribosylamine, on the carboxyl carbon. It has been postulated by us that this reaction occurs in a concerted manner with the formation of a termolecular transition state of the reactants on the enzyme surface. This type of enzyme, for want of a better name, has been called a "kinosynthase." Adoption of the term kinosynthase (or kinosynthetase) for this class of enzymes, however, should not be contingent on the ultimate solution of the mechanism of this reaction.

In the purine biosynthetic reactions there are two other important mechanisms for the introduction of nitrogen either into the ring or into the substituted positions on the ring. They involve either the utilization of the nitrogen of aspartic acid or the amide nitrogen of glutamine. There are two reactions of purine biosynthesis with which aspartic acid metabolism is concerned. These reactions involve the introduction of nitrogen into the N–1 position of the purine ring and into the extracyclic amino group at the 6 position of adenylic acid. These reactions resemble the syn-

thesis of argininosuccinic acid (76) except in the detail of the
product of nucleoside triphosphate utilization. In both these reversible reactions of purine biosynthesis a carbon-to-nitrogen bond

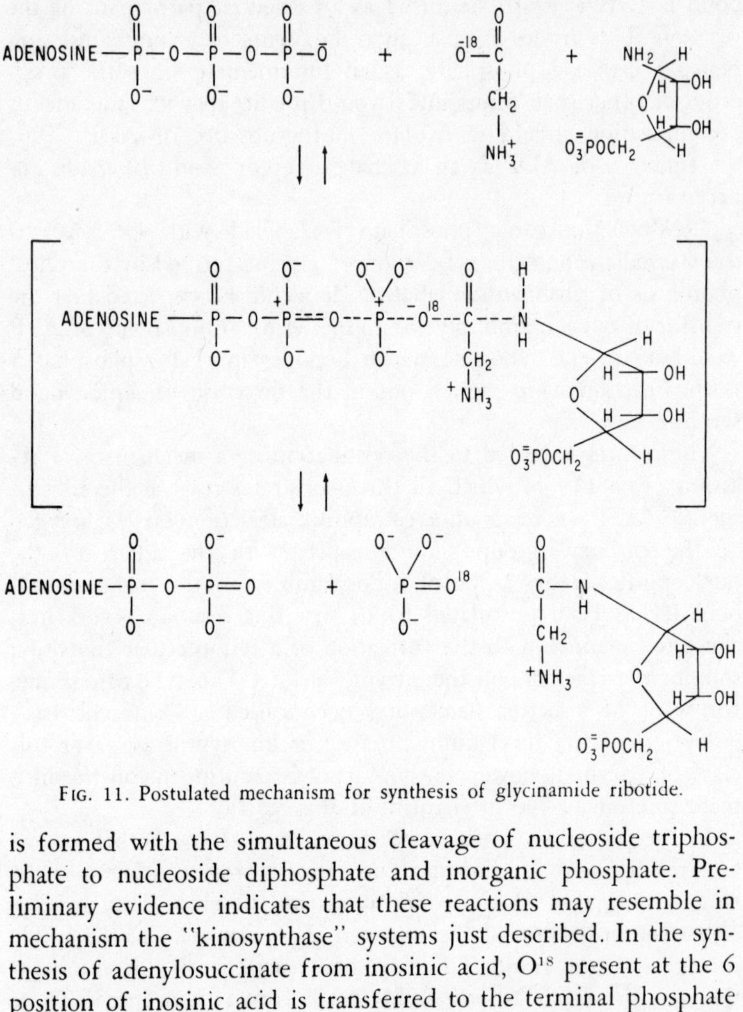

FIG. 11. Postulated mechanism for synthesis of glycinamide ribotide.

is formed with the simultaneous cleavage of nucleoside triphosphate to nucleoside diphosphate and inorganic phosphate. Preliminary evidence indicates that these reactions may resemble in
mechanism the "kinosynthase" systems just described. In the synthesis of adenylosuccinate from inosinic acid, O^{18} present at the 6
position of inosinic acid is transferred to the terminal phosphate
of the nucleoside triphosphate (62). In the breakdown of 5-
amino-4-imidazole-N-succinocarboxamide ribotide to 5-amino-4-
imidazolecarboxylic acid and aspartic acid, it is necessary to in-

clude ADP in the reaction system to obtain splitting of the carbon-to-nitrogen bond either in the presence of orthophosphate or when orthophosphate is replaced by arsenate.

The second part of the reactions leading to the introduction of nitrogen atoms from aspartic acid by the two steps just indicated require the removal of the carbon chain of aspartic acid from the purine intermediate as fumaric acid. At the present time it is believed that the enzyme *adenylosuccinase,* the catalyst of reaction 16, will carry out both functions. Adenine-requiring mutants of *Neurospora crassa* (53, 69), *E. coli,* and *S. typhimurium* (70) which lack adenylosuccinase also lack the ability to split 5-amino-4-imidazole-*N*-succinocarboxamide ribotide to 5-amino-4-imidaz-olecarboxamide ribotide and fumaric acid. Since both adenylo-succinate and the succinocarboxamide ribotide are substrates for the enzyme, they both inhibit the splitting of the other.

There are three reactions in purine biosynthesis which require glutamine as a nitrogen donor. Although being similar in many respects, they have certain important differences. The first reaction involves the substitution of the pyrophosphate group at the 1 position of 5-phosphoribosylpyrophosphate with an amino group. The second is a complex process involving the reaction of formyl-glycinamide ribotide with glutamine and ATP to yield formyl-glycinamidine ribotide, glutamic acid, ADP, and inorganic phosphate. In the third reaction xanthylic acid is aminated by glutamine to yield guanylic acid with a splitting of a phospho-anhydride bond of ATP. The products, however, are adenylic acid and pyrophosphate rather than ADP and orthophosphate. All three of the reactions are essentially irreversible. The incubation of the systems with the products of the reactions with either the pyrophosphate or phosphate labeled with P^{32} does not lead to the formation of radioactive ATP, nor is radioactivity from labeled glutamic acid exchanged into glutamine. Likewise, all three reactions are inhibited to varying extents by the glutamine antagonists, azaserine (*O*-diazoacetyl-L-serine) or 6-diazo-5-oxo-L-norleucine (Fig. 12) (47, 66, 77). Of the three, the second reaction is by far most sensitive to these inhibitors. The inhibitor and the substrate, glutamine, compete for the enzyme site, but the inhibitor may react with the enzyme to cause irreversible inactivation. This finding has now led to the possibility of using these antagonists, when properly labeled with C^{14}, as markers of the site on the enzyme which is concerned with the process of amide transfer. The enzyme which catalyzes formylglycinamidine ribotide formation has now been extensively purified by Dr. Robert

$$NH_2—CO—CH_2—CH_2—CHNH_2—COOH$$
GLUTAMINE

$$\overset{-}{N}=\overset{+}{N}=CH—CO—O—CH_2—CHNH_2—COOH$$
AZASERINE

$$\overset{-}{N}=\overset{+}{N}=\text{:}CH—CO—CH_2—CH_2—CHNH_2—COOH$$
6-DIAZO-5-OXO-NORLEUCINE

FIG. 12. Glutamine antagonists, L-azaserine and 6-diazo-5-oxo-L-norleucine.

Herrmann. He has found, together with Dr. Richard Day, that a small amount of radioactive azaserine becomes tightly bound by the enzyme when enzyme and radioactive azaserine are incubated together. We are hoping that enzymatic digestion of the enzyme will yield radioactive polypeptides the identification of which will give some clue as to the chemical composition of the area of the enzyme where azaserine binds and hence where amide transfer reactions are catalyzed. The structure of the inhibitor has an important bearing on its action on the enzyme. Thus, the D forms of either inhibitor are inactive, as is a homolog, 5-diazo-4-oxo-L-norvaline.

These studies serve as a reminder that if one phase of the problem, the identification of the intermediates of purine biosynthesis, is concluding, another phase is opening. The studies of structure and function of enzymes are problems of absorbing interest. Undoubtedly these enzymes of purine biosynthesis are extremely complex multifunctional proteins which coordinate the utilization of the energy of phosphoanhydride bonds of ATP (or in one case GTP) in the synthesis of the carbon-to-nitrogen bonds of the heterocyclic purine ring.

In summing up, we can now calculate that seven moles of ATP are required for the synthesis of inosinic acid from formate, CO_2, glycine, ribose-5-phosphate, glutamine, and aspartic acid. Five moles are directly used in the reactions of purine synthesis themselves and two are required for the activation of formate as a derivative of tetrahydrofolic acid. It must also be remembered that the synthesis of glutamine from glutamic acid and ammonia also requires the participation of ATP. The calculation of the energy cost for the synthesis of a mole of inosinic acid therefore depends upon the point at which one starts. However, from the precursors just mentioned and with the assumption the cleavage of a phosphoanhydride bond liberates 8000 calories (78), the energy cost would be in the neighborhood of 8000 × 7 or 56,000 calories per mole.

REFERENCES

1. Wiener, H. (1902). *Beitr. chem. Physiol. u. Pathol.* **2**, 42.
2. Barnes, F. W., Jr., and Schoenheimer, R. (1943). *J. Biol. Chem.* **151**, 123.
3. Bloch, K. (1946). *J. Biol. Chem.* **165**, 477.
4. Tesar, C., and Rittenberg, D. (1947). *J. Biol. Chem.* **170**, 35.
5. Edson, N. L., Krebs, H. A., and Model, A. (1936). *Biochem. J.* **30**, 1380.
6. Örström, Å., Örström, M., and Krebs, H. A. (1939). *Biochem. J.* **33**, 990
7. Sonne, J. C., Buchanan, J. M., and Delluva, A. M. (1946). *J. Biol. Chem.* **166**, 395.
8. Buchanan, J. M., and Sonne, J. C. (1946). *J. Biol. Chem.* **166**, 781.
9. Sonne, J. C., Buchanan, J. M., and Delluva, A. M. (1948). *J. Biol. Chem.* **173**, 69.
10. Buchanan, J. M., Sonne, J. C., and Delluva, A. M. (1948). *J. Biol. Chem.* **173**, 81.
11. Karlsson, J. L., and Barker, H. A. (1949). *J. Biol. Chem.* **177**, 597.
12. Shemin, D., and Rittenberg, D. (1947). *J. Biol. Chem.* **167**, 875.
13. Brandenberger, H. (1954). *Biochim. et Biophys. Acta* **15**, 108.
14. Hartman, S. C., and Fellig, J. (1955). *J. Am. Chem. Soc.* **77**, 1051.
15. Greenberg, G. R. (1948). *Arch. Biochem.* **19**, 337.
16. Greenberg, G. R. (1951). *J. Biol. Chem.* **190**, 611.
17. Schulman, M. P., and Buchanan, J. M. (1951). *Federation Proc.* **10**, 244.
18. Schulman, M. P., Sonne, J. C., and Buchanan, J. M. (1952). *J. Biol. Chem.* **196**, 499.
19. Greenberg, G. R. (1951). *Federation Proc.* **10**, 192.
20. Sonne, J. C., Lin, I., and Buchanan, J. M. (1956). *J. Biol. Chem.* **220**, 369.
21. Sonne, J. C., Lin, I., and Buchanan, J. M. (1953). *J. Am. Chem. Soc.* **75**, 1516.
22. Levenberg, B., Hartman, S. C., and Buchanan, J. M. (1956). *J. Biol. Chem.* **220**, 379.
23. Stetten, M. R., and Fox, C. L., Jr. (1945). *J. Biol. Chem.* **161**, 333.

24. Shive, W., Ackermann, W. W., Gordon, M., Getzendaner, M. E., and Eakin, R. E. (1947). *J. Am. Chem. Soc.* **69**, 725.

25. Miller, C. S., Gurin, S., and Wilson, D. W. (1950). *Science* **112**, 654.

26. Schulman, M. P., Buchanan, J. M., and Miller, C. S. (1950). *Federation Proc.* **9**, 225.

27. Buchanan, J. M., and Schulman, M. P. (1952). *J. Biol. Chem.* **196**, 513.

28. Greenberg, G. R. (1954). *Federation Proc.* **13**, 745.

29. Greenberg, G. R., and Spilman, E. L. (1956). *J. Biol. Chem.* **219**, 411.

30. Greenberg, G. R. (1956). *J. Biol. Chem.* **219**, 423.

31. Flaks, J. G., Warren, L., and Buchanan, J. M. (1957). *J. Biol. Chem.* **228**, 215.

32. Korn, E. D., and Buchanan, J. M. (1955). *J. Biol. Chem.* **217**, 183.

33. Flaks, J. G., Erwin, M. J., and Buchanan, J. M. (1957). *J. Biol. Chem.* **228**, 201.

34. Kalckar, H. M. (1947). *J. Biol. Chem.* **167**, 477.

35. Kornberg, A., and Pricer, W. E., Jr. (1951). *J. Biol. Chem.* **193**, 481.

36. Williams, W. J., and Buchanan, J. M. (1953). *J. Biol. Chem.* **203**, 583.

37. Korn, E. D., Remy, C. N., Wasilejko, H. C., and Buchanan, J. M. (1955). *J. Biol. Chem.* **217**, 875.

38. Remy, C. N., Remy, W. T., and Buchanan, J. M. (1955). *J. Biol. Chem.* **217**, 885.

39. Kornberg, A., Lieberman, I., and Simms, E. S. (1955). *J. Biol. Chem.* **215**, 389.

40. Goldthwait, D. A., Peabody, R. A., and Greenberg, G. R. (1954). *J. Am. Chem. Soc.* **76**, 5258.

41. Hartman, S. C., Levenberg, B., and Buchanan, J. M. (1956). *J. Biol. Chem.* **221**, 1057.

42. Peabody, R. A., Goldthwait, D. A., and Greenberg, G. R. (1956). *J. Biol. Chem.* **221**, 1071.

43. Hartman, S. C., Levenberg, B., and Buchanan, J. M. (1955). *J. Am. Chem. Soc.* **77**, 501.

44. Hartman, S. C., and Buchanan, J. M. (1958). *J. Biol. Chem.* **233**, 451.

45. Hartman, S. C., and Buchanan, J. M. (1958). *J. Biol. Chem.* **233**, 456.

46. Goldthwait, D. A., Greenberg, G. R., and Peabody, R. A. (1955). *Biochim. et Biophys. Acta* **18**, 148.

47. Goldthwait, D. A. (1956). *J. Biol. Chem.* **222**, 1051.

48. Bratton, A. C., and Marshall, E. K., Jr. (1939). *J. Biol. Chem.* **128**, 537.

49. Levenberg, B., and Buchanan, J. M. (1957). *J. Biol. Chem.* **224**, 1005.

50. Levenberg, B., and Buchanan, J. M. (1957). *J. Biol. Chem.* **224**, 1019.

51. Melnick, I., and Buchanan, J. M. (1957). *J. Biol. Chem.* **225**, 157.

52. Lukens, L. N., and Buchanan, J. M. (1957). *J. Am. Chem. Soc.* **79**, 1511.

53. Miller, R. W., Lukens, L. N., and Buchanan, J. M. (1957). *J. Am. Chem. Soc.* **79**, 1513.

54. Shive, W. (1950). *Ann. N.Y. Acad. Sci.* **52**, 1212.

55. Greenberg, G. R., Jaenicke, L., and Silverman, M. (1955). *Biochim. et Biophys. Acta* **17**, 589.

56. Flaks, J. G., Erwin, M. J., and Buchanan, J. M. (1957). *J. Biol. Chem.* **229**, 603.
57. Warren, L., Flaks, J. G., and Buchanan, J. M. (1957). *J. Biol. Chem.* **229**, 627.
58. Rabinowitz, J. C., and Pricer, W. E., Jr. (1956). *J. Am. Chem. Soc.* **78**, 5702.
59. Warren, L., and Buchanan, J. M. (1957). *J. Biol. Chem.* **229**, 613.
60. Hartman, S. C., and Buchanan, J. M. (1959). *J. Biol. Chem.* **234**, 1812.
61. Abrams, R., and Bentley, M. (1955). *J. Am. Chem. Soc.* **77**, 4179.
62. Lieberman, I. (1956). *J. Biol. Chem.* **223**, 327.
63. Carter, C. E., and Cohen, L. H. (1956). *J. Biol. Chem.* **222**, 17.
64. Lagerkvist, U. (1958). *J. Biol. Chem.* **233**, 138.
65. Lagerkvist, U. (1958). *J. Biol. Chem.* **233**, 143.
66. Abrams, R., and Bentley, M. (1959). *Arch. Biochem. Biophys.* **79**, 91.
67. Moyed, H. S., and Magasanik, B. (1957). *J. Biol. Chem.* **226**, 351.
68. Magasanik, B., Moyed, H. S., and Gehring, L. B. (1957). *J. Biol. Chem.* **226**, 339.
69. Giles, N. H., Partridge, C. W. H., and Nelson, N. J. (1957). *Proc. Natl. Acad. Sci. U. S.* **43**, 305.
70. Gots, J. S., and Gollub, E. G. (1957). *Proc. Natl. Acad. Sci. U. S.* **43**, 826.
71. Love, S. H., and Gots, J. S. (1955). *J. Biol. Chem.* **212**, 647.
72. Revel, H. R. B., and Magasanik, B. (1958). *J. Biol. Chem.* **233**, 439.
73. Speck, J. F. (1949). *J. Biol. Chem.* **179**, 1405.
74. Snoke, J. E., and Bloch, K. (1955). *J. Biol. Chem.* **213**, 825.
75. Varner, J. E., and Webster, G. C. (1955). *Plant Physiol.* **30**, 393.
76. Ratner, S., and Petrack, B. (1956). *Arch. Biochem. Biophys.* **65**, 582.
77. Levenberg, B., and Melnick, I., and Buchanan, J. M. (1957). *J. Biol. Chem.* **225**, 163.
78. Benzinger, T. H., and Herns, R. (1956). *Proc. Natl. Acad. Sci. U. S.* **42**, 896.

References

Aleem, M. I. H. (1970). Oxidation of inorganic nitrogen compounds. *Ann. Rev. Plant Physiol.*, **21**, 67–90.

Allen, M. B., and C. B. van Niel (1952). Experiments on bacterial denitrification. *J. Bacteriol.*, **64**, 397–412.

Auhagen, E. (1933). *Biochem. Z.*, **258**, 330.

Baas-Becking, L. G. M., and G. S. Parks (1927). Energy relations in the metabolism of autotrophic bacteria. *Physiol. Rev.* **7**, 85–106.

Baddiley, J. (1955). The structure of coenzyme A. *Advan. Enzymol.*, **16**, 1–22.

Barnett, J. A., and H. L. Kornberg (1960). The utilization by yeasts of acids of the tricarboxylic acid cycle. *J. Gen. Microbiol.*, **23**, 65–82.

Bassham, J. A., A. A. Benson, L. D. Kay, A. E. Harris, A. T. Wilson, and M. Calvin (1954). The path of carbon in photosynthesis. XXI. The cyclic regeneration of carbon dioxide acceptor. *J. Amer. Chem. Soc.*, **76**, 1760–1770.

Beijerinck, W. M. (1895). Über *Spirillum desulfuricans* als Ursache von Sulfatreduktion. *Zentra. Bakteriol,* II. Abt., **1**, 1–9.

———(1895). Über *Spirillum desulfuricans* als Ursache von Sulfatreduktion (Fortsetzung). *Zentra. Bakteriol,* II. Abt., **1**, 49–59.

———(1904) Über die Bakterien, welche sich im Dunkeln mit Kohlensäure als Kohlenstoffquelle ernähren konnen. *Zentra. Bakteriol.*, II. Abt., **11**, 593–599.

Bloch, K., and O. Hayaishi (eds.) (1966). *Biological and Chemical Aspects of Oxygenases.* Maruzen Co. Ltd., Tokyo.

Block, R. J., E. J. Durrum and G. Zweig (1958). *A Manual of Paper Chromatography and Electrophoresis.* Academic Press, Inc., New York.

Braunstein, A. E., and M. G. Kritzmann (1937). Über den Ab und Aufbau von Aminosäuren durch Umaminierung. *Enzymologia*, **2**, 129–146.

Brock, T. D. (1961). *Milestones in Microbiology.* Prentice-Hall, Inc., Englewood Cliffs, N.J.

Bryson, V. (1959). *Microbiology Yesterday and Today.* Institute for Microbiol., Rutgers, The State University, New Brunswick, N.J.

Buchner, E. (1897). Alkoholische Gärung ohne Hefezellen. (Zweite Mitt.). *Ber. Deut. Chem. Ges. (Chem. Ber.)*, **30**, 1110–1113.

———(1898). Über zellenfreie Gärung. *Ber. Deut. Chem. Ges. (Chem. Ber.)*, **31**, 568–574.

———(1900). Zymase aus getöteter Hefe. *Ber. Deut. Chem. Ges. (Chem. Ber.)*, **33**, 3307–3310.

———, and W. Antoni (1905). Weitere Versuche über die zellfreie Gärung. *Z. Physiol. Chem.*, **44**, 206–228.

———, and W. Antoni (1905). Existiert ein Coenzym für die Zymase? *Z. Physiol. Chem.*, **46**, 136–154.

———, and F. Duchacek (1909). Über fraktionierte Fällung des Hefepresssaftes. *Biochem. Z.*, **15**, 221–253.

———, and E. Haehn (1909). Über das Spiel der Enzyme des Hefepresssaftes. *Biochem. Z.*, **19**, 191–218.

————, and R. Hoffmann (1907). Einige Versuche mit Hefepresssaft, *Biochem. Z.*, **4**, 215–234.

————, and F. Klatter (1908). Über das Koenzym des Hefepresssaftes. *Biochem. Z.*, **8**, 520–557.

————, and J. Meisenheimer (1904). Die chemischen Vorgänge bei der alkoholischen Gärung. *Ber. Deut. Chem. Ges. (Chem. Ber.)*, **37**, 417–428.

————, and J. Meisenheimer (1905). Die chemischen Vorgänge bei der alkoholischen Gärung (Zweite Mitt.). *Ber. Deut. Chem. Ges. (Chem. Ber.)*, **38**, 620–630.

————, and J. Meisenheimer (1906). Die chemischen Vorgänge bei der alkoholischen Gärung. (Dritte Mitt.). *Ber. Deut. Chem. Ges. (Chem. Ber.)*, **39**, 3201–3218.

————, J. Meisenheimer, and H. Schade (1906). Zur Vergärung des Zuckers ohne Enzyme. *Ber. Deut. Chem. Ges. (Chem. Ber.)*, **39**, 4217–4231.

————, and J. Meisenheimer (1908). Über Buttersäuregärung. *Ber. Deut. Chem. Ges. (Chem. Ber.)*, **41**, 1410–1419.

————, and J. Meisenheimer (1910). Die chemischen Vorgänge bei der alkoholischen Gärung (4. Mitt.) *Ber. Deut. Chem. Ges. (Chem. Ber.)*, **43**, 1773–1795.

————, and J. Meisenheimer (1912). Die chemischen Vorgänge bei der alkoholischen Gärung (V. Mitt.). *Ber. Deut. Chem. Ges. (Chem. Ber.)*, **45**, 1633–1643.

————, and R. Rapp (1897). Alkoholische Gärung ohne Hefezellen. (Dritte Mitt.). *Ber. Deut. Chem. Ges. (Chem. Ber.)*, **30**, 2668–2678.

————, and R. Rapp (1898). Alkoholische Gärung ohne Hefezellen. (Vierte Mitt.). *Ber. Deut. Chem. Ges. (Chem. Ber.)*, **31**, 209–217.

————, and R. Rapp (1898). Alkoholische Gärung ohne Hefezellen. (V. Mitt.). *Ber. Deut. Chem. Ges. (Chem. Ber.)*, **31**, 1084–1090.

————, and R. Rapp (1898). Alkoholische Gärung ohne Hefezellen. (VI. Mitt.). *Ber. Deut. Chem. Ges. (Chem. Ber.)*, **31**, 1090–1094.

————, and R. Rapp (1898). Alkoholische Gärung ohne Hefezellen. (VII. Mitt.). *Ber. Deut. Chem. Ges. (Chem. Ber.)*, **31**, 1531–1533.

————, and R. Rapp (1899). Alkoholische Gärung ohne Hefezellen (VIII. Mitt.). *Ber. Deut. Chem. Ges. (Chem. Ber.)*, **32**, 127–137.

————, and R. Rapp (1899). Alkoholische Gärung ohne Hefezellen (IX. Mitt.). *Ber. Deut. Chem. Ges. (Chem. Ber.)*, **32**, 2086–2094.

————, and R. Rapp (1901). Alkoholische Gärung ohne Hefezellen (X. Mitt.). *Ber. Deut. Chem. Ges. (Chem. Ber.)*, **34**, 1523–1530.

Butlin, K. R., and J. R. Postgate (1956). Formation enzymatique de sulfure à partir de substrats minéraux par les microorganismes, In *La Biochimie du Soufre,* pp. 61–73. Centre National de la Recherche Scientifique, Paris.

————, M. E. Adams, and M. Thomas (1949). The isolation and cultivation of sulphate-reducing bacteria. *J. Gen. Microbiol.*, **3**, 46–59.

Calvin, M., C. Heidelberger, J. C. Reid, B. M. Tolbert, and P. E. Yankwich (1949). *Isotopic Carbon. Techniques in Its Measurement and Chemical Manipulation.* John Wiley & Sons, Inc., New York.

Campbell, J. R., R. A. Smith, and B. A. Eagles (1953). A deviation from the conventional tricarboxylic acid cycle in *Pseudomonas aeruginosa. Biochim. Biophys. Acta,* **11**, 594.

Campbell, L. L., and J. R. Postgate (1965). Classification of the spore-forming sulphate-reducing bacteria. *Bacteriol. Rev.*, **29**, 359.

Carson, S. F. (1948). Design and interpretation of carbon isotope experiments in bacterial metabolism. *Cold Spring Harbor Symp. Quant. Biol.*, **13**, 75–80.

————, and S. Ruben (1940). CO_2 assimilation by propionic acid bacteria studied by the use of radioactive carbon. *Proc. Natl. Acad. Sci. U.S.*, **26**, 418.

Collins, J. F., and H. L. Kornberg (1960). The metabolism of C_2-compounds in microorganisms. 4. Synthesis of cell materials from acetate by *Aspergillus niger. Biochem. J.,* **77**, 430–438.

Cori, O., and F. Lipmann (1952). The primary oxidation product of enzymatic glucose 6-phosphate oxidation. *J. Biol. Chem.*, **194**, 417–425.

Davis, B. D. (1955). Intermediates in amino acid biosynthesis. *Advan. Enzymol.*, **16**, 247–312.

Dickens, F. (1936). Mechanisms of carbohydrate oxidation. *Nature,* **138**, 1057.

————(1938). Oxidation of phosphohexonate and pentose phosphoric acids by yeast enzymes. I. Oxidation of phosphohexonate. II. Oxidation of pentose phosphoric acids. *Biochem. J.*, **32**, 1626–1644.

————(1938). Yeast fermentation of pentose phosphoric acids. *Biochem. J.*, **32**, 1645–1653.

Dische, Z. (1936/37). Mit dem Hauptoxydoreduktionsprozess der Blutglykolyse gekoppelte Synthese der Adenosinetriphosphorsäure. *Enzymologia*, **1**, 288–310.

Doetsch, R. N. (1960). *Microbiology, Historical Contribution from 1776–1908.* Rutgers University Press, New Brunswick, N.J.

Dorfman, A., S. Berkman, and S. A. Koser (1942). Pantothenic acid in the metabolism of *Proteus morganii. J. Biol. Chem.*, **144**, 393–400.

Drysdale, G. R., and H. A. Lardy (1953). Fatty acid oxidation by a soluble enzyme system from mitochondria. *J. Biol. Chem.*, **202**, 119–136.

Dubos, R. J. (1950). *Louis Pasteur.* Little, Brown and Company, Boston.

Euler, H. v. (1905). Chemische Dynamik der zellfreien Gärung. *Z. Physiol. Chem.*, **44**, 53–73.

————, and H. Backstrom (1912). Zur Kenntnis der Hefegärung (2. Mitteilung). *Z. Physiol. Chem.*, **77**, 394–401.

————, and Th. Berggren (1912). Über die primäre Umwandlung der Hexosen bei der alkoholischen Gärung. *Z. Gärungsphysiol.*, **1**, 203–218.

————, and A. Fodor (1911). Über ein Zwischenprodukt der alkoholischen Gärung. *Biochem. Z.*, **36**, 401–410.

————, and Y. Funke (1912). Über die Spaltung der Kohlenhydratphosphorsäure-ester. *Z. Physiol. Chem.*, **77**, 488–496.

————, and S. Heintze (1918). Über die Rolle der Phosphate bei der alkoholischen Gärung. *Z. Physiol. Chem.*, **102**, 252–261.

————, and D. Johansson (1913). Über die Reaktionsphasen der alkoholischen Gärung. *Z. Physiol. Chem.*, **85**, 192–208.

————, and G. Lundequist (1911). Zur Kenntnis der Hefegärung. *Z. Physiol. Chem.*, **71**, 97–112.

————, and K. Myrbäck (1923). Gärungs-Co-Enzyme (Co-Zymase) der Hefe. I. *Z. Physiol. Chem.*, **131**, 179–203.

————, and K. Myrbäck (1923). Gärungs-Co-Enzyme (Co-Zymase) der Hefe. II. *Z. Physiol. Chem.*, **133**, 260–278.

————, and K. Myrbäck (1924). Gärungs-Co-Enzyme (Co-Zymase) der Hefe. III. *Z. Physiol. Chem.*, **136**, 107–129.

————, and K. Myrbäck (1924). Gärungs-Co-Enzyme (Co-Zymase) der Hefe. V. *Z. Physiol. Chem.*, **139**, 15–23.

————, and K. Myrbäck (1924). Gärungs-Co-Enzyme (Co-Zymase) der Hefe. VI. *Z. Physiol. Chem.*, **139**, 281–306.

————, and E. Brunius (1926). Beziehung zwischen Gesamtumsatz der Kohlenhydrate und ihrer enzymatischen Phosphorylierung. *Z. Physiol. Chem.*, **160**, 242–245.

————, and K. Myrbäck (1927). Bildung und Zerfall der Hexose-diphsophorsäure bei der alkoholischen Gärung. *Z. Physiol. Chem.*, **167**, 236–244.

————, H. J. Ohlson, and D. Johansson (1917). Über Zwischenreaktionen bei der alkoholischen Gärung. *Biochem. Z.*, **84**, 402–406.

Feigl, F. (1966). *Spot Tests in Organic Analysis.* Elsevier Publishing Co., Amsterdam.

Goldschmidt, E. P., I. Yall, and H. Koffler (1956). Biochemistry of filamentous fungi. IV. The significance of the tricarboxylic acid cycle in the oxidation of acetate. *J. Bacteriol.*, **72**, 436–446.

Grafflin, A. L., and D. E. Green (1948). Studies on the cyclophorase system. II. The complete oxidation of fatty acids. *J. Biol. Chem.*, **176**, 95–115.

Gregory, J. D., and P. W. Robbins (1960). Metabolism of sulfur compounds. *Ann. Rev. Biochem.*, **29**, 347–364.

Grossman, J. P., and J. R. Postgate (1953). Cultivation of sulphate-reducing bacteria. *Nature*, **171**, 600–602.

Gunsalus, I. C., B. L. Horecker, and W. A. Wood (1955). Pathways of carbohydrate metabolism in microorganisms. *Bacteriol. Rev.,* **19**, 79–128.

Harden, A. (1917). Fermentation by dried yeast preparations. *Biochem. J.,* **19**, 477–483.

———(1932). *Alcoholic fermentation.* 4th ed. The Longman Group, London.

———, and F. R. Henley (1927). The equation of alcoholic fermentation. *Biochem. J.,* **21**, 1216–1223.

———, and F. R. Henley (1929). The equation of alcoholic fermentation. II. *Biochem. J.,* **23**, 230–236.

———, and D. Norris (1912). The bacterial production of acetylmethylcarbinol and 2,3-butylene-glycol from various substances. *Proc. Royal Soc.,* **84B**, 492–499.

———, and R. Robison (1914). A new phosphoric ester obtained by the aid of yeast juice (Preliminary note). *Proc. Chem. Soc.,* **30**, 16–17.

———, and W. J. Young (1906). The alcoholic ferment of yeast juice. *Proc. Royal Soc.,* **77B**, 405–420.

———, and W. J. Young (1909). The alcoholic ferment of yeast juice. Part IV. The fermentation of glucose, mannose, and fructose by yeast juice. *Proc. Royal Soc.,* **81B**, 336–347.

———, and W. J. Young (1910). The function of phosphates in alcoholic fermentation. *Zentra. Bakteriol.,* II. Abt., **26**, 178–184.

———, and W. J. Young (1912). Der Mechanismus der alkoholischen Gärung. *Biochem. Z.,* **40**, 458–478.

Hayaishi, O. (1966). Crystalline oxygenase of Pseudomonads. *Bacteriol. Rev.,* **30**, 720–731.

Herbst, R. M., and L. L. Engel (1934). A reaction between $^d\alpha$-ketonic acids and $^d\alpha$-amino acids. *J. Biol. Chem.,* **107**, 505–512.

Hevesy, G. (1938). The application of isotopic indicators in biological research. *Enzymologia,* **5**, 138–157.

Hills, G. M. (1943). Experiments on the function of pantothenate in bacterial metabolism. *Biochem. J.,* **37**, 418–425.

Horecker, B. L. (1961/62). Interdependent pathways of carbohydrate metabolism. *Harvey Lectures,* **57**, 35–61.

———, and P. Z. Smyrniotis (1952). The fixation of carbon dioxide in 6-phosphogluconic acid. *J. Biol. Chem.,* **196**, 135–142.

Kalnitzky, G., and C. H. Werkman (1942). Fixation of CO_2 by a cell-free extract of *Escherichia coli. J. Bacteriol.,* **44**, 256–257.

———, and C. H. Werkman. (1943). The anaerobic dissimilation of pyruvate by a cell-free extract of *Escherichia coli. Arch. Biochem.,* **2**, 113–124.

Kamp, A. F., J. W. M. LaRiviere, and W. Verhoeven (1959). *Albert Jan Kluyver. His Life and Work.* North-Holland Pub. Co., Amsterdam.

Kaserer, H. (1906). Über die Oxydation des Wasserstoffes und des Methans durch Mikroorganismen. *Zentra. Bakteriol.,* II. Abt., **15**, 573–576.

Keil, F. (1912). Beiträge zur Physiologie der farblosen Schwefelbakterien, *Beitr. Biol. Pflanz.,* II, 302–335.

King, T. E., H. S. Mason, and M. Morrison, (eds.).(1965). *Oxidases and Related Redox Systems.* John Wiley & Sons, Inc., New York.

Korkes, S., J. R. Stern, I. C. Gunsalus, and S. Ochoa (1950). Enzymatic synthesis of citrate from pyruvate and oxalacetate. *Nature,* **169**, 439–440.

———, A. DelCampillo, I. C. Gunsalus, and S. Ochoa (1951). Enzymatic synthesis of citric acid. IV. Pyruvate as acetyl donor. *J. Biol. Chem.,* **193**, 721–735.

Kornberg, H. L. (1957). Acetate metabolism in acetate-grown *Pseudomonas. Biochem. J.,* **66**, 13 P.

———(1958). The metabolism of C_2-compounds in microorganisms. 1. The incorporation of 2-^{14}C acetate by *Pseudomonas fluorescens,* and by a Corynebacterium, grown on ammonium acetate. *Biochem. J.,* **68**, 535–542.

———, and J. F. Collins (1958). The glyoxylate cycle in *Aspergillus niger. Biochem. J.,* **68**, 3–4 P.

———, and S. R. Elsden (1961). The metabolism of 2-carbon compounds by microorganisms. *Advan. Enzymol.,* **23**, 401–470.

———, and N. B. Madsen (1957). Synthesis of C_4-dicarboxylic acids from acetate by a "glyoxylate bypass" of the tricarboxylic acid cycle. *Biochim. Biophys. Acta,* **24**, 651–653.

————, and N. B. Madsen (1957). Formation of C₄-dicarboxylic acids from acetate by *Pseudomonas* KB 1. *Biochem. J.*, **66**, 13 P.

————, and N. B. Madsen (1958). The metabolism of C₂-compounds in microorganisms. 3. Synthesis of malate from acetate via the glyoxylate cycle. *Biochem. J.*, **68**, 549–557.

————, and J. R. Quayle (1958). The metabolism of C₂-compounds in microorganisms. 2. The effect of carbon dioxide on the incorporation of ¹⁴C-acetate by acetate-grown *Pseudomonas* KB 1. *Biochem. J.*, **68**, 542–549.

————, A. M. Gotto, and P. Lund (1958). Effect of growth substrates on isocitratase formation by *Pseudomonas ovalis* Chester. *Nature*, **182**, 1430–1431.

————, P. J. R. Phizackerley, and J. R. Sadler (1959). Synthesis of cell constituents from acetate by *Escherichia coli*. *Biochem. J.*, **72**, 32–33 P.

————, P. J. R. Phizackerley, and J. R. Sadler (1960). The metabolism of C₂-compounds in microorganisms. 5. Biosynthesis of cell materials from acetate in *Escherichia coli*. *Biochem. J.*, **77**, 438–445.

Kovachevich, R., and W. A. Wood (1955). Carbohydrate metabolism by *Pseudomonas fluorescens*. III. Purification and properties of a 6-phosphogluconate dehydrase. *J. Biol. Chem.*, **213**, 745–756.

————, and W. A. Wood (1955). Carbohydrate metabolism by *Pseudomonas fluorescens*. IV. Purification and properties of 2-keto-3-deoxy-6-phosphogluconate aldolase. *J. Biol. Chem.*, **213**, 757–767.

Krebs, H. A. (1934). Metabolism of amino acids. III. Deamination of amino acids. *Biochem. J.*, **29**, 1620–1644.

————(1943). The intermediary stages in the biological oxidation of carbohydrate. *Advan. Enzymol.*, **3**, 191–252.

————, S. Gurin, and L. V. Eggleston (1952). The pathway of oxidation of acetate in baker's yeast. *Biochem. J.*, **51**, 614–628.

Lebedev, A. v. (1909). Versuche zur Aufklärung des zellfreien Gärungsprozesses mit Hilfe des Ultrafilters. *Biochem. Z.*, **20**, 114–125.

————(1911). Über den Mechanismus der alkoholischen Gärung. *Ber. Deut. Chem. Ges. (Chem. Ber.)*, **44**, 2932–2942.

————(1911). Extraction de la zymase par simple macération. *Compt. Rend.*, **152**, 49–51.

————(1911). Sur l'extraction de la zymase. *Compt. Rend.*, **152**, 1129.

————(1912). Über den Mechanismus der alkoholischen Gärung. *Biochem. Z.*, **46**, 483–489.

————(1913). Über den kinetischen Verlauf der alkoholischen Gärung. *Z. Gärungsphysiol.*, **2**, 104–106.

————(1926). Trennung der Oxydoreduktase vom Zymasekomplex. *Z. Physiol. Chem.*, **156**, 153–158.

————(1927). Über die Zucker- und Brenztraubensäuregärung. *Biochem. Z.*, **186**, 376–377.

Lees, H. (1960). Energy metabolism in chemolithotrophic bacteria. *Ann. Rev. Microbiol.*, **14**, 83–98.

Lehninger, A. L. (1944). The relationship of adenosine polyphosphates to fatty acid oxidation in homogenized liver preparations. *J. Biol. Chem.*, **157**, 365–381.

————(1945). On the activation of fatty acid oxidation. *J. Biol. Chem.*, **161**, 435–451.

————(1945). Fatty acid oxidation and the tricarboxylic acid cycle. *J. Biol. Chem.*, **161**, 413–414.

————(1946). A quantitative study of the products of fatty acid oxidation in liver suspensions. *J. Biol. Chem.*, **164**, 291–306.

Lipmann, F. (1936). Fermentation of phosphogluconic acid. *Nature*, **138**, 588–589.

————(1937). Die Dehydrierung der Brenztraubensäure. *Eyzymologia*, **4**, 65–72.

————(1939). An analysis of the pyruvic acid oxidation system. *Cold Springs Harbor Symp. Quant. Biol.*, **7**, 248–257.

————(1940). A phosphorylated oxidation product of pyruvic acid. *J. Biol. Chem.*, **134**, 463–464.

————(1941). Metabolic generation and utilization of phosphate bond energy. *Advan. Enzymol.*, **1**, 99–162.

————(1944). Enzymatic synthesis of acetyl-phosphate. *J. Biol. Chem.*, **155**, 55–70.

————(1945). Acetylation of sulfanilamides by liver homogenates and extracts. *J. Biol. Chem.*, **160**, 173–190.

————(1954). Development of the acetylation problem, a personal account. *Science*, **120**, 855–865.

————, and L. C. Tuttle (1944). Acetyl-phosphate: chemistry, determination and synthesis. *J. Biol. Chem.*, **153**, 571–582.

————, and L. C. Tuttle (1944). Keto acid formation through the reversal of the phosphoroclastic reaction. *J. Biol. Chem.*, **154**, 725–726.

————, N. O. Kaplan, G. D. Novelli, L. C. Tuttle, and B. M. Guirard (1947). Coenzyme for acetylation, a pantothenic acid derivative. *J. Biol. Chem.*, **167**, 869–870.

Lipmann, J. G., S. A. Waksman, and J. S. Joffe (1921). The oxidation of sulfur by soil microorganisms. *Soil Sci.*, **12**, 475–489.

Lohmann, K. (1933). Über Phosphorylierung und Dephosphorylierung. Bildung der natürlichen Hexosemonophosphorsäure aus ihren Komponenten. *Biochem. Z.*, **262**, 137–151.

————, and O. Meyerhof (1934). Über die enzymatische Umwandlung von Phosphoglycerinsäure in Brenztraubensäure und Phosphorsäure. *Biochem. Z.*, **273**, 60–72.

Lynen, F. (1953). Acetyl coenzyme A and the fatty acid cycle. *Harvey Lectures*, **48**, 210–244.

McElroy, W. D., and B. H. Glass, (eds.) (1956). *Symposium on Inorganic Nitrogen Metabolism.* The John Hopkins University Press, Baltimore.

Marmur, J., and F. Schlenk (1951). Glycolaldehyde and glycolaldehyde phosphate as reaction components in enzymatic pentose formation. *Arch. Biochem. Biophys.*, **31**, 154–155.

Meister, A. (1955). Transamination. *Advan. Enzymol.*, **16**, 185–246.

Meyerhof, O. (1916). Untersuchungen über den Atmungsvorgang nitrifizierender Bakterien. I. Die Atmung des Nitratbildners. *Pflügers Arch. Ges. Physiol.*, **164**, 353–427.

————(1916). Untersuchungen über den Atmungsvorgang nitrifizierender Bakterien. II. Beeinflussung der Atmung des Nitratbildners durch chemische Substanzen. *Pflügers Arch. Ges. Physiol.*, **165**, 239–284.

————(1916). Untersuchungen über den Atmungsvorgang nitrifizierender Bakterien. III. Die Atmung des Nitritbildners und ihre Beeinflussung durch chemische Substanzen. *Pflügers Arch. Ges. Physiol.*, **166**, 240–280.

————(1918). Über das Gärungscoferment im Tierkörper. 2. Mitt. *Hoppe-Seylers Z. Physiol. Chem.*, **102**, 1–32.

————(1918). Über das Vorkommen des Cofermentes der alkoholischen Hefegärung im Muskelgewebe und seine mutmaßliche Bedeutung im Atmungsmechanismus (Vorläufige Mitt.). *Hoppe-Seylers Z. Physiol. Chem.*, **101**, 165–175.

————(1918). Zur Kinetik der zellfreien Gärung. *Hoppe-Seylers Z. Physiol. Chem.*, **102**, 185–225.

————(1935). Über die Kinetik der umkehrbaren Reaktion zwischen Hexosediphosphorsäure und Dioxyacetonphosphorsäure. *Biochem. Z.*, **277**, 77–96.

————(1942). Intermediate carbohydrate metabolism. In *A Symposium on Respiratory Enzymes*, pp. 3–15. University of Wisconsin Press, Madison, Wis.

————(1945). The origin of the reaction of Harden and Young in cell free alcoholic fermentation. *J. Biol. Chem.*, **157**, 105–119.

————(1949). Further studies of the Harden–Young effect in alcoholic fermentation of yeast preparation. *J. Biol. Chem.*, **180**, 575–586.

————, and W. Kiessling (1935). Über die Isolierung der isomeren Phosphoglycerinsäuren (Glycerin-2-phosphorsäure und Glycerinsäure-3-phosphorsäure) aus Gäransätzen und ihr enzymatisches Gleichgewicht. *Biochem. Z.*, **276**, 239–253.

————, and K. Lohmann (1934). Über die enzymatische Gleichgewichtsreaktion zwischen Hexosediphosphorsäure und Dioxyacetonphosphorsäure. *Nature*, **22**, 220.

————, K. Lohmann, and P. Schuster (1936). Über die Aldolase, ein Kohlenstoff-verknüpfendes Ferment. I. Aldolkondensation von Dioxyacetonphosphorsäure mit Acetaldehyde. *Biochem. Z.*, **286**, 301–318.

————, K. Lohmann, and P. Schuster (1936). Über die Aldolase, ein Kohlenstoff-verknüpfendes Ferment. II. Aldolkondensationen von Dioxyacetonphosphorsäure mit Glycerinaldehyde. *Biochem. Z.*, **286**, 319–335.

Moat, A. G., and H. Friedman (1960). The biosynthesis and interconversion of purines and their derivatives. *Bacteriol. Rev.*, **24**, 309–339.

Nason, A. (1962). Symposium on metabolism of inorganic compounds. II. Enzymatic pathways of nitrate, nitrite and hydroxylamine metabolism. *Bacteriol. Rev.*, **26**, 16–41.

———, and H. Takahashi (1958). Inorganic nitrogen metabolism. *Ann. Rev. Microbiol.*, **12**, 203–246.

Nathanson, A. (1902). Über eine neue Gruppe von Schwefelbakterien und ihren Stoffwechsel. *Mitt. Zool. Sta. Neapel*, **15**, 665–680.

Neuberg, C. (1915). Fortgesetzte Untersuchungen über Carboxylase und andere Hefefermente. *Biochem. Z.*, **71**, 1–103.

———(1918). Überführung der Fructose-diphosphorsäure in Fructose-monophosphorsäure. *Biochem. Z.*, **88**, 432–436.

———(1920). Die physikalisch-chemische Betrachtung der Gärungsvorgänge. *Biochem. Z.*, **105**, 306.

———, and A. Gottschalk (1925). Über Apozymase und Cozymase. Zur Lehre von der Phosphorylierung. *Biochem. Z.*, **161**, 244–256.

———, and A. Hildesheimer (1911). Über zuckerfreie Hefegärungen. I. *Biochem. Z.*, **31**, 170–176.

———, and L. Karczag (1911). Über zuckerfreie Hefegärungen. IV. Carboxylase, ein neues Enzym der Hefe. *Biochem. Z.*, **36**, 68–75.

———, and L. Karczag (1911). Über zuckerfreie Hefegärungen. V. Zur Kenntnis der Carboxylase. *Biochem. Z.*, **36**, 76–81.

———, and J. Kerb (1914). Zur Frage der Bildung von Acetaldehyde bei Hefegärungen. *Ber. Deut. Chem. Ges. (Chem. Ber.)*, **47**, 2730–2732.

———, and M. Kobel (1928). Phosphorylierung und alkoholische Zuckerspaltung. *Liebig's Ann.*, **465**, 272–282.

———, and M. Kobel (1930). Über den Verlauf der Brenztraubensäurebildung bei der Hefegärung. *Biochem. Z.*, **219**, 490–494.

———, and A. May (1923). Die Bilanz der Brenztraubensäuregärung. *Biochem. Z.*, **140**, 299–313.

———, and C. Oppenheimer (1925). Zur Nomenklatur der Gärungsfermente und Oxydasen. *Biochem. Z.*, **166**, 450–453.

———, and E. Reinfurth (1918). Die Festlegung der Aldehydstufe bei der alkoholischen Gärung. Ein experimenteller Beweis der Acetaldehyd-Brenztraubensäuretheorie. *Biochem. Z.*, **89**, 365–414.

———, and L. Tir (1911). Über zuckerfreie Hefegärungen. II. *Biochem. Z.*, **32**, 323–331.

———, E. Farber, A. Levite, and E. Schwenk (1917). Über die Hexosephosphorsäure, ihre Zusammensetzung und die Frage ihrer Rolle bei der alkoholischen Gärung, sowie über das Verhalten der Dreikohlenstoffzucker zu Hefen. *Biochem. Z.*, **83**, 244–268.

Nilsson, R., and F. Alm (1940). Zur Kenntnis der alkoholischen Gärung in dem intakten Fermentsystem der Hefezellen, und in desorganisierten Zymasesystemen. III. Die Bedeutung der Zellstruktur für den harmonischen Gärverlauf. *Biochem. Z.*, **304**, 285–317.

———, and J. Westerberg (1940). Zur Kenntnis der alkoholischen Gärung in dem intakten Fermentsystem der Hefezellen, und in desorganisierten Zymasesystemen. IV. *Biochem. Z.*, **308**, 255–265.

Nisman, B. (1954). The Stickland reaction. *Bacteriol. Rev.*, **18**, 16–42.

———, M. Reynaud, and G. N. Cohen (1948). Extension of the Stickland reaction to several bacterial species. *Arch. Biochem.*, **16**, 473–474.

Novelli, G. D., and F. Lipmann (1947). Bacterial conversion of pantothenic acid into coenzyme A (acetylation) and its relation to pyruvic oxidation. *Arch. Biochem.*, **14**, 23–27.

———, and F. Lipmann (1947). The involvement of coenzyme A in acetate oxidation in yeast. *J. Biol. Chem.*, **171**, 833–834.

———, and F. Lipmann (1950). The catalytic function of CoA in citric acid synthesis. *J. Biol. Chem.*, **182**, 213–228.

Ochoa, S., J. R. Stern, and M. C. Schneider (1951). Enzymatic synthesis of citric acid. II. Crystalline condensing enzyme. *J. Biol. Chem.*, **193**, 691–702.

Olson, J. A. (1954). The d-isocitric lyase system: the formation of glyoxylic and succinic acids from D-isocitric acid. *Nature*, **174**, 695–696.

Parnas, J. K. (1938). Über die enzymatischen Phosphorylierungen in der alkoholischen Gärung und in der Muskelglykogenolyse. *Enzymologia,* **5**, 166–184.

———, P. Ostern, and T. Mann (1935). Über die Verkettung der chemischen Vorgänge im Muskel. II. *Biochem. Z.*, **275**, 74–86.

Peck, H. D., Jr. (1960). Adenosine 5′-phosphosulfate as an intermediate in the oxidation of thiosulfate by *Thiobacillus thioparus. Proc. Natl. Acad. Sci. U.S.*, **46**, 1053–1057.

———, (1962). Symposium on metabolism of inorganic compounds. V. Comparative metabolism of inorganic sulfur compounds in microorganisms. *Bacteriol. Rev.*, **26**, 67–94.

Peters, R. A. (1936). Pyruvic acid oxidation in brain. I. Vitamin B_1 and the pyruvate oxidase in pigeon's brain. *Biochem. J.*, **30**, 2206–2218.

Postgate, J. R. (1951). On the nutrition of *Desulphovibrio desulphuricans. J. Gen. Microbiol.*, **5**, 714–724.

———(1953). On the nutrition of *Desulphovibrio desulphuricans:* a correction. *J. Gen. Microbiol.*, **9**, 440–444.

———(1956). Cytochrome c_3 and desulphoriridin; pigments of the anaerobe *Desulphoribrio desulphuricans. J. Gen. Microbiol.*, **14**, 545–572.

———(1959). Sulphate reduction by bacteria. *Ann Rev. Microbiol.*, **13**, 505.

———(1965). Recent advances in the study of the sulphate-reducing bacteria. *Bacteriol. Rev.*, **29**, 425.

Pratt, E. F., and R. J. Williams (1939). The effects of pantothenic acid on respiratory activity. *J. Gen. Physiol.*, **22**, 637–647.

Quastel, J. H. (1928). The study of "resting" or non-proliferating bacteria. *J. Hyg.*, **28**, 139–146.

———, and P. G. Scholefield (1951). Biochemistry of nitrification in soil. *Bacteriol. Rev.*, **15**, 1–53.

———, and M. D. Whetham (1925). Dehydrogenations produced by resting bacteria. I. *Biochem. J.*, **19**, 520–531.

———, and M. D. Whetham (1925). Dehydrogenations produced by resting bacteria. II. *Biochem. J.*, **19**, 645–651.

———, and W. R. Woolridge (1928). Some properties of the dehydrogenating enzymes of bacteria. *Biochem. J.*, **22**, 689–702.

Racker, E. (1954). Alternative pathways of glucose and fructose metabolism. *Advan. Enzymol.* **15**, 141–182.

Robison, R. (1922). A new phosphoric ester produced by the action of yeast juice on hexoses. *Biochem. J.*, **16**, 809–824.

Santer, M., and W. Vishniac (1955). CO_2 incorporation by extracts of *Thiobacillus thioparus. Biochim. Biophys. Acta*, **18**, 157–158.

Saz, H. J. (1954). The enzymic formation of glyoxylates and succinate from tricarboxylic acids. *Biochem. J.*, **58**, xx–xxi.

Schlegel, H. G. (1954). Die Rolle des molekularen Wasserstoffs im Stoffwechsel der Mikroorganismen. *Arch. Mikrobiol.*, **20**, 293–322.

———(1960). Die wasserstoffoxydierenden Bakterien. *Handbuch Pflanzenphysiol.*, **5**, 687–714.

———(1966). Physiology and biochemistry of Knallgasbacteria. *Advan. Comp. Physiol. Biochem.*, **2**, 185–236.

Schloesing, J. J. T., and A. Müntz (1877). Sur la nitrification par les ferments organisés. *Compt. Rend.*, **85**, 1018.

———, and A. Müntz (1878). Recherches sur la nitrification par les ferments organises. *Compt. Rend.*, **86**, 891.

———, and A. Müntz (1879). Recherches sur la nitrification. *Compt. Rend.*, **89**, 1074.

Smith, R. A., and I. C. Gunsalus (1955). Distribution and formation of isocitritase. *Nature*, **175**, 774–775.

Söhngen, N. L. (1906). Über Bakterien, welche Methan als Kohlenstoffnahrung und Energie-quelle gebrauchen. *Zentra. Bakteriol.*, II. Abt., **15**, 513–517.

——(1913). Benzin, Petroleum, Paraffinöl und Paraffin als Kohlenstoff- und Energiequelle für Mikroben. *Zentra. Bakteriol.*, II. Abt., **37**, 595–609.

——(1913). Einfluss von Kolloiden auf mikrobiologische Prozesse. *Zentra. Bakteriol.*, II. Abt., **38**, 621–647.

Stadtman, E. R. (1952). The purification and properties of phosphotransacetylase. *J. Biol. Chem.*, **196**, 527–534.

——(1952). The net enzymatic synthesis of acetyl coenzyme A. *J. Biol. Chem.*, **196**, 535–546.

Stern, J. R., and S. Ochoa (1949). Enzymatic synthesis of citric acid by condensation of acetate and oxalacetate. *J. Biol. Chem.*, **179**, 491–492.

——, and S. Ochoa (1952). Enzymatic synthesis of citric acid. V. Reaction of acetyl coenzyme A. *J. Biol. Chem.*, **198**, 313–321.

——, B. Shapiro, and S. Ochoa (1950). Synthesis and breakdown of citric acid with crystal-line condensing enzyme. *Nature*, **166**, 403–404.

——, B. Shapiro, E. R. Stadtman, and S. Ochoa (1951). Enzymatic synthesis of citric acid. III. Reversibility and mechanism. *J. Biol. Chem.*, **193**, 703–720.

Stickland, L. H. (1935). The reduction of proline by *C. sporogenes. Biochem. J.*, **29**, 288–290.

——(1935). The oxidation of alanine by *C. sporogenes. Biochem. J.*, **29**, 889–896.

——(1935). The reduction of glycine by *C. sporogenes. Biochem. J.*, **29**, 896–898.

Störmer, K. (1908). Über die Wirkung des Schwefelkohlenstoffes and ähnlicher Stoffe auf den Boden. *Zentra. Bakteriol.*, II. Abt., **20**, 282–286.

Suzuki, I., and C. H. Werkman (1958).Chemoautotrophic carbon dioxide fixation by ex-tracts of *Thiobacillus thiooxydans*. II. Formation of phosphoglyceric acid. *Arch. Biochem. Bio-phys.*, **77**, 112–113.

Taniguchi, S. (1961). Comparative biochemistry of nitrate metabolism. *Z. Allgem. Mikrobiol.*, **1**, 341.

Teague, P. C. and R. J. Williams (1942). Pantothenic acid and the utilization of glucose by living and cell-free systems. *J. Gen. Physiol.*, **25**, 777–783.

Trudinger, P. A. (1955). Phosphoglycerate formation from pentose phosphate by extracts of *Thiobacillus denitrificans. Biochim. Biophys. Acta*, **18**, 581–582.

——(1956). Fixation of carbon dioxide by extracts of the strict autotroph *Thiobacillus denitri-ficans. Biochem. J.*, **64**, 274–286.

——(1967). The metabolism of inorganic sulphur compounds by thiobacilli. *Rev. Pure Appl. Chem.*, **17**, 1–24.

Umbreit, W. W., R. H. Burris, and J. F. Stauffer (1964). *Manometric Techniques*, 4th ed. Burgess Publishing Company, Minneapolis.

Utter, M. F., and C. H. Werkman (1943). Role of phosphate in the anaerobic dissimilation of pyruvic acid. *Arch. Biochem.*, **2**, 491–492.

——, C. H. Werkman, and F. Lipmann (1944). Reversibility of the phosphoroclastic split of pyruvate. *J. Biol. Chem.*, **154**, 723–724.

——, F. Lipmann, and C. H. Werkman (1945). Reversibility of the phosphoroclastic split of pyruvate. *J. Biol. Chem.*, **158**, 521–531.

Vallery-Radot, R. (1960). *The Life of Pasteur.* Dover Publications Inc., New York.

Van Niel, C. B. (1931). On the morphology and physiology of the purple and green sulphur bacteria. *Arch. Mikrobiol.*, **3**, 1–112.

Vishniac, W., and M. Santer (1957). The thiobacilli. *Bacteriol. Rev.*, **21**, 195–213.

——, and P. A. Trudinger (1962). Symposium on autotrophy. V. Carbon dioxide fixation and substrate oxidation in the chemosynthetic sulfur and hydrogen bacteria. *Bacteriol. Rev.*, **26**, 168–175.

Waksman, S. A. (1922). Microorganisms concerned in the oxidation of sulfur in the soil. IV. A solid medium for the isolation and cultivation of *Thiobacillus thiooxidans. J. Bacteriol.*, **7**, 605–608.

————(1922). Microorganisms concerned in the oxidation of sulfur in the soil. V. Bacteria oxidizing sulfur under acid and alkaline conditions. *J. Bacteriol.*, **7**, 609–616.

————(1953). *Sergei N. Winogradsky.* Rutgers University Press, New Brunswick, N. J.

————, and J. S. Joffee (1921). The oxidation of sulfur by microorganisms. *Proc. Soc. Exptl. Biol. Med.*, **18**, 1–3.

————, and J. S. Joffee (1921). Acid production by a new sulfur-oxidizing bacterium. *Science*, **53**, 216.

————, and J. S. Joffee (1922). Microorganisms concerned in the oxidation of sulfur in the soil. II. *Thiobacillus thiooxidans*, a new sulfur-oxidizing organism isolated from the soil. *J. Bacteriol.*, **7**, 239–256.

————, and R. L. Starkey (1923). On the growth and respiration of sulfur-oxidizing bacteria. *J. Gen. Physiol.*, **5**, 285–310.

Warburg, O., and W. Christian (1933). Über das gelbe Oxydationsferment. *Biochem. Z.*, **257**, 492.

————, and W. Christian (1936). Verbrennung von Robison–Ester durch Triphospho-Pyridin-Nucleotid. *Biochem. Z.*, **287**, 440–441.

————, and W. Christian (1937). Abbau von Robison–Ester durch Triphospho-Pyridin-Nucleotid. *Biochem. Z.*, **292**, 287–295.

Warrington, R. (1878). On nitrification. *J. Chem. Soc.*, **33**, 44–51.

————(1879). On nitrification. Part II. *J. Chem. Soc.*, **35**, 429–456.

————(1883). On nitrification. Part III. *J. Chem. Soc.*, **45**, 637–672.

Winogradsky, S. (1888). *Beiträge zur Morphologie und Physiologie der Schwefelbakterien.* A. Felix, Leipzig.

————(1888). Über Eisenbakterien. *Botan. Zeitung*, **46**, 261–270.

————(1889). Recherches physiologiques sur les sulfobactéries. *Ann. Inst. Pasteur*, **3**, 49–60.

————(1890). Recherches sur les organismes de la nitrification. *Ann. Inst. Pasteur*, **4**, 215–231.

————(1890). Recherches sur les organismes de la nitrification. *Ann. Inst. Pasteur*, **4**, 257–275.

————(1890). Recherches sur les organismes de la nitrification. *Ann. Inst. Pasteur*, **4**, 760–771.

————(1890). Recherches sur les organismes de la nitrification. *Ann. Inst. Pasteur*, **5**, 92–100.

————(1890). Recherches sur les organismes de la nitrification. *Ann. Inst. Pasteur*, **5**, 577–616.

Winslow, C. E. (1950). Some leaders and landmarks in the history of microbiology. *Bacteriol. Rev.*, **14**, 99–110.

Wong, D. T. O., and S. J. Ajl (1957). Significance of the malate synthetase reaction in bacteria. *Science*, **126**, 1013–1014.

Wood, H. G. (1946). The fixation of carbon dioxide and the interrelationship of the tricarboxylic acid cycle. *Physiol. Rev.*, **26**, 198–246.

Wood, W. A., and R. F. Schwerdt (1953). Carbohydrate oxidation by *Pseudomonas fluorescens*. I. The mechanism of glucose and gluconic acid oxidation. *J. Biol. Chem.*, **201**, 501–511.

————, and R. F. Schwerdt (1954). Carbohydrate oxidation by *Pseudomonas fluorescens*. II. Mechanism of hexosephosphate oxidation. *J. Biol. Chem.*, **206**, 625–635.

————, and C. H. Werkman (1936). Mechanisms of glucose dissimilation by the propionic acid bacteria. *Biochem. J.*, **30**, 618.

————, C. H. Werkman, A. Hemingway, and A. O. Nier (1940). Heavy carbon as a tracer in heterotrophic carbon dioxide assimilation. *J. Biol. Chem.*, **139**, 365.

Zobell, C. E. (1946). Action of microorganisms on hydrocarbons. *Bacteriol. Rev.*, **10**, 1–40.

————(1950). Assimilation of hydrocarbons by microorganisms. *Advan. Enzymol.*, **10**, 443–486.

Author Citation Index

Kaplan, N. O., 158, 176, 183, 265, 406
Karczag, L., 407
Karlsson, J. L., 283, 397
Karström, H., 278
Kaserer, H., 404
Katagiri, M., 292
Kaufman, S., 199
Kay, L. D., 401
Keighley, G., 371
Keil, F., 338, 404
Keilin, D., 288
Kelsey, M., 316
Kendal, L. P., 288
Kendall, A. I., 147
Kennedy, E. P., 199, 200
Kerb, J., 407
Keresztesy, J. C., 172
Kertesz, D., 287
Keskin, H., 199
Khouvine, Y., 241
Kida, S., 319
Kiessling, W., 117, 128, 406
Kimoto, N., 288
King, E. J., 142
King, H. K., 320, 337
King, T. E., 176, 404
Klatter, F., 402
Klein, R. M., 288
Kleinzeller, A., 199
Kluyver, A. J., 278
Knappe, J., 352
Knight, T. E., 337, 338
Knoop, F., 168, 199, 205
Knowles, P. F., 319
Knox, W. E., 200, 283
Kobel, M., 158, 407
Koch, R., 231
Koffler, H., 403
Kogut, M., 205
Korkes, S., 200, 404
Korn, E. D., 398
Kornberg, A., 200, 398
Kornberg, H. L., 205, 401, 402, 404
Koser, S. A., 403
Kovachevich, R., 405
Krafft, H., 128
Krampitz, L. O., 183, 351
Krebs, H. A., 158, 168, 205, 338, 397, 405
Kritzmann, M. G., 401
Kubowitz, F., 288
Kulka, R. G., 351
Kuno, S., 320
Kurahashi, K., 205, 351

Kurihara, N., 320
Kutscher, W., 168, 171

Lacroute, F., 319
Lafferty, R., 258
Lagerkvist, U., 399
Lampen, J. O., 158
Lardy, H. A., 199, 351, 403
LaRiviere, J. W. M., 404
Lars, J., 317
Laugham, 371
Lax, S. R., 320
Leaver, F. W., 351
Lebedev, A. v., 405
Lederberg, J., 371
Lederer, E., 315, 318
Lees, H., 405
Lehninger, A. L., 199, 200, 405
Leifer, E., 371
Lein, J., 371
Leistner, E., 318, 321
Leloir, L. F., 199, 200
Lenfant, M., 318
Lennox, E. S., 321
Lerner, A. B., 288
Lester, G., 318
Lester, R. L., 318
Letters, R., 265
Levenberg, B., 397, 398, 399
Levin, J. G., 318, 319
Levintow, L., 176
Levite, A., 407
Lieberman, I., 398, 399
Lieske, R., 363
Lin, E. C. C., 320
Lin, I., 397
Lindner, P., 77
Lingens, F., 319
Link, G. K. K., 288
Lipmann, F., 176, 183, 199, 200, 265, 351, 352, 402, 405, 407, 409
Lipmann, J. G., 406
Littlefield, J. W., 200
Ljunggren, 168
Locher, L. M., 176
Lohmann, C., 128
Lohmann, K., 115, 117, 128, 158, 406
Long, M. V., 205
Lorch, E., 352
Lord, R., 318
Lorence, J. H., 319
Love, S. H., 399
Lowy, P. H., 371

415

Oda, Y., 283
Ohlmeyer, P., 158
Ohlson, H. J., 403
Olivier, 216
Olsen, R. K., 319
Olson, J. A., 205, 408
Onoprienko, I., 292
Oppenheimer, C., 407
Orshansky, J., 351
Örström, Å., 397
Örström, M., 397
Ortiz, P. J., 352
Östberg, O., 168
Ostern, P., 147, 408

Parnas, J. K., 128, 408
Parson, W. W., 319, 320
Partington, J. R., 256
Partridge, C. W. H., 318, 399
Paskhina, T. S., 283
Payen, 28
Peabody, R. A., 398
Peanasky, R., 351
Peck, H. D., Jr., 408
Pendergast, J., 199
Pennella, P., 315
Peters, R. A., 171, 408
Peters, W. J., 320
Peterson, E. W., 292
Petrack, B., 399
Phares, E. F., 351, 352
Phillips, P. G., 317
Phizackerly, P. J. R., 405
Pittard, J., 316, 317, 318, 320, 321
Plauchud, 216
Podoski, E. P., 205
Polglase, W. J., 320
Pollak, H., 168
Pomerantz, S. H., 351
Popják, G., 200
Posner, H. S., 292
Postgate, J. R., 256, 402, 403, 408
Pratt, B. C., 316
Pratt, E. F., 408
Price, S. A., 318
Pricer, W. E., Jr., 398, 399
Proctor, C. M., 258
Pucher, G. W., 168
Pun, W. T., 320

Quastel, J. H., 338, 408
Quayle, J. R., 241, 405

Rabinowitz, J. C., 399
Racker, E., 158, 241, 408
Raff, F., 158
Raistrick, H., 158
Rapp, R., 402
Rappoport, D. A., 158
Ratledge, C., 320
Ratner, S., 399
Rauen, H., 168
Ravel, J. M., 317, 320
Raw, I., 200
Reich, E., 317
Reichert, E., 200
Reid, E. E., 199
Reid, J. C., 402
Reinfurth, E., 407
Remy, C. N., 398
Remy, W. T., 398
Revel, H. R. B., 399
Reynaud, M., 407
Rey-Pailhade, J. de, 77
Ringelmann, E., 352
Rittenberg, D., 200, 397
Rittenberg, S. C., 256
Rivera, A., 317, 320
Robbins, E. A., 265
Robbins, P. W., 265, 403
Roberts, E. A. H., 288
Robison, R., 141, 142, 404, 408
Roepke, R. R., 371
Rose, I. A., 351
Rosenthal, C., 200
Roth, L. J., 287
Rothberg, S., 292
Rothschild, J., 320
Roy, A. B., 265
Ruben, S., 402
Rudney, H., 319, 320
Rueff, L., 200
Rüegg, R., 318
Ruehle, A. E., 172

Sadler, J. R., 405
Sakami, W., 199, 371
Salton, M. R. J., 320
Samuel, O., 315
Sanadi, D. R., 200
Sanderson, K. E., 320
Santer, M., 408, 409
Sato, K., 319
Saz, H. J., 205, 408
Schade, H., 402
Schaffner, C. P., 317

419

Subject Index

421